SOME DRUGS AND HERBAL PRODUCTS

VOLUME 108

This publication represents the views and expert opinions of an IARC Working Group on the Evaluation of Carcinogenic Risks to Humans, which met in Lyon, 4–11 June 2013

Lyon, France - 2016

IARC MONOGRAPHS ON THE EVALUATION OF CARCINOGENIC RISKS TO HUMANS

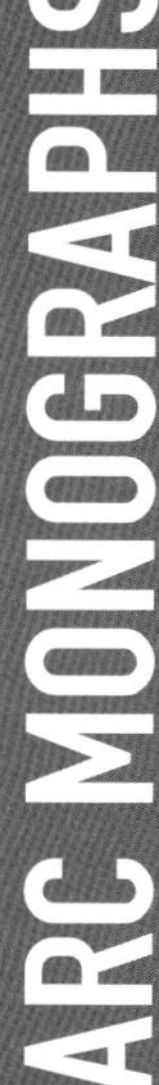

International Agency for Research on Cancer

World Health Organization

IARC MONOGRAPHS

In 1969, the International Agency for Research on Cancer (IARC) initiated a programme on the evaluation of the carcinogenic risk of chemicals to humans involving the production of critically evaluated monographs on individual chemicals. The programme was subsequently expanded to include evaluations of carcinogenic risks associated with exposures to complex mixtures, lifestyle factors and biological and physical agents, as well as those in specific occupations. The objective of the programme is to elaborate and publish in the form of monographs critical reviews of data on carcinogenicity for agents to which humans are known to be exposed and on specific exposure situations; to evaluate these data in terms of human risk with the help of international working groups of experts in carcinogenesis and related fields; and to indicate where additional research efforts are needed. The lists of IARC evaluations are regularly updated and are available on the Internet at http://monographs.iarc.fr/.

This programme has been supported since 1982 by Cooperative Agreement U01 CA33193 with the United States National Cancer Institute, Department of Health and Human Services. Additional support has been provided since 1986 by the European Commission Directorate-General for Employment, Social Affairs, and Inclusion, initially by the Unit of Health, Safety and Hygiene at Work, and since 2014 by the European Union Programme for Employment and Social Innovation "EaSI" (2014–2020) (for further information please consult: http://ec.europa.eu/social/easi). Support has also been provided since 1992 by the United States National Institute of Environmental Health Sciences, Department of Health and Human Services. The contents of this volume are solely the responsibility of the Working Group and do not necessarily represent the official views of the United States National Cancer Institute, the United States National Institute of Environmental Health Sciences, the United States Department of Health and Human Services, or the European Commission.

Published by the International Agency for Research on Cancer,
150 cours Albert Thomas, 69372 Lyon Cedex 08, France

©International Agency for Research on Cancer, 2016
On-line publication, 15 September 2015 (see Corrigenda)

Distributed by WHO Press, World Health Organization, 20 Avenue Appia, 1211 Geneva 27, Switzerland
(tel.: +41 22 791 3264; fax: +41 22 791 4857; email: bookorders@who.int).

Publications of the World Health Organization enjoy copyright protection in accordance with the provisions
of Protocol 2 of the Universal Copyright Convention. All rights reserved.

Corrigenda to the IARC Monographs are published online at http://monographs.iarc.fr/ENG/Publications/corrigenda.php
To report an error, please contact: editimo@iarc.fr

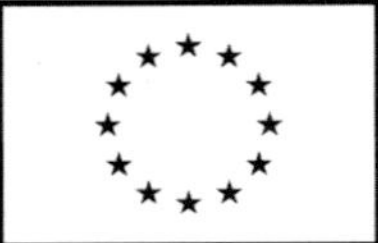
Co-funded by the European Union

The International Agency for Research on Cancer welcomes requests for permission to reproduce or translate its publications, in part or in full. Requests for permission to reproduce or translate IARC publications – whether for sale or for non-commercial distribution – should be addressed to the IARC Communications Group at: publications@iarc.fr.

The designations employed and the presentation of the material in this publication do not imply the expression of any opinion whatsoever on the part of the Secretariat of the World Health Organization concerning the legal status of any country, territory, city, or area or of its authorities, or concerning the delimitation of its frontiers or boundaries.

The mention of specific companies or of certain manufacturers' products does not imply that they are endorsed or recommended by the World Health Organization in preference to others of a similar nature that are not mentioned. Errors and omissions excepted, the names of proprietary products are distinguished by initial capital letters.

The IARC Monographs Working Group alone is responsible for the views expressed in this publication.

IARC Library Cataloguing in Publication Data

Some drugs and herbal products / IARC Working Group on the Evaluation of Carcinogenic Risks to Humans (2013: Lyon, France)

(IARC monographs on the evaluation of carcinogenic risks to humans ; volume 108)

1. Carcinogens – pharmacology 2. Drug-Related Side Effects and Adverse Reactions – drug effects 3. Plant Preparations – adverse effects 4. Pharmaceutical Preparations – adverse effects 5. Plants, Medicinal – adverse effects
6. Cell Transformation, Neoplastic – drug effects
I. IARC Working Group on the Evaluation of Carcinogenic Risks to Humans
II. Series

ISBN 978 92 832 0146 5   (NLM Classification: W1)
ISSN 1017-1606

PRINTED IN FRANCE

CONTENTS

NOTE TO THE READER

The term 'carcinogenic risk' in the *IARC Monographs* series is taken to mean that an agent is capable of causing cancer. The *Monographs* evaluate cancer hazards, despite the historical presence of the word 'risks' in the title.

Inclusion of an agent in the *Monographs* does not imply that it is a carcinogen, only that the published data have been examined. Equally, the fact that an agent has not yet been evaluated in a *Monograph* does not mean that it is not carcinogenic. Similarly, identification of cancer sites with *sufficient evidence* or *limited evidence* in humans should not be viewed as precluding the possibility that an agent may cause cancer at other sites.

The evaluations of carcinogenic risk are made by international working groups of independent scientists and are qualitative in nature. No recommendation is given for regulation or legislation.

Anyone who is aware of published data that may alter the evaluation of the carcinogenic risk of an agent to humans is encouraged to make this information available to the Section of IARC Monographs, International Agency for Research on Cancer, 150 cours Albert Thomas, 69372 Lyon Cedex 08, France, in order that the agent may be considered for re-evaluation by a future Working Group.

Although every effort is made to prepare the *Monographs* as accurately as possible, mistakes may occur. Readers are requested to communicate any errors to the Section of IARC Monographs, so that corrections can be reported in future volumes.

LIST OF PARTICIPANTS

Members[1]

Bruce C. Baguley

Auckland Cancer Society Research Centre
University of Auckland
Auckland
New Zealand

Frederick A. Beland

National Center for Toxicological Research
Food and Drug Administration
Jefferson, AR
USA

Joseph M. Betz (Subgroup chair, Exposure Data)

Office of Dietary Supplements
National Institutes of Health
Rockville, MD
USA

Robert J. Biggar

Queensland University of Technology
Brisbane
Australia

Esperanza J. Carcache de Blanco

College of Pharmacy
Ohio State University
Columbus, OH
USA

Michael L. Cunningham [retired]

National Institute of Environmental Health Sciences
Chapel Hill, NC
USA

---

[1] Working Group Members and Invited Specialists serve in their individual capacities as scientists and not as representatives of their government or any organization with which they are affiliated. Affiliations are provided for identification purposes only. Invited Specialists do not serve as Meeting Chair or Subgroup Chair, draft text that pertains to the description or interpretation of cancer data, or participate in the evaluations.

Each participant was asked to disclose pertinent research, employment, and financial interests. Current financial interests and research and employment interests during the past 4 years or anticipated in the future are identified here. Minor pertinent interests are not listed and include stock valued at no more than US $1000 overall, grants that provide no more than 5% of the research budget of the expert's organization and that do not support the expert's research or position, and consulting or speaking on matters not before a court or government agency that does not exceed 2% of total professional time or compensation. All grants that support the expert's research or position and all consulting or speaking on behalf of an interested party on matters before a court or government agency are listed as significant pertinent interests.

June K. Dunnick

Toxicology Branch
National Institute of Environmental Health
Sciences
Research Triangle Park, NC
USA

Lei Guo

National Center for Toxicological Research
Food and Drug Administration
Jefferson, AR
USA

Charles William Jameson (Subgroup Chair,
Cancer in Experimental Animals)

CWJ Consulting, LLC
Cape Coral, FL
USA

Margaret Karagas (Subgroup Chair, Cancer in
Humans)

Section of Biostatistics and Epidemiology
Dartmouth Medical School
Lebanon, NH
USA

Trudy L. Knight

Institute of Occupational Environmental
Medicine
University of Birmingham
Birmingham
United Kingdom

Dirk W. Lachenmeier

Ministry of Rural Region and Consumer
Protection Baden-Württemberg
Stuttgart
Germany

Ruth M. Lunn

National Toxicology Program
National Institute of Environmental Health
Sciences
Research Triangle Park, NC
USA

M. Matilde Marques (Subgroup Chair,
Mechanistic and Other Relevant Data)

Department of Chemical and Biological
Engineering
Technical University of Lisbon
Lisbon
Portugal

David L. McCormick

IIT Research Institute
Chicago, IL
USA

Sonal Singh

Department of Epidemiology
Johns Hopkins School of Medicine and Public
Health
Baltimore, MD
USA

Saranjit Singh [unable to attend]

> Department of Pharmaceutical Analysis
> National Institute of Pharmaceutical
> Education and Research
> Punjab
> India

Bernard W. Stewart (Overall Chair)

> Cancer Control Program
> South Eastern Sydney Public Health Unit
> Randwick
> Australia

Chin-Hsiao Tseng [2]

> College of Medicine
> Taiwan University
> Taipei
> Taiwan, China

Hiroyuki Tsuda

> Nanotoxicology Project
> Nagoya City University
> Nagoya
> Japan

Kristine L. Witt [unable to attend]

> National Toxicology Program
> National Institute of Environmental Health
> Sciences
> Research Triangle Park, NC
> USA

Shufeng Zhou

> College of Pharmacy
> University of South Florida
> Tampa, FL
> USA

Invited specialist

Randall S. Stafford [3]

> Program on Prevention Outcomes and
> Practices
> Stanford Prevention Research Center
> Stanford, CA
> USA

Representatives

> None

Observers

David Alexander [4] [unable to attend]

> Williams Kherkher Hart Boundas, LLP
> League City, Texas
> USA

Andrea Bertocco [5]

> Global Products Science & Safety EMEA
> Herbalife Europe Limited
> Uxbridge
> England

---

[2] Chin-Hsiao Tseng received non-significant honoraria for serving on advisory boards and presentations from pharmaceutical companies, including Bristol-Myers-Squibb Company, Eli Lilly and Company, and Takeda Pharmaceutical Company Limited.

[3] Randall S. Stafford provided expert testimony (ceased in 2011) for Mylan Pharmaceuticals, Morgantown, WV, manufacturer of generic drugs, including hydrochlorothiazide containing drugs.

[4] David Alexander represents clients who claim they have been injured by the drug pioglitazone. He is employed and sponsored by Williams Kherkher Hart Boundas, LLP, Houston Texas, USA.

[5] Andrea Bertocco is employed by Herbalife, where he served as regulatory Manager for Herbalife products containing Aloe vera, Goldenseal and Ginkgo biloba. He is sponsored by Herbalife Europe Limited, United Kingdom.

Paul Dolin [6]

> Takeda Global Research & Development
> Centre (Europe) Ltd
> London
> England

Olaf Kelber [7]

> World Self-Medication Industry
> Steigerwald Arzneimittelwerk GmbH
> Darmstadt
> Germany

Egon Koch [8]

> World Self-Medication Industry
> Dr. Willmar Schwabe GmbH & Co. KG
> Karlsruhe
> Germany

IARC Secretariat

> Melina Arnold
> Robert Baan (*Senior Visiting Scientist*)
> Helen Bailey
> Lamia Benbrahim-Tallaa (*Rapporteur Mechanistic and Other Relevant Data*)
> Véronique Bouvard (*Rapporteur Exposure Data*)
> Fatiha El Ghissassi (*Rapporteur Mechanistic and Other Relevant Data*)
> Akram Ghantous

Yann Grosse (*Responsible Officer, Rapporteur Cancer in Experimental Animals*)
Neela Guha (*Rapporteur Cancer in Humans*)
Kate Z. Guyton
Béatrice Lauby-Secretan (*Rapporteur Exposure Data*)
Ho-Sun Lee
Dana Loomis (*Rapporteur Cancer in Humans*)
Heidi Mattock (*Scientific Editor*)
Douglas Puricelli Perin
Mónica S. Sierra
Kurt Straif (*Head of Programme*)
Jiri Zavadil

Administrative Assistance

> Sandrine Egraz
> Brigitte Kajo
> Michel Javin
> Annick Leroux
> Helene Lorenzen-Augros

Production Team

> Elisabeth Elbers
> Solène Quennehen
> Dorothy Russell

---

[6] Paul Dolin is employed and sponsored by Takeda Pharmaceutical Company Limited, Europe, manufacturing pioglitazone-containing and other pharmaceutical drugs. He holds stock of pharmaceutical companies marketing drugs that are reviewed at this meeting.

[7] Olaf Kelber is employed by Steigerwald Arzneimittelwerk GmbH, Darmstadt, Germany, manufacturing herbal medicines. He is sponsored by the World-Self-Medication Industry (WSMI), France.

[8] Egon Koch is employed by Dr. Wilmar Schwabe GmbH & Co KG, Karlsruhe, Germany. He provides expert testimony with respect to the commercialization of Ginkgo biloba extracts. He is sponsored by the World-Self-Medication Industry (WSMI), France.

PREAMBLE

The Preamble to the *IARC Monographs* describes the objective and scope of the programme, the scientific principles and procedures used in developing a *Monograph*, the types of evidence considered and the scientific criteria that guide the evaluations. The Preamble should be consulted when reading a *Monograph* or list of evaluations.

A. GENERAL PRINCIPLES AND PROCEDURES

1. Background

Soon after IARC was established in 1965, it received frequent requests for advice on the carcinogenic risk of chemicals, including requests for lists of known and suspected human carcinogens. It was clear that it would not be a simple task to summarize adequately the complexity of the information that was available, and IARC began to consider means of obtaining international expert opinion on this topic. In 1970, the IARC Advisory Committee on Environmental Carcinogenesis recommended '...that a compendium on carcinogenic chemicals be prepared by experts. The biological activity and evaluation of practical importance to public health should be referenced and documented.' The IARC Governing Council adopted a resolution concerning the role of IARC in providing government authorities with expert, independent, scientific opinion on environmental carcinogenesis. As one means to that end, the Governing Council recommended that IARC should prepare monographs on the evaluation of carcinogenic risk of chemicals to man, which became the initial title of the series.

In the succeeding years, the scope of the programme broadened as *Monographs* were developed for groups of related chemicals, complex mixtures, occupational exposures, physical and biological agents and lifestyle factors. In 1988, the phrase 'of chemicals' was dropped from the title, which assumed its present form, *IARC Monographs on the Evaluation of Carcinogenic Risks to Humans*.

Through the *Monographs* programme, IARC seeks to identify the causes of human cancer. This is the first step in cancer prevention, which is needed as much today as when IARC was established. The global burden of cancer is high and continues to increase: the annual number of new cases was estimated at 10.1 million in 2000 and is expected to reach 15 million by 2020 (Stewart & Kleihues, 2003). With current trends in demographics and exposure, the cancer burden has been shifting from high-resource countries to low- and medium-resource countries. As a result of *Monographs* evaluations, national health agencies have been able, on scientific grounds, to take measures to reduce human exposure to carcinogens in the workplace and in the environment.

The criteria established in 1971 to evaluate carcinogenic risks to humans were adopted by the Working Groups whose deliberations resulted in the first 16 volumes of the *Monographs* series. Those criteria were subsequently updated by further ad hoc Advisory Groups (IARC, 1977, 1978, 1979, 1982, 1983, 1987, 1988, 1991; Vainio et al., 1992; IARC, 2005, 2006).

The Preamble is primarily a statement of scientific principles, rather than a specification of working procedures. The procedures through which a Working Group implements these principles are not specified in detail. They usually involve operations that have been established as being effective during previous *Monograph* meetings but remain, predominantly, the prerogative of each individual Working Group.

2. Objective and scope

The objective of the programme is to prepare, with the help of international Working Groups of experts, and to publish in the form of *Monographs*, critical reviews and evaluations of evidence on the carcinogenicity of a wide range of human exposures. The *Monographs* represent the first step in carcinogen risk assessment, which involves examination of all relevant information to assess the strength of the available evidence that an agent could alter the age-specific incidence of cancer in humans. The *Monographs* may also indicate where additional research efforts are needed, specifically when data immediately relevant to an evaluation are not available.

In this Preamble, the term 'agent' refers to any entity or circumstance that is subject to evaluation in a *Monograph*. As the scope of the programme has broadened, categories of agents now include specific chemicals, groups of related chemicals, complex mixtures, occupational or environmental exposures, cultural or behavioural practices, biological organisms and physical agents. This list of categories may expand as causation of, and susceptibility to, malignant disease become more fully understood.

A cancer 'hazard' is an agent that is capable of causing cancer under some circumstances, while a cancer 'risk' is an estimate of the carcinogenic effects expected from exposure to a cancer hazard. The *Monographs* are an exercise in evaluating cancer hazards, despite the historical presence of the word 'risks' in the title. The distinction between hazard and risk is important, and the *Monographs* identify cancer hazards even when risks are very low at current exposure levels, because new uses or unforeseen exposures could engender risks that are significantly higher.

In the *Monographs*, an agent is termed 'carcinogenic' if it is capable of increasing the incidence of malignant neoplasms, reducing their latency, or increasing their severity or multiplicity. The induction of benign neoplasms may in some circumstances (see Part B, Section 3a) contribute to the judgement that the agent is carcinogenic. The terms 'neoplasm' and 'tumour' are used interchangeably.

The Preamble continues the previous usage of the phrase 'strength of evidence' as a matter of historical continuity, although it should be understood that *Monographs* evaluations consider studies that support a finding of a cancer hazard as well as studies that do not.

Some epidemiological and experimental studies indicate that different agents may act at different stages in the carcinogenic process, and several different mechanisms may be involved. The aim of the *Monographs* has been, from their inception, to evaluate evidence of carcinogenicity at any stage in the carcinogenesis process, independently of the underlying mechanisms. Information on mechanisms may, however, be used in making the overall evaluation (IARC, 1991; Vainio et al., 1992; IARC, 2005, 2006; see also Part B, Sections 4 and 6). As mechanisms of carcinogenesis are elucidated, IARC convenes international scientific conferences to determine whether a broad-based consensus has emerged on how specific mechanistic data can be used in an evaluation of human carcinogenicity. The results of such conferences are reported in IARC Scientific Publications, which, as long as they still reflect the current state of scientific knowledge, may guide subsequent Working Groups.

Although the *Monographs* have emphasized hazard identification, important issues may also involve dose–response assessment. In many cases, the same epidemiological and experimental studies used to evaluate a cancer hazard can also be used to estimate a dose–response relationship. A *Monograph* may undertake to estimate dose–response relationships within the range of the available epidemiological data, or it may compare the dose–response information from experimental and epidemiological studies. In some cases, a subsequent publication may be prepared by a separate Working Group with expertise in quantitative dose–response assessment.

The *Monographs* are used by national and international authorities to make risk assessments, formulate decisions concerning preventive measures, provide effective cancer control programmes and decide among alternative options for public health decisions. The evaluations of IARC Working Groups are scientific, qualitative judgements on the evidence for or against carcinogenicity provided by the available data. These evaluations represent only one part of the body of information on which public health decisions may be based. Public health options vary from one situation to another and from country to country and relate to many factors, including different socioeconomic and national priorities. Therefore, no recommendation is given with regard to regulation or legislation, which are the responsibility of individual governments or other international organizations.

3. Selection of agents for review

Agents are selected for review on the basis of two main criteria: (a) there is evidence of human exposure and (b) there is some evidence or suspicion of carcinogenicity. Mixed exposures may occur in occupational and environmental settings and as a result of individual and cultural habits (such as tobacco smoking and dietary practices). Chemical analogues and compounds with biological or physical characteristics similar to those of suspected carcinogens may also be considered, even in the absence of data on a possible carcinogenic effect in humans or experimental animals.

The scientific literature is surveyed for published data relevant to an assessment of carcinogenicity. Ad hoc Advisory Groups convened by IARC in 1984, 1989, 1991, 1993, 1998 and 2003 made recommendations as to which agents should be evaluated in the *Monographs* series. Recent recommendations are available on the *Monographs* programme web site (http://monographs.iarc.fr). IARC may schedule other agents for review as it becomes aware of new scientific information or as national health agencies identify an urgent public health need related to cancer.

As significant new data become available on an agent for which a *Monograph* exists, a re-evaluation may be made at a subsequent meeting, and a new *Monograph* published. In some cases it may be appropriate to review only the data published since a prior evaluation. This can be useful for updating a database, reviewing new data to resolve a previously open question or identifying new tumour sites associated with a carcinogenic agent. Major changes in an evaluation (e.g. a new classification in Group 1 or a determination that a mechanism does not operate in humans, see Part B, Section 6) are more appropriately addressed by a full review.

4. Data for the *Monographs*

Each *Monograph* reviews all pertinent epidemiological studies and cancer bioassays in experimental animals. Those judged inadequate or irrelevant to the evaluation may be cited but not summarized. If a group of similar studies is not reviewed, the reasons are indicated.

Mechanistic and other relevant data are also reviewed. A *Monograph* does not necessarily cite all the mechanistic literature concerning the agent being evaluated (see Part B, Section 4). Only those data considered by the Working Group to be relevant to making the evaluation are included.

With regard to epidemiological studies, cancer bioassays, and mechanistic and other relevant data, only reports that have been published or accepted for publication in the openly available scientific literature are reviewed. The same publication requirement applies to studies originating from IARC, including meta-analyses or pooled analyses commissioned by IARC in advance of a meeting (see Part B, Section 2c). Data from government agency reports that are publicly available are also considered. Exceptionally, doctoral theses and other material that are in their final form and publicly available may be reviewed.

Exposure data and other information on an agent under consideration are also reviewed. In the sections on chemical and physical properties, on analysis, on production and use and on occurrence, published and unpublished sources of information may be considered.

Inclusion of a study does not imply acceptance of the adequacy of the study design or of the analysis and interpretation of the results, and limitations are clearly outlined in square brackets at the end of each study description (see Part B). The reasons for not giving further consideration to an individual study also are indicated in the square brackets.

5. Meeting participants

Five categories of participant can be present at *Monograph* meetings.

(a)   The Working Group

The Working Group is responsible for the critical reviews and evaluations that are developed during the meeting. The tasks of Working Group Members are: (i) to ascertain that all appropriate data have been collected; (ii) to select the data relevant for the evaluation on the basis of scientific merit; (iii) to prepare accurate summaries of the data to enable the reader to follow the reasoning of the Working Group; (iv) to evaluate the results of epidemiological and experimental studies on cancer; (v) to evaluate data relevant to the understanding of mechanisms of carcinogenesis; and (vi) to make an overall evaluation of the carcinogenicity of the exposure to humans. Working Group Members generally have published significant research related to the carcinogenicity of the agents being reviewed, and IARC uses literature searches to identify most experts. Working Group Members are selected on the basis of (a) knowledge and experience and (b) absence of real or apparent conflicts of interests. Consideration is also given to demographic diversity and balance of scientific findings and views.

(b)   Invited Specialists

Invited Specialists are experts who also have critical knowledge and experience but have a real or apparent conflict of interests. These experts are invited when necessary to assist in the Working Group by contributing their unique knowledge and experience during subgroup and plenary discussions. They may also contribute text on non-influential issues in the section on exposure, such as a general description of data on production and use (see Part B, Section 1). Invited Specialists do not serve as meeting chair or subgroup chair, draft text that pertains to the description or interpretation of cancer data, or participate in the evaluations.

(c) Representatives of national and international health agencies

Representatives of national and international health agencies often attend meetings because their agencies sponsor the programme or are interested in the subject of a meeting. Representatives do not serve as meeting chair or subgroup chair, draft any part of a *Monograph,* or participate in the evaluations.

(d) Observers with relevant scientific credentials

Observers with relevant scientific credentials may be admitted to a meeting by IARC in limited numbers. Attention will be given to achieving a balance of Observers from constituencies with differing perspectives. They are invited to observe the meeting and should not attempt to influence it. Observers do not serve as meeting chair or subgroup chair, draft any part of a *Monograph,* or participate in the evaluations. At the meeting, the meeting chair and subgroup chairs may grant Observers an opportunity to speak, generally after they have observed a discussion. Observers agree to respect the Guidelines for Observers at *IARC Monographs* meetings (available at http://monographs.iarc.fr).

(e) The IARC Secretariat

The IARC Secretariat consists of scientists who are designated by IARC and who have relevant expertise. They serve as rapporteurs and participate in all discussions. When requested by the meeting chair or subgroup chair, they may also draft text or prepare tables and analyses.

Before an invitation is extended, each potential participant, including the IARC Secretariat, completes the WHO Declaration of Interests to report financial interests, employment and consulting, and individual and institutional research support related to the subject of the meeting. IARC assesses these interests to determine whether there is a conflict that warrants some limitation on participation. The declarations are updated and reviewed again at the opening of the meeting. Interests related to the subject of the meeting are disclosed to the meeting participants and in the published volume (Cogliano et al., 2004).

The names and principal affiliations of participants are available on the *Monographs* programme web site (http://monographs.iarc.fr) approximately two months before each meeting. It is not acceptable for Observers or third parties to contact other participants before a meeting or to lobby them at any time. Meeting participants are asked to report all such contacts to IARC (Cogliano et al., 2005).

All participants are listed, with their principal affiliations, at the beginning of each volume. Each participant who is a Member of a Working Group serves as an individual scientist and not as a representative of any organization, government or industry.

6. Working procedures

A separate Working Group is responsible for developing each volume of *Monographs*. A volume contains one or more *Monographs*, which can cover either a single agent or several related agents. Approximately one year in advance of the meeting of a Working Group, the agents to be reviewed are announced on the *Monographs* programme web site (http://monographs.iarc.fr) and participants are selected by IARC staff in consultation with other experts. Subsequently, relevant biological and epidemiological data are collected by IARC from recognized sources of information on carcinogenesis, including data storage and retrieval systems such as PubMed. Meeting participants who are asked to prepare preliminary working papers for specific sections are expected to supplement the IARC literature searches with their own searches.

Industrial associations, labour unions and other knowledgeable organizations may be asked to provide input to the sections on production and use, although this involvement is not required as a general rule. Information on production and trade is obtained from governmental, trade and market research publications and, in some cases, by direct contact with industries. Separate production data on some agents may not be available for a variety of reasons (e.g. not collected or made public in all producing countries, production is small). Information on uses may be obtained from published sources but is often complemented by direct contact with manufacturers. Efforts are made to supplement this information with data from other national and international sources.

Six months before the meeting, the material obtained is sent to meeting participants to prepare preliminary working papers. The working papers are compiled by IARC staff and sent, before the meeting, to Working Group Members and Invited Specialists for review.

The Working Group meets at IARC for seven to eight days to discuss and finalize the texts and to formulate the evaluations. The objectives of the meeting are peer review and consensus. During the first few days, four subgroups (covering exposure data, cancer in humans, cancer in experimental animals, and mechanistic and other relevant data) review the working papers, develop a joint subgroup draft and write summaries. Care is taken to ensure that each study summary is written or reviewed by someone not associated with the study being considered. During the last few days, the Working Group meets in plenary session to review the subgroup drafts and develop the evaluations. As a result, the entire volume is the joint product of the Working Group, and there are no individually authored sections.

IARC Working Groups strive to achieve a consensus evaluation. Consensus reflects broad agreement among Working Group Members, but not necessarily unanimity. The chair may elect to poll Working Group Members to determine the diversity of scientific opinion on issues where consensus is not readily apparent.

After the meeting, the master copy is verified by consulting the original literature, edited and prepared for publication. The aim is to publish the volume within six months of the Working Group meeting. A summary of the outcome is available on the *Monographs* programme web site soon after the meeting.

B. SCIENTIFIC REVIEW AND EVALUATION

The available studies are summarized by the Working Group, with particular regard to the qualitative aspects discussed below. In general, numerical findings are indicated as they appear in the original report; units are converted when necessary for easier comparison. The Working Group may conduct additional analyses of the published data and use them in their assessment of the evidence; the results of such supplementary analyses are given in square brackets. When an important aspect of a study that directly impinges on its interpretation should be brought to the attention of the reader, a Working Group comment is given in square brackets.

The scope of the *IARC Monographs* programme has expanded beyond chemicals to include complex mixtures, occupational exposures, physical and biological agents, lifestyle factors and other potentially carcinogenic exposures. Over time, the structure of a *Monograph* has evolved to include the following sections:

Exposure data
Studies of cancer in humans
Studies of cancer in experimental animals
Mechanistic and other relevant data
Summary
Evaluation and rationale

In addition, a section of General Remarks at the front of the volume discusses the reasons the agents were scheduled for evaluation and some key issues the Working Group encountered during the meeting.

This part of the Preamble discusses the types of evidence considered and summarized in each section of a *Monograph*, followed by the scientific criteria that guide the evaluations.

1. Exposure data

Each *Monograph* includes general information on the agent: this information may vary substantially between agents and must be adapted accordingly. Also included is information on production and use (when appropriate), methods of analysis and detection, occurrence, and sources and routes of human occupational and environmental exposures. Depending on the agent, regulations and guidelines for use may be presented.

(a)   General information on the agent

For chemical agents, sections on chemical and physical data are included: the Chemical Abstracts Service Registry Number, the latest primary name and the IUPAC systematic name are recorded; other synonyms are given, but the list is not necessarily comprehensive. Information on chemical and physical properties that are relevant to identification, occurrence and biological activity is included. A description of technical products of chemicals includes trade names, relevant specifications and available information on composition and impurities. Some of the trade names given may be those of mixtures in which the agent being evaluated is only one of the ingredients.

For biological agents, taxonomy, structure and biology are described, and the degree of variability is indicated. Mode of replication, life cycle, target cells, persistence, latency, host response and clinical disease other than cancer are also presented.

For physical agents that are forms of radiation, energy and range of the radiation are included. For foreign bodies, fibres and respirable particles, size range and relative dimensions are indicated.

For agents such as mixtures, drugs or lifestyle factors, a description of the agent, including its composition, is given.

Whenever appropriate, other information, such as historical perspectives or the description of an industry or habit, may be included.

(b)   Analysis and detection

An overview of methods of analysis and detection of the agent is presented, including their sensitivity, specificity and reproducibility. Methods widely used for regulatory purposes are emphasized. Methods for monitoring human exposure are also given. No critical evaluation or recommendation of any method is meant or implied.

(c)   Production and use

The dates of first synthesis and of first commercial production of a chemical, mixture or other agent are provided when available; for agents that do not occur naturally, this information may allow a reasonable estimate to be made of the date before which no human exposure to the agent could have occurred. The dates of first reported occurrence of an exposure are also provided when available. In addition, methods of synthesis used in past and present commercial production and different methods of production, which may give rise to different impurities, are described.

The countries where companies report production of the agent, and the number of companies in each country, are identified. Available data on production, international trade and uses are obtained for representative regions. It should not, however, be inferred that those areas or nations are necessarily the sole or major sources or users of the agent. Some identified uses may not be current or major applications, and the coverage is not necessarily comprehensive. In the case of drugs, mention of their therapeutic uses does not necessarily represent current practice nor does it imply judgement as to their therapeutic efficacy.

(d)   Occurrence and exposure

Information on the occurrence of an agent in the environment is obtained from data derived from the monitoring and surveillance of levels in occupational environments, air, water, soil, plants, foods and animal and human tissues. When available, data on the generation, persistence and bioaccumulation of the agent are also included. Such data may be available from national databases.

Data that indicate the extent of past and present human exposure, the sources of exposure, the people most likely to be exposed and the factors that contribute to the exposure are reported. Information is presented on the range of human exposure, including occupational and environmental exposures. This includes relevant findings from both developed and developing countries. Some of these data are not distributed widely and may be available from government reports and other sources. In the case of mixtures, industries, occupations or processes, information is given about all agents known to be present. For processes, industries and occupations, a historical description is also given, noting variations in chemical composition, physical properties and levels of occupational exposure with date and place. For biological agents, the epidemiology of infection is described.

(e)   Regulations and guidelines

Statements concerning regulations and guidelines (e.g. occupational exposure limits, maximal levels permitted in foods and water, pesticide registrations) are included, but they may not reflect the most recent situation, since such limits are continuously reviewed and modified. The absence of information on regulatory status for a country should not be taken to imply that that country does not have regulations with regard to the exposure. For biological agents, legislation and control, including vaccination and therapy, are described.

2.   Studies of cancer in humans

This section includes all pertinent epidemiological studies (see Part A, Section 4). Studies of biomarkers are included when they are relevant to an evaluation of carcinogenicity to humans.

(a)   Types of study considered

Several types of epidemiological study contribute to the assessment of carcinogenicity in humans — cohort studies, case–control studies, correlation (or ecological) studies and intervention studies. Rarely, results from randomized trials may be available. Case reports and case series of cancer in humans may also be reviewed.

Cohort and case–control studies relate individual exposures under study to the occurrence of cancer in individuals and provide an estimate of effect (such as relative risk) as the main measure of association. Intervention studies may provide strong evidence for making causal inferences, as exemplified by cessation of smoking and the subsequent decrease in risk for lung cancer.

In correlation studies, the units of investigation are usually whole populations (e.g. in particular geographical areas or at particular times), and cancer frequency is related to a summary measure of the exposure of the population to the agent under study. In correlation studies, individual exposure is not documented, which renders this kind of study more prone to confounding. In some circumstances, however, correlation studies may be more informative than analytical study designs (see, for example, the *Monograph* on arsenic in drinking-water; IARC, 2004).

In some instances, case reports and case series have provided important information about the carcinogenicity of an agent. These types of study generally arise from a suspicion, based on clinical experience, that the concurrence of two events — that is, a particular exposure and occurrence of a cancer — has happened rather more frequently than would be expected by chance. Case reports and case series usually lack complete ascertainment of cases in any population, definition or enumeration of the population at risk and estimation of the expected number of cases in the absence of exposure.

The uncertainties that surround the interpretation of case reports, case series and correlation studies make them inadequate, except in rare instances, to form the sole basis for inferring a causal relationship. When taken together with case–control and cohort studies, however, these types of study may add materially to the judgement that a causal relationship exists.

Epidemiological studies of benign neoplasms, presumed preneoplastic lesions and other end-points thought to be relevant to cancer are also reviewed. They may, in some instances, strengthen inferences drawn from studies of cancer itself.

(b)   *Quality of studies considered*

It is necessary to take into account the possible roles of bias, confounding and chance in the interpretation of epidemiological studies. Bias is the effect of factors in study design or execution that lead erroneously to a stronger or weaker association than in fact exists between an agent and disease. Confounding is a form of bias that occurs when the relationship with disease is made to appear stronger or weaker than it truly is as a result of an association between the apparent causal factor and another factor that is associated with either an increase or decrease in the incidence of the disease. The role of chance is related to biological variability and the influence of sample size on the precision of estimates of effect.

In evaluating the extent to which these factors have been minimized in an individual study, consideration is given to several aspects of design and analysis as described in the report of the study. For example, when suspicion of carcinogenicity arises largely from a single small study, careful consideration is given when interpreting subsequent studies that included these data in an enlarged population. Most of these considerations apply equally to case–control, cohort and correlation studies. Lack of clarity of any of these aspects in the reporting of a study can decrease its credibility and the weight given to it in the final evaluation of the exposure.

First, the study population, disease (or diseases) and exposure should have been well defined by the authors. Cases of disease in the study population should have been identified in a way that was independent of the exposure of interest, and exposure should have been assessed in a way that was not related to disease status.

Second, the authors should have taken into account — in the study design and analysis — other variables that can influence the risk of disease and may have been related to the exposure of interest. Potential confounding by such variables should have been dealt with either in the design of the study, such as by matching, or in the analysis, by statistical adjustment. In cohort studies, comparisons with local rates of disease may or may not be more appropriate than those with national rates. Internal comparisons of frequency of disease among individuals at different levels of exposure are also desirable in cohort studies, since they minimize the potential for confounding related to the difference in risk factors between an external reference group and the study population.

Third, the authors should have reported the basic data on which the conclusions are founded, even if sophisticated statistical analyses were employed. At the very least, they should have given the numbers of exposed and unexposed cases and controls in a case–control study and the numbers of cases observed and expected in a cohort study. Further tabulations by time since exposure began and other temporal factors are also important. In a cohort study, data on all cancer sites and all causes of death should have been given, to reveal the possibility of reporting bias. In a case–control study, the effects of investigated factors other than the exposure of interest should have been reported.

Finally, the statistical methods used to obtain estimates of relative risk, absolute rates of cancer, confidence intervals and significance tests, and to adjust for confounding should have been clearly stated by the authors. These methods have been reviewed for case–control studies (Breslow & Day, 1980) and for cohort studies (Breslow & Day, 1987).

(c)   Meta-analyses and pooled analyses

Independent epidemiological studies of the same agent may lead to results that are difficult to interpret. Combined analyses of data from multiple studies are a means of resolving this ambiguity, and well conducted analyses can be considered. There are two types of combined analysis. The first involves combining summary statistics such as relative risks from individual studies (meta-analysis) and the second involves a pooled analysis of the raw data from the individual studies (pooled analysis) (Greenland, 1998).

The advantages of combined analyses are increased precision due to increased sample size and the opportunity to explore potential confounders, interactions and modifying effects that may explain heterogeneity among studies in more detail. A disadvantage of combined analyses is the possible lack of compatibility of data from various studies due to differences in subject recruitment, procedures of data collection, methods of measurement and effects of unmeasured co-variates that may differ among studies. Despite these limitations, well conducted combined analyses may provide a firmer basis than individual studies for drawing conclusions about the potential carcinogenicity of agents.

IARC may commission a meta-analysis or pooled analysis that is pertinent to a particular *Monograph* (see Part A, Section 4). Additionally, as a means of gaining insight from the results of multiple individual studies, ad hoc calculations that combine data from different studies may be conducted by the Working Group during the course of a *Monograph* meeting. The results of such original calculations, which would be specified in the text by presentation in square brackets, might involve updates of previously conducted analyses that incorporate the results of more recent studies or de-novo analyses. Irrespective of the source of data for the meta-analyses and pooled analyses, it is important that the same criteria for data quality be applied as those that would be applied to individual studies and to ensure also that sources of heterogeneity between studies be taken into account.

(d)   Temporal effects

Detailed analyses of both relative and absolute risks in relation to temporal variables, such as age at first exposure, time since first exposure, duration of exposure, cumulative exposure, peak exposure (when appropriate) and time since cessation of exposure, are reviewed and summarized when available. Analyses of temporal relationships may be useful in making causal inferences. In addition, such analyses may suggest whether a carcinogen acts early or late in the process of carcinogenesis, although, at best, they allow only indirect inferences about mechanisms of carcinogenesis.

(e) Use of biomarkers in epidemiological studies

Biomarkers indicate molecular, cellular or other biological changes and are increasingly used in epidemiological studies for various purposes (IARC, 1991; Vainio et al., 1992; Toniolo et al., 1997; Vineis et al., 1999; Buffler et al., 2004). These may include evidence of exposure, of early effects, of cellular, tissue or organism responses, of individual susceptibility or host responses, and inference of a mechanism (see Part B, Section 4b). This is a rapidly evolving field that encompasses developments in genomics, epigenomics and other emerging technologies.

Molecular epidemiological data that identify associations between genetic polymorphisms and interindividual differences in susceptibility to the agent(s) being evaluated may contribute to the identification of carcinogenic hazards to humans. If the polymorphism has been demonstrated experimentally to modify the functional activity of the gene product in a manner that is consistent with increased susceptibility, these data may be useful in making causal inferences. Similarly, molecular epidemiological studies that measure cell functions, enzymes or metabolites that are thought to be the basis of susceptibility may provide evidence that reinforces biological plausibility. It should be noted, however, that when data on genetic susceptibility originate from multiple comparisons that arise from subgroup analyses, this can generate false-positive results and inconsistencies across studies, and such data therefore require careful evaluation. If the known phenotype of a genetic polymorphism can explain the carcinogenic mechanism of the agent being evaluated, data on this phenotype may be useful in making causal inferences.

(f) Criteria for causality

After the quality of individual epidemiological studies of cancer has been summarized and assessed, a judgement is made concerning the strength of evidence that the agent in question is carcinogenic to humans. In making its judgement, the Working Group considers several criteria for causality (Hill, 1965). A strong association (e.g. a large relative risk) is more likely to indicate causality than a weak association, although it is recognized that estimates of effect of small magnitude do not imply lack of causality and may be important if the disease or exposure is common. Associations that are replicated in several studies of the same design or that use different epidemiological approaches or under different circumstances of exposure are more likely to represent a causal relationship than isolated observations from single studies. If there are inconsistent results among investigations, possible reasons are sought (such as differences in exposure), and results of studies that are judged to be of high quality are given more weight than those of studies that are judged to be methodologically less sound.

If the risk increases with the exposure, this is considered to be a strong indication of causality, although the absence of a graded response is not necessarily evidence against a causal relationship. The demonstration of a decline in risk after cessation of or reduction in exposure in individuals or in whole populations also supports a causal interpretation of the findings.

Several scenarios may increase confidence in a causal relationship. On the one hand, an agent may be specific in causing tumours at one site or of one morphological type. On the other, carcinogenicity may be evident through the causation of multiple tumour types. Temporality, precision of estimates of effect, biological plausibility and coherence of the overall database are considered. Data on biomarkers may be employed in an assessment of the biological plausibility of epidemiological observations.

Although rarely available, results from randomized trials that show different rates of cancer among exposed and unexposed individuals provide particularly strong evidence for causality.

When several epidemiological studies show little or no indication of an association between an exposure and cancer, a judgement may be made that, in the aggregate, they show evidence of lack of carcinogenicity. Such a judgement requires first that the studies meet, to a sufficient degree, the standards of design and analysis described above. Specifically, the possibility that bias, confounding or misclassification of exposure or outcome could explain the observed results should be considered and excluded with reasonable certainty. In addition, all studies that are judged to be methodologically sound should (a) be consistent with an estimate of effect of unity for any observed level of exposure, (b) when considered together, provide a pooled estimate of relative risk that is at or near to unity, and (c) have a narrow confidence interval, due to sufficient population size. Moreover, no individual study nor the pooled results of all the studies should show any consistent tendency that the relative risk of cancer increases with increasing level of exposure. It is important to note that evidence of lack of carcinogenicity obtained from several epidemiological studies can apply only to the type(s) of cancer studied, to the dose levels reported, and to the intervals between first exposure and disease onset observed in these studies. Experience with human cancer indicates that the period from first exposure to the development of clinical cancer is sometimes longer than 20 years; latent periods substantially shorter than 30 years cannot provide evidence for lack of carcinogenicity.

3. Studies of cancer in experimental animals

All known human carcinogens that have been studied adequately for carcinogenicity in experimental animals have produced positive results in one or more animal species (Wilbourn et al., 1986; Tomatis et al., 1989). For several agents (e.g. aflatoxins, diethylstilbestrol, solar radiation, vinyl chloride), carcinogenicity in experimental animals was established or highly suspected before epidemiological studies confirmed their carcinogenicity in humans (Vainio et al., 1995). Although this association cannot establish that all agents that cause cancer in experimental animals also cause cancer in humans, it is biologically plausible that agents for which there is *sufficient evidence of carcinogenicity* in experimental animals (see Part B, Section 6b) also present a carcinogenic hazard to humans. Accordingly, in the absence of additional scientific information, these agents are considered to pose a carcinogenic hazard to humans. Examples of additional scientific information are data that demonstrate that a given agent causes cancer in animals through a species-specific mechanism that does not operate in humans or data that demonstrate that the mechanism in experimental animals also operates in humans (see Part B, Section 6).

Consideration is given to all available long-term studies of cancer in experimental animals with the agent under review (see Part A, Section 4). In all experimental settings, the nature and extent of impurities or contaminants present in the agent being evaluated are given when available. Animal species, strain (including genetic background where applicable), sex, numbers per group, age at start of treatment, route of exposure, dose levels, duration of exposure, survival and information on tumours (incidence, latency, severity or multiplicity of neoplasms or preneoplastic lesions) are reported. Those studies in experimental animals that are judged to be irrelevant to the evaluation or judged to be inadequate (e.g. too short a duration, too few animals, poor survival; see below) may be omitted. Guidelines for conducting long-term carcinogenicity experiments have been published (e.g. OECD, 2002).

Other studies considered may include: experiments in which the agent was administered in the presence of factors that modify carcinogenic effects (e.g. initiation–promotion studies, co-carcinogenicity studies and studies in genetically modified animals); studies in which the end-point was not cancer but a defined precancerous lesion; experiments on the carcinogenicity of known metabolites and derivatives; and studies of cancer in non-laboratory animals (e.g. livestock and companion animals) exposed to the agent.

For studies of mixtures, consideration is given to the possibility that changes in the physicochemical properties of the individual substances may occur during collection, storage, extraction, concentration and delivery. Another consideration is that chemical and toxicological interactions of components in a mixture may alter dose–response relationships. The relevance to human exposure of the test mixture administered in the animal experiment is also assessed. This may involve consideration of the following aspects of the mixture tested: (i) physical and chemical characteristics, (ii) identified constituents that may indicate the presence of a class of substances and (iii) the results of genetic toxicity and related tests.

The relevance of results obtained with an agent that is analogous (e.g. similar in structure or of a similar virus genus) to that being evaluated is also considered. Such results may provide biological and mechanistic information that is relevant to the understanding of the process of carcinogenesis in humans and may strengthen the biological plausibility that the agent being evaluated is carcinogenic to humans (see Part B, Section 2f).

(a) Qualitative aspects

An assessment of carcinogenicity involves several considerations of qualitative importance, including (i) the experimental conditions under which the test was performed, including route, schedule and duration of exposure, species, strain (including genetic background where applicable), sex, age and duration of follow-up; (ii) the consistency of the results, for example, across species and target organ(s); (iii) the spectrum of neoplastic response, from preneoplastic lesions and benign tumours to malignant neoplasms; and (iv) the possible role of modifying factors.

Considerations of importance in the interpretation and evaluation of a particular study include: (i) how clearly the agent was defined and, in the case of mixtures, how adequately the sample characterization was reported; (ii) whether the dose was monitored adequately, particularly in inhalation experiments; (iii) whether the doses, duration of treatment and route of exposure were appropriate; (iv) whether the survival of treated animals was similar to that of controls; (v) whether there were adequate numbers of animals per group; (vi) whether both male and female animals were used; (vii) whether animals were allocated randomly to groups; (viii) whether the duration of observation was adequate; and (ix) whether the data were reported and analysed adequately.

When benign tumours (a) occur together with and originate from the same cell type as malignant tumours in an organ or tissue in a particular study and (b) appear to represent a stage in the progression to malignancy, they are usually combined in the assessment of tumour incidence (Huff et al., 1989). The occurrence of lesions presumed to be preneoplastic may in certain instances aid in assessing the biological plausibility of any neoplastic response observed. If an agent induces only benign neoplasms that appear to be end-points that do not readily undergo transition to malignancy, the agent should nevertheless be suspected of being carcinogenic and requires further investigation.

(b) Quantitative aspects

The probability that tumours will occur may depend on the species, sex, strain, genetic background and age of the animal, and on the dose, route, timing and duration of the exposure. Evidence of an increased incidence of neoplasms with increasing levels of exposure strengthens the inference of a causal association between the exposure and the development of neoplasms.

The form of the dose–response relationship can vary widely, depending on the particular agent under study and the target organ. Mechanisms such as induction of DNA damage or inhibition of repair, altered cell division and cell death rates and changes in intercellular communication are important determinants of dose–response relationships for some carcinogens. Since many chemicals require metabolic activation before being converted to their reactive intermediates, both metabolic and toxicokinetic aspects are important in determining the dose–response pattern. Saturation of steps such as absorption, activation, inactivation and elimination may produce nonlinearity in the dose–response relationship (Hoel et al., 1983; Gart et al., 1986), as could saturation of processes such as DNA repair. The dose–response relationship can also be affected by differences in survival among the treatment groups.

(c) Statistical analyses

Factors considered include the adequacy of the information given for each treatment group: (i) number of animals studied and number examined histologically, (ii) number of animals with a given tumour type and (iii) length of survival. The statistical methods used should be clearly stated and should be the generally accepted techniques refined for this purpose (Peto et al., 1980; Gart et al., 1986; Portier & Bailer, 1989; Bieler & Williams, 1993). The choice of the most appropriate statistical method requires consideration of whether or not there are differences in survival among the treatment groups; for example, reduced survival because of non-tumour-related mortality can preclude the occurrence of tumours later in life. When detailed information on survival is not available, comparisons of the proportions of tumour-bearing animals among the effective number of animals (alive at the time the first tumour was discovered) can be useful when significant differences in survival occur before tumours appear. The lethality of the tumour also requires consideration: for rapidly fatal tumours, the time of death provides an indication of the time of tumour onset and can be assessed using life-table methods; non-fatal or incidental tumours that do not affect survival can be assessed using methods such as the Mantel-Haenzel test for changes in tumour prevalence. Because tumour lethality is often difficult to determine, methods such as the Poly-K test that do not require such information can also be used. When results are available on the number and size of tumours seen in experimental animals (e.g. papillomas on mouse skin, liver tumours observed through nuclear magnetic resonance tomography), other more complicated statistical procedures may be needed (Sherman et al., 1994; Dunson et al., 2003).

Formal statistical methods have been developed to incorporate historical control data into the analysis of data from a given experiment. These methods assign an appropriate weight to historical and concurrent controls on the basis of the extent of between-study and within-study variability: less weight is given to historical controls when they show a high degree of variability, and greater weight when they show little variability. It is generally not appropriate to discount a tumour response that is significantly increased compared with concurrent controls by arguing that it falls within the range of historical controls, particularly when historical controls show high between-study variability and are, thus, of little relevance to the current experiment. In analysing results for uncommon tumours, however, the analysis may be improved by considering historical control data, particularly when between-study variability is low. Historical controls should be selected to resemble the concurrent controls as closely as possible with respect to species, gender and strain, as well as other factors such as basal diet and general laboratory environment, which may affect tumour-response rates in control animals (Haseman et al., 1984; Fung et al., 1996; Greim et al., 2003).

Although meta-analyses and combined analyses are conducted less frequently for animal experiments than for epidemiological studies due to differences in animal strains, they can be useful aids in interpreting animal data when the experimental protocols are sufficiently similar.

4. Mechanistic and other relevant data

Mechanistic and other relevant data may provide evidence of carcinogenicity and also help in assessing the relevance and importance of findings of cancer in animals and in humans. The nature of the mechanistic and other relevant data depends on the biological activity of the agent being considered. The Working Group considers representative studies to give a concise description of the relevant data and issues that they consider to be important; thus, not every available study is cited. Relevant topics may include toxicokinetics, mechanisms of carcinogenesis, susceptible individuals, populations and life-stages, other relevant data and other adverse effects. When data on biomarkers are informative about the mechanisms of carcinogenesis, they are included in this section.

These topics are not mutually exclusive; thus, the same studies may be discussed in more than one subsection. For example, a mutation in a gene that codes for an enzyme that metabolizes the agent under study could be discussed in the subsections on toxicokinetics, mechanisms and individual susceptibility if it also exists as an inherited polymorphism.

(a)   Toxicokinetic data

Toxicokinetics refers to the absorption, distribution, metabolism and elimination of agents in humans, experimental animals and, where relevant, cellular systems. Examples of kinetic factors that may affect dose–response relationships include uptake, deposition, biopersistence and half-life in tissues, protein binding, metabolic activation and detoxification. Studies that indicate the metabolic fate of the agent in humans and in experimental animals are summarized briefly, and comparisons of data from humans and animals are made when possible. Comparative information on the relationship between exposure and the dose that reaches the target site may be important for the extrapolation of hazards between species and in clarifying the role of in-vitro findings.

(b)   Data on mechanisms of carcinogenesis

To provide focus, the Working Group attempts to identify the possible mechanisms by which the agent may increase the risk of cancer. For each possible mechanism, a representative selection of key data from humans and experimental systems is summarized. Attention is given to gaps in the data and to data that suggests that more than one mechanism may be operating. The relevance of the mechanism to humans is discussed, in particular, when mechanistic data are derived from experimental model systems. Changes in the affected organs, tissues or cells can be divided into three non-exclusive levels as described below.

(i) Changes in physiology

Physiological changes refer to exposure-related modifications to the physiology and/or response of cells, tissues and organs. Examples of potentially adverse physiological changes include mitogenesis, compensatory cell division, escape from apoptosis and/or senescence, presence of inflammation, hyperplasia, metaplasia and/or preneoplasia, angiogenesis, alterations in cellular adhesion, changes in steroidal hormones and changes in immune surveillance.

(ii) Functional changes at the cellular level

Functional changes refer to exposure-related alterations in the signalling pathways used by cells to manage critical processes that are related to increased risk for cancer. Examples of functional changes include modified activities of enzymes involved in the metabolism of xenobiotics, alterations in the expression of key genes that regulate DNA repair, alterations in cyclin-dependent kinases that govern cell cycle progression, changes in the patterns of post-translational modifications of proteins, changes in regulatory factors that alter apoptotic rates, changes in the secretion of factors related to the stimulation of DNA replication and transcription and changes in gap–junction-mediated intercellular communication.

(iii) Changes at the molecular level

Molecular changes refer to exposure-related changes in key cellular structures at the molecular level, including, in particular, genotoxicity. Examples of molecular changes include formation of DNA adducts and DNA strand breaks, mutations in genes, chromosomal aberrations, aneuploidy and changes in DNA methylation patterns. Greater emphasis is given to irreversible effects.

The use of mechanistic data in the identification of a carcinogenic hazard is specific to the mechanism being addressed and is not readily described for every possible level and mechanism discussed above.

Genotoxicity data are discussed here to illustrate the key issues involved in the evaluation of mechanistic data.

Tests for genetic and related effects are described in view of the relevance of gene mutation and chromosomal aberration/aneuploidy to carcinogenesis (Vainio et al., 1992; McGregor et al., 1999). The adequacy of the reporting of sample characterization is considered and, when necessary, commented upon; with regard to complex mixtures, such comments are similar to those described for animal carcinogenicity tests. The available data are interpreted critically according to the end-points detected, which may include DNA damage, gene mutation, sister chromatid exchange, micronucleus formation, chromosomal aberrations and aneuploidy. The concentrations employed are given, and mention is made of whether the use of an exogenous metabolic system in vitro affected the test result. These data are listed in tabular form by phylogenetic classification.

Positive results in tests using prokaryotes, lower eukaryotes, insects, plants and cultured mammalian cells suggest that genetic and related effects could occur in mammals. Results from such tests may also give information on the types of genetic effect produced and on the involvement of metabolic activation. Some end-points described are clearly genetic in nature (e.g. gene mutations), while others are associated with genetic effects (e.g. unscheduled DNA synthesis). In-vitro tests for tumour promotion, cell transformation and gap–junction intercellular communication may be sensitive to changes that are not necessarily the result of genetic alterations but that may have specific relevance to the process of carcinogenesis. Critical appraisals of these tests have been published (Montesano et al., 1986; McGregor et al., 1999).

Genetic or other activity manifest in humans and experimental mammals is regarded to be of greater relevance than that in other organisms. The demonstration that an agent can induce gene and chromosomal mutations in mammals in vivo indicates that it may have carcinogenic activity. Negative results in tests for mutagenicity in selected tissues from animals treated in vivo provide less weight, partly because they do not exclude the possibility of an effect in tissues other than those examined. Moreover, negative results in short-term tests with genetic end-points cannot be considered to provide evidence that rules out the carcinogenicity of agents that act through other mechanisms (e.g. receptor-mediated effects, cellular toxicity with regenerative cell division, peroxisome proliferation) (Vainio et al., 1992). Factors that may give misleading results in short-term tests have been discussed in detail elsewhere (Montesano et al., 1986; McGregor et al., 1999).

When there is evidence that an agent acts by a specific mechanism that does not involve genotoxicity (e.g. hormonal dysregulation, immune suppression, and formation of calculi and other deposits that cause chronic irritation), that evidence is presented and reviewed critically in the context of rigorous criteria for the operation of that mechanism in carcinogenesis (e.g. Capen et al., 1999).

For biological agents such as viruses, bacteria and parasites, other data relevant to carcinogenicity may include descriptions of the pathology of infection, integration and expression of viruses, and genetic alterations seen in human tumours. Other observations that might comprise cellular and tissue responses to infection, immune response and the presence of tumour markers are also considered.

For physical agents that are forms of radiation, other data relevant to carcinogenicity may include descriptions of damaging effects at the physiological, cellular and molecular level, as for chemical agents, and descriptions of how these effects occur. 'Physical agents' may also be considered to comprise foreign bodies, such as surgical implants of various kinds, and poorly soluble fibres, dusts and particles of various sizes, the pathogenic effects of which are a result of their physical presence in tissues or body cavities. Other relevant data for such materials may include characterization of cellular, tissue and physiological reactions to these materials and descriptions of pathological conditions other than neoplasia with which they may be associated.

(c)   Other data relevant to mechanisms

A description is provided of any structure–activity relationships that may be relevant to an evaluation of the carcinogenicity of an agent, the toxicological implications of the physical and chemical properties, and any other data relevant to the evaluation that are not included elsewhere.

High-output data, such as those derived from gene expression microarrays, and high-throughput data, such as those that result from testing hundreds of agents for a single end-point, pose a unique problem for the use of mechanistic data in the evaluation of a carcinogenic hazard. In the case of high-output data, there is the possibility to overinterpret changes in individual end-points (e.g. changes in expression in one gene) without considering the consistency of that finding in the broader context of the other end-points (e.g. other genes with linked transcriptional control). High-output data can be used in assessing mechanisms, but all end-points measured in a single experiment need to be considered in the proper context. For high-throughput data, where the number of observations far exceeds the number of end-points measured, their utility for identifying common mechanisms across multiple agents is enhanced. These data can be used to identify mechanisms that not only seem plausible, but also have a consistent pattern of carcinogenic response across entire classes of related compounds.

(d)   Susceptibility data

Individuals, populations and life-stages may have greater or lesser susceptibility to an agent, based on toxicokinetics, mechanisms of carcinogenesis and other factors. Examples of host and genetic factors that affect individual susceptibility include sex, genetic polymorphisms of genes involved in the metabolism of the agent under evaluation, differences in metabolic capacity due to life-stage or the presence of disease, differences in DNA repair capacity, competition for or alteration of metabolic capacity by medications or other chemical exposures, pre-existing hormonal imbalance that is exacerbated by a chemical exposure, a suppressed immune system, periods of higher-than-usual tissue growth or regeneration and genetic polymorphisms that lead to differences in behaviour (e.g. addiction). Such data can substantially increase the strength of the evidence from epidemiological data and enhance the linkage of in-vivo and in-vitro laboratory studies to humans.

(e)   Data on other adverse effects

Data on acute, subchronic and chronic adverse effects relevant to the cancer evaluation are summarized. Adverse effects that confirm distribution and biological effects at the sites of tumour development, or alterations in physiology that could lead to tumour development, are emphasized. Effects on reproduction, embryonic and fetal survival and development are summarized briefly. The adequacy of epidemiological studies of reproductive outcome and genetic and related effects in humans is judged by the same criteria as those applied to epidemiological studies of cancer, but fewer details are given.

5. Summary

This section is a summary of data presented in the preceding sections. Summaries can be found on the *Monographs* programme web site (http://monographs.iarc.fr).

(a)   Exposure data

Data are summarized, as appropriate, on the basis of elements such as production, use, occurrence and exposure levels in the workplace and environment and measurements in human tissues and body fluids. Quantitative data and time trends are given to compare exposures in different occupations and environmental settings. Exposure to biological agents is described in terms of transmission, prevalence and persistence of infection.

(b)   Cancer in humans

Results of epidemiological studies pertinent to an assessment of human carcinogenicity are summarized. When relevant, case reports and correlation studies are also summarized. The target organ(s) or tissue(s) in which an increase in cancer was observed is identified. Dose–response and other quantitative data may be summarized when available.

(c)   Cancer in experimental animals

Data relevant to an evaluation of carcinogenicity in animals are summarized. For each animal species, study design and route of administration, it is stated whether an increased incidence, reduced latency, or increased severity or multiplicity of neoplasms or preneoplastic lesions were observed, and the tumour sites are indicated. If the agent produced tumours after prenatal exposure or in single-dose experiments, this is also mentioned. Negative findings, inverse relationships, dose–response and other quantitative data are also summarized.

(d)   Mechanistic and other relevant data

Data relevant to the toxicokinetics (absorption, distribution, metabolism, elimination) and the possible mechanism(s) of carcinogenesis (e.g. genetic toxicity, epigenetic effects) are summarized. In addition, information on susceptible individuals, populations and life-stages is summarized. This section also reports on other toxic effects, including reproductive and developmental effects, as well as additional relevant data that are considered to be important.

6. Evaluation and rationale

Evaluations of the strength of the evidence for carcinogenicity arising from human and experimental animal data are made, using standard terms. The strength of the mechanistic evidence is also characterized.

It is recognized that the criteria for these evaluations, described below, cannot encompass all of the factors that may be relevant to an evaluation of carcinogenicity. In considering all of the relevant scientific data, the Working Group may assign the agent to a higher or lower category than a strict interpretation of these criteria would indicate.

These categories refer only to the strength of the evidence that an exposure is carcinogenic and not to the extent of its carcinogenic activity (potency). A classification may change as new information becomes available.

An evaluation of the degree of evidence is limited to the materials tested, as defined physically, chemically or biologically. When the agents evaluated are considered by the Working Group to be sufficiently closely related, they may be grouped together for the purpose of a single evaluation of the degree of evidence.

(a) Carcinogenicity in humans

The evidence relevant to carcinogenicity from studies in humans is classified into one of the following categories:

Sufficient evidence of carcinogenicity: The Working Group considers that a causal relationship has been established between exposure to the agent and human cancer. That is, a positive relationship has been observed between the exposure and cancer in studies in which chance, bias and confounding could be ruled out with reasonable confidence. A statement that there is *sufficient evidence* is followed by a separate sentence that identifies the target organ(s) or tissue(s) where an increased risk of cancer was observed in humans. Identification of a specific target organ or tissue does not preclude the possibility that the agent may cause cancer at other sites.

Limited evidence of carcinogenicity: A positive association has been observed between exposure to the agent and cancer for which a causal interpretation is considered by the Working Group to be credible, but chance, bias or confounding could not be ruled out with reasonable confidence.

Inadequate evidence of carcinogenicity: The available studies are of insufficient quality, consistency or statistical power to permit a conclusion regarding the presence or absence of a causal association between exposure and cancer, or no data on cancer in humans are available.

Evidence suggesting lack of carcinogenicity: There are several adequate studies covering the full range of levels of exposure that humans are known to encounter, which are mutually consistent in not showing a positive association between exposure to the agent and any studied cancer at any observed level of exposure. The results from these studies alone or combined should have narrow confidence intervals with an upper limit close to the null value (e.g. a relative risk of 1.0). Bias and confounding should be ruled out with reasonable confidence, and the studies should have an adequate length of follow-up. A conclusion of *evidence suggesting lack of carcinogenicity* is inevitably limited to the cancer sites, conditions and levels of exposure, and length of observation covered by the available studies. In addition, the possibility of a very small risk at the levels of exposure studied can never be excluded.

In some instances, the above categories may be used to classify the degree of evidence related to carcinogenicity in specific organs or tissues.

When the available epidemiological studies pertain to a mixture, process, occupation or industry, the Working Group seeks to identify the specific agent considered most likely to be responsible for any excess risk. The evaluation is focused as narrowly as the available data on exposure and other aspects permit.

(b)   Carcinogenicity in experimental animals

Carcinogenicity in experimental animals can be evaluated using conventional bioassays, bioassays that employ genetically modified animals, and other in-vivo bioassays that focus on one or more of the critical stages of carcinogenesis. In the absence of data from conventional long-term bioassays or from assays with neoplasia as the end-point, consistently positive results in several models that address several stages in the multistage process of carcinogenesis should be considered in evaluating the degree of evidence of carcinogenicity in experimental animals.

The evidence relevant to carcinogenicity in experimental animals is classified into one of the following categories:

Sufficient evidence of carcinogenicity: The Working Group considers that a causal relationship has been established between the agent and an increased incidence of malignant neoplasms or of an appropriate combination of benign and malignant neoplasms in (a) two or more species of animals or (b) two or more independent studies in one species carried out at different times or in different laboratories or under different protocols. An increased incidence of tumours in both sexes of a single species in a well conducted study, ideally conducted under Good Laboratory Practices, can also provide *sufficient evidence*.

A single study in one species and sex might be considered to provide *sufficient evidence of carcinogenicity* when malignant neoplasms occur to an unusual degree with regard to incidence, site, type of tumour or age at onset, or when there are strong findings of tumours at multiple sites.

Limited evidence of carcinogenicity: The data suggest a carcinogenic effect but are limited for making a definitive evaluation because, e.g. (a) the evidence of carcinogenicity is restricted to a single experiment; (b) there are unresolved questions regarding the adequacy of the design, conduct or interpretation of the studies; (c) the agent increases the incidence only of benign neoplasms or lesions of uncertain neoplastic potential; or (d) the evidence of carcinogenicity is restricted to studies that demonstrate only promoting activity in a narrow range of tissues or organs.

Inadequate evidence of carcinogenicity: The studies cannot be interpreted as showing either the presence or absence of a carcinogenic effect because of major qualitative or quantitative limitations, or no data on cancer in experimental animals are available.

Evidence suggesting lack of carcinogenicity: Adequate studies involving at least two species are available which show that, within the limits of the tests used, the agent is not carcinogenic. A conclusion of *evidence suggesting lack of carcinogenicity* is inevitably limited to the species, tumour sites, age at exposure, and conditions and levels of exposure studied.

(c)   Mechanistic and other relevant data

Mechanistic and other evidence judged to be relevant to an evaluation of carcinogenicity and of sufficient importance to affect the overall evaluation is highlighted. This may include data on preneoplastic lesions, tumour pathology, genetic and related effects, structure–activity relationships, metabolism and toxicokinetics, physicochemical parameters and analogous biological agents.

The strength of the evidence that any carcinogenic effect observed is due to a particular mechanism is evaluated, using terms such as 'weak', 'moderate' or 'strong'. The Working Group then assesses whether that particular mechanism is likely to be operative in humans. The strongest indications that a particular mechanism operates in humans derive from data on humans or biological specimens obtained from exposed humans. The data may be considered to be especially relevant if they show that the agent in question has caused changes in exposed humans that are on the causal pathway to carcinogenesis. Such data may, however, never become available, because it is at least conceivable that certain compounds may be kept from human use solely on the basis of evidence of their toxicity and/or carcinogenicity in experimental systems.

The conclusion that a mechanism operates in experimental animals is strengthened by findings of consistent results in different experimental systems, by the demonstration of biological plausibility and by coherence of the overall database. Strong support can be obtained from studies that challenge the hypothesized mechanism experimentally, by demonstrating that the suppression of key mechanistic processes leads to the suppression of tumour development. The Working Group considers whether multiple mechanisms might contribute to tumour development, whether different mechanisms might operate in different dose ranges, whether separate mechanisms might operate in humans and experimental animals and whether a unique mechanism might operate in a susceptible group. The possible contribution of alternative mechanisms must be considered before concluding that tumours observed in experimental animals are not relevant to humans. An uneven level of experimental support for different mechanisms may reflect that disproportionate resources have been focused on investigating a favoured mechanism.

For complex exposures, including occupational and industrial exposures, the chemical composition and the potential contribution of carcinogens known to be present are considered by the Working Group in its overall evaluation of human carcinogenicity. The Working Group also determines the extent to which the materials tested in experimental systems are related to those to which humans are exposed.

(d)   Overall evaluation

Finally, the body of evidence is considered as a whole, to reach an overall evaluation of the carcinogenicity of the agent to humans.

An evaluation may be made for a group of agents that have been evaluated by the Working Group. In addition, when supporting data indicate that other related agents, for which there is no direct evidence of their capacity to induce cancer in humans or in animals, may also be carcinogenic, a statement describing the rationale for this conclusion is added to the evaluation narrative; an additional evaluation may be made for this broader group of agents if the strength of the evidence warrants it.

The agent is described according to the wording of one of the following categories, and the designated group is given. The categorization of an agent is a matter of scientific judgement that reflects the strength of the evidence derived from studies in humans and in experimental animals and from mechanistic and other relevant data.

Group 1: The agent is carcinogenic to humans.

This category is used when there is *sufficient evidence of carcinogenicity* in humans. Exceptionally, an agent may be placed in this category when evidence of carcinogenicity in humans is less than *sufficient* but there is *sufficient evidence of carcinogenicity* in experimental animals and strong evidence in exposed humans that the agent acts through a relevant mechanism of carcinogenicity.

Group 2.

This category includes agents for which, at one extreme, the degree of evidence of carcinogenicity in humans is almost *sufficient*, as well as those for which, at the other extreme, there are no human data but for which there is evidence of carcinogenicity in experimental animals. Agents are assigned to either Group 2A (*probably carcinogenic to humans*) or Group 2B (*possibly carcinogenic to humans*) on the basis of epidemiological and experimental evidence of carcinogenicity and mechanistic and other relevant data. The terms *probably carcinogenic* and *possibly carcinogenic* have no quantitative significance and are used simply as descriptors of different levels of evidence of human carcinogenicity, with *probably carcinogenic* signifying a higher level of evidence than *possibly carcinogenic*.

Group 2A: The agent is probably carcinogenic to humans.

This category is used when there is *limited evidence of carcinogenicity* in humans and *sufficient evidence of carcinogenicity* in experimental animals. In some cases, an agent may be classified in this category when there is *inadequate evidence of carcinogenicity* in humans and *sufficient evidence of carcinogenicity* in experimental animals and strong evidence that the carcinogenesis is mediated by a mechanism that also operates in humans. Exceptionally, an agent may be classified in this category solely on the basis of *limited evidence of carcinogenicity* in humans. An agent may be assigned to this category if it clearly belongs, based on mechanistic considerations, to a class of agents for which one or more members have been classified in Group 1 or Group 2A.

Group 2B: The agent is possibly carcinogenic to humans.

This category is used for agents for which there is *limited evidence of carcinogenicity* in humans and less than *sufficient evidence of carcinogenicity* in experimental animals. It may also be used when there is *inadequate evidence of carcinogenicity* in humans but there is *sufficient evidence of carcinogenicity* in experimental animals. In some instances, an agent for which there is *inadequate evidence of carcinogenicity* in humans and less than *sufficient evidence of carcinogenicity* in experimental animals together with supporting evidence from mechanistic and other relevant data may be placed in this group. An agent may be classified in this category solely on the basis of strong evidence from mechanistic and other relevant data.

Group 3: The agent is not classifiable as to its carcinogenicity to humans.

This category is used most commonly for agents for which the evidence of carcinogenicity is *inadequate* in humans and *inadequate* or *limited* in experimental animals.

Exceptionally, agents for which the evidence of carcinogenicity is *inadequate* in humans but *sufficient* in experimental animals may be placed in this category when there is strong evidence that the mechanism of carcinogenicity in experimental animals does not operate in humans.

Agents that do not fall into any other group are also placed in this category.

An evaluation in Group 3 is not a determination of non-carcinogenicity or overall safety. It often means that further research is needed, especially when exposures are widespread or the cancer data are consistent with differing interpretations.

Group 4: The agent is probably not carcinogenic to humans.

This category is used for agents for which there is *evidence suggesting lack of carcinogenicity* in humans and in experimental animals. In some instances, agents for which there is *inadequate evidence of carcinogenicity* in humans but *evidence suggesting lack of carcinogenicity* in experimental animals, consistently and strongly supported by a broad range of mechanistic and other relevant data, may be classified in this group.

(e)   Rationale

The reasoning that the Working Group used to reach its evaluation is presented and discussed. This section integrates the major findings from studies of cancer in humans, studies of cancer in experimental animals, and mechanistic and other relevant data. It includes concise statements of the principal line(s) of argument that emerged, the conclusions of the Working Group on the strength of the evidence for each group of studies, citations to indicate which studies were pivotal to these conclusions, and an explanation of the reasoning of the Working Group in weighing data and making evaluations. When there are significant differences of scientific interpretation among Working Group Members, a brief summary of the alternative interpretations is provided, together with their scientific rationale and an indication of the relative degree of support for each alternative.

References

Bieler GS & Williams RL (1993). Ratio estimates, the delta method, and quantal response tests for increased carcinogenicity. *Biometrics*, 49: 793–801. doi:10.2307/2532200 PMID:8241374

Breslow NE & Day NE (1980). Statistical methods in cancer research. Volume I - The analysis of case-control studies. *IARC Sci Publ*, 32: 5–338. PMID:7216345

Breslow NE & Day NE (1987). Statistical methods in cancer research. Volume II–The design and analysis of cohort studies. *IARC Sci Publ*, 82: 1–406. PMID:3329634

Buffler P, Rice J, Baan R *et al.* (2004). Workshop on Mechanisms of Carcinogenesis: Contributions of Molecular Epidemiology. Lyon, 14–17 November 2001. Workshop report. *IARC Sci Publ*, 157: 1–27. PMID:15055286

Capen CC, Dybing E, Rice JM, Wilbourn JD (1999). Species Differences in Thyroid, Kidney and Urinary Bladder Carcinogenesis. Proceedings of a consensus conference. Lyon, France, 3–7 November 1997. *IARC Sci Publ*, 147: 1–225.

Cogliano V, Baan R, Straif K *et al.* (2005). Transparency in IARC Monographs. *Lancet Oncol*, 6: 747. doi:10.1016/S1470-2045(05)70380-6

Cogliano VJ, Baan RA, Straif K *et al.* (2004). The science and practice of carcinogen identification and evaluation. *Environ Health Perspect*, 112: 1269–1274. doi:10.1289/ehp.6950 PMID:15345338

Dunson DB, Chen Z, Harry J (2003). A Bayesian approach for joint modeling of cluster size and subunit-specific outcomes. *Biometrics*, 59: 521–530. doi:10.1111/1541-0420.00062 PMID:14601753

Fung KY, Krewski D, Smythe RT (1996). A comparison of tests for trend with historical controls in carcinogen bioassay. *Can J Stat*, 24: 431–454. doi:10.2307/3315326

Gart JJ, Krewski D, Lee PN *et al.* (1986). Statistical methods in cancer research. Volume III–The design and analysis of long-term animal experiments. *IARC Sci Publ*, 79: 1–219. PMID:3301661

Greenland S (1998). Meta-analysis. In: *Modern Epidemiology*. Rothman KJ, Greenland S, editors. Philadelphia: Lippincott Williams & Wilkins, pp. 643–673

Greim H, Gelbke H-P, Reuter U *et al.* (2003). Evaluation of historical control data in carcinogenicity studies. *Hum Exp Toxicol*, 22: 541–549. doi:10.1191/0960327103ht394oa PMID:14655720

Haseman JK, Huff J, Boorman GA (1984). Use of historical control data in carcinogenicity studies in rodents. *Toxicol Pathol*, 12: 126–135. doi:10.1177/019262338401200203 PMID:11478313

Hill AB (1965). The environment and disease: Association or causation? *Proc R Soc Med*, 58: 295–300. PMID:14283879

Hoel DG, Kaplan NL, Anderson MW (1983). Implication of nonlinear kinetics on risk estimation in carcinogenesis. *Science*, 219: 1032–1037. doi:10.1126/science.6823565 PMID:6823565

Huff JE, Eustis SL, Haseman JK (1989). Occurrence and relevance of chemically induced benign neoplasms in long-term carcinogenicity studies. *Cancer Metastasis Rev*, 8: 1–22. doi:10.1007/BF00047055 PMID:2667783

IARC (1977). *IARC Monographs Programme on the Evaluation of the Carcinogenic Risk of Chemicals to Humans*. Preamble (IARC Intern Tech Rep No. 77/002)

IARC (1978). *Chemicals with Sufficient Evidence of Carcinogenicity in Experimental Animals* – IARC Monographs *Volumes 1–17* (IARC Intern Tech Rep No. 78/003)

IARC (1979). *Criteria to Select Chemicals for* IARC Monographs (IARC Intern Tech Rep No. 79/003)

IARC (1982). Chemicals, industrial processes and industries associated with cancer in humans (IARC Monographs, Volumes 1 to 29). *IARC Monogr Eval Carcinog Risk Chem Hum Suppl*, 4: 1–292.

IARC (1983). *Approaches to Classifying Chemical Carcinogens According to Mechanism of Action* (IARC Intern Tech Rep No. 83/001)

IARC (1987). Overall evaluations of carcinogenicity: an updating of IARC Monographs volumes 1 to 42. *IARC Monogr Eval Carcinog Risks Hum Suppl*, 7: 1–440. PMID:3482203

IARC (1988). *Report of an IARC Working Group to Review the Approaches and Processes Used to Evaluate the Carcinogenicity of Mixtures and Groups of Chemicals* (IARC Intern Tech Rep No. 88/002)

IARC (1991). *A Consensus Report of an IARC Monographs Working Group on the Use of Mechanisms of Carcinogenesis in Risk Identification* (IARC Intern Tech Rep No. 91/002)

IARC (2005). *Report of the Advisory Group to Recommend Updates to the Preamble to the* IARC Monographs (IARC Intern Rep No. 05/001)

IARC (2006). *Report of the Advisory Group to Review the Amended Preamble to the* IARC Monographs (IARC Intern Rep No. 06/001)

IARC (2004). Some drinking-water disinfectants and contaminants, including arsenic. *IARC Monogr Eval Carcinog Risks Hum*, 84: 1–477. PMID:15645577

McGregor DB, Rice JM, Venitt S, editors (1999). The use of short- and medium-term tests for carcinogens and data on genetic effects in carcinogenic hazard evaluation. Consensus report. *IARC Sci Publ*, 146: 1–536.

Montesano R, Bartsch H, Vainio H *et al.*, editors (1986). Long-term and short-term assays for carcinogenesis—a critical appraisal. *IARC Sci Publ*, 83: 1–564.

OECD (2002). *Guidance Notes for Analysis and Evaluation of Chronic Toxicity and Carcinogenicity Studies* (Series on Testing and Assessment No. 35), Paris: OECD

Peto R, Pike MC, Day NE *et al.* (1980). Guidelines for simple, sensitive significance tests for carcinogenic effects in long-term animal experiments. *IARC Monogr Eval Carcinog Risk Chem Hum Suppl*, 2: 311–426. PMID:6935185

Portier CJ & Bailer AJ (1989). Testing for increased carcinogenicity using a survival-adjusted quantal response test. *Fundam Appl Toxicol*, 12: 731–737. doi:10.1016/0272-0590(89)90004-3 PMID:2744275

Sherman CD, Portier CJ, Kopp-Schneider A (1994). Multistage models of carcinogenesis: an approximation for the size and number distribution of late-stage clones. *Risk Anal*, 14: 1039–1048. doi:10.1111/j.1539-6924.1994.tb00074.x PMID:7846311

Stewart BW, Kleihues P, editors (2003). *World Cancer Report,* Lyon: IARC

Tomatis L, Aitio A, Wilbourn J, Shuker L (1989). Human carcinogens so far identified. *Jpn J Cancer Res*, 80: 795–807. PMID:2513295

Toniolo P, Boffetta P, Shuker DEG *et al.*, editors (1997). Proceedings of the workshop on application of biomarkers to cancer epidemiology. Lyon, France, 20–23 February 1996. *IARC Sci Publ*, 142: 1–318.

Vainio H, Magee P, McGregor D, McMichael A, editors (1992). Mechanisms of carcinogenesis in risk identification. IARC Working Group Meeting. Lyon, 11–18 June 1991. *IARC Sci Publ*, 116: 1–608.

Vainio H, Wilbourn JD, Sasco AJ *et al.* (1995). [Identification of human carcinogenic risks in IARC monographs.] *Bull Cancer*, 82: 339–348. PMID:7626841

Vineis P, Malats N, Lang M *et al.*, editors (1999). Metabolic Polymorphisms and Susceptibility to Cancer. *IARC Sci Publ*, 148: 1–510. PMID:10493243

Wilbourn J, Haroun L, Heseltine E *et al.* (1986). Response of experimental animals to human carcinogens: an analysis based upon the IARC Monographs programme. *Carcinogenesis*, 7: 1853–1863. doi:10.1093/carcin/7.11.1853 PMID:3769134

GENERAL REMARKS

1. Introduction

This one-hundred-and-eighth volume of the *IARC Monographs* includes evaluations of the carcinogenic hazard to humans of exposure to 14 herbal products or pharmaceutical drugs. None of these, except hydrochlorothiazide, have been previously evaluated by the Working Group.

Hydrochlorothiazide – a pharmaceutical drug – was considered in 1989 by an *IARC Monographs* Working Group (IARC, 1990), and was evaluated as *not classifiable as to its carcinogenicity to humans* (Group 3) based on *inadequate evidence* for carcinogenicity in humans and in experimental animals.

A summary of the findings of this meeting appears in The *Lancet Oncology* (Grosse *et al.*, 2013).

Among the agents that are known to cause cancer in humans specifically, there are several pharmaceuticals and other drugs. Volume 100A of the *IARC Monographs* (IARC, 2012) reviewed pharmaceuticals that in previous evaluations had been categorized as *carcinogenic to humans* (Group 1), primarily on the basis of epidemiological evidence for causation. In respect of specific chemical carcinogens, the number of agents classified as *carcinogenic to humans* that are therapeutic drugs is second only to the number of agents that have been identified in the context of occupational exposures.

Apart from pharmaceutical drugs that are industrially produced agents identified with a specific therapeutic usage, a major aspect of the use of drugs worldwide involves herbal products. Estimates from WHO indicate that 80% of the world's population has used herbal products as medicines. Use of the term "herbal medicine" is arbitrary in many contexts. In particular, a wide variety of pharmaceutical drugs, that is, agents recognized as having a particular pharmacological mode of action and associated clinical benefit, are derived from plants or other natural sources. This category of agent is likewise represented in previous *IARC Monographs*; and one – aristolochic acid – has been classified as a Group 1 agent (IARC, 2012).

Pharmaceutical drugs are subject to strict regulation in most countries, and their availability is highly restricted. This may not be the case with materials used in the preparation of herbal medicines. The therapeutic benefit of such herbal products may have been recognized in certain communities for centuries. Moreover, herbal products are available in several regulatory paradigms, ranging from foods and dietary supplements to cosmetics and over-the-counter (non-prescription) and prescription drugs. Worldwide, this means that product quality and composition may vary from country to country and within countries, even when different products bear the same name. In addition, the use of particular herbal products may vary markedly between countries and between communities within a country.

2. Exposure to herbal products and pharmaceuticals

Herbal products are complex mixtures that originate from biological sources. Unlike single-entity pharmaceuticals, plants contain thousands of primary and secondary metabolic constituents. In addition, raw materials are inherently variable because their chemical composition depends on factors such as geographical origin, weather, harvesting practices, while the chemical composition of the finished herbal products may not match that of the parent plants, and products frequently contain multiple botanical ingredients.

Discussions of exposure to natural products can be complicated by several factors. The first is the market category in which the product falls. Herbal products can be sold as conventional foods or food additives (e.g. flavouring or colouring agents), as dietary supplements, as cosmetic ingredients, or as herbal medicines (various national regulatory schemes may classify these as natural health products, therapeutic goods, phytomedicines, herbal medicinal products, traditional medicines, or conventional drugs). There may also be use of self-collected plants that are not marketed products.

Herbal medicine preparations are herbal products and consequently constitute complex mixtures. The biological impact, and specifically the carcinogenicity of complex mixtures, may be addressed by consideration of information concerning the mixture, and its variability in different contexts, and also by consideration of information concerning biologically active components within such mixtures. Information relevant to possible carcinogenicity may be most adequately addressed with reference either to the mixture or to the active component(s). Therefore, some *Monographs* in the present volume are specified with reference to the plant itself, i.e. *Aloe vera*, *Ginkgo biloba*, goldenseal, or kava. Other *Monographs* are specified with reference to individual components known to occur in particular plants, as is the case for pulegone and digoxin. Certain previous *IARC Monographs* evaluations are immediately relevant to the present evaluations to the extent that they involve components (e.g. quercetin for *Ginkgo biloba*, anthraquinones for *Aloe vera*) or metabolites (e.g. phenobarbital for primidone) of agents considered in the present volume.

Over the past several decades, there has been a revolution in the production, sale, and use of herbal products. In the 1970s, botanicals were largely sifted, cut, or powdered plant material in the form of a tablet, capsule, tea, or tincture. More recently, herbal products are often derived from intensely processed, carefully controlled organic extracts of plant material that have been spray-dried onto a solid carrier or diluent and then formed into a hard or soft capsule or tablet. The goal of many such processes is to create "standardized" extracts adjusted to contain consistent amounts of selected compounds of interest. Unfortunately, most standardized extracts focus on one or a handful of the thousands of constituents of the whole plant, so that even standardized extracts that are created using different processing techniques (e.g. different solvents, different ratios of plant to solvent) may achieve the desired levels of the desired chemical constituents while being otherwise chemically dissimilar. Attempts to compare herbal products by viewing the entire phytochemical fingerprint are beginning to appear, but these techniques have not yet had time to have an impact on the market or the publicly available scientific literature (van Beek & Montoro, 2009).

There are several advantages to using such highly processed raw materials. These include the ability to produce dosage forms that are more uniform in their composition, and the ability to preferentially concentrate the desirable constituents of a plant while leaving behind undesirable constituents. Because products are frequently referred to generically by the name of the plant in marketing and consumer-use surveys, it is difficult to differentiate between exposure to the crude plant material or to unique, highly processed proprietary extracts that differ significantly from both the plant source and from other proprietary products. In countries where there is pre-market review and product licensing, products must often conform to published compositional standards, such as those in the United States Pharmacopoeia or the European Pharmacopoeia; and similarly named products marketed in this regulatory environment are likely to be relatively similar to each other in composition, but may be very dissimilar from products that do not meet such standards.

In addition to the broad variability in composition of herbal products that are available to consumers, problems in interpreting published scientific studies of herbal products have been reported. Wolsko *et al.* (2005) performed a systematic review of the "Materials and Methods" sections of 81 published studies on herbal products. They noted that only 12 (15%) of the studies reported any kind of quantitative chemical analysis of the study material, and that only 8 (10%) of those reporting analysis reported results of the analysis. In addition, only 40 of the studies (49%) provided the Latin binomial name of the study material, only 8 (10%) identified the part of the plant used, and only 23 (28%) described the extraction/processing method used to create the product. A larger review by Gagnier *et al.* (2011) reported similar findings. To prevent such problems in future studies, Swanson (2002) and Gagnier *et al.* (2006) have published guidelines for the reporting of studies on natural products.

While some organizations that conduct safety studies adhere to or surpass the above guidelines when selecting test articles or designing studies, it would be useful if these guidelines became standard practice, as the reproducibility and reliability of safety studies would be greatly enhanced. Unfortunately, while such recommendations are useful, selecting the article to be tested from among dozens or hundreds of products with similar or identical names but widely divergent compositions remains a major obstacle.

As with most herbal products, there may be some controversy surrounding generalizability of conclusions for a commercial entity, because commercial products are very diverse in terms of processing, composition, and intended use. Attempts to identify the predominant form of an herbal product in the market place are pure conjecture in the absence of data. This is a recurring theme for all discussions on herbal products.

The ability of the Working Group to gauge the extent of global exposure to herbal products was very limited, since the quality and quantity of data available were inconsistent across countries. Having better information on patterns of use and on product composition would provide a means to prioritize the herbal products considered in this volume for such activities as policy formulation or further research needs.

While the available information on exposure to pharmaceuticals was more abundant and accessible than that on herbal products, limitations remain. For the most part, information on prescribing patterns outside the USA was not available to the Working Group. In addition, published studies indicated that patterns of adherence and persistence are suboptimal for medications used to manage or treat chronic conditions. And while prescribing patterns are available for some drugs, such data do not exist for over-the-counter drugs; consequently, exposure estimates must be made using means similar to those used to estimate exposure to herbal products (e.g. *Aloe vera*, for which over-the-counter use is difficult to quantify), namely sales data and consumer use surveys. Although not widely available or widely accessible, such data for over-the-counter drugs is more informative than for herbal products sold as foods or dietary supplements because drug products with similar names are required to be similar in composition.

As indicated above, exposure can generally be much more accurately measured for pharmaceuticals than for other agents, and therapeutic doses used in humans are often closer to those tested in experimental animals. Nonetheless, characterizing the true nature of exposure to drugs in relation to carcinogenicity is complicated by the variability in adherence to drugs and their varying patterns of use – intermittent versus continuous.

Exposure to herbal products or pharmaceutical drugs may occur as a consequence of occupational exposure of people involved in production or manufacture of these agents. Exposure may also occur as a result of water pollution by these agents. Generally, levels of occupational or environmental exposure are much lower than levels of exposure experienced by people using the respective herbal products or drugs. Almost no information was available to the Working Group concerning occupational or environmental circumstances of exposure to the agents evaluated in this volume.

3. Epidemiological studies of populations using drugs

The *Monograph* on digoxin exemplifies the complications in drug nomenclature that may arise due to differences in professional practice and disciplines (e.g. manufacturer, medical professional). As explained therein, the term "digitalis" as used with reference to chemical specifications may refer to a plant extract, while the same word in a medical therapeutic context may refer to a particular category of agents (e.g. digoxin, digitoxin). Such incongruities not only contribute to potential misunderstanding of data; in an immediate sense, they may complicate adoption of a particular term as the appropriate identification of the subject of a *Monograph*

and/or the subject of evaluation statements adopted within a particular *Monograph*. In some instances, studies may generate epidemiological data that refer to the use of particular classes of drug, rather than particular individual drugs. Interpretation of such data to infer effects attributable to particular drugs, such as pioglitazone, rosiglitazone and hydrochlorothiazide, and the small number of available epidemiological studies, may render this task difficult or almost impossible.

Historically, in *IARC Monographs* evaluations for which relevant epidemiological data were available, determination of causality on the basis of associations reported in epidemiological studies has always been recognized as both challenging and of critical importance. In general terms, this subject is addressed in the Preamble to the *IARC Monographs*, and the matters raised in that context are fundamental to all such epidemiological data. In the specific case of epidemiological findings in relation to pharmaceutical drugs, it is self-evident that the exposed individuals are not a representative sample of the community, but rather are individuals identified by a diagnosis in consequence of which they have received the drug in question. At one extreme, increased risk of cancer in such individuals may be caused by the drug they have received. At the other extreme, an association between increased risk of cancer and use of a particular drug may be totally independent of causality and arise for several reasons: because patients with a particular disease are at greater risk of malignancy; because patients with a particular disease are more liable than the community in general to be exposed to an independent factor that causes or is correlated with increased risk of cancer; or because the symptoms of an undiagnosed cancer may also prompt the use of a drug, which can subsequently be suspected as its cause. An additional problem is that patients commonly receive more than one drug, and determination of the carcinogenicity of any single drug may be difficult.

4. Extrapolating from specific scientific findings

While historically, multiple studies of carcinogenicity in experimental animals may have been conducted on a single test agent in several independent laboratories, today the massive expense involved in rigorous testing for carcinogenicity in experimental animals often means that only one or two well conducted studies of carcinogenicity (often in one strain of rat and/or one strain of mouse, and typically involving males and females) may be available in the peer-reviewed literature or from government agency reports that are publicly available. As indicated in the Preamble, such studies, ideally conducted under good laboratory practice, may be able to establish *sufficient evidence* of carcinogenicity in experimental animals, depending upon the nature of results obtained.

Again, in relation to "single studies" as outlined above, when the test agent is a complex mixture, exemplified, for example, by an herbal product, it may not be possible to assume that the agent being tested is identical to either the material marketed under the same name and/or material tested in other studies that might otherwise be understood to indicate possible mechanism(s) of carcinogenesis or to exclude particular mechanism(s) of carcinogenesis.

As indicated in the Preamble, the *IARC Monographs* evaluations are wholly dependent on publicly available data that are exemplified by published research results in the peer-reviewed literature. This information comprises only a subset of data on pharmaceutical drugs, specifically excluding "commercial in-confidence" findings of the type provided by industry to national or multinational regulatory authorities in the context of applications to market particular drugs. The initiatives of the European Medicines Agency and other organizations to make such data publicly available are properly noted in this context.

5. Considerations beyond hazard identification

Many (if not most) regulatory decisions concerning putative carcinogens necessitate consideration not only of perceived hazard, but also of potential benefit. It is crucial, therefore, that regulatory decisions affecting drug availability include assessment not only of potential carcinogenicity (and other adverse effects), but also of the health benefits derived from their usage.

References

Gagnier JJ, Boon H, Rochon P, Moher D, Barnes J, Bombardier C; CONSORT Group(2006). Recommendations for reporting randomized controlled trials of herbal interventions: Explanation and elaboration. *J Clin Epidemiol*, 59(11):1134–49. doi:10.1016/j.jclinepi.2005.12.020 PMID:17027423

Gagnier JJ, Moher D, Boon H, Beyene J, Bombardier C (2011). Randomized controlled trials of herbal interventions underreport important details of the intervention. *J Clin Epidemiol*, 64(7):760–9. doi:10.1016/j.jclinepi.2010.10.005 PMID:21208777

Grosse Y, Loomis D, Lauby-Secretan B, El Ghissassi F, Bouvard V, Benbrahim-Tallaa L *et al.* International Agency for Research on Cancer Monograph Working Group (2013). Carcinogenicity of some drugs and herbal products. *Lancet Oncol*, 14(9):807–8. doi:10.1016/S1470-2045(13)70329-2 PMID:24058961

IARC (1990). Hydrochlorothiazide. *IARC Monogr Eval Carcinog Risks Hum*, 50:293–305. PMID:2292804

IARC (2012). Pharmaceuticals. Volume 100 A. A review of human carcinogens. *IARC Monogr Eval Carcinog Risks Hum*, 100:Pt A: 1–401. PMID:23189749

Swanson CA (2002). Suggested guidelines for articles about botanical dietary supplements. *Am J Clin Nutr*, 75(1):8–10. PMID:11756054

van Beek TA, Montoro P (2009). Chemical analysis and quality control of *Ginkgo biloba* leaves, extracts, and phytopharmaceuticals. *J Chromatogr A*, 1216(11):2002–32. doi:10.1016/j.chroma.2009.01.013 PMID:19195661

Wolsko PM, Solondz DK, Phillips RS, Schachter SC, Eisenberg DM (2005). Lack of herbal supplement characterization in published randomized controlled trials. *Am J Med*, 118(10):1087–93. doi:10.1016/j.amjmed.2005.01.076 PMID:16194636

1. Exposure Data

The first record of human use of *Aloe vera* is in Sumerian hieroglyphics engraved on clay tablets during the Mesopotamia civilization circa 2200 BC, in which it is described as a laxative. Use of aloe in ancient times is also documented in Egypt, Greece, and China. *Aloe vera* was cultivated on the islands of Barbados and Curacao in the Caribbean by Spain and the Netherlands, and was sold in various parts of Europe during the 17th century (Park & Jo, 2006). Commercial cultivation of *Aloe vera* in the USA began in the 1920s in Florida (Grindlay & Reynolds, 1986). Although *Aloe vera* originated in the warm, dry climates of Africa, the plant is readily adaptable and grows worldwide (Steenkamp & Stewart, 2007).

Use of *Aloe vera* gel extracts in health foods and beverages, and moisturizing cosmetics, began during the 1970s, starting in the USA and parts of Europe (Park & Jo, 2006). Historically, *Aloe vera* was used topically to heal wounds and for various skin conditions, and orally as a laxative (Steenkamp & Stewart, 2007). The dried latex of other *Aloe* species, such as *Aloe ferox Miller* (Cape aloe or bitter aloe) has also been used as a laxative (EMA, 2006). Today, *Aloe vera* is also used as a folk or traditional remedy for a variety of conditions and is found in some dietary supplements and food products. *Aloe vera* gel can be found in hundreds of skin products, including lotions and sunblocks (NCCAM, 2012).

A glossary of commonly used terms for *Aloe vera* products is provided in Table 1.1.

1.1 Identification of the agent

1.1.1 *Botanical data*

(a) *Nomenclature*

For details on botanical nomenclature, see Newton (2004).

Chem. Abstr. Serv. Reg. No.: 8001-97-6

Chem. Abstr. Name: Aloe barbadensis

Botanical name: *Aloe vera* (L.) *Burm. f.* (synonym, *Aloe barbadensis*, *Aloe humilis Blanco*, *Aloe indica Royle*, nomen nudum, *Aloe perfoliata* var. *vera* L., *Aloe vulgaris Lam.*) (GRIN, 2013).

Family: Xanthorrhoeaceae

Genus: Aloe

Plant part: Leaf

Common names: *Aloe vera*; *Aloe vera* Linné; True aloe; *Aloe barbadensis*; Barbados aloe; Curaçao aloe; Mediterranean aloe; Ghritakumari; Lu Hui; Luhui, etc.

From WHO (1999), Eur Ph (2008), O'Neil *et al.* (2006), SciFinder (2013), IASC (2013a), Boudreau *et al.* (2013a).

Table 1.1 Definition of terms commonly used in the Aloe industry

Term	Definition
Leaf	The part of the *Aloe vera* plant used in commerce, where processing is begun without stripping off the rind.
Whole leaf	Historically used to describe products derived from the entire leaf that were filtered/purified. However, use of this terminology without adequate additional descriptors is not recommended. This terminology is now seen on products or in reference to raw material where the entire leaf is used as a starting ingredient to create *Aloe vera* juice.
Decolorized whole leaf	A process, usually involving filtration with activated charcoal, that clarifies the liquid aloe mass.
Inner leaf	Plant part used to describe the clear, central parenchymatous tissues of the aloe leaf.
Aloe latex	Brown, yellow-brown, or occasionally red exudate found between the rind and inner leaf. Also called "sap," it contains several constituents, but most notably anthraquinones.
Anthraquinone	An organic compound primarily found in the aloe latex, whose structure serves as the basic building block for several naturally occurring plant pigments. The substance is commonly used for laxative purposes.
Gel	Liquid product typically derived from the inner leaf.
Juice	Liquid product derived from *Aloe vera* leaf [the Working Group noted that the term "juice" is used arbitrarily and may either apply to products from the latex or from the gel].

Adapted from IASC (2009)

(b) Description

Aloes are perennial succulents or xerophytes; they can adapt to habitats with low or erratic water availability, are characterized by the capacity to store large volumes of water in their tissue, and are able to use crassulacean acid metabolism, an adaptation to the photosynthetic pathway that involves the formation of malic acid (Boudreau *et al.*, 2013a). Aloe plants, such as *Aloe vera* (Fig. 1.1), all have green fleshy leaves covered by a thick cuticle or rind, under which is a thin vascular layer covering an inner clear pulp (Boudreau *et al.*, 2013a; Fig. 1.2) The leaves are 30–50 cm in length and 10 cm in width at the base, pea-green in colour (when young spotted with white), and with bright yellow tubular flowers 25–35 cm in length arranged in a slender loose spike (WHO, 1999).

The vascular bundles, located within the leaf pulp, transport (i) water and minerals from the roots to the leaves; (ii) synthesized materials to the roots; and (iii) latex along the margins of the leaf for storage (Ni *et al.*, 2004; Fig. 1.2). The number of vascular bundles varies depending on the size of the leaves and the age of the plant (Ni *et al.*, 2004).

Aloe vera plants contain two major liquid materials (Fig. 1.2): first, a bitter yellow latex located under the strongly cutinized epidermis of the leaves in the vascular layer and containing a high concentration of anthraquinone compounds, which has been used throughout the centuries as a cathartic and for medicinal purges; and, second, a clear mucilaginous gel produced by the thin-walled tubular cells in the inner central zone (parenchyma) that has been used since ancient times to treat burns and other wounds, where it is thought to increase the rate of healing and reduce the risk of infection (Joseph & Raj, 2010). A third liquid may also be obtained by macerating the whole leaf.

[Both the scientific and the lay literature (e.g. on internet sites) are extremely inconsistent when referring to products obtained from *Aloe vera*. The problem starts with the fact that the three types of liquids that are obtained from *Aloe vera* leaves are interchangeably referred to as "Aloe juice," which has caused confusion in the literature. For disambiguation reasons, the term "Aloe juice" should be restricted – if used at all – to the latex material of the pericycle, which is in accordance with the pharmacopoeial definitions

Fig. 1.1 *Aloe vera* (L.) Burm. F, plant and flower

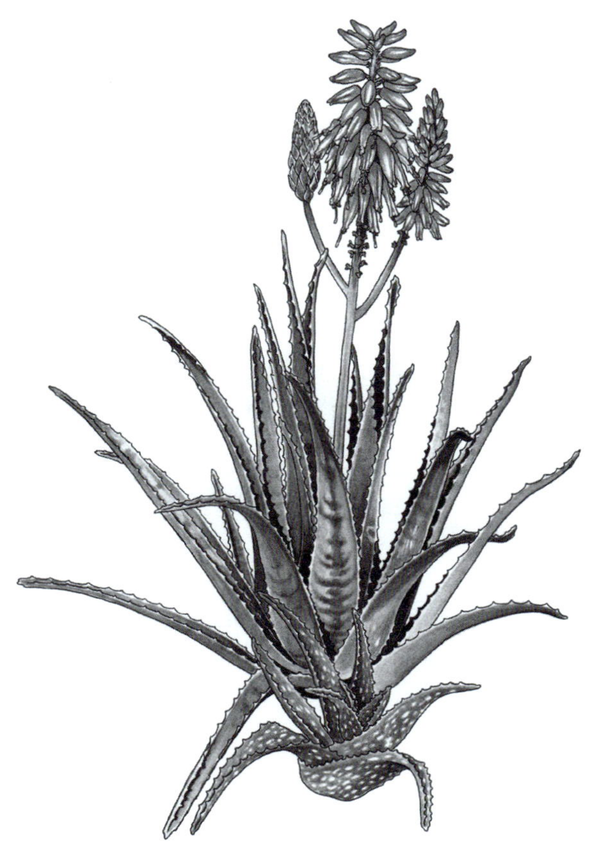

From Spohn (2013)
© Roland Spohn

(WHO, 1999; Eur Ph, 2008; JP XVI, 2011); and the inner leaf liquid material should be referred to as "gel" (WHO, 1999). Interchangable terms found in the literature for the "gel" are inner pulp, mucilage tissue, mucilaginous gel, mucilaginous jelly, inner gel, and leaf parenchyma tissue (Hamman, 2008).]

1.1.2 Chemical constituents and their properties

A review of the chemistry of *Aloe vera* was provided by Reynolds (2004), and a summary of the chemical constituents of *Aloe vera* is provided in Table 1.2.

The main feature of the *Aloe vera* plant is its high water content, ranging from 99% to 99.5%, while the remaining 0.5–1.0% solid material is reported to contain over 200 different potentially active compounds, including vitamins, minerals, enzymes, simple and complex polysaccharides, phenolic compounds, and organic acids (Boudreau *et al.*, 2013a; Rodríguez *et al.*, 2010).

In compositional studies on the structural components of leaf portions of the *Aloe vera* plant, the rind was found to compose 20–30% and the pulp 70–80% of the whole leaf weight. On a dry-weight basis, the rind and pulp contain 2.7% and 4.2% lipids, and 6.3% and 7.3% proteins, respectively (Femenia *et al.*, 1999). The percentages of soluble sugars (11.2% and 16.5%), primarily as glucose, and the percentages of ash (13.5% and 15.4%), in particular calcium, were relatively high in the rind and pulp, respectively. Non-starch polysaccharides and lignin represented the bulk of each leaf fraction and were found to be 62.3% and 57.6% of the dry weight of the rind and pulp, respectively (Boudreau *et al.*, 2013a). Acetylated mannan is the primary polysaccharide in *Aloe vera* gel (Ni *et al.*, 2004). Other chemical constituents of *Aloe vera* include lectins such as aloctins A and B (Kuzuya *et al.*, 2004).

The physical and chemical constituents of the products derived from *Aloe vera* plants differ depending on the source (e.g. part of the plant), the species of the plant, the climate conditions, seasonal and grower influences (Boudreau *et al.*, 2013a), and processing techniques (Waller *et al.*, 2004).

1.1.3 Technical and commercial products

Three types of *Aloe vera* extracts can be distinguished –gel extract, whole leaf extract, and decolorized whole leaf extract (Boudreau *et al.*, 2013a), and a fourth type of commercial material is available as dried latex, which has

Fig. 1.2 Schematic representation of the *Aloe vera* plant, showing a cross-section through a leaf

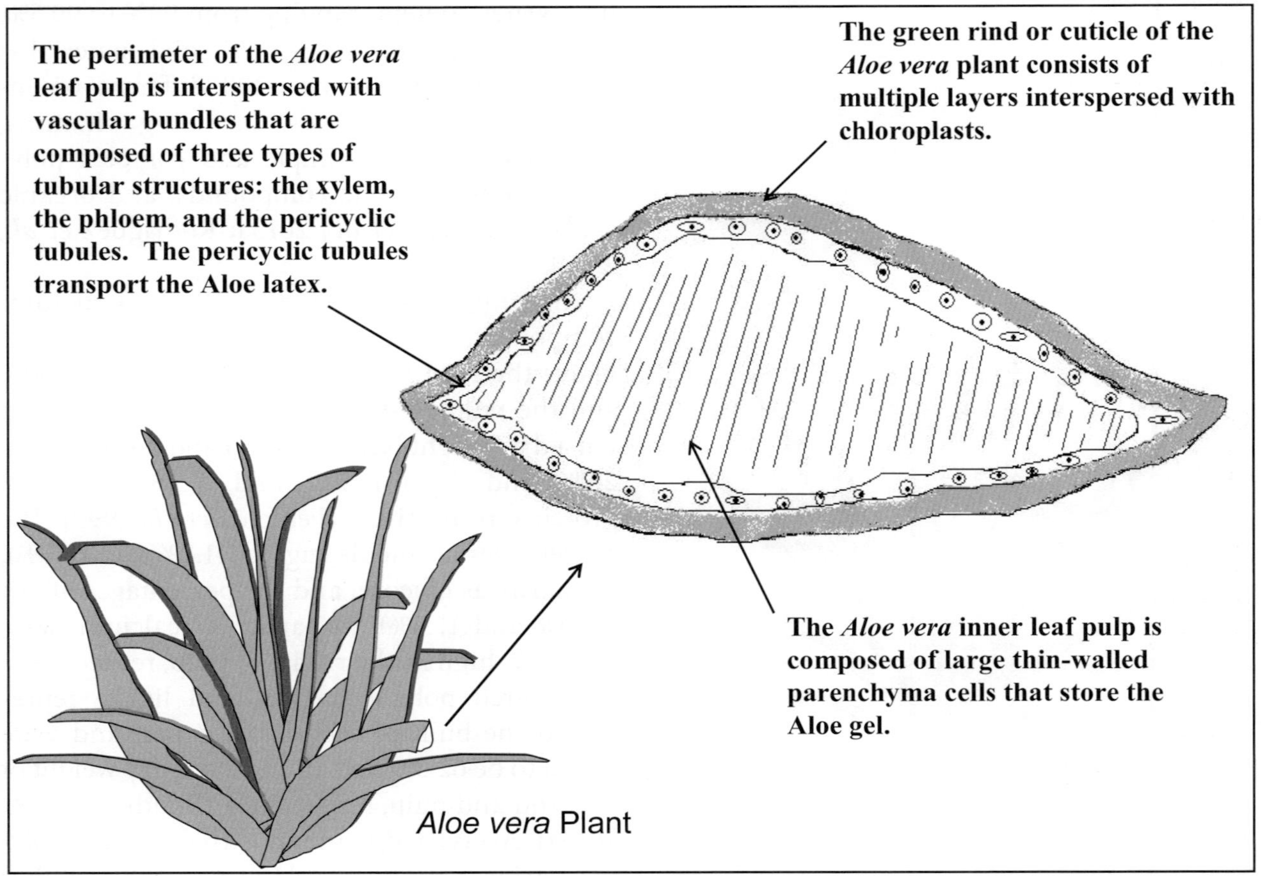

From Boudreau *et al.* (2013a)

been traditionally used as the laxative (Eur Ph, 2008).

(a) Aloe vera *gel extract*

The inner leaf pulp of the *Aloe vera* plant contains large, thin-walled cells that produce gel, the clear, mucilaginous, and aqueous extract of the inner central area of the leaf pulp (Fig. 1.2). *Aloe vera* gel serves as the water and energy storage component of the plant. The mechanical extrusion of the mucilaginous gel from the inner leaf pulp gives a 70% yield with a water content of 99–99.5% (Femenia *et al.*, 1999).

Polysaccharides in *Aloe vera* gel consist of linear chains of glucose and mannose molecules, and, because there is considerably more mannose present than glucose, the molecules are referred to as polymannans. These linear chains range in size from a few to several thousand monosaccharide molecules. The major polysaccharide, acetylated mannan, is composed of one or more polymers of various chain lengths with molecular weights ranging from 30 to 40 kDa or greater, and consisting of repeating units of glucose and mannose in a 1:3 ratio (Channe Gowda *et al.*, 1979; Mandal & Das, 1980; Yaron, 1993; Femenia *et al.*, 1999; Boudreau *et al.*, 2013a; Fig. 1.3). Chemically preserved fresh *Aloe vera* gel stored at room temperature or incubated at 40 °C for 48 hours exhibited degradation in its

Table 1.2 Summary of chemical constituents of *Aloe vera* products

Class	Compounds
Anthraquinones/anthrones	Aloe-emodin, aloetic acid, anthranol, aloin A and B (or collectively known as barbaloin), isobarbaloin, emodin, ester of cinnamic acid
Carbohydrates	Pure mannan, acetylated mannan, acetylated glucomannan, glucogalactomannan, galactan, galactogalacturan, arabinogalactan, galactoglucoarabinomannan, pectic substance, xylan, cellulose
Chromones	8-*C*-Glucosyl-(2′-*O*-cinnamoyl)-7-*O*-methylaloediol A, 8-*C*-glucosyl-(*S*)-aloesol, 8-*C*-glucosyl-7-*O*-methyl-(*S*)-aloesol, 8-*C*-glucosyl-7-*O*-methylaloediol, 8-*C*-glucosyl-noreugenin, isoaloeresin D, isorabaichromone, neoaloesin A
Enzymes	Alkaline phosphatase, amylase, carboxypeptidase, catalase, cyclooxidase, cyclooxygenase, lipase, oxidase, phosphoenolpyruvate carboxylase, superoxide dismutase
Minerals	Calcium, chlorine, chromium, copper, iron, magnesium, manganese, potassium, phosphorous, sodium, zinc
Lipids and miscellaneous organic compounds	Arachidonic acid, γ-linolenic acid, steroids (campestrol, cholesterol, β-sitosterol), triglycerides, triterpenoid, gibberillin, lignins, potassium sorbate, salicylic acid, uric acid
Amino acids	Alanine, arginine, aspartic acid, glutamic acid, glycine, histidine, hydroxyproline, isoleucine, leucine, lysine, methionine, phenylalanine, proline, threonine, tyrosine, valine
Proteins	Lectins, lectin-like substance
Saccharides	Mannose, glucose, *L*-rhamnose, aldopentose
Vitamins	B1, B2, B6, C, β-carotene, choline, folic acid, α-tocopherol

Adapted from Hamman (2008)

rheological properties, a decrease in the content and composition of polysaccharides, and a substantial increase in the mannose:glucose ratio, from 2.9 in the fresh gel to 13.4 in the incubated gel (Yaron, 1993).

(b) Aloe vera *whole leaf extract*

The *Aloe vera* whole leaf extract (sometimes referred to as whole leaf *Aloe vera* juice, Aloe juice or nondecolorized whole leaf extract), is the aqueous extract of the whole leaf with lignified fibres removed. The whole leaf extract contains both the gel from the inner parenchyma leaf pulp and the latex. The restricted distribution of the bitter latex within the margins of the leaves of the *Aloe vera* plant suggests that this thin layer is the primary site of secondary metabolites biosynthesis: compounds that do not function directly in plant growth and development and serve as a plant defence strategy (Boudreau *et al.*, 2013a). A wide variety of secondary compounds have been isolated from the *Aloe vera* latex (Reynolds, 2004). The isolated compounds are largely phenolic in nature, and many are anthraquinone *C*-glycosides, anthrones, and free anthraquinones (Park *et al.*, 1998). The levels of anthraquinone *C*-glycosides in *Aloe vera* latex are quite variable; however, they may constitute up to 30% of the dry weight of the latex (Groom & Reynolds, 1987). *Aloe vera* latex contains four major *C*-glycosyl constituents: aloin A, aloin B, aloesin, and aloeresin A (Fig. 1.3; Saccù *et al.*, 2001). Aloin A, a *C*-glycosyl anthrone, also referred to as barbaloin, is the major component of aloe latex. Aloin A and its epimer, aloin B, also referred to as isobarbaloin, have a 9-anthrone skeleton and a β-D-glucopyranosyl substituent. Aloesin, also known as aloeresin B, is a 5-methyl chromone with an 8-β-D-glucopyranosyl substituent, and aloeresin A is a 5-methyl chromone with an 8-β-D-glucopyranosyl-2-*O*-*trans*-*p*-coumarol substituent. Several other *C*-glycosyl-chromones and anthrones have been isolated from *Aloe vera*, including aloe-emodin, the anthraquinone of barbaloin and isobarbaloin (Boudreau *et al.*, 2013a).

Fig. 1.3 Chemicals present in gel and latex prepared from *Aloe vera*

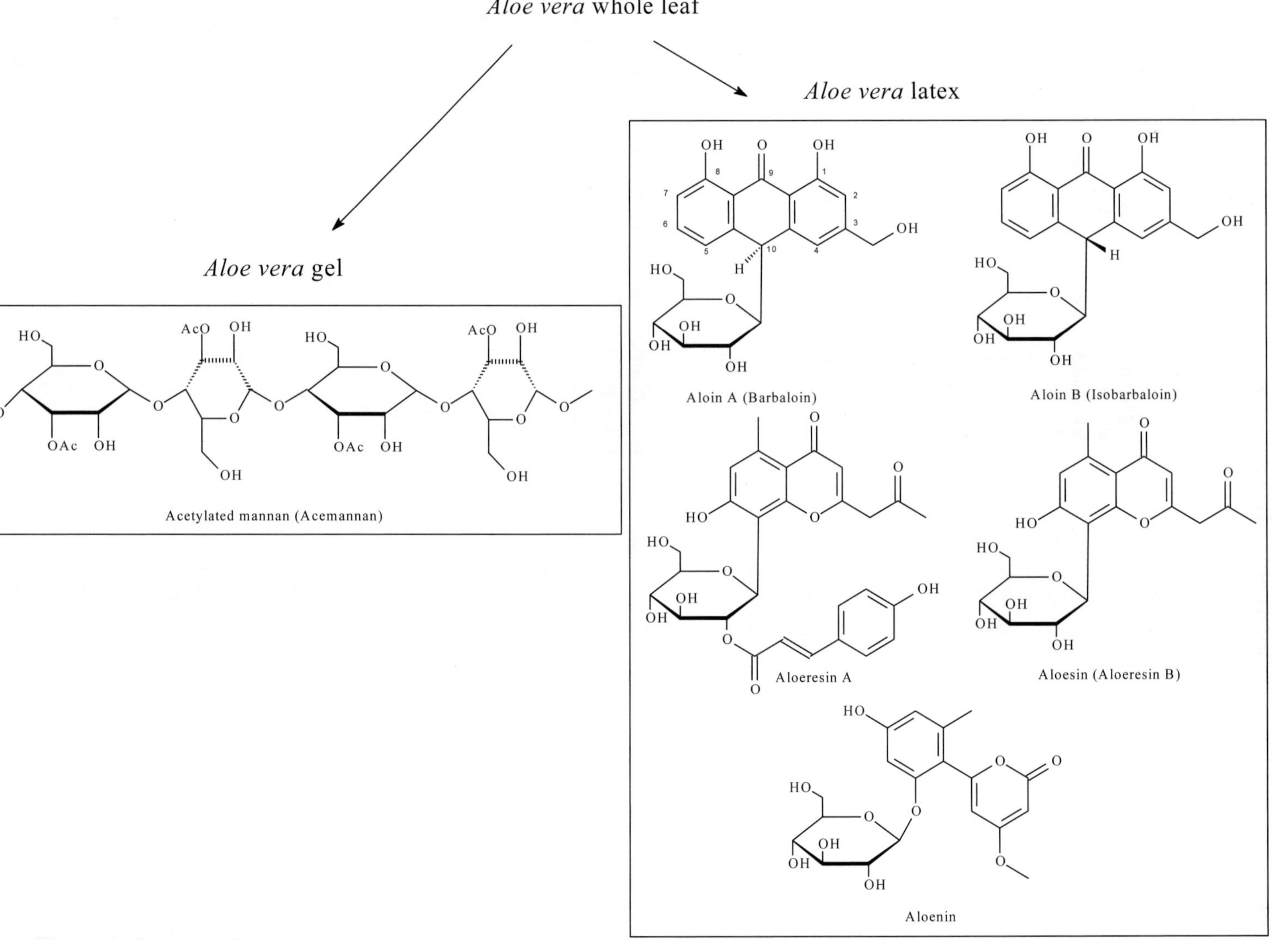

Ac, acetyl group
From Boudreau *et al.* (2013a)

The occurrence in *Aloe vera* latex of endogenous free anthraquinones and anthrones results from oxidative processes acting on the glycosides rather than from metabolic synthesis (Boudreau *et al.*, 2013a). In addition, the latex from *Aloe vera* contains several aromatic compounds, such as aldehydes and ketones (Saccù *et al.*, 2001). The sugar moiety in aloins is D-glucose, and studies indicate that carbon atom 1 of the D-glucose moiety is linked directly to carbon atom 10 of the anthracene ring in a β-configuration (Fig. 1.3). The carbon–carbon bond is quite resistant to acid and alkaline conditions; however, the intestinal microflora of humans and animals have been shown to cleave the β-*C*-glucosyl bond, although considerable variation in response among animal species occurs. Cleavage of the β-*C*-glucosyl bond results in the formation of aloe-emodin, the cathartic principle of the latex, and other free anthraquinones and anthrones (Boudreau *et al.*, 2013a; see Section 4.1.1b). In commercial products containing whole leaf extract, a rapid deterioration of aloin was detected during storage, especially at higher temperatures (Pellizzoni *et al.*, 2011).

(c) Aloe vera *decolorized whole leaf extract*

Activated carbon treatment of the *Aloe vera* whole leaf extract is used to remove bitterness and colour caused by the anthraquinone components of *the* latex. This results in a product termed "decolorized whole leaf extract" that has quite different properties from the whole leaf extract. *Aloe vera* decolorized whole leaf extract is also referred to as "whole leaf *Aloe vera* gel" (Boudreau *et al.*, 2013a). Dentali (2013) noted that an industry standard for aloin content of decolorized *Aloe vera* whole leaf extract is < 10 ppm. Sehgal *et al.* (2013) reported results of toxicological assessment of a commercial decolorized whole leaf extract that contained approximately Aloin A at 0.9 ppm, Aloin B at 1.3 ppm, and aloe-emodin at 0.2 ppm. A decolorized *Aloe vera* whole leaf extract assessed for safety by Shao

et al. (2013) was reported to contain combined Aloin A and Aloin B at < 0.1 ppm.

Although *Aloe vera* gel and the decolorized whole leaf extract are similar in that each contain little or no latex anthraquinones, carbon adsorption changes the physical and chemical properties of the whole leaf extract. *Aloe vera* decolorized whole leaf extract differs from the gel in that it exhibits a degradation in rheological properties and a loss of approximately 19–23% of the complex polysaccharide content (Pelley *et al.*, 1998).

(d) *Dried* Aloe vera *latex (pharmaceutical material)*

The dried *Aloe vera* latex is the solidified liquid originating in the cells of the pericycle and adjacent leaf parenchyma, and flowing spontaneously from the cut leaf, allowed to dry with or without the aid of heat (WHO, 1999). The material is used for medicinal purposes and its composition is specified in several official pharmacopoeias (see Section 1.6).

1.2 Analysis

For *Aloe vera* sold for medicinal purposes, analyses are defined in pharmacopoeial monographs (see Section 1.6). Most of the published analytical methods (Table 1.3) deal with the determination of the anthraquinone compounds in the latex, and fewer and mostly qualitative methods are available for authentication.

To carry out an exhaustive quality control of commercial *Aloe vera* gel products (e.g. for food or cosmetic uses), the following analyses should be carried out: (i) investigation of authenticity; (ii) test for identification of additives (to control the labelling or regulatory limits); and (iii) determination of the aloin content (Lachenmeier *et al.*, 2005; Rodríguez *et al.*, 2010). The investigation of authenticity aims at confirming the amount of *Aloe vera* in the preparation; adulteration

Table 1.3 Selected methods of analysis of *Aloe vera* constituents in various matrices

Sample matrix	Analyte/purpose of analysis	Sample preparation	Assay method	Detection limit	Reference
Urine	Aloin/detection of laxative abuse	Glucuronidase, SPE	HPTLC	10–20 mg/L	Perkins & Livesey (1993)
Urine	Aloe-emodin/detection of laxative abuse	Glucuronidase, Extraction with chloroform/isopropanol 9+1	HPLC/UV	0.015 mg/L	Stolk & Hoogtanders (1999)
Serum	Aloin/pharmacokinetic study	Extraction with ethyl acetate	TLC	0.033 mg/L	Ishii *et al.* (1987)
Plasma	Aloe-emodin/pharmacokinetic study	Dichloromethane extraction	HPLC/FD	4.5 µg/L	Zaffaroni *et al.* (2003)
Aloe leave exudates	Aloin/taxonomy	Methanolic solution	HPLC/UV	NA	Groom & Reynolds (1987)
Aloe vera gel	13 phenolic compounds/quality control and standardization	Liquid–liquid extraction	HPLC/UV	NA	Kim & Park (2006)
Aloe vera products	Acetylated polysaccharides, glucose, malic acid, lactic acid, and acetic acid/quality control	None (dissolve in D_2O)	NMR	< 0.05 µg/L	Jiao *et al.* (2010)
Aloe extracts and commercial formulations	Aloe-emodin/identity confirmation	Preparative TLC	HPLC/UV and FD	UV: 3 µg/L FD: 0.8 µg/L	Mandrioli *et al.* (2011)
Aloe vera plants	Metabolite profiling/metabolomics	Extraction with methanol. Derivatization with MSTFA for GC-IT-MS analysis	GC-IT-MS and UPLC-Q-TOF-MS	NA	Lee *et al.* (2012)
Aloe vera leaves	Aloin derivatives/regulatory control	Ultrasound-assisted extraction in methanol	HPLC-DAD, HPLC-MS, UPLC	3–10 mg/L	Azaroual *et al.* (2012)
Pharmaceutical formulations	*Aloe vera* polysaccharides/control for adulteration or degradation	None (dissolve in D_2O)	NMR	2 g/L	Davis & Goux (2009)
Cosmetics	Mannose/determination of quantity of *Aloe* in product	Extraction with diethyl ether and hydrolysis with sulfuric acid	HPTLC	3% of *Aloe vera* in cosmetic product	Geisser & Kratz (2010)
Aloe species	Aloin derivatives/authenticity control	Methanolic extraction	HPLC/UV	< 0.05 mg/L	Okamura *et al.* (1996)
Aloe exudate	Volatiles/flavour characterization for beverage industry	Ethanol 40% for HPLC, HS sampling for GC	HPLC, HS-GC/MS	NA	Saccù *et al.* (2001)

Table 1.3 (continued)

Sample matrix	Analyte/purpose of analysis	Sample preparation	Assay method	Detection limit	Reference
Aloe vera beverages	Profiling for identity, adulteration, dilution	None	HPTLC, HS-SPME-GC/MS	NA	Lachenmeier *et al.* (2005)
Aloe species	13 Phenolic compounds/seasonal variation	Extraction with ethanol	HPLC/UV	NA	Park *et al.* (1998)
Commercial aloe products	High molecular-weight polysaccharides	Dilution with water and 0.2 M NaCl	SEC	NA	Turner *et al.* (2004)
Commercial aloe products	Aloe-emodin, aloin A	Extraction with ethyl acetate/methanol 9+1	HPLC/MS	Aloin-A, 1 µg/L; Aloe emodin, 2.5 µg/L	Elsohly *et al.* (2007)
Commercial aloe products	Aloin A, aloin B	Extraction with ethanol/water (90+10)	HPLC	0.06 mg/L	Ramírez Durón *et al.* (2008)

DAD, diode array detector; FD, fluorescence detection; GC, gas chromatography; HPLC, high-performance liquid chromatography; HPTLC, high-performance thin-layer chromatography; HS, headspace; IT; ion trap; MS, mass spectrometry; MSTFA, *N*-methyl-*N*-(trimethylsilyl)trifluoroacetamide; NA, not applicable; NMR, nuclear magnetic resonance spectroscopy; Q-TOF, quadrupole-time of flight; SEC, size-exclusion chromatography; SPE, solid-phase extraction; SPME, solid-phase microextraction; TLC, thin-layer chromatography; UPLC, ultra-performance liquid chromatography; UV, ultraviolet has been a major concern as a consequence of the high cost of the raw materials. Common adulterants have included maltodextrin in *Aloe vera* gel, powder or water in the liquid preparations (Pelley *et al.*, 1998). Many authors have reviewed the considerable available amount of literature for analysis and authenticity control of *Aloe vera*. Besides various chromatographic approaches, nuclear magnetic resonance spectroscopy appears to be the method of choice for this purpose (Table 1.3). Common additives found in *Aloe vera* gel preparations, which can be detected by chromatographic methods, include preservatives such as benzoic acid and sorbic acid, or antioxidants such as ascorbic acid (Lachenmeier *et al.*, 2005). Several methods to control the gel material for contamination with aloin are available (see review by Rodríguez *et al.* (2010) and Table 1.3).

1.3 Use

1.3.1 Indications

(a) Medicinal use

The *Aloe vera* plant has been used in folk medicine for more than 2000 years, and it remains an important component of traditional medicine in many contemporary cultures, such as China, India, the Caribbean, and Japan (Grindlay & Reynolds, 1986). *Aloe vera* first gained popularity in the USA in the 1930s with reports of successful use of freshly cut leaves in treating X-ray burns (Ulbricht *et al.*, 2007). Both classes of *Aloe vera* leaf products, gel and latex, are reported to possess a wide range of pharmaceutical activities.

WHO lists the short-term treatment of occasional constipation as a use for *Aloe vera* latex that is supported by clinical data (WHO, 1999). The well established cathartic properties of anthraquinone glycosides provide strong evidence in support of the laxative properties of *Aloe vera* (Ulbricht *et al.*, 2007). The European Medicines

Agency also found that the therapeutic indication as an "herbal product for short-term use in cases of occasional constipation" is a well established use of *Aloe vera* latex (EMA, 2006).

For the gel, WHO identified no uses supported by clinical data. Traditional uses include the external treatment of minor wounds and inflammatory skin disorders. The gel may be used in the treatment of minor skin irritations, including burns, bruises, and abrasions (WHO, 1999).

In recent times, the oral consumption of *Aloe vera* has been promoted as prophylaxis and therapy for a variety of unrelated systemic conditions. The scientific literature yields little to substantiate claims of usefulness for systemic conditions by the ingestion of *Aloe vera* (Boudreau *et al.*, 2013a).

Aloe vera may be used in veterinary medicine as laxative or in topical applications, e.g. in udder disinfectants (Leon, 2003).

(b) Food use

Aloe vera extracts may be used in beverages as bitter flavouring agent (O'Neil *et al.*, 2006). Food products include health and soft drinks, yoghurts, jams, instant tea granules, candies, alcoholic beverages, and ice cream (Ahlawat & Khatkar, 2011). *Aloe vera* may also be used in food supplements (Steenkamp & Stewart, 2007). The Dietary Supplements Label Database lists 43 products that contain *Aloe vera* as an active ingredient in amounts of 0.33 to 750 mg per capsule (NLM, 2012). *Aloe vera* whole leaf extract (which combines both the gel and latex) and *Aloe vera* decolorized whole leaf extract (from which most of the latex components have been removed) are popular as dietary supplements for various systemic ailments. The anthraquinone components of these products appear to vary significantly in their content of aloe-emodin and aloin A, the major anthraquinone constituent of *Aloe vera* latex. (Elsohly *et al.*, 2007) evaluated 53 liquid and 30 semisolid and solid aloe-based commercial products. The liquid samples all contained either aloe-emodin or aloin A at ≤ 10 ppm, with many having no detectable levels of either of the two compounds. Unlike liquid products, many solid and semisolid products (11 out of 30) contained one or both of the compounds, aloe-emodin and aloin A, at ≥ 10 ppm.

(c)   Cosmetic use

The gel may be used as emollient and moisturizer in cosmetics and personal care products (O'Neil *et al.*, 2006). The gel is used in the cosmetics industry as a hydrating ingredient in liquids, creams, sun lotions, shaving creams, lip balms, healing ointments, and face packs (WHO, 1999). Other products containing *Aloe vera* include after-shave gel, mouthwash, hair tonic, shampoo, and skin-moistening gel (Newton, 2004).

Aloe vera may be used in cosmetics for marketing reasons (i.e. to impart a touch of "nature" to the product) rather than for actual effects, and the content may be normally kept at a low level (Committee of Experts on Cosmetic Products, 2008).

A study on skin hydration found that a single application of a cosmetic formulation containing > 0.25% of a commercial freeze-dried *Aloe vera* gel 200:1 concentrate improved the water content of the stratum corneum (Dal'Belo *et al.*, 2006). However, the concentrations of *Aloe vera* raw materials in cosmetics vary widely from 0.1% or less up to 20% (Cosmetic Ingredient Review Expert Panel, 2007).

Anthraquinone-rich *Aloe vera* extracts may function as absorbers of ultraviolet radiation in suncreens, because anthraquinones absorb ultraviolet radiation (Committee of Experts on Cosmetic Products, 2008). Regulatory authorities in Germany have proposed that cosmetic products for which claims are made regarding *Aloe vera* should contain at least 5 g of *Aloe vera* per 100 g of product (Kratz, 2009).

1.3.2 Dosage

For medicinal use as a laxative, the correct individual dose is the smallest amount required to produce a soft-formed stool. For adults and children aged more than 10 years, the dose is 40–110 mg of the dried latex, corresponding to 10–30 mg of hydroxyanthraquinones per day, or 100 mg as a single dose in the evening (WHO, 1999). The European Medicines Agency suggests a maximum daily dose of hydroxyanthracene glycosides of 30 mg, and that the correct individual dose is the smallest required to produce a comfortable soft-formed motion (EMA, 2006). As for other laxatives, there is potential for abuse of *Aloe vera* latex (Perkins & Livesey, 1993; Stolk & Hoogtanders, 1999). It is difficult to estimate rates of laxative abuse, and more so for cases of abuse attributable to *Aloe vera* alone.

For medicinal use of *Aloe vera* gel, 25 to 100 mL per day of a 4.5:1 gel concentrate was suggested as typical oral dose range in adults (Morgan *et al.*, 2005). The International Aloe Science Council recommended a total daily consumption of *Aloe vera* of 2–8 fluid ounces (59–237 mL) of single-strength leaf gel (IASC, 2013b). For topical use, pure *Aloe vera* gel is often used liberally on the skin. Hydrophilic cream of 0.5% (by weight) of a 50% ethanol extract of *Aloe vera*, three times per day for five consecutive days per week has been used for treatment of genital herpes and psoriasis vulgaris (Ulbricht *et al.*, 2007).

1.4   Production, sales, and consumption

1.4.1 Production

(a)   Production process

Aloe vera grows best in dry chalky soil or in a sandy loam (Grindlay & Reynolds, 1986). While the plant needs warm semi-tropical conditions, overexposure to sun results in stunted plants with low gel yield. Therefore, *Aloe vera* is commonly interplanted with other crops, such as fruit trees. The quality of *Aloe vera* plant products varies considerably due to differences in growing, harvesting, processing, and storage techniques (Boudreau *et al.*, 2013a), and may also depend on the regulatory regime under which the product is sold (see Section 1.6).

Mexico, followed by the rest of Latin America, China, Thailand, and the USA were described as main producing countries (Rodríguez *et al.*, 2010). *Aloe vera* has become an important plant crop in Arizona and in the Rio Grande valley of southern Texas (Boudreau *et al.*, 2013a).

The production processes for *Aloe vera* products include various steps such as crushing, grinding or pressing, filtration, decolorization, stabilization, heat processing, and may be followed by addition of preservatives and stabilizers. A complete overview of production was provided by Ahlawat & Khatkar (2011). The technology for processing of *Aloe vera* gel was reviewed by Ramachandra & Rao (2008).

Harvesting of the leaves of the *Aloe vera* plant is generally performed by hand, with the leaves cut from the base of the plant (Grindlay & Reynolds, 1986). Individual leaves are wrapped, crated, and transported to processing plants. Ideally, the leaves are processed within a few hours after harvesting, as temperature, light, air, and humidity can affect the stability of the plant components (Paez *et al.*, 2000). At the processing step, the leaves may be cleaned with water and a mild chlorine solution (Grindlay & Reynolds, 1986).

Aloe vera gel from the fillet of the inner leaf pulp is obtained either by manual removal of the outer layers of the leaf with a knife or by machine. Either method can be flawed and has the potential to contaminate the gel with latex (Grindlay & Reynolds, 1986). This process yields crude *Aloe vera* gel. High quality gel appears opaque, slightly off-white in colour, and is viscous (Vogler & Ernst, 1999).

Aloe vera whole leaf extract is obtained by grinding the whole fresh leaves, without removal of the rind. Extraneous material and lignified fibres are then removed by homogenizing and filtering the crude gel or whole leaf extracts (Yaron, 1993). Since various amounts of latex and rind may be present in the whole leaf extracts, the extracts may appear yellow to yellow-green in colour.

Activated carbon adsorption to produce *Aloe vera* decolorized whole leaf extract is the first processing step where an extract is intentionally subjected to chemical alteration. *Aloe vera* decolorized whole leaf has lower rheological values than the gel and has a lower content of complex carbohydrates than either gel or whole leaf extracts (Pelley *et al.*, 1998).

The processed extracts are difficult to keep stable, a problem that may cause differences in product potency; therefore, the gel or whole leaf extracts can undergo a stabilization process before being bottled. This process may involve pasteurization, ultraviolet stabilization, chemical oxidation with hydrogen peroxide, addition of chemical preservatives and additives, or concentration, and/or drying (Boudreau *et al.*, 2013a).

(b) Production volume

In the cosmetic industry, *Aloe vera* ingredients hold a prominent position at the top of the list showing the relative frequency of use of plant ingredients within formulations filed with the United States Food and Drug Administration (FDA) (Committee of Experts on Cosmetic Products, 2008).

1.4.2 Sales

According to the 2012 Nutrition Business Journal Annual Report, *Aloe vera* was 20th among best-selling dietary supplements in the USA. There has been a general upward trend in sales from US$ 31 million in 2000 to US$

Fig. 1.4 Sales of dietary supplements containing *Aloe vera* in the USA

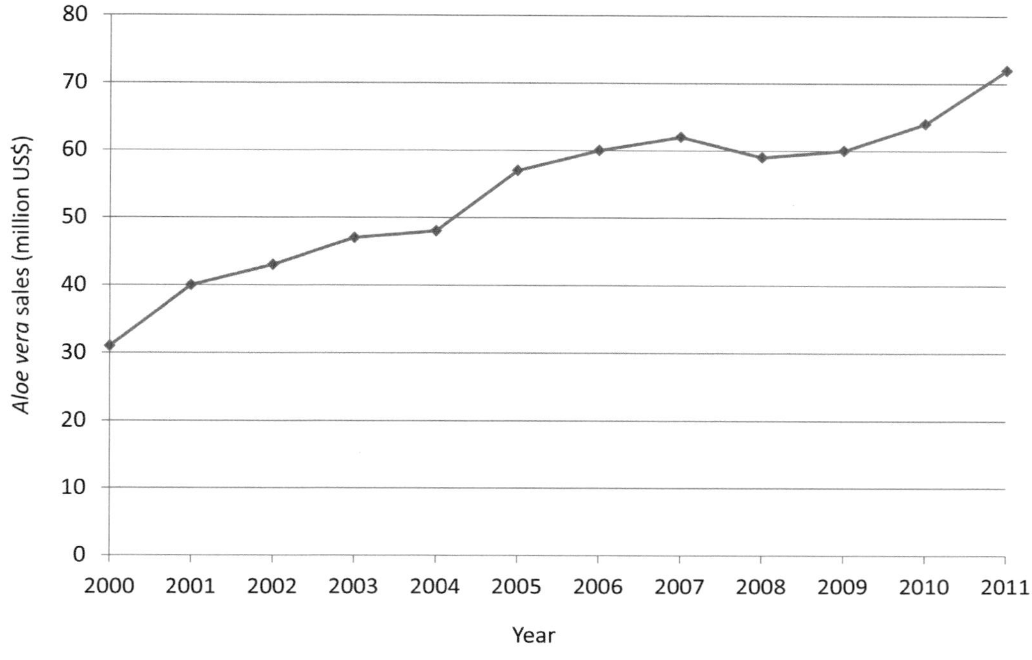

Compiled by the Working Group from data in Nutrition Business Journal (2010, 2012).

72 million in 2011 (Fig. 1.4; Nutrition Business Journal, 2010, 2012).

In 2006, the industry size for *Aloe* species raw material was estimated to be about US$ 125 million worldwide, while the industry for finished products containing *Aloe vera* was around US$ 110 billion (Ahlawat & Khatkar, 2011).

Global sales of *Aloe* species products in 2012 totalled US$ 351 million, according to IMS Health MIDAS data. Most products were reported as derived from *Aloe vera* (90%). Substantial sales as a dietary supplement were reported in Brazil (US$ 74 million), Indonesia (US$ 50 million), India (US$ 34 million), USA (US$ 29 million), the Russian Federation (US$ 19 million), Japan (US$ 15 million), and Mexico (US$ 12 million) (IMS Health, 2012).

1.4.3 Consumption

Consumers of products specified in Section 1.3 are exposed to *Aloe vera*. While the occasional short-term use of the latex as a laxative may allow exposure to be estimated for use in that context, it is unclear whether or not the gel products or liquid preparations are used over the short or long-term.

According to a representative survey conducted by the National Health and Nutrition Examination Survey from 1999 to 2010 (NHANES, 2010), the consumption of dietary supplements containing *Aloe vera* in the USA (prevalence of use in the past 30 days among adults in the USA) was 0.3% in 1999–2006 and 0.1% in 2007–2010 [figures calculated by the Working Group from publicly available data; due to the small use, the coefficient of variation is > 30%, so that the data for *Aloe vera* are less reliable than for other herbs]. In the context of complementary and alternative medicine, use

Table 1.4 Regulations for different *Aloe vera* products

Regulation	WHO Monograph on Selected Medicinal Plants (1999)[a]		Japanese Pharmacopoeia Sixteenth Edition (2011)[b]	European Pharmacopoeia 7.0 (2008)[c]	The International Aloe Science Council (2013)[d]
Regulated Aloe product	Dried juice	Gel	Dried juice	Concentrated and dried juice	Raw materials for use in products for oral consumption
Content	Min. 28% of hydroxyanthracene derivatives, expressed as aloin		Min. 4% aloin (dried material)	Min. 28% of hydroxyanthracene derivatives, expressed as aloin (dried drug)	Max. 10 ppm (aloin A + B)
Identity tests	Macroscopic and microscopic examinations, solvent solubility; TLC		Colour reactions with sodium tetraborate and nitric acid; TLC	TLC; fluorescence with disodium tetraborate; colour reaction with bromine water	Min. 5% acetylated mannan content by dry weight. Organoleptic standards: Aloe solids in single strength juice (1% in leaf juice and 0.5% for inner leaf juice) Malic acid and glucose must be present at a minimum Whole leaf marker (isocitrate). Max. 5% for inner leaf by dry weight.
Moisture	Max. 12% for Curacao or Barbados Aloe	Contains 98.5% water			
Total ash	Max. 2%		Max. 2%	Max. 2%	< 40%
Loss on drying			Max. 12%	Max. 12%	
Foreign substances/ contaminants	Limits for certain microorganisms, absence of adulterants such as black catechu, pieces of iron, and stones; limits for certain pesticides, heavy metals, and radioactive residues	Limits for certain microorganisms, pesticides, heavy metals, radioactive residues	Two different purity tests are specified		Microbiologicals (pathogens, lactic acid, mould, yeast), heavy metals, maltodextrin
Extract content	Min. 50% (water-soluble extract), max. 10% (alcohol-insoluble extract)		Min. 40% (water-soluble extract)		

[a] WHO (1999)
[b] Eur Ph (2008)
[c] JP XVI (2011)
[d] IASC (2013b)

max., maximum; min., minimum; TLC, thin-layer chromatography of *Aloe vera* has been reported in 8.5–13.8% of people in predominantly Hispanic populations in the southern USA; according to surveys, it is also used frequently by 10.8%, 10.3%, and 7.6% of adults in Australia, Italy, and Jamaica, respectively (Ngo *et al.*, 2010).

1.5　Occupational exposure

No specific studies on occupational exposure were identified. It can be assumed that workers in the production of *Aloe vera* may be exposed, as well as workers in pharmaceutical, cosmetic, and food industries that use *Aloe vera* as an ingredient.

1.6　Regulations and guidelines

Products made with various components of *Aloe vera* (aloin, aloe-emodin, and barbaloin) were at one time regulated by the FDA as oral over-the-counter (OTC) laxatives (NCCAM, 2012). In 2002, the FDA promulgated a regulation stating that the stimulant laxative ingredient *Aloe vera* in over the counter (OTC) drug products is not "generally recognized as safe and effective" or is misbranded (FDA, 2002). Because the companies that manufactured such products did not provide the necessary safety data, the FDA required that all OTC *Aloe vera* laxative products be removed from the USA market or reformulated (NCCAM, 2012). [The Working Group noted that currently no medicinal OTC *Aloe vera* products are available in the USA, unlike Europe where some medicinal *Aloe vera* products are still available.]

According to FDA regulations, *Aloe vera* may be safely used as a flavouring in foods as defined in 21CFR172.510. The Environmental Protection Agency (EPA) classified *Aloe vera* gel as a List 3 substance (inerts of unknown toxicity), and also listed *Aloe vera* gel as an inert ingredient of pesticide products (SciFinder, 2013).

A published tabulation of acceptable levels of natural flavourings by the Flavor and Extract Manufacturers' Association indicates that an acceptable level of *Aloe vera* extract is 5–2000 ppm. No distinction is given for the part of the plant or type of plant extract used to produce the extract used as a flavouring additive (Duke & Beckstrom-Sternberg, 1994).

For cosmetic uses, many of the manufacturers of *Aloe vera* gel take care to supply an ingredient containing anthraquinones at no more than 50 ppm (Committee of Experts on Cosmetic Products, 2008). This maximum level was also demanded in a safety assessment of the cosmetic industry (Cosmetic Ingredient Review Expert Panel, 2007).

Aloe vera is specified in several official pharmacopoeias, and an industry quality standard of the International Aloe Science Council is also available (Table 1.4). An American Herbal Pharmacopoeia on "Aloe vera leaf, Aloe vera leaf juice, Aloe vera inner leaf juice" was provided (AHP, 2012).

2.　Cancer in Humans

No data were available to the Working Group.

3.　Cancer in Experimental Animals

3.1　Studies of carcinogenicity

Whole leaf extract of *Aloe barbadensis* Miller [*Aloe vera*] was tested for carcinogenicity by oral administration (drinking-water) in one study in mice and one study in rats.

3.1.1　Mouse

In a 2-year study of carcinogenicity, groups of 48 male and 48 female B6C3F$_1$ mice (age, 6–7 weeks) were given drinking-water containing 0 (controls), 1.0%, 2.0%, or 3.0% (wt/wt) whole leaf extract of *Aloe barbadensis* Miller [*Aloe vera*] for 104 weeks. The average content of aloin A and aloe-emodin of the whole leaf test material was 6.40 and 0.071 mg/g respectively. The doses of whole leaf extract were equivalent to average daily doses of approximately 0, 2.9, 7.0, or 11.8 g/kg body weight (bw) in males; and 0, 2.2, 6.3, or 11.8 g/kg bw in females (Boudreau *et al.*, 2013a). Survival of exposed groups was similar to that of controls. There was no significantly increased incidence of any tumour type in male or female mice. Whole leaf extract increased the incidence of goblet cell hyperplasia in the intestine of male and female mice (Table 3.1).

3.1.2 Rat

In a 2-year study of carcinogenicity, groups of 48 male and 48 female F344/N rats were given drinking-water containing whole leaf extract of *Aloe barbadensis* Miller [*Aloe vera*] at 0 (controls), 0.5%, 1.0%, or 1.5% (wt/wt) for 104 weeks. The average content of aloin A and aloe-emodin of the whole leaf test material was 6.40 and 0.071 mg/g, respectively. The doses of whole leaf extract were equivalent to average daily doses of approximately 0, 0.2, 0.6, or 1.1 g/kg bw in males and 0, 0.3, 0.7, or 1.3 g/kg bw in females (Boudreau *et al.*, 2013a). Survival of exposed groups was similar to that of controls. Whole leaf extract caused increased incidences of adenoma and carcinoma of the large intestine (colon and caecum) in males and females. Other treatment-related lesions included hyperplasia and/or inflammation in the mesenteric lymph node, forestomach, small intestine, and large intestine in males and females (Table 3.1). [The Working Group noted that large intestine tumours are rare spontaneous neoplasms in F344/N rats.]

3.2 Photo-co-carcinogenicity studies

Mouse

There has been one study reported in which *Aloe barbadensis* Miller [*Aloe vera*] test articles were studied by dermal application in mice.

Groups of 36 male and 36 female Crl:SKH-1 (*hr/hr*) hairless mice (age, 8 weeks) received topical applications of control cream or creams containing: 3% or 6% (w/w) gel; 3% or 6% (w/w) whole leaf extract; 3% or 6% (w/w) decolorized whole leaf extract; or 7.46 or 74.6 µg/g of aloe-emodin to the dorsal skin region, for 5 days per week, for up to 40 weeks. After application of the cream in the morning, mice were exposed to filtered solar simulated light (SSL) at 0 (0.00 mJ.CIE/cm² per day) or 0.6 (13.70 mJ.CIE/cm² per day) minimal erythema doses of light (NTP, 2010). The minimal erythema dose is defined as the minimal amount of radiation that causes slight erythema within 24 hours after irradiation (Table 3.2). The mice were killed after a recovery/observation period of 12 weeks.

At 52 weeks, there was no significant increase in the incidence of skin neoplasms in any group receiving any of the four creams containing *Aloe* preparations without exposure to SSL. [The Working Group noted that the duration of the experiment, 1 year, was too short to consider this arm of the experiment as a full carcinogenicity study.]

There was no treatment-related increase in the incidence of skin neoplasms in any groups receiving any of the four creams containing *Aloe* preparations followed by SSL when compared with the groups receiving control cream followed by SSL. Almost all mice in groups exposed to SSL presented with skin neoplasms due to SSL exposure. [As a result, the primary experimental end-point was multiplicity of skin tumours.]

There was a significant enhancing effect of *Aloe* gel cream or of aloe-emodin cream on the photocarcinogenic activity of SSL in female mice, and there was a significant enhancing effect of the cream containing whole leaf extract, or cream containing decolorized whole leaf extract, on the photocarcinogenic activity of SSL in male and female mice, based on an increase in the multiplicity of squamous cell papilloma, carcinoma or carcinoma in situ (combined) (NTP, 2010).

Table 3.1 Studies of carcinogenicity in mice and rats given *Aloe vera* by oral administration

Species, strain (sex) Duration Reference	Dosing regimen Animals/group at start	Incidence of tumours	Significance	Comments
Mouse, B6C3F$_1$ (M, F) 104 wk Boudreau *et al.* (2013a)	Whole leaf extract of *Aloe barbadensis* Miller [*Aloe vera*]: 0 (control), 1.0%, 2.0%, or 3.0% (w/w) in drinking-water (estimated to be 0, 2.9, 7.0, or 11.8 g/kg bw (M); 0, 2.2, 6.3, or 11.8 g/kg bw (F) 48 M and 48 F/group (age, 6–7 wk)	No significantly increased incidence of any tumour type		Aloin A content, 6.40 mg/g whole leaf test material Aloin-emodin content, 0.071 mg/g whole leaf.
Rat, F344/N (M, F) 104 wk Boudreau *et al.* (2013a)	Whole leaf extract of *Aloe barbadensis* Miller [*Aloe vera*]: 0 (control), 0.5%, 1.0%, or 1.5% (w/w) in drinking-water (estimated to be 0, 0.2, 0.6, or 1.1 g whole leaf/kg bw (M); 0, 0.3, 0.7, 1.3 g whole leaf/kg bw (F) 48 M and 48 F/group (age, 6–7 wk)	All large intestine (colon and caecum) adenoma: M: 0/47 (0%)[#], 0/48 (0%), 26/48 (54%)*, 23/48 (48%)* F: 0/48 (0%)[#], 0/48 (0%), 6/48 (13%)**, 13/48 (27%)* All large intestine (colon and caecum) carcinoma: M: 0/47 (0%)[#], 0/48 (0%), 10/48 (21%)*, 14/48 (29%)* F: 0/48 (0%)[##], 0/48 (0%), 3/48 (6%), 4/48 (8%)** All large intestine (colon and caecum) adenoma or carcinoma (combined): M: 0/47 (0%)[#], 0/48 (0%), 28/48 (58%)*, 31/48 (65%)* F: 0/48 (0%)[#], 0/48 (0%), 8/48 (17%)***, 15/48 (31%)*	[#] $P \leq 0.001$ (trend) [##] $P \leq 0.01$ (trend) * $P \leq 0.001$ ** $P < 0.05$ *** $P \leq 0.01$	Aloin A content, 6.40 mg/g whole leaf. Aloin-emodin content, 0.071 mg/g whole leaf

bw, body weight; F, female; M, male; wk, week; w, weight

Table 3.2 Co-carcinogenicity studies in SKH-1 mice given *Aloe vera* or aloe-emodin by skin application followed by exposure to simulated solar light

Species, strain (sex) Duration Reference	Dosing regimen Animals/group at start	Overall age-adjusted tumour multiplicity	Significance	Comments
Mouse, Crl:SKH-1 (*hr/hr*) hairless (M, F) 52 wk NTP (2010)	*Aloe vera* gel cream at 0%, 3%, or 6% (w/w) + SSL (13.70 mJ•CIE/cm² per day). Cream applied in the morning; SSL in the afternoon. 5 d per wk for 40 wk, followed by 12-wk recovery/observation period 36 M and 36 F/group (age 8 wk)	Squamous cell papilloma, squamous cell carcinoma in situ, and/or squamous cell carcinoma of the skin: M: 5.8 (4.7–7.2), 6.8 (5.6–8.4), 7.1 (5.8–8.7) F: 6.4 (5.3–7.6)*, 9.2 (7.8–10.8)**, 8.1 (6.9–9.6)***	* $P < 0.05$ (trend) ** $P = 0.006$ *** $P < 0.05$	No significant increase in the incidence of skin neoplasms in any group receiving creams containing *Aloe vera* preparations without exposure to SSL
Mouse, Crl:SKH-1 (*hr/hr*) hairless (M, F) 52 wk NTP (2010)	Whole leaf *Aloe vera* cream at 0%, 3%, or 6% (w/w) + SSL (13.70 mJ•CIE/cm² per day). Cream applied in the morning; SSL in the afternoon. 5 d per wk for 40 wk, followed by 12-wk recovery/observation period 36 M and 36 F/group (age 8 wk)	Squamous cell papilloma, squamous cell carcinoma in situ, and/or squamous cell carcinoma of the skin: M: 5.8* (4.7–7.2), 6.4 (5.2–7.9), 8.4** (6.8–10.3) F: 6.4* (5.3–7.6), 8.7** (7.4–10.3), 7.7 (6.5–9.1)	* $P < 0.05$ (trend) ** $P < 0.05$	
Mouse, Crl:SKH-1 (*hr/hr*) hairless (M, F) 52 wk NTP (2010)	Decolorized whole leaf *Aloe vera* cream at 0%, 3%, or 6% (w/w) + SSL (13.70 mJ•CIE/cm² per day). Cream applied in the morning; SSL in the afternoon. 5 d per wk for 40 wk, followed by 12-wk recovery/observation period 36 M and 36 F/group (age 8 wk)	Squamous cell papilloma, squamous cell carcinoma in situ, and/or squamous cell carcinoma of the skin: M: 5.8 (4.6–7.3), 8.0* (6.5–9.9), 6.4 (5.2 –8.0) F: 6.4** (5.2–7.7), 10.0*** (8.4–12.0), 9.3**** (7.8–11.1)	* $P < 0.05$ ** $P = 0.007$ (trend) *** $P = 0.002$ **** $P = 0.007$	
Mouse, Crl:SKH-1 (*hr/hr*) hairless (M, F) 52 wk NTP (2010)	Aloe-emodin cream at 0, 7.46, or 74.6 µg/g + SSL (13.70 mJ•CIE/cm² per day). Cream applied in the morning; SSL in the afternoon. 5 d per wk for 40 wk, followed by 12 wk recovery/observation period 36 M and 36 F/group (age, 8 wk)	Squamous cell papilloma, squamous cell carcinoma in situ, and/or squamous cell carcinoma of the skin: M: 5.8 (4.7–7.2), 6.3 (5.1–7.8), 7.1 (5.8–8.7) F: 6.4* (5.3–7.7) 7.9 (6.6–9.4), 8.9** (7.5–10.6)	* $P < 0.05$ (trend) ** $P < 0.05$	

bw, body weight; CIE, Commission Internationale de l'Eclairage [International Commission on Illumination]; d, day; F, female; M, male; SSL, simulated solar light; wk, week

4. Mechanistic and Other Relevant Data

In reviewing studies relevant to the possible carcinogenicity of *Aloe vera*, the Working Group noted that attributing appropriate weight to individual studies was complicated by the consideration that, despite the terminology used, the material tested may not have been identical across various studies and/or may not have been identical to the material that was studied in experimental animals, as described in Section 3 of this *Monograph*.

4.1 Absorption, distribution, metabolism, and excretion

4.1.1 Humans

There were no reports of studies to determine the absorption, distribution, metabolism, or excretion of topically applied *Aloe vera* gel, whole leaf extract or decolorized whole leaf extract in experimental animals or humans.

Aloe vera whole leaf extract is composed of gel and latex. *Aloe vera* gel contains non-starch polysaccharides of high molecular weight (the major one being acemannan) that are composed of sugar moieties linked by β-1,4-glycosyl bonds (Fig. 1.3 in Section 1). *Aloe vera* latex contains the anthrone *C*-glycosides aloin A (barbaloin) and aloin B (isobarbaloin) that are linked by β-glycosyl bonds to D-glucopyranose. Other *C*-glycosides found in *Aloe vera* latex include aloesin (aloeresin B) and aloeresin A in which the glycosyl linkage is to the benzo ring of benzopyran-4-one (Boudreau & Beland, 2006). Aloenin, an *O*-β-glucoside, is also a component of *Aloe vera* latex (Hirata *et al.*, 1981; Matsuda *et al.*, 2008).

(a) Components of Aloe vera gel: metabolism ex vivo

Incubation of acemannan (aloemannan; molecular weight > 400 kDa) labelled with fluoresceinyl isothiocyanate (FITC) with a suspension of fresh human faeces for 5 days gave two metabolites, with molecular weights of 10 and 30 kDa, in 1% yield, meaning that aloemannan is catabolized by human intestinal bacteria (Yagi *et al.*, 1999).

(b) Components of Aloe vera latex

Orally ingested anthrone *C*-glycosides (*i.e.* aloin A and aloin B) pass intact through the upper portion of the gastrointestinal tract and upon reaching the lower gastrointestinal tract are cleaved to aloe-emodin-9-anthrone by human *Eubacterium* sp. BAR given to germ-free rats (Che *et al.*, 1991; Hattori *et al.*, 1993; Akao *et al.*, 1996). The free aglycone is then absorbed, undergoes oxidation, and is excreted in the urine as rhein, as was shown in three volunteers receiving *Aloe vera* or barbaloin (Vyth & Kamp, 1979; Fig. 4.1).

4.1.2 Experimental systems

(a) Components of Aloe vera gel

In beagle dogs, the oral administration of radiolabelled acemannan at a dose of 20 mg/kg body weight (bw) per day for 3 months resulted in peak blood concentrations at 4–6 hours and a half-life of > 48 hours (Fogleman *et al.*, 1992).

Male ddY mice were given FITC-labelled acemannan (aloemannan; molecular weight, 500 kDa) at a dose of 120 mg/kg bw by gavage, and urinary and faecal excretion was monitored for 48 hours. Of the administered dose, 95% was excreted in the faeces, with > 90% occurring within 24 hours. Only 0.3% of the material was found in the urine. In both urine and faeces, FITC-labelled acemannan was converted to substances of low molecular weight (< 9 kDa).

Fig. 4.1 Metabolites of aloin A and aloin B

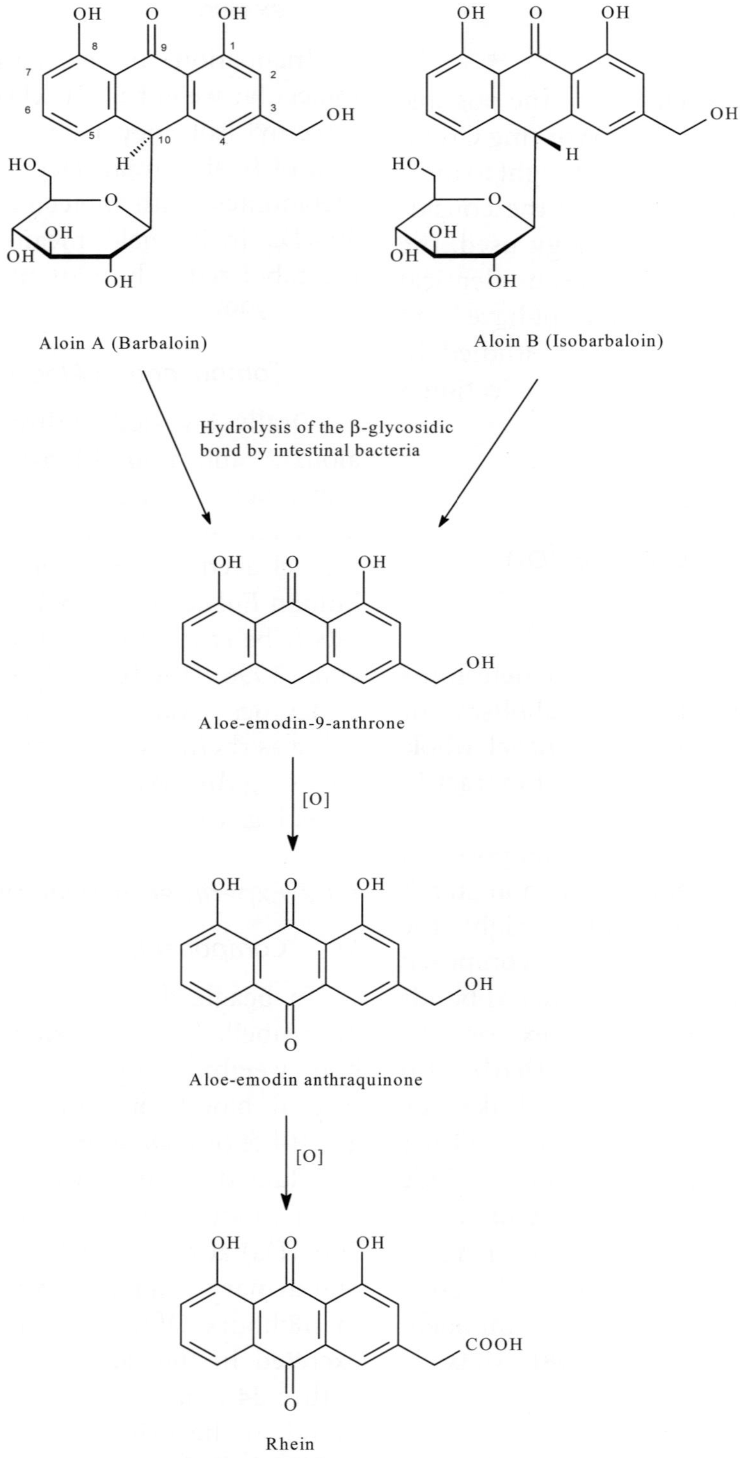

Aloin A and B are constituents of *Aloe vera* whole leaf latex.
Compiled by the Working Group.

FITC-labelled acemannan was also administered to mice by intravenous injection at a dose of 120 mg/kg bw. Of the administered dose, 73% was excreted in the urine, with > 60% occurring within 24 hours; 13% of the material was found in the faeces. In both urine and faeces, FITC-labelled acemannan was converted to substances of low molecular weight (10–70 kDa in urine; 5 kDa in faeces) (Yagi *et al.*, 1999).

(b) Components of Aloe vera latex

In male Wistar rats, oral administration of aloin A (barbaloin; 100 mg/kg bw) resulted in maximum serum concentrations of aloin A [340 ng/mL; ~0.8 µM, based upon the molecular weight of aloin A of 404 Da] 1.5 hours after administration, followed by a decrease in concentration, with aloin A still detectable 6 hours after dosing (Ishii *et al.*, 1987).

The ability to cleave anthrone *C*-glycosides varies among species; free anthrones are detected in faecal contents from humans and rats, but not mice or guinea-pigs (Dreessen & Lemli, 1988; Hattori *et al.*, 1988).

In male and female Brown-Norway rats, oral administration of [14C]aloe-emodin (4.5 mg/kg bw) resulted in maximum blood concentrations [~350 ng/mL; ~1.3 µM, based upon the molecular weight of aloe-emodin of 270 Da] 2 hours after dosing, and a terminal half-life of elimination of approximately 50 hours. Seven metabolites were detected in the plasma. These were characterized as aloe-emodin, rhein, an unidentified aglycone, and conjugates of these aglycones. Approximately 20% of the radiolabel was eliminated in the urine, primarily as aloe-emodin, rhein, and their conjugates. More than 75% of the radiolabel was excreted in the faeces and nearly all of this was aloe-emodin. At early time-points (< 48 hours), a great majority of the radiolabel was associated with the gastrointestinal tract. At later time-points (i.e. 96 hours), the highest levels of radioactivity were found in the kidney and liver.

This material was characterized as aloe-emodin, rhein, and their conjugates (Lang, 1993).

Intracaecal administration of [14C]rhein to male Wistar rats resulted in 37% of the radioactivity being excreted in the urine and 53% in the faeces. The highest tissue concentrations were found in the kidney (De Witte & Lemli, 1988).

The oral administration of [14C]-labelled aloenin to rats resulted in the faecal and urinary excretion of the aglycone 4-methoxy-6-(2,4-dihydroxy-6-methylphenyl)-2-pyrone (Hirata *et al.*, 1981).

4.1.3 Alterations in enzymes involved in metabolism

Incubation of the human colon carcinoma cell line LS180 with *Aloe vera* juice resulted in a significant increase in the expression of *CYP1A2*, *CYP3A4*, and multidrug resistance 1 genes (Brandin *et al.*, 2007).

Commercial preparations of *Aloe vera* were tested for their ability to inhibit the activities of CYP3A4 and CYP2D6 in vitro. Inhibition was observed with half maximal inhibitory concentrations IC_{50} in the range 8–43 mg/mL, concentrations that were probably sufficiently high as to preclude any significant inhibition in vivo (Djuv & Nilsen, 2012). Rhein was shown to inhibit CYP1A2, CYP2C9, CYP2D6, CYP2E1, and CYP3A activities in rat liver microsomes, with K_i in the range of 10–74 µM (Tang *et al.*, 2009).

4.2 Genetic and related effects

4.2.1 Humans

No data were available to the Working Group.

4.2.2 Experimental systems

(a)   DNA damage

An *Aloe vera* whole leaf extract induced single-strand breaks in pUC 9.1 plasmid DNA, and this was associated with decreased transformation efficiency of the plasmid (Table 4.1; Paes-Leme *et al.*, 2005).

Aloe-emodin and/or rhein induced DNA damage in NPC-039 and NPC-076 human nasopharyngeal carcinoma cells and SCC-4 human tongue cancer cells, as measured by comet assays (Table 4.2; Lin *et al.*, 2007, 2010; Chen *et al.*, 2010).

(b)   End-points associated with DNA damage

In addition to inducing DNA damage (as indicated by comet assays), aloe-emodin significantly inhibited expression of genes associated with DNA damage and repair: ataxia telangiectasia mutated (*ATM*), ataxia telangiectasia and Rad3-related (*ATR*), *14–3-3σ*, breast cancer 1, early onset (*BRCA1*), and DNA-dependent serine/threonine protein kinase (*DNA-PK*) in SCC-4 human tongue squamous cancer cells (Chen *et al.*, 2010). Aloe-emodin also induced the formation of reactive oxygen species (ROS) in SCC-4 cells, which was accompanied by S-phase cell-cycle arrest, apoptosis, and several molecular markers associated with apoptosis (Chiu *et al.*, 2009). Rhein induced the formation of ROS in NPC-039 human nasopharyngeal carcinoma cells, SCC-4 human tongue squamous cancer cells, and A-549 human lung cancer cells, which was accompanied by apoptosis and several molecular markers associated with apoptosis (Lin *et al.*, 2007; Hsia *et al.* 2009; Lai *et al.*, 2009).

Aloe-emodin induced DNA damage in mouse lymphoma L5178 cells, as measured by comet assay (Table 4.2; Müller *et al.*, 1996).

(c)   Gene mutation

Extracts in water, ethanol or methanol of *Aloe ferox* Mill., stabilized *Aloe vera* gel, *Aloe vera* whole leaf extract, *Aloe vera* decolorized whole leaf extract, *Aloe vera* gel, acemannan, and aloin were tested in *Salmonella typhimurium* reverse mutation assays, *Bacillus subtilis* rec-assays, and/or SOS DNA damage-repair assays. With the exception of the *Bacillus subtilis* rec-assay with water extracts of *Aloe ferox* Mill., all gave negative results (Table 4.1; Table 4.2; Brown & Dietrich, 1979; Morimoto *et al.*, 1982; Boudreau *et al.*, 2013a; Sehgal *et al.*, 2013a, b).

Aloe-emodin was mutagenic in reversion assays with various strains of *Salmonella typhimurium*, at the *Tk*[+/−] locus in mouse lymphoma L5178Y cells, and the *Gpt* locus in AS52 Chinese hamster cells (Table 4.2; Brown *et al.*, 1977; Brown & Dietrich, 1979; Westendorf *et al.*, 1990; Heidemann *et al.*, 1996; Müller *et al.*, 1996; Müller & Stopper, 1999; Nesslany *et al.*, 2009).

Mutation analysis of eight adenomas and four carcinomas from the large intestine of F344 rats given drinking-water containing an *Aloe vera* whole leaf extract (Boudreau *et al.*, 2013a, b) indicated four point mutations in exons 1 and 2 of the *Kras* gene and four point mutations in exon 2 of the *Ctnnb1* gene (Table 4.1; Pandiri *et al.*, 2011).

(d)   Other genotoxicity end-points

Aloe vera inner leaf fillet Qmatrix® did not induce chromosomal aberration in Chinese hamster lung cells in vitro; micronuclei were not formed in bone-marrow cells of mice treated orally in vivo (Williams *et al.*, 2010; Table 4.1).

Aloe-emodin induced unscheduled DNA synthesis in primary hepatocytes from male Wistar rats, micronucleus formation in mouse lymphoma L5178Y cells and TK6 human lymphoblastoid cells, and chromosomal aberrations in Chinese hamster ovary cells. Aloe-emodin also inhibited topoisomerase II, gave positive results in comet assays in mouse lymphoma L5178Y cells, SCC-4 human tongue cancer cells, and NPC-039 human nasopharyngeal carcinoma cells, and transformed C3H/M2 mouse cells (Table 4.2; Heidemann *et al.*, 1996; Müller *et al.*, 1996; Müller & Stopper, 1999; Lin *et al.*, 2010).

Table 4.1 Genetic and related effects of *Aloe vera* preparations

Test system	Results		Dose (LED or HID)	*Aloe vera* preparation	Reference
	Without exogenous metabolic system	With exogenous metabolic system			
In vitro					
Single-strand breaks in pUC 9.1 plasmid DNA	+	NT	3 µg/mL	Whole leaf extract	Paes-Leme *et al.* (2005)
Bacillus subtilis rec-assay	+	NT	6 mg/disk	*Aloe ferox* Mill. water extract	Morimoto *et al.* (1982)
Bacillus subtilis rec-assay	–	NT	6 mg/disk	*Aloe ferox* Mill. methanol extract	Morimoto *et al.* (1982)
Salmonella typhimurium, TA98, TA100, reverse mutation	–	–	10 mg/plate[a]	*Aloe ferox* Mill. water extract	Morimoto *et al.* (1982)
Salmonella typhimurium, TA98, TA100, reverse mutation	–	–	10 mg/plate[b]	*Aloe ferox* Mill. methanol extract	Morimoto *et al.* (1982)
Salmonella typhimurium, TA100, reverse mutation	–	–	NR	Stabilized gel; aloin A and aloin B, ≤ 10 ppm; in some instances, material was sterilized by filtration or autoclaving	Sehgal *et al.* (2013a)
Salmonella typhimurium, TA98, TA100, TA1535, TA1537, reverse mutation	–	–	10 mg/plate	Qmatrix° inner leaf fillet; aloin, < 10 ppm	Williams *et al.* (2010)
Salmonella typhimurium, TA98, TA100, reverse mutation	–	–	6 mg/plate	Whole leaf extract	Boudreau *et al.* (2013a)
Salmonella typhimurium, TA98, TA100, reverse mutation	–	–	6 mg/plate	Decolorized whole leaf extract	Boudreau *et al.* (2013a)
Salmonella typhimurium, TA97, TA98, TA100, TA1535, reverse mutation	–	–	10 mg/plate	Gel	Boudreau *et al.* (2013a)
Salmonella typhimurium, TA98, TA100, reverse mutation	–	–	21 × initial concentration	Decolorized whole leaf extract; aloin A & aloin B, ~1 ppm. Material sterilized by filtration.	Sehgal *et al.* (2013b)
Escherichia coli, WP2 *uvrA*/pKM101	–	–	6 mg/plate	Whole leaf extract	Boudreau *et al.* (2013a)
Escherichia coli, WP2 *uvrA*/pKM101	–	–	6 mg/plate	Decolorized whole leaf extract	Boudreau *et al.* (2013a)
Escherichia coli, WP2 *uvrA*/pKM101	–	–	3 mg/plate	Gel	Boudreau *et al.* (2013a)
Escherichia coli, SOS DNA damage repair assay	–	–	10 × initial concentration	Stabilized gel; aloin A and aloin B, ≤ 10 ppm	Sehgal *et al.* (2013a)

Table 4.1 (continued)

Test system	Results		Dose (LED or HID)	*Aloe vera* preparation	Reference
	Without exogenous metabolic system	With exogenous metabolic system			
Escherichia coli, SOS DNA damage repair assay	–	–	21 × initial concentration	Decolorized whole leaf extract; aloin A and aloin B, ~1 ppm. Material sterilized by filtration.	Sehgal *et al.* (2013b)
Chromosomal aberrations, Chinese hamster lung cells	–	–	10 mg/plate	Qmatrix˚ inner leaf fillet; aloin,< 10 ppm	Williams *et al.* (2010)
In vivo					
Micronucleus formation, male ICR mice, bone-marrow cells	–	NT	5000 mg/kg bw, po	Qmatrix˚ inner leaf fillet; aloin,< 10 ppm	Williams *et al.* (2010)
Gene mutations in exon 1 and 2 of *Kras* gene in large intestine adenomas and carcinomas, F344 rats	+	NT	1%	Whole leaf preparation	Pandiri *et al.* (2011)
Gene mutations in exon 2 of *Ctnnb1* gene in large intestine adenomas and carcinomas, F344 rats	+	NT	1%	Whole leaf preparation	Pandiri *et al.* (2011)

+, positive; –, negative; LED, lowest effective dose; HID, highest ineffective dose; NR, not reported; NT, not tested; po, per oral

[a] Toxic in TA98, without exogenous metabolic system, and in TA100, with or without exogenous metabolic system

[b] Toxic in TA98, without exogenous metabolic system

Table 4.2 Genetic and related effects of constituents of *Aloe vera*

Constituent Test system	Results		Dose (LED or HID)	Reference
	Without exogenous metabolic system	With exogenous metabolic system		
Acemannan				
Salmonella typhimurium reverse mutation *in vitro*	–	–	800 µL/plate	Fogleman et al. (1992)
Aloin				
Salmonella typhimurium, TA1535, TA100, TA1537, TA1538, TA98, TA100FR50, reverse mutation in vitro	–	–	250 µg/plate	Brown & Dietrich (1979)
Aloe-emodin in vitro				
Salmonella typhimurium, TA1537, reverse mutation	+	–	100 µg/plate	Brown et al. (1977), Brown & Dietrich (1979)
Salmonella typhimurium, TA1535, TA100, TA1538, TA98, TA100FR50, reverse mutation	–	–	250 µg/plate	Brown et al. (1977), Brown & Dietrich (1979)
Salmonella typhimurium, TA1537, TA102, TA1538, TA98, TA1978, reverse mutation	+[a]	+[b]	10 µg/plate	Westendorf et al. (1990)
Salmonella typhimurium, TA98, TA100, TA1535, TA1537, TA1538, reverse mutation	+[c]	+[d]	10 µg/plate	Heidemann et al. (1996)
Salmonella typhimurium, TA1537, TA98, TA100, reverse mutation	+	+	0.62 µg/plate	Nesslany et al. (2009)
Unscheduled DNA synthesis, male Wistar rat primary hepatocytes	+	NT	25 µg/mL	Westendorf et al. (1990)
Gene mutation, Chinese hamster lung V79 cells, 8-azaguanine resistance	(+)	NT	10 µg/mL	Westendorf et al. (1990)
Gene mutation, Chinese hamster lung V79 cells, *Hprt* locus, 6-thioguanine resistance	–	–	350 µg/mL	Heidemann et al. (1996)
Gene mutation, Chinese hamster lung V79 cells, *Hprt* locus, 6-thioguanine resistance	–	–	350 µg/mL	Brusick & Mengs (1997)
Gene mutation, mouse lymphoma L5178Y cells, $Tk^{+/-}$ locus, trifluorothymidine resistance	+	NT	37 µM	Müller et al. (1996)
Gene mutation, mouse lymphoma L5178Y cells, $Tk^{+/-}$ locus, trifluorothymidine resistance	+[e]	NT	100 µM	Müller & Stopper (1999)
Gene mutation, AS52 Chinese hamster cells, *Gpt* locus	+	NT	28 µM	Müller et al. (1996)
Micronucleus formation, mouse lymphoma L5178Y cells	+	NT	37 µM	Müller et al. (1996)
Micronucleus formation, TK6 human lymphoblastoid cells	+	+	3.12 µg/mL	Nesslany et al. (2009)
Chromosomal aberrations, Chinese hamster ovary cells	+	+	18.75 µg/mL	Heidemann et al. (1996)
Topoisomerase II inhibition, decatenation of kDNA[f]	+	NT	1 mM	Müller et al. (1996)
Topoisomerase II inhibition, decatenation of kDNA[f]	+	NT	741 µM[g]	Müller & Stopper (1999)
DNA damage, comet assay, mouse lymphoma L5178Y cells	+	NT	55 µM	Müller et al. (1996)
DNA fragmentation, comet assay, SCC-4 human tongue cancer cells	+	NT	100 µM	Chen et al. (2010)

Table 4.2   (continued)

Constituent Test system	Results		Dose (LED or HID)	Reference
	Without exogenous metabolic system	With exogenous metabolic system		
DNA fragmentation, comet assay, NPC-039 & NPC-076 human nasopharyngeal carcinoma cells	+	NT	60 µM	Lin et al. (2010)
Cell transformation, C3H/M2 mouse fibroblast cells	+	NT	3 µg/mL	Westendorf et al. (1990)
Aloe-emodin in vivo				
Chromosomal aberrations, Wistar rats, bone-marrow cells	–	NT	200 mg/kg bw, po	Heidemann et al. (1996)
Micronucleus formation, polychromatic erythrocytes, NMRI mice, bone-marrow cells	–	NT	1500 mg/kg bw, po	Heidemann et al. (1996)
Spot test in F1 offspring of NMRI female mice, X DBA male mice	–	NT	2000 mg/kg bw, po[h]	Heidemann et al. (1996)
Unscheduled DNA synthesis, hepatocytes of Wistar rats treated in vivo	–	NT	1000 mg/kg bw, po	Heidemann et al. (1996)
DNA damage, comet assay, male OF1 mice, kidney and colon, treated in vivo	+	NT	500 mg/kg bw, po	Nesslany et al. (2009)
Rhein				
Salmonella typhimurium, TA1537, TA102, TA1538, TA98, TA1978, reverse mutation	–	(+)[i]	NR	Westendorf et al. (1990)
Unscheduled DNA synthesis, male Wistar rat primary hepatocytes	–	NT	NR	Westendorf et al. (1990)
Gene mutation, Chinese hamster lung V79 cells, 8-azaguanine resistance	–	NT	NR	Westendorf et al. (1990)
DNA fragmentation, comet assay, NPC-039 human nasopharyngeal carcinoma cells	+	NT	180 µM	Lin et al. (2007)
DNA fragmentation, comet assay, SCC-4 human cancer tongue cells	+	NT	50 µM	Chen et al. (2010)
Cell transformation, C3H/M2 mouse cells	–	NT	NR	Westendorf et al. (1990)
Cell transformation, C3H/M2 mouse fibroblast cells	–	NT	10 µg/mL	Wölfle et al. (1990)

+, positive; (+), weakly positive; –, negative; bw, body weight; HID, highest ineffective dose; LED, lowest effective dose; NR, not reported; NT, not tested; po, oral

[a] Not positive in TA102

[b] Not positive in TA102 or TA1978

[c] Positive only in TA98, TA1537, and TA1538

[d] Positive only in TA1538

[e] Mutations associated with loss of heterozygosity.

[f] kDNA, kinetoplast DNA, a catenated network of mitochondrial DNA rings isolated from *Crithidia fasciculate*.

[g] IC_{50} = 741 ± 272 µM, represents the concentration at which the catalytic activity of the topoisomerase II was reduced to 50%.

[h] The mother mice were treated on day 9 of the pregnancy.

[i] In TA1537 only.

Rhein gave positive results in comet assays in SCC-4 human tongue cancer cells and NPC-039 human nasopharyngeal carcinoma cells (Table 4.2; Lin *et al.*, 2007; Chen *et al.*, 2010).

4.3 Toxic effects and other mechanistic data

[The Working Group noted that the following studies would have been strengthened by the inclusion of positive controls, and *Aloe vera* whole leaf was not included for comparison.]

Short-term studies were conducted in which technical-grade acemannan (acemannan, 78%) was fed to male and female Sprague-Dawley rats at doses up to 2000 mg/kg bw per day for 6 months, and to male and female beagle dogs at doses up to 1500 mg/kg bw per day for 90 days. There were no significant gross or microscopic lesions in either species that could be associated with the dietary administration of acemannan (Fogleman *et al.*, 1992).

Short-term studies were conducted in which *Aloe vera* gel (designated "process A aloe") or charcoal-treated *Aloe vera* gel (designated "process B aloe") were fed to male F344 rats at dietary concentrations of 1% or 10% for up to 7 months [corresponding to doses of *Aloe vera* gel of ~0.33 and 3.3 g per kg bw per day]. Gross and microscopic histopathological analyses indicated that there were no significant differences between the control rats and rats fed either of the *Aloe vera* preparations (Herlihy *et al.*, 1998).

Male F344 rats were given drinking-water containing *Aloe vera* gel at a concentration of 1% [~0.2 g/kg bw per day], or charcoal-treated *Aloe vera* gel at 1% [~0.2 g/kg bw per day], or charcoal-treated *Aloe vera* whole leaf at 0.02% [amount consumed could not be determined] for 30 months. None of the treatments caused any obvious histopathological changes (Ikeno *et al.*, 2002).

Male and female Sprague-Dawley rats were treated by gavage with an *Aloe vera* preparation designated Qmatrix® at a dose of 0, 500, 1000, or 2000 mg/kg bw per day for 90 days. This material was prepared from *Aloe vera* inner leaf fillets and was further treated to reduce the aloin content to < 10 ppm. At necroscopy, there were no gross or histopathological alterations that could be ascribed to treatment with *Aloe vera* (Williams *et al.*, 2010).

Short-term studies were conducted in which charcoal-treated *Aloe vera* gel (designated "Aloe juice") was fed to male and female B6C3F₁ mice at a dose of 350–540 mg per day for 13 weeks. At necropsy, no significant differences were observed between mice fed Aloe juice and the control mice. Likewise, histopathological examination of the livers revealed no treatment-related lesions (Sehgal *et al.*, 2013a).

Male and female Wistar Hannover rats fed whole leaf powder from *Aloe arborescens* Miller var. *natalensis* Berger at a dietary concentration of 0%, 0.16%, 0.8%, or 4% [corresponding to doses of whole leaf powder of 0, 99, 486, and 2447 mg per kg bw per day] for 1 or 2 years showed severe sinus dilatation and yellowish pigmentation of the ileocaecal lymph nodes, as well as yellow-brown pigmentation of the renal tubules. Rats from the 2-year study also showed pigmentation, epithelial thickening, and atypical hyperplasia of the large intestine (Matsuda *et al.*, 2008; Yokohira *et al.*, 2009).

Male and female F344Du rats given drinking-water containing *Aloe vera* decolorized whole leaf juice at 0%, 0.5%, 1%, or 2% [corresponding to doses of decolorized whole leaf juice of 0, 565, 1201, and 2382 mg per kg bw per day] for 3 months. No alterations were detected upon histopathological examination of the caecum and colon (Shao *et al.*, 2013).

Male and female B6C3F₁ mice were given an *Aloe vera* decolorized whole leaf extract to which had been added a high-molecular-weight *Aloe vera* polysaccharide designated Aloesorb, by gavage, twice in 24 hours. The material was administered at 1% of the mouse body weight [the absolute amount of the decolorized whole leaf extract administered could not be determined] and the mice were monitored for up to 14 days after treatment. No adverse effects were detected. The same *Aloe* preparation was also mixed in the diet at a concentration of 100 g/kg and fed to male and female F344 rats for 3 months [total amount administered, 10 g of decolorized whole leaf extract per g bw]. Histopathological examination of the caecum, colon, and rectum indicated no significant alterations (Sehgal *et al.*, 2013b).

Male and female F344/N rats exposed to drinking-water containing *Aloe vera* whole leaf extract at 1%, 2%, or 3% [corresponding to whole leaf extract at approximately 1.2, 2.4, and 3.6 g per kg bw per day] for 13 weeks, or *Aloe vera* whole leaf extract at 0.5%, 1.0%, or 1.5% [corresponding to whole leaf extract at 0.25, 0.65, and 1.2 g per kg bw per day] for 2 years, had dose-related increases in the incidence and severity of goblet cell and lymph node hyperplasia in the large intestine. Goblet cell hyperplasia also occurred in the large intestine of B6C3F$_1$ mice given drinking-water containing *Aloe vera* whole leaf extract at 1%, 2%, or 3% [corresponding to whole leaf extract at 2.55, 6.65, and 11.8 g per kg bw per day] for 13 weeks, but with lesser severity than that observed in rats (Boudreau *et al.*, 2013a, b).

Aloe vera Liliaceae was extracted with 95% ethanol, the solvent was evaporated, and the residue was administered in the drinking-water at a dose of 100 mg/kg bw to male Swiss albino mice for 3 months. Of the treated mice, 30% (6/20) died compared with 10% (2/20) of the control mice, a difference that was not statistically significant. Mice treated with the *Aloe vera* preparation had an increased incidence ($P < 0.01$) of sperm abnormalities, including megacephaly, flat head, swollen acrosome, and rotated head (Shah *et al.*, 1989). [The identity of the material being tested was not certain.]

4.4 Other mechanistic data

Gastrointestinal transit times were measured in B6C3F$_1$ mice and F344/N rats given drinking-water containing *Aloe vera* whole leaf extract (aloin A, 14.1–15.9 mg per g of extract), *Aloe vera* decolorized whole leaf extract (aloin A, 0.06–0.2 mg per g of extract), or *Aloe vera* gel (aloin A, 1.1–1.4 mg per g of gel) for 14 days. Without treatment, B6C3F$_1$ mice have shorter transit times than F344/N rats. *Aloe vera* whole leaf extract decreased transit times in the rats, but not in mice. A decrease in gastrointestinal transit times was also observed in a 13-week study in F344/N rats, but not B6C3F$_1$ mice, receiving *Aloe vera* whole leaf extract (Boudreau *et al.*, 2013a, b).

Molecular pathways shown to be important in human colorectal carcinogenesis, including mitogen-activated protein kinases *MAPK*, *WNT*, and transforming growth factor *TGF-β* signalling pathways, were also altered in adenomas and carcinomas of the large intestine in F344 rats given drinking-water containing *Aloe vera* whole leaf preparations at 1% and 1.5% (Pandiri *et al.*, 2011).

Aloe vera whole leaf preparations were incubated with pure and mixed human gut-bacteria cultures. The *Aloe vera* preparations possessed bacteriogenic activity and altered the production of acetic acid, butyric acid, and propionic acid (Pogribna *et al.*, 2008).

4.5 Susceptibility

No data were available to the Working Group.

4.6 Mechanistic considerations

Upon oral ingestion, *Aloe vera* components pass through the upper portion of the gastrointestinal tract; upon reaching the lower gastrointestinal tract, the anthrone *C*-glycosides aloin A and aloin B are converted by the intestinal microflora to aloe-emodin-9-anthrone, which undergoes sequential oxidation to aloe-emodin and rhein (Fig. 4.1). Likewise, intestinal microflora metabolize acemannan to smaller compounds by cleavage of the β-1$\rightarrow$4 linkages.

The oral administration of *Aloe vera* whole leaf preparation induces hyperplasia of the large intestine in mice and rats, and adenomas and carcinomas of the large intestine in rats. Rats dosed orally with acemannan for up to 6 months did not display any treatment-related pathological changes. Likewise, rats given *Aloe vera* gel orally, and mice and rats given charcoal-treated *Aloe vera* gel did not show any treatment-related non-neoplastic or neoplastic lesions.

Aloe vera preparations, acemannan, and aloin A do not display genotoxic activity in bacterial assays for mutagenesis and/or other assays for genotoxicity. In contrast, aloe-emodin is mutagenic in *Salmonella typhimurium* reversion assays, induces unscheduled DNA synthesis, gene mutations, micronucleus formation, and chromosomal aberrations, inhibits topoisomerase II, and gives positive results in comet assays. These data suggest that the neoplastic response observed with *Aloe vera* is a consequence of the conversion of the anthrone *C*-glycosides to aloe-emodin, which by itself or in combination with other *Aloe vera* components is responsible for the development of adenomas and carcinomas in the large intestine.

In the 2-year bioassays with *Aloe vera* whole leaf preparations, mice were exposed to nearly 10 times more test material (on a per kg bw basis) than rats. In spite of this higher exposure, the mice did not develop adenoma or carcinoma of the large intestine, which may be due to the fact that the intestinal bacteria in mice are less efficient than the intestinal bacteria of rats in converting aloin A and aloin B to aloe-emodin anthrone and subsequently aloe-emodin. In addition, mice have shorter gastrointestinal tracts and faster gastrointestinal transit times than rats, which could contribute to the lack of a tumour response in mice.

Although the carcinogenicity of *Aloe vera* appears to be dependent upon the presence of the anthraquinone fraction, in particular aloe-emodin, the mechanism by which this fraction causes intestinal tumours is presently unknown. The administration of *Aloe vera* whole leaf preparations to rats induced non-neoplastic lesions (i.e. goblet cell hyperplasia) that are not observed with other *Aloe vera* preparations (e.g. *Aloe vera* gel, decolorized gel, or decolorized whole leaf). These non-neoplastic changes may result in the formation of ROS that could promote neoplastic progression. Aloe-emodin has been shown to generate ROS after incubation with human cells in vitro, probably as a result of its anthraquinone structure. Aloe-emodin also contains a benzylic hydroxy moiety that has the potential to undergo esterification (e.g. sulfation) to a reactive electrophile that could bind to DNA. This pathway does not appear to have been investigated. The incubation of *Aloe vera* whole leaf preparations with human intestinal microflora results in an increased production of short-chain fatty acids. The impact of this increased production is presently not clear. Although the mechanism by which *Aloe vera* whole leaf preparations induce intestinal neoplasms in rats is not fully understood, it is clear that the molecular pathways observed in the intestinal neoplasms induced in rats by *Aloe vera* whole leaf preparations are also observed in human colorectal cancers.

5. Summary of Data Reported

5.1 Exposure data

Aloe vera, also known as *Aloe barbadensis*, is a perennial succulent plant with green fleshy leaves. The leaves contain two types of liquids: a yellow bitter latex under the skin, and a viscous gel in the inner section. Commercial products are made from processed leaves. Four major types of processed products were identified: whole leaf extract; decolorized whole leaf extract; inner-leaf gel; and dried bitter latex. Decolorization removes pigments and anthraquinones from the whole leaf extract. The dried latex has medicinal uses as a laxative. The other forms are used in foods, dietary supplements, beverages, and cosmetic products. Exposure data, where they exist, do not identify the nature of products containing *Aloe vera* used by consumers.

5.2 Human carcinogenicity data

No data were available to the Working Group.

5.3 Animal carcinogenicity data

Whole leaf extract of *Aloe vera* was tested for carcinogenicity after oral administration in one 2-year study in mice, and one 2-year study in rats.

In male and female rats, drinking-water containing whole leaf extract of *Aloe vera* caused significantly increased incidences of adenoma of the large intestine (colon and caecum) and carcinoma of the large intestine (colon and caecum), tumours rarely developed spontaneously in rats.

In the 2-year study in mice, there was no significantly increased incidence of any type of tumours in males or females given drinking-water containing whole leaf extract of *Aloe vera*.

In a study of photo-co-carcinogenesis with simulated sunlight, four articles were studied by skin application in hairless mice: three test articles containing *Aloe vera* that included gel, whole leaf extract, and decolorized whole leaf extract; and an aloe-emodin preparation. Almost all mice exposed to simulated sunlight developed skin neoplasms. No increase in the incidence of skin neoplasms was observed in the groups receiving any of the four test articles applied as a cream followed by simulated sunlight when compared with the group receiving control cream followed by simulated sunlight. There was a significant enhancing effect of *Aloe vera* gel cream or aloe-emodin cream on the photocarcinogenic activity of simulated sunlight in female mice based on an increase in the multiplicity of squamous cell papilloma, carcinoma or carcinoma in situ (combined). There was a significant enhancing effect of the whole leaf extract cream or decolorized whole leaf extract cream on the photocarcinogenic activity of simulated sunlight in both male and female mice, based on an increase in the multiplicity of squamous cell papilloma, carcinoma or carcinoma in situ (combined).

5.4 Mechanistic and other relevant data

The *C*-glycosides aloin A and aloin B, which are components of *Aloe vera* latex, are converted to aloe-emodin-9-anthrone by bacteria present in the gastrointestinal tract of rats and humans. Aloe-emodin-9-anthrone undergoes sequential oxidation to aloe-emodin and rhein. Preparations of *Aloe vera*, acemannan, and aloin A, do not display genotoxic activity in assays for mutagenesis in bacteria and/or other assays for genotoxicity. In contrast, aloe-emodin has genotoxic activity. These data suggest that the neoplastic response observed with *Aloe vera* is a consequence of the conversion of the anthrone *C*-glycosides to aloe-emodin, which by itself or in combination with other components of *Aloe vera* is responsible for the adenomas and carcinomas in the large intestine of rats.

6. Evaluation

6.1 Cancer in humans

There is inadequate evidence in humans for the carcinogenicity of *Aloe vera*.

6.2 Cancer in experimental animals

There is *sufficient evidence* in experimental animals for the carcinogenicity of whole leaf extract of *Aloe vera*.

6.3 Overall evaluation

Whole leaf extract of *Aloe vera* is *possibly carcinogenic to humans (Group 2B)*.

References

Ahlawat KS & Khatkar BS (2011). Processing, food applications and safety of aloe vera products: a review. *J Food Sci Technol*, 48(5):525–33. doi:10.1007/s13197-011-0229-z PMID:23572784

AHP; American Herbal Pharmacopoeia (2012). Aloe Vera Leaf, Aloe Vera Leaf Juice, Aloe Vera Inner Leaf Juice. Scotts Valley (CA): American Herbal Pharmacopoeia.

Akao T, Che Q-M, Kobashi K, Hattori M, Namba T (1996). A purgative action of barbaloin is induced by Eubacterium sp. strain BAR, a human intestinal anaerobe, capable of transforming barbaloin to aloe-emodin anthrone. *Biol Pharm Bull*, 19(1):136–8. doi:10.1248/bpb.19.136 PMID:8820926

Azaroual L, Liazid A, Barbero GF, Brigui J, Palma M, Barroso CG (2012). Improved chromatographic methods for determination of bioactive compounds from *Aloe vera* leaves. *ISRN Chromatography*, 2012:1–7. doi:10.5402/2012/609095

Boudreau MD & Beland FA (2006). An evaluation of the biological and toxicological properties of Aloe barbadensis (miller), Aloe vera. *J Environ Sci Health C Environ Carcinog Ecotoxicol Rev*, 24(1):103–54. doi:10.1080/10590500600614303 PMID:16690538

Boudreau MD, Beland FA, Nichols JA, Pogribna M (2013a). Toxicology and carcinogenesis studies of a noncolorized whole leaf extract of Aloe barbadensis Miller (Aloe vera) in F344/N rats and B6C3F1 mice (drinking water study). *Natl Toxicol Program Tech Rep Ser*, 577(577):1–266. PMID:24042237

Boudreau MD, Mellick PW, Olson GR, Felton RP, Thorn BT, Beland FA (2013b). Clear evidence of carcinogenic activity by a whole-leaf extract of Aloe barbadensis miller (aloe vera) in F344/N rats. *Toxicol Sci*, 131(1):26–39. doi:10.1093/toxsci/kfs275 PMID:22968693

Brandin H, Viitanen E, Myrberg O, Arvidsson A-K (2007). Effects of herbal medicinal products and food supplements on induction of CYP1A2, CYP3A4 and MDR1 in the human colon carcinoma cell line LS180. *Phytother Res*, 21(3):239–44. doi:10.1002/ptr.2057 PMID:17163579

Brown JP & Dietrich PS (1979). Mutagenicity of anthraquinone and benzanthrone derivatives in the Salmonella/microsome test: activation of anthraquinone glycosides by enzymic extracts of rat cecal bacteria. *Mutat Res*, 66(1):9–24. doi:10.1016/0165-1218(79)90003-X PMID:370585

Brown JP, Dietrich PS, Brown RJ (1977). Frameshift mutagenicity of certain naturally occurring phenolic compounds in the 'Salmonella/microsome' test: activation of anthraquinone and flavonol glycosides by gut bacterial enzymes [proceedings]. *Biochem Soc Trans*, 5(5):1489–92. PMID:336434

Brusick D & Mengs U (1997). Assessment of the genotoxic risk from laxative senna products. *Environ Mol Mutagen*, 29(1):1–9. doi:10.1002/(SICI)1098-2280(1997)29:1<1::AID-EM1>3.0.CO;2-J PMID:9020301

Channe Gowda D, Neelisiddaiah B, Anjaneyalu YV (1979). Structural studies of polysaccharides from *Aloe vera*. *Carbohydr Res*, 72:201–5. doi:10.1016/S0008-6215(00)83936-1

Che Q-M, Akao T, Hattori M, Kobashi K, Namba T (1991). Isolation of a human intestinal bacterium capable of transforming barbaloin to aloe-emodin anthrone. *Planta Med*, 57(1):15–9. doi:10.1055/s-2006-960007 PMID:2062951

Chen Y-Y, Chiang S-Y, Lin J-G, Yang JS, Ma YS, Liao CL et al. (2010). Emodin, aloe-emodin and rhein induced DNA damage and inhibited DNA repair gene expression in SCC-4 human tongue cancer cells. *Anticancer Res*, 30(3):945–51. PMID:20393018

Chiu T-H, Lai W-W, Hsia T-C, Yang JS, Lai TY, Wu PP et al. (2009). Aloe-emodin induces cell death through S-phase arrest and caspase-dependent pathways in human tongue squamous cancer SCC-4 cells. *Anticancer Res*, 29(11):4503–11. PMID:20032398

Committee of Experts on Cosmetic Products (2008). Aloe extracts with anthraquinones. Active ingredients used in cosmetics: safety survey. Strasbourg, France: Council of Europe Publishing; pp. 9–27.

Cosmetic Ingredient Review Expert Panel (2007). Final report on the safety assessment of AloeAndongensis Extract, Aloe Andongensis Leaf Juice,aloe Arborescens Leaf Extract, Aloe Arborescens Leaf Juice, Aloe Arborescens Leaf Protoplasts, Aloe Barbadensis Flower Extract, Aloe Barbadensis Leaf, Aloe Barbadensis Leaf Extract, Aloe Barbadensis Leaf Juice,aloe Barbadensis Leaf Polysaccharides, Aloe Barbadensis Leaf Water, Aloe Ferox Leaf Extract, Aloe Ferox Leaf Juice, and Aloe Ferox Leaf Juice Extract. *Int J Toxicol*, 26(1):Suppl 2: 1–50. doi:10.1080/10915810701351186 PMID:17613130

Dal'Belo SE, Gaspar LR, Maia Campos PM (2006). Moisturizing effect of cosmetic formulations containing Aloe vera extract in different concentrations assessed by skin bioengineering techniques. *Skin Res Technol*, 12(4):241–6. doi:10.1111/j.0909-752X.2006.00155.x PMID:17026654

Davis B & Goux WJ (2009). Single-laboratory validation of an NMR method for the determination of aloe vera polysaccharide in pharmaceutical formulations. *J AOAC Int*, 92(6):1607–16. PMID:20166576

De Witte P & Lemli J (1988). Excretion and distribution of [14C]rhein and [14C]rhein anthrone in rat. *J Pharm Pharmacol*, 40(9):652–5. doi:10.1111/j.2042-7158.1988.tb05330.x PMID:2907037

Dentali S (2013). "Nondecolorized" essential qualifier for NTP aloe vera study material. *Toxicol Sci*, 133(2):342 doi:10.1093/toxsci/kft072 PMID:23492813

Djuv A & Nilsen OG (2012). Aloe vera juice: IC$_{50}$ and dual mechanistic inhibition of CYP3A4 and CYP2D6. *Phytother Res*, 26(3):445–51. PMID:21842479

Dreessen M & Lemli J (1988). Studies in the field of drugs containing anthraquinone derivatives. XXXVI. The metabolism of cascarosides by intestinal bacteria. *Pharm Acta Helv*, 63(9-10):287–9. PMID:3237734

Duke JA & Beckstrom-Sternberg SM (1994). "Acceptable" Levels of Flavoring Ingredients? *Developmental Food Science*, 34:741–757.

Elsohly MA, Gul W, Avula B, Khan IA (2007). Determination of the anthraquinones aloe-emodin and aloin-A by liquid chromatography with mass spectrometric and diode array detection. *J AOAC Int*, 90(1):28–42. PMID:17373434

EMA (2006). Community herbal monograph on Aloe barbadensis MILLER and on Aloe (various species, mainly Aloe ferox MILLER and its hybrids). London, UK: European Medicines Agency.

Eur Ph; European Pharmacopoeia (2008). European pharmacopoeia. 7.0. Strasbourg, France: European Directorate for the Quality of Medicines & HealthCare.

FDA; Food and Drug Administration (2002). Status of certain additional over-the-counter drug category II and III active ingredients. *Fed Regist*, 67(90):31125–7. Availabe from: http://www.fda.gov/downloads/Drugs/DevelopmentApprovalProcess/DevelopmentResources/Over-the-CounterOTCDrugs/StatusofOTCRulemakings/ucm094018.pdf. PMID:12001972

Femenia A, Sanchez E, Simal S, Rosselló C (1999). Compositional features of polysacchardies from *Aloe vera* (Aloe barbadensis Miller) plant tissues. *Carbohydr Polym*, 39(2):109–17. doi:10.1016/S0144-8617(98)00163-5

Fogleman RW, Shellenberger TE, Balmer MF, Carpenter RH, McAnalley BH (1992). Subchronic oral administration of acemannan in the rat and dog. *Vet Hum Toxicol*, 34(2):144–7. PMID:1509675

Geisser J & Kratz E (2010). Determination of *Aloe vera* gel in cosmetics. *CBS Camag Bibliography Service*, 104:13–15.

GRIN; Germplasm Resources Information Network (2013). National Germplasm Resources Laboratory, Beltsville (Md): USDA. Available from: http://www.ars-grin.gov/cgi-bin/npgs/html/genform.pl, accessed 5 June 2013

Grindlay D & Reynolds T (1986). The Aloe vera phenomenon: a review of the properties and modern uses of the leaf parenchyma gel. *J Ethnopharmacol*, 16(2-3):117–51. doi:10.1016/0378-8741(86)90085-1 PMID:3528673

Groom QJ & Reynolds T (1987). Barbaloin in aloe species. *Planta Med*, 53(4):345–8. doi:10.1055/s-2006-962735 PMID:17269040

Hamman JH (2008). Composition and applications of Aloe vera leaf gel. *Molecules*, 13(8):1599–616. doi:10.3390/molecules13081599 PMID:18794775

Hattori M, Akao T, Kobashi K, Namba T (1993). Cleavages of the O- and C-glucosyl bonds of anthrone and 10,10′-bianthrone derivatives by human intestinal bacteria. *Pharmacology*, 47:Suppl 1: 125–33. doi:10.1159/000139851 PMID:8234419

Hattori M, Kanda T, Shu Y-Z, Akao T, Kobashi K, Namba T (1988). Metabolism of barbaloin by intestinal bacteria. *Chem Pharm Bull (Tokyo)*, 36(11):4462–6. doi:10.1248/cpb.36.4462 PMID:3246014

Heidemann A, Völkner W, Mengs U (1996). Genotoxicity of aloeemodin in vitro and in vivo. *Mutat Res*, 367(3):123–33. doi:10.1016/0165-1218(95)00084-4 PMID:8600368

Herlihy JT, Bertrand HA, Kim JD, Ikeno Y, Yu BP (1998). Effects of *Aloe vera* ingestion in the rat I. Growth, food and fluid intake and serum chemistry. *Phytother Res*, 12(3):183–8. doi:10.1002/(SICI)1099-1573(199805)12:3<183::AID-PTR219>3.0.CO;2-Q

Hirata T, Sakano S, Suga T (1981). Biotransformation of aloenin, a bitter glucoside constituent of Aloe arborescens, by rats. *Experientia*, 37(12):1252–3. doi:10.1007/BF01948341 PMID:7035211

Hsia T-C, Yang J-S, Chen G-W, Chiu TH, Lu HF, Yang MD et al. (2009). The roles of endoplasmic reticulum stress and Ca2+ on rhein-induced apoptosis in A-549 human lung cancer cells. *Anticancer Res*, 29(1):309–18. PMID:19331167

IASC (2009). IASC Labeling Guidance. Silver Spring (MD): International Aloe Science Council. Available from: http://www.iasc.org/pdfs/10_0405_IASC_Labeling_Guidance_Definitions.pdf.

IASC (2013a). The nomenclature of Aloe vera. Silver Spring (MD): International Aloe Science Council. Available from: http://www.iasc.org/Aloe_Taxonomy.pdf, accessed 3 June 2014.

IASC (2013b). Aloe vera quality standard. Silver Spring (MD), USA: International Aloe Science Council. Available from: http://iasc.org/pdfs/AloeVeraQualityStandard.pdf, accessed 3 June 2014.

Ikeno Y, Hubbard GB, Lee S, Yu BP, Herlihy JT (2002). The influence of long-term Aloe vera ingestion on age-related disease in male Fischer 344 rats. *Phytother Res*, 16(8):712–8. doi:10.1002/ptr.1022 PMID:12458471

IMS Health (2012). Multinational Integrated Data Analysis (MIDAS). Worldwide Sales of Selected Products. Plymouth Meeting, Pennsylvania: IMS Health

Ishii Y, Tanizawa H, Takino Y (1987). Determination of barbaloin in rat serum. *Chem Pharm Bull (Tokyo)*, 35(11):4642–4. doi:10.1248/cpb.35.4642 PMID:3442898

Jiao P, Jia Q, Randel G, Diehl B, Weaver S, Milligan G (2010). Quantitative 1H-NMR spectrometry method for quality control of Aloe vera products. *J AOAC Int*, 93(3):842–8. PMID:20629385

Joseph B & Raj SJ (2010). Pharmacognostic and phytochemical properties of *Aloe vera* Linn–an overview. *International Journal of Pharmaceutical Sciences Review and Research*, 4:106–110.

JP XVI, The Japanese Pharmacopoeia (2011). The Japanese Pharmacopoeia. 16th ed. English Version, Tokyo, Japan: Ministry of Health, Labour and Welfare.

Kim KH, Park JH (2006). Quality control and standardization of Aloe products. In: Park YI, Lee SK, editors. New Perspectives on Aloe. New York (NY), USA: Springer Science and Business Media; pp. 169–189

Kratz E (2009). *Aloe vera*. Evidence of active content. *Cossma*, 10:12–13.

Kuzuya H, Shimpo K, Beppu H (2004). Aloe lectins and their activities. In: Reynolds T, editor. Aloes: The genus Aloe. 38th ed. Boca Raton (FL), USA: CRC Press; pp. 88–110

Lachenmeier K, Kuepper U, Musshoff F *et al.* (2005). Quality control of *Aloe vera* beverages. *Electronic Journal of Environmental, Agricultural and Food Chemistry*, 4:1033–1042.

Lai W-W, Yang J-S, Lai K-C, Kuo CL, Hsu CK, Wang CK *et al.* (2009). Rhein induced apoptosis through the endoplasmic reticulum stress, caspase- and mitochondria-dependent pathways in SCC-4 human tongue squamous cancer cells. *In Vivo*, 23(2):309–16. PMID:19414420

Lang W (1993). Pharmacokinetic-metabolic studies with 14C-aloe emodin after oral administration to male and female rats. *Pharmacology*, 47:Suppl 1: 110–9. doi:10.1159/000139849 PMID:8234417

Lee S, Do SG, Kim SY, Kim J, Jin Y, Lee CH (2012). Mass spectrometry-based metabolite profiling and antioxidant activity of Aloe vera (Aloe barbadensis Miller) in different growth stages. *J Agric Food Chem*, 60(45):11222–8. doi:10.1021/jf3026309 PMID:23050594

Leon L (2003). The medicinal plant Aloe. *Ganzheitliche Tiermedizin*, 17:138–143.

Lin M-L, Chen S-S, Lu Y-C, Liang RY, Ho YT, Yang CY *et al.* (2007). Rhein induces apoptosis through induction of endoplasmic reticulum stress and Ca2+-dependent mitochondrial death pathway in human nasopharyngeal carcinoma cells. *Anticancer Res*, 27:5A: 3313–22. PMID:17970076

Lin M-L, Lu Y-C, Chung J-G, Li YC, Wang SG, N G SH *et al.* (2010). Aloe-emodin induces apoptosis of human nasopharyngeal carcinoma cells via caspase-8-mediated activation of the mitochondrial death pathway. *Cancer Lett*, 291(1):46–58. doi:10.1016/j.canlet.2009.09.016 PMID:19942342

Mandal G & Das A (1980). Structure of the D-galactan isolated from Aloe barbadensis Miller. *Carbohydr Res*, 86(2):247–57. doi:10.1016/S0008-6215(00)85902-9

Mandrioli R, Mercolini L, Ferranti A, Fanali S, Raggi MA (2011). Determination of aloe emodin in *Aloe vera* extracts and commercial formulations by HPLC with tandem UV absorption and fluorescence detection. *Food Chem*, 126(1):387–93. doi:10.1016/j.foodchem.2010.10.112

Matsuda Y, Yokohira M, Suzuki S, Hosokawa K, Yamakawa K, Zeng Y *et al.* (2008). One-year chronic toxicity study of Aloe arborescens Miller var. natalensis Berger in Wistar Hannover rats. A pilot study. *Food Chem Toxicol*, 46(2):733–9. doi:10.1016/j.fct.2007.09.107 PMID:17981383

Morgan M, Bone K, Mills S et al. (2005). Aloe. Safety monograph. In: Mills S, Bone K, editors. The essential guide to herbal safety. St. Louis (MO), USA: Elsevier Churchill Livingstone; pp. 233–240

Morimoto I, Watanabe F, Osawa T, Okitsu T, Kada T (1982). Mutagenicity screening of crude drugs with Bacillus subtilis rec-assay and Salmonella/microsome reversion assay. *Mutat Res*, 97(2):81–102. doi:10.1016/0165-1161(82)90007-3 PMID:6804865

Müller SO & Stopper H (1999). Characterization of the genotoxicity of anthraquinones in mammalian cells. *Biochim Biophys Acta*, 1428(2-3):406–14. doi:10.1016/S0304-4165(99)00064-1 PMID:10434060

Müller SO, Eckert I, Lutz WK, Stopper H (1996). Genotoxicity of the laxative drug components emodin, aloe-emodin and danthron in mammalian cells: topoisomerase II mediated? *Mutat Res*, 371(3-4):165–73. doi:10.1016/S0165-1218(96)90105-6 PMID:9008718

NCCAM (2012). Aloe vera. Bethesda (MD): National Center for Complementary and Alternative Medicine. Available from: http://nccam.nih.gov/health/aloevera, accessed 5 June 2014.

Nesslany F, Simar-Meintières S, Ficheux H, Marzin D (2009). Aloe-emodin-induced DNA fragmentation in the mouse in vivo comet assay. *Mutat Res*, 678(1):13–9. doi:10.1016/j.mrgentox.2009.06.004 PMID:19559101

Newton LE (2004). Aloes in habitat. In: Reynolds T, editor. Aloes: the genus Aloe. Boca Raton (FL), USA: CRC Press; pp. 3–14

Ngo MQ, Nguyen NN, Shah SA (2010). Oral aloe vera for treatment of diabetes mellitus and dyslipidemia. *Am J Health Syst Pharm*, 67(21):1804–11, 1806, 1808 passim. doi:10.2146/ajhp100182 PMID:20966143

NHANES (2010). National Health and Nutrition Examination Survey (1999–2010). Atlanta (GA):

Centers for Disease Control and Prevention. Available from: http://www.cdc.gov/nchs/nhanes.htm; accessed 5 June 2014.

Ni Y, Turner D, Yates KM, Tizard I (2004). Isolation and characterization of structural components of Aloe vera L. leaf pulp. *Int Immunopharmacol*, 4(14):1745–55. doi:10.1016/j.intimp.2004.07.006 PMID:15531291

NLM (2012). Products that contain active ingredient - Aloe vera. Dietary supplements labels database. United States National Library of Medicine. Available from: http://www.dsld.nlm.nih.gov/dsld/; accessed 5 June 2014.

NTP; National Toxicology Program (2010). Photocarcinogenesis study of aloe vera [CAS NO. 481–72–1(Aloe-emodin)] in SKH-1 mice (simulated solar light and topical application study). *Natl Toxicol Program Tech Rep Ser*, 553(553):7–33, 35–97, 99–103 passim. PMID:21031007

Nutrition Business Journal (2010). NBJ's Supplement Business Report. An analysis of markets, trends, competition and strategy in the U.S. dietary supplement industry. New York (NY), USA: Penton Media, Inc.

Nutrition Business Journal (2012). NBJ's Supplement Business Report. An analysis of markets, trends, competition and strategy in the U.S. dietary supplement industry. . New York (NY), USA: Penton Media, Inc. Available from: http://newhope360.com/2012-supplement-business-report; accessed 5 June 2014.

O'Neil MJ, Heckelman PE, Koch CB et al. (2006). The Merck Index - An Encyclopedia of Chemicals, Drugs, and Biologicals. 14th Ed. Version 14.6. Whitehouse Station (NJ), USA: Merck & Co., Inc.

Okamura N, Asai M, Hine N, Yagi A (1996). High-performance liquid chromatographic determination of phenolic compounds in *Aloe* species. *J Chromatogr A*, 746(2):225–31. doi:10.1016/0021-9673(96)00342-1

Paes-Leme AA, Motta ES, De Mattos JCP, Dantas FJ, Bezerra RJ, Caldeira-de-Araujo A (2005). Assessment of Aloe vera (L.) genotoxic potential on Escherichia coli and plasmid DNA. *J Ethnopharmacol*, 102(2):197–201. doi:10.1016/j.jep.2005.06.013 PMID:16054315

Paez A, Michael Gebre G, Gonzalez ME, Tschaplinski TJ (2000). Growth, soluble carbohydrates, and aloin concentration of Aloe vera plants exposed to three irradiance levels. *Environ Exp Bot*, 44(2):133–9. doi:10.1016/S0098-8472(00)00062-9 PMID:10996366

Pandiri AR, Sills RC, Hoenerhoff MJ, Peddada SD, Ton TV, Hong HH et al. (2011). Aloe vera non-decolorized whole leaf extract-induced large intestinal tumors in F344 rats share similar molecular pathways with human sporadic colorectal tumors. *Toxicol Pathol*, 39(7):1065–74. doi:10.1177/0192623311422081 PMID:21937742

Park MK, Park JH, Kim NY, Shin YG, Choi YS, Lee JG et al. (1998). Analysis of 13 phenolic compounds in *Aloe* species by high performance liquid chromatography. *Phytochem Anal*, 9(4):186–91. doi:10.1002/(SICI)1099-1565(199807/08)9:4<186::AID-PCA406>3.0.CO;2-#

Park YI, Jo TH (2006). Perspectives of industrial application of *Aloe vera*. In: Park YI, Lee SK, editors. New Perspectives on Aloe. New York (NY), USA: Springer Science+Business Media; pp. 191–200

Pelley RP, Martini WJ, Liu DQ et al. (1998). Multiparameter analysis of commercial "*Aloe vera*" materials and comparison to Aloe barbadensis Miller extracts. *Subtropical Plant Science*, 50:1–14.

Pellizzoni M, Molinari GP, Lucini L (2011). Stability of the main Aloe fractions and Aloe-based commercial products under different storage conditions *Agrochimica*, 5:288–296.

Perkins SL & Livesey JF (1993). A rapid high-performance thin-layer chromatographic urine screen for laxative abuse. *Clin Biochem*, 26(3):179–81. doi:10.1016/0009-9120(93)90023-Y PMID:8330386

Pogribna M, Freeman JP, Paine D, Boudreau MD (2008). Effect of Aloe vera whole leaf extract on short chain fatty acids production by Bacteroides fragilis, Bifidobacterium infantis and Eubacterium limosum. *Lett Appl Microbiol*, 46(5):575–80. doi:10.1111/j.1472-765X.2008.02346.x PMID:18363656

Ramachandra CT & Rao PS (2008). Processing of *Aloe vera* leaf gel: a review. *Am J Agric Biol Sci*, 3(2):502–10. doi:10.3844/ajabssp.2008.502.510

Ramírez Durón R, Ceniceros Almaguer L, Cavazos Rocha NC, Silva Flores PG, De Torres NW (2008). Comparison of high-performance liquid chromatographic and thin-layer chromatographic methods for determination of aloin in herbal products containing Aloe vera. *J AOAC Int*, 91(6):1265–70. PMID:19202785

Reynolds T (2004). Aloe chemistry. In: Reynolds T, editor. Aloes: The genus Aloe. 38th Ed. Boca Raton (FL), USA: CRC Press; pp. 39–74

Rodríguez ER, Martín JD, Romero CD (2010). Aloe vera as a functional ingredient in foods. *Crit Rev Food Sci Nutr*, 50(4):305–26. doi:10.1080/10408390802544454 PMID:20301017

Saccù D, Bogoni P, Procida G (2001). Aloe exudate: characterization by reversed phase HPLC and headspace GC-MS. *J Agric Food Chem*, 49(10):4526–30. doi:10.1021/jf010179c PMID:11599983

SciFinder (2013). CAS Registry Number 8001–97–6. Columbus (OH). USA: Chemical Abstracts Service, American Chemical Society. Accessed: 15 January 2013

Sehgal I, Winters WD, Scott M, David A, Gillis G, Stoufflet T et al. (2013b). Toxicologic assessment of a commercial decolorized whole leaf aloe vera juice, lily of the desert filtered whole leaf juice with aloesorb. *J Toxicol*, Epub802453 doi:10.1155/2013/802453 PMID:23554812

Sehgal I, Winters WD, Scott M, Kousoulas K (2013). An in vitro and in vivo toxicologic evaluation of a stabilized aloe vera gel supplement drink in mice. *Food*

Chem Toxicol, 55:363–70. doi:10.1016/j.fct.2013.01.012 PMID:23376510

Sehgal I, Winters WD, Scott M, Kousoulas K (2013a). An in vitro and in vivo toxicologic evaluation of a stabilized aloe vera gel supplement drink in mice. *Food Chem Toxicol*, 55:363–70. doi:10.1016/j.fct.2013.01.012 PMID:23376510

Shah AH, Qureshi S, Tariq M, Ageel M (1989). Toxicity studies on six plants used in the traditional Arab system of medicine. *Phytother Res*, 3(1):25–9. doi:10.1002/ptr.2650030107

Shao A, Broadmeadow A, Goddard G, Bejar E, Frankos V (2013). Safety of purified decolorized (low anthraquinone) whole leaf Aloe vera (L) Burm. f. juice in a 3-month drinking water toxicity study in F344 rats. *Food Chem Toxicol*, 57:21–31. doi:10.1016/j.fct.2013.03.002 PMID:23500775

Spohn R (2013). Water colour of Aloe vera. Available from: http://www.spohns.de/heilpflanzenillus/aloevera.html; accessed 28 May 2014.

Steenkamp V & Stewart MJ (2007). Medicinal applications and toxicological activities of *Aloe* products. *Pharmaceutical Biology*, 45(5):411–20. doi:10.1080/13880200701215307

Stolk LM & Hoogtanders K (1999). Detection of laxative abuse by urine analysis with HPLC and diode array detection. *Pharm World Sci*, 21(1):40–3. doi:10.1023/A:1008647424809 PMID:10214668

Tang JC, Yang H, Song XY, Song XH, Yan SL, Shao JQ *et al.* (2009). Inhibition of cytochrome P450 enzymes by rhein in rat liver microsomes. *Phytother Res*, 23(2):159–64. doi:10.1002/ptr.2572 PMID:18814214

Turner CE, Williamson DA, Stroud PA, Talley DJ (2004). Evaluation and comparison of commercially available Aloe vera L. products using size exclusion chromatography with refractive index and multi-angle laser light scattering detection. *Int Immunopharmacol*, 4(14):1727–37. doi:10.1016/j.intimp.2004.07.004 PMID:15531289

Ulbricht C, Armstrong J, Basch E, Basch S, Bent S, Dacey C *et al.* (2007). An evidence-based systematic review of Aloe vera by the natural standard research collaboration. *J Herb Pharmacother*, 7(3-4):279–323. doi:10.1080/15228940802153339 PMID:18928148

Vogler BK & Ernst E (1999). Aloe vera: a systematic review of its clinical effectiveness. *Br J Gen Pract*, 49(447):823–8. PMID:10885091

Vyth A & Kamp PE (1979). Detection of anthraquinone laxatives in the urine. *Pharm Weekbl*, 1(1):456–9. doi:10.1007/BF02293250

Waller TA, Pelley RP, Strickland FM (2004). Industrial processing and quality control of Aloe barbadensis (Aloe vera) gel. In: Reynolds T, editor. Aloes: The genus Aloe. 38th Ed. Boca Raton (FL), USA: CRC Press; pp. 139–205

Westendorf J, Marquardt H, Poginsky B, Dominiak M, Schmidt J, Marquardt H (1990). Genotoxicity of naturally occurring hydroxyanthraquinones. *Mutat Res*, 240(1):1–12. doi:10.1016/0165-1218(90)90002-J PMID:2294411

WHO (1999). Aloe and Aloe vera gel. WHO Monographs on selected medicinal plants. Vol. 1. Geneva, Switzerland: World Health Organization; pp. 33–49 (available from http://apps.who.int/medicinedocs/en/d/Js2200e/5.html)

Williams LD, Burdock GA, Shin E, Kim S, Jo TH, Jones KN *et al.* (2010). Safety studies conducted on a proprietary high-purity aloe vera inner leaf fillet preparation, Qmatrix. *Regul Toxicol Pharmacol*, 57(1):90–8. doi:10.1016/j.yrtph.2010.01.002 PMID:20096744

Wölfle D, Schmutte C, Westendorf J, Marquardt H (1990). Hydroxyanthraquinones as tumor promoters: enhancement of malignant transformation of C3H mouse fibroblasts and growth stimulation of primary rat hepatocytes. *Cancer Res*, 50(20):6540–4. PMID:2208114

Yagi A, Nakamori J, Yamada T, Iwase H, Tanaka T, Kaneo Y *et al.* (1999). In vivo metabolism of aloemannan. *Planta Med*, 65(5):417–20. doi:10.1055/s-1999-14018 PMID:10418327

Yaron A (1993). Characterization of *Aloe vera* gel before and after autodegradation, and stabilization of the natural fresh gel. *Phytother Res*, 7(7):11 doi:10.1002/ptr.2650070706

Yokohira M, Matsuda Y, Suzuki S, Hosokawa K, Yamakawa K, Hashimoto N *et al.* (2009). Equivocal colonic carcinogenicity of Aloe arborescens Miller var. natalensis berger at high-dose level in a Wistar Hannover rat 2-y study. *J Food Sci*, 74(2):T24–30. doi:10.1111/j.1750-3841.2009.01070.x PMID:19323775

Zaffaroni M, Mucignat C, Pecere T, Zagotto G, Frapolli R, D'Incalci M *et al.* (2003). High-performance liquid chromatographic assay for the determination of Aloe Emodin in mouse plasma. *J Chromatogr B Analyt Technol Biomed Life Sci*, 796(1):113–9. doi:10.1016/j.jchromb.2003.08.012 PMID:14552822

1. Exposure Data

Goldenseal (*Hydrastis canadensis* L.) was traditionally used by native Americans as a medicinal remedy and as a colouring agent (Sinclair & Catling, 2000; McKenna & Plotnikoff, 2010). In his *Collections for an Essay Towards a Materia Medica of the United States,* the American botanist Benjamin Smith Barton first mentioned the medicinal use of *H. canadensis* by the Cherokee (Hobbs, 1990). Today, the main application of *H. canadensis* is for the prevention and treatment of skin disorders, dyspepsia, gastritis, peptic ulcer, colitis, anorexia, menorrhagia, dysmenorrhoea, sinusitis, mucosal inflammation, and other inflammatory conditions or infectious diseases (BHMA, 1983; BHMA, 1992; NTP, 2010; Sun *et al.*, 2009; McKenna & Plotnikoff, 2010).

1.1 Identification of the agent and its major constituents

1.1.1 Botanical data

(a) Nomenclature

Chem. Abstr. Serv. Reg. No.: 84603-60-1

Chem. Abstr. Name: Golden seal root

Botanical name: *Hydrastis canadensis* L. (Fig. 1.1)

Family: *Ranunculaceae*

Genus: *Hydrastis*

Plant part: Root

Common names: Hydrastis; Golden seal; Yellow Indian plant; Yellow seal

(b) Description

Goldenseal is a perennial plant, which grows naturally in eastern USA and Canada (AHP, 2001; Zieger & Tice, 1997). Goldenseal has one long-trunked basal leaves, a single stem, and two smaller leaves attached to the flowering stem. Usually, the plant has two rounded, lobed, and double-toothed leaves on a forked branch, with one being larger than the other. The plant has a knotted yellow rhizome and a solitary terminal flower with three white sepals and many greenish-white stamens in clusters, while the fruit is small and red raspberry-like (Zieger & Tice, 1997; AHP, 2001). The plant grows up to about 1 foot in height [30.5 cm] (Palmer, 1975; Duke, 2002).

1.1.2 Chemical constituents and their properties

The major constituents of goldenseal root are isoquinoline alkaloids such as hydrastine (1.5–4%), berberine (2.5%), canadine (0.5%), and other alkaloids (see Fig. 1.2; BHMA, 1992). Berberine is usually found in the roots of goldenseal as a sulfate with a yield of 5000–60 000 ppm (HSDB, 1997). Hydrastine is also found in goldenseal in concentrations of 15 000–40 000 ppm (NTP, 2010). Junio *et al.* (2011) have also identified sideroxylin, 8-desmethyl-sideroxylin, and

Fig. 1.1 Goldenseal (*Hydrastis canadensis* L.), showing leaves, root, flower and seed

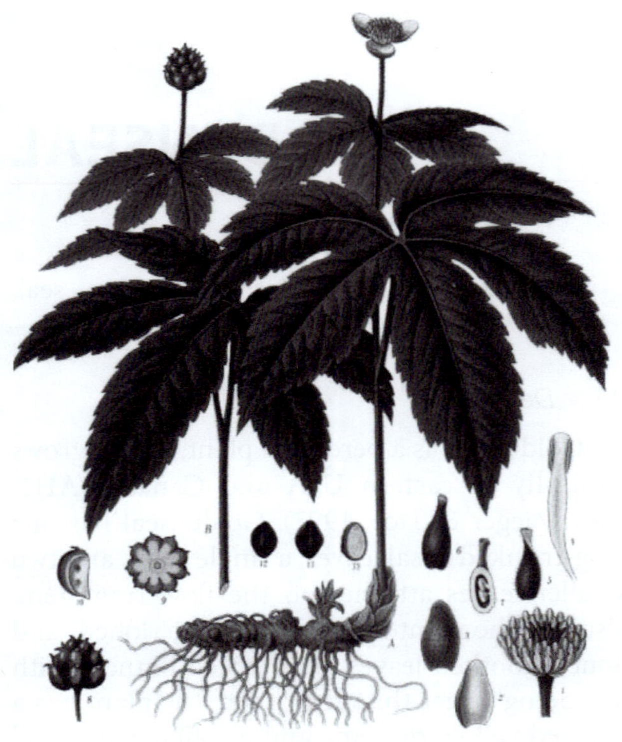

From Koehler's Medicinal-Plants (1887)

6-desmethyl-sideroxylin. Chemical Abstract Registry (CAS) number, International Union of Pure and Applied Chemistry (IUPAC) names and some physical properties of goldenseal major alkaloids are presented below (American Chemical Society, 2014; Zieger & Tice, 1997).

(a) Berberine

Chem. Abstr. Serv. Reg. No.: 2086-83-1

IUPAC name: 7,8,13,13α-Tetradehydro-9,10-dimethoxy-2,3-(methylenedioxy)berbinium

Description: Yellow solid with a melting point of 145 °C and slowly soluble in water (O'Neil, 2013).

(b) Hydrastine

Chem. Abstr. Serv. Reg. No.: 60594-55-0

IUPAC name: 1(3*H*)-Isobenzofuranone, 6,7-dimethoxy-3-(5,6,7,8-tetrahydro-6-methyl-1,3-dioxolo[4,5-*g*]isoquinolin-5-yl)-

Description: Solid with a melting point of 132 °C and highly soluble in acetone and benzene; insoluble in water (O'Neil, 2013).

(c) Canadine

Chem. Abstr. Serv. Reg. No.: 522-97-4

IUPAC name: 6*H*-benzo[*g*]-1,3-benzodioxolo[5,6-α]quinolizine, 5,8,13,13α-tetrahydro-9,10-dimethoxy-(13αS)

Description: Yellow pale solid with a melting point of 172 °C and soluble in methanol (O'Neil, 2013).

(d) Others

Other goldenseal components of the flavonoid class include:

- sideroxylin (CAS No., 3122-87-0; IUPAC name, 4',5-dihydroxy-7-methoxy-6,8-dimethylflavone)
- 8-desmethyl-sideroxylin (CAS No., 80621-54-1; IUPAC name, 4*H*-1-benzopyran-4-one, 5-hydroxy-2-(4-hydroxyphenyl)-7-methoxy-6-methyl-)
- 6-desmethyl-sideroxylin (CAS No., 1194721-03-3; IUPAC name, 4*H*-1-benzopyran-4-one, 5-hydroxy-2-(4-hydroxyphenyl)-7-methoxy-8-methyl-).

For structural and molecular formulae and relative molecular mass, see Huang & Johnston (1990), Junio *et al.* (2011), Li *et al.* (2011), and Fig. 1.2.

1.1.3 Technical and commercial products

Official technical products are goldenseal root, powdered goldenseal root, and powdered goldenseal root extract (NTP, 2010; USP, 2013). Other minor technical products may include powdered goldenseal leaf and its derived extracts, as well as fluid extracts (Mikkelsen & Ash, 1988; Oldfield, 2005; NTP, 2010).

Powdered goldenseal root and leaf products are available as capsules and teas in combination with other herbs, in some over-the-counter (OTC) herbal supplements (Mikkelsen & Ash, 1988; Zieger & Tice, 1997; AHP, 2001). Goldenseal is also found in eardrops, feminine cleansing products, cold/flu remedies, allergy relief products, laxative products, and aids to digestion (Zieger & Tice, 1997; AHP, 2001). Chemical derivatives of purified major components of goldenseal, such as berberine hydrochloride and berberine bisulfate, are found in some commercial eyewash formulations (Zeiger & Tice, 1997). Hydrastine, another derivative, is commercially available in the form of (–)-hydrastine and used as an ingredient in some decongestant nose sprays and feminine hygiene products (Zeiger & Tice, 1997; Huang & Johnston, 1990).

As a consequence of the high cost of genuine goldenseal, some commercial products contain little or no goldenseal plant material (Govindan & Govindan, 2000). *Coptis chinensis* has been sold in place of "Chinese goldenseal" and has been found as an adulterant of goldenseal (Brown & Roman, 2008). Moreover, other species that contain berberine, such as *Coptis japonica*, *Berberis aquifolium*, *Berberis* spp., *Rumex* spp., and *Xanthorhiza simplicissima,* have been used to adulterate goldenseal (Brown & Roman, 2008; Pengelly, 2012).

1.2 Analysis

Botanical identity and composition are confirmed by macroscopic and microscopic examinations of rhizome and root, as well as by thin-layer chromatography (TLC) (USP, 2013). TLC identification tests for the major goldenseal alkaloids are reported in the United States Pharmacopeia: a dry extract from roots and rhizomes contains at least 2% hydrastine and 2.5% berberine calculated on a dried basis; a standardized developing solvent system includes ethyl acetate, butyl alcohol, formic acid, and water (5:3:1:1); chromatogram analysis with ultraviolet (UV) light at 365 nm demonstrates a lemon-yellow fluorescence for berberine and a blue-white fluorescence for hydrastine (USP, 2013). Content of the most active alkaloids is determined by high-performance liquid chromatography (HPLC) using a mobile phase composed of 0.1 M monobasic potassium phosphate and acetonitrile (60:40) (USP, 2013). An official HPLC/UV method for hydrastine and berberine in goldenseal has been published (Brown & Roman, 2008), but other HPLC methods have also been developed (Abourashed & Khan, 2001).

Additional analyses report on the use of goldenseal and illicit drugs. Goldenseal may prevent the detection of illicit drugs (such as tetrahydrocanabinol and barbiturates) in urine by inducing their rapid elimination (Mikkelsen & Ash, 1988; Hamon, 1990; Schwarzhoff & Cody, 1993).

1.3 Use

1.3.1 Indications and applications

(a) Medicinal use

Native Americans used goldenseal to treat common conditions such as wounds, ulcers, digestive disorders, cancer, and skin and eye ailments (Hamon, 1990; Hobbs, 1990). Over the years, goldenseal has been used to treat a variety of digestive and haemorrhagic disorders. When

Fig. 1.2 Selected alkaloids and flavonoids from goldenseal

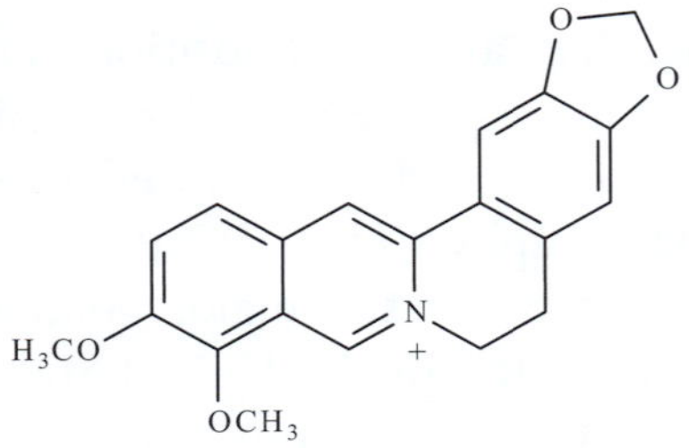

RMM, relative molecular mass
Compiled by the Working Group

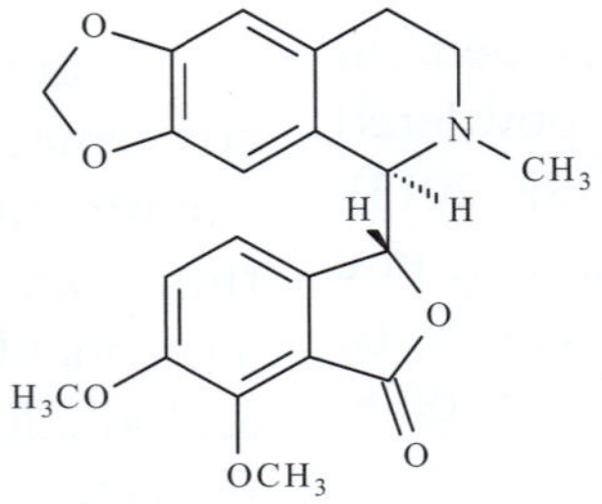

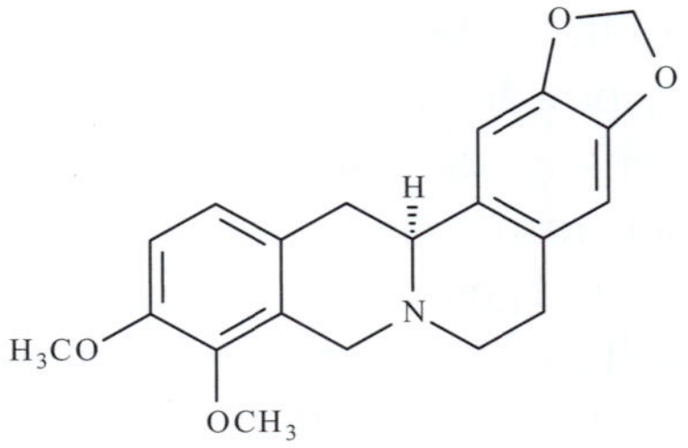

applied topically, it is thought to possess slight antiseptic, astringent, and haemostatic qualities (NTP, 2010).

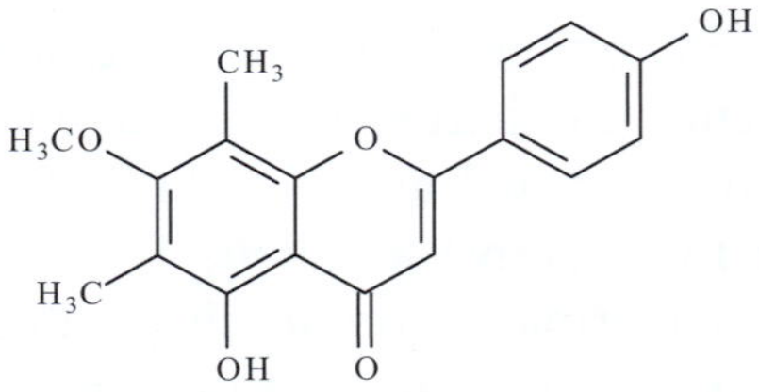

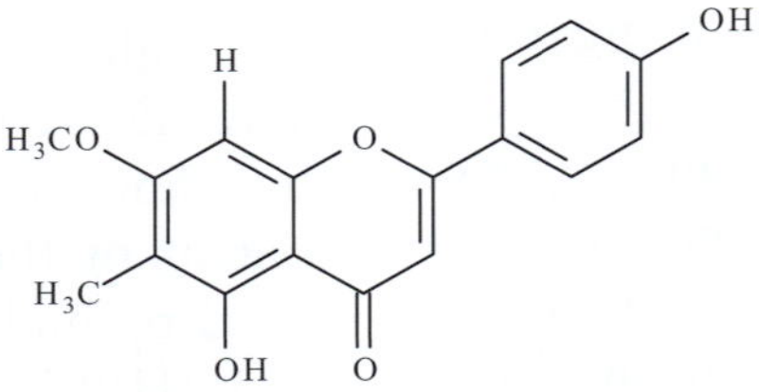

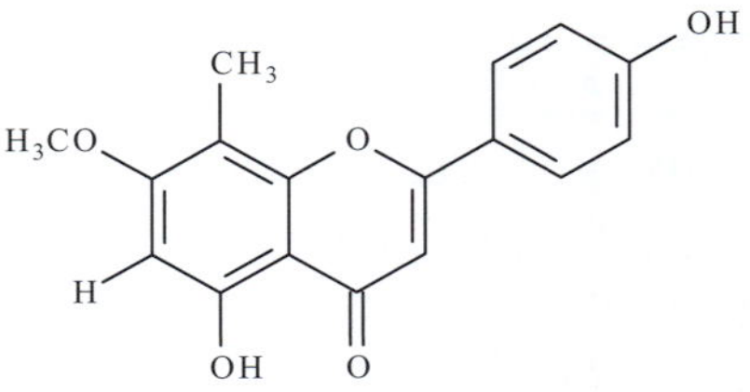

Some OTC dietary supplements containing goldenseal are used as to treat menstrual disorders, minor sciatica, rheumatic and muscular pain (Hamon, 1990), allergy symptoms, cold and flu symptoms, motion sickness and nausea, earaches and ear infections, and chronic diarrhoea from protozoal, fungal, and bacterial infections (Zieger & Tice, 1997; AHP, 2001; Hwang *et al.*, 2003). Goldenseal has also been used in combination with dietary vitamins and minerals in an attempt to treat symptoms of AIDS (Zieger & Tice, 1997). It is also claimed to have the ability to cleanse the body from mucus, toxins, and waste (Zieger & Tice, 1997).

Berberine, a major goldenseal alkaloid, has been used as a bitter tonic, diaphoretic, and antipyretic (Kulkarni *et al.*, 1972), for the treatment of skin diseases, liver diseases, eye infections, diarrhoea, cholera, giardiasis, amoebiasis, and dermal leishmaniasis (Choudhry *et al.*, 1972; Kulkarni *et al.*, 1972; Martin *et al.*, 1978; Sabir *et al.*, 1978; Khin-Maung-U *et al.*, 1985; Vennerstrom *et al.*, 1990; Chi *et al.*, 1994; Müller *et al.*, 1995). Berberine appears to control psoriasis through its ability to inhibit hyperproliferation (Müller *et al.*, 1995). The evidence on the efficacy of berberine in treating peptic ulcers and hyperacidity, and malaria, is conflicting (Sabir *et al.*, 1978; Vennerstrom & Klayman, 1988).

Some other pharmacological properties that have been identified for berberine include antiplatelet, anticerebral ischaemia, vasodilation, and anti-arrythmia (Peng *et al.*, 1997). Berberine is thought to increase ileal contractility and acetylcholine retention by cholinesterase activity and is believed to be the active ingredient of *Coptis* rhizome, used to treat amnesia (Peng *et al.*, 1997).

A clinical trial using berberine suggested that it is effective in improving cardiac performance in patients with heart failure (Marin-Neto *et al.*, 1988). Berberine appears to exercise a direct depressive effect on myocardial, vascular, and smooth musculature (Sabir & Bhide, 1971; Creasey, 1977, 1979). Berberine may also have anticholinesterolase activity (Sabir & Bhide, 1971). It is also suggested that berberine exerts anticancer activities both in vitro and in vivo through different mechanisms (Sun *et al.*, 2009).

Hydrastine, another major goldenseal alkaloid, is claimed to be an abortifacient, antibiotic, antiuterotic, antivaginitic, bactericide, central nervous system depressant, choleretic, convulsant, haemostat, hypertensive, hypotensive, pesticide, sedative, uterotonic, and vasoconstrictor (NTP, 2010).

(b) Medical research

In medical research, berberine is used as a fluorescent stain for cells, chromosomes, and energized mitochondria (Borodina *et al.*, 1979; Ridler & Jennings, 1983; Mikeš & Dadák, 1983; Mikeš & Yaguzhinskij, 1985; Kim *et al.*, 1990).

1.3.2 Dosage

As a dietary supplement, goldenseal can be given at a wide range of doses: decoction of dried roots, 0.5–10 g three times per day; alcoholic tincture, 2–4 mL three times per day; and fluid extract, 0.3–10 mL three times per day (Newall *et al.*, 1996; Zieger & Tice, 1997; AHP, 2001; McKenna & Plotnikoff, 2010). OTC preparations of goldenseal are available in doses of 100 mg up to 470 mg (Zieger & Tice, 1997; AHP, 2001).

1.4 Production, sales, and consumption

1.4.1 Production

No data on production processes or volumes were available to the Working Group.

1.4.2 Sales

According to data from 2012 IMS Health MIDAS, worldwide sales of goldenseal root (*Hydrastis canadensis*) as a dietary supplement in pharmaceutical outlets totalled US$ 25 million. Appreciable sales occurred in Germany (US$ 8 million), France (US$ 5 million), and the United States (US$ 5 million) (IMS Health, 2012). Other countries known to sell products containing goldenseal include Canada.

According to the 2012 Nutrition Business Journal Report, goldenseal was the 37th best-selling herb in the USA in 2011. Following a decline from US$ 40 million in 2003, sales have remained constant (NBJ, 2012a, b). According to data from the United States National Health and Nutrition Examination Survey, there has been a decline in the prevalence of goldenseal use as follows: 1999–2002 (0.6%), 2003–2006 (0.3%), and 2007–2010 (0.2%), with similar data for males and females. These data showed a large coefficient of variation and caution should be used in interpretation (CDC, 2013).

1.4.3 Consumption

Goldenseal is consumed orally as a tea and in capsules, applied dermally as a skin lotion, applied to the eye as eyewash, to the ear as eardrops, and applied as a vaginal douche (Zieger & Tice, 1997; Hamon, 1990; AHP, 2001; NTP, 2010). Exposure to hydrastine also occurs when used in decongestant nose sprays and feminine hygiene products (Zeiger & Tice, 1997).

1.5 Occupational exposure

No data were available to the Working Group. Workers on goldenseal plantations and in goldenseal processing plants are probably exposed.

1.6 Regulations and guidelines

According to the 1994 Dietary Supplement Health and Education Act (DSHEA) in the USA, goldenseal is considered a dietary supplement under the general umbrella of "foods" (FDA, 1994). In the USA, dietary supplements put on the market before 15 October 1994 do not require proof of safety; however, the labelling recommendations for dietary supplements include warnings, dosage recommendations, and substantiated "structure or function" claims. The product label must declare prominently that the claims have not been evaluated by the Food and Drug Administration, and bear the statement "This product is not intended to diagnose, treat, cure, or prevent any disease" (Croom & Walker, 1995).

The Natural Medicines Comprehensive Database ranks goldenseal as a "possibly safe" dietary supplement when used at a single dose, and at recommended oral dosages for short-term administration (NCCAM, 2012; NMCD, 2013).

In Canada, goldenseal is a Natural Health Product (a form of OTC drug) and requires a product license (pre-market authorization) to be sold (Goldenseal Buccal, 2010). Goldenseal (*H. canadensis*) is also regulated as an endangered species under Appendix II of the Convention on International Trade in Endangered Species of Wild Fauna and Flora (CITES, 2006).

2. Cancer in Humans

No data were available to the Working Group.

3. Cancer in Experimental Animals

See Table 3.1

Goldenseal (*H. canadensis*) root powder was tested for carcinogenicity by oral administration in one study in mice and one study in rats.

3.1 Mouse

In a 2-year study of carcinogenicity, groups of 50 male and 50 female B6C3F$_1$ mice (age, 5–6 weeks) were fed ad libitum with diet containing well-characterized goldenseal root powder (*H. canadensis*) shown to contain all the major alkaloids characteristic of goldenseal (berberine, hydrastine and canadine) at a concentration of 0 (control), 3000, 9000, or 25 000 ppm. Concentrations were equivalent to average daily doses of goldenseal root powder of approximately 0, 375, 1120, or 3275 mg/kg body weight (bw) for males and 0, 330, 1000, or 2875 mg/kg bw for females (NTP, 2010). Survival of the females at 9000 ppm was lower than that of controls. At 105–106 weeks, goldenseal root powder caused a significant positive trend in the incidence of hepatoblastoma, and of hepatocellular adenoma, in males. There were no significant increases in the incidence of tumours in female mice. The incidence of liver eosinophilic foci was significantly increased in males at the intermediate and highest doses, and in all exposed females.

3.2 Rat

In a 2-year study of carcinogenicity, groups of 50 male and 50 female F344/N rats (age, 5–6 weeks) were fed ad libitum with diet containing a well-characterized goldenseal root powder (*H. canadensis*) shown to contain all the major alkaloids (berberine, hydrastine and canadine) characteristic of goldenseal at a concentration of 0 (control), 3000, 9000, or 25 000 ppm. Concentrations were equivalent to average daily

Table 3.1 Studies of carcinogenicity with goldenseal root powder in mice and rats

Species, strain (sex) Duration Reference	Dosing regimen Animals/group at start	Incidence of tumours	Significance	Comments
Mouse, B6C3F$_1$ (M, F) 105–106 wk NTP (2010)	Goldenseal root powder (*H. canadensis*): 0 (control), 3000, 9000, or 25 000 ppm in feed, corresponding to 0, 375, 1120, or 3275 mg/kg bw (M); 0, 330, 1000, or 2875 mg/kg bw (F) 50 M and 50 F/group (age, 5–6-wk)	Hepatoblastoma: 1/50 (2%)*, 2/50 (4%), 1/50 (25), 6/50 (12%) (M)[a] Hepatocellular adenoma: 22/50 (44%)**, 16/50 (32%), 23/50 (46%), 29/50 (58%) (M) 3/50 (6%), 6/50 (12%), 7/50 (14%), 7/50 (14%) (F) Hepatocellular carcinoma: 8/50 (16%), 14/50 (28%), 15/50 (30%), 12/50 (24%) (M)	*P = 0.030 (trend test) **P = 0.016	Major alkaloids content: berberine, 3.89%; hydrastine, 2.8%; and canadine, 0.17%
Rat, F344/N (M, F) 105–106 wk NTP (2010)	Goldenseal root powder (*H. canadensis*): 0 (control), 3000, 9000, or 25 000 ppm in feed: 0, 135, 400, or 1175 mg/kg bw (M); 0, 150, 470, 1340 mg/kg bw (F) 50 M and 50 F/group (age, 5–6 wk)	Hepatocellular adenoma: 1/50 (2%)*, 1/50 (2%), 2/50 (4%), 10/50 (20%)** (M) 0/50 (0%)*, 0/50 (05), 1/50 (2%), 8/50 (16%)** (F)[b] Hepatocellular carcinoma: 0/50 (0%), 0/50 (0%), 0/50 (0%), 1/50 (2%) (M)[c] Hepatocellular adenoma or carcinoma (combined): 1/50 (2%)*, 1/50 (2%), 2/50 (4%), 11/50 (22%)*** (M)[d]	*P < 0.001 (trend test) **P ≤ 0.004 ***P < 0.001	Major alkaloids content: berberine, 3.89%; hydrastine, 2.8%; and canadine, 0.17%

[a] Historical incidence of hepatoblastoma (includes multiple) (mean ± standard deviation) for feed studies in untreated control male mice: 1/250 (0.4% ± 0.9%); range, 0–2%; all routes: 48/1447 (3.3% ± 6.4%); range, 0–34%.

[b] Historical incidence of hepatocellular adenoma (mean ± standard deviation) for feed studies in untreated control female rats: 4/250 (1.6% ± 2.2%); range, 0–4%; all routes: 16/1350 (1.2% ± 2.6%); range, 0–12%

[c] Historical incidence of hepatocellular carcinoma in untreated control male rats: 1/1250 (all routes)

[d] Historical incidence of hepatocellular adenoma or carcinoma (mean ± standard deviation) for feed studies in untreated control male rats: 7/300 (2.3% ± 2.3%); range, 0–6%; all routes: 22/1399 (1.6% ± 1.7%); range, 0–6%

bw, body weight; F, female; M, male; wk, week

doses of goldenseal root powder of approximately 0, 135, 400, or 1175 mg/kg bw to males and 0, 150, 470, or 1340 mg/kg bw for females (NTP, 2010). Survival of the females at 9000 ppm was greater than that of controls. At 105–106 weeks, goldenseal root powder caused increased incidences of hepatocellular adenoma in males and females at the highest dose. One male rat at the highest dose also developed a rare hepatocellular carcinoma. There was a treatment-related statistically significant increase in the incidence of liver eosinophilic foci in male and female rats. [The Working Group noted that hepatocellular tumours are uncommon tumours in F344/N rats and that evidence from studies reported in the literature showed that hepatocellular adenomas may progress to malignant tumours in F344/N rats.]

4. Mechanistic and Other Relevant Data

4.1 Absorption, distribution, metabolism, and excretion

4.1.1 Humans

Goldenseal contains berberine and hydrastine (see Section 1). Most data on the carcinogenicity of goldenseal came from studies with berberine. In 11 healthy subjects treated orally with a single dose of goldenseal (2.7 g) containing 78 mg of hydrastine and 132 mg of berberine, both berberine and hydrastine were absorbed from the gastrointestinal tract, and their phase I and II metabolites were rapidly detected in the plasma and urine (Gupta $et\ al.$, 2010). The maximal plasma concentration (C_{max}) of hydrastine was 225 ± 100 ng/mL, the time to C_{max} (T_{max}) was 1.5 ± 0.3 hours, and the area under the curve (AUC) was 6.4 ± 4.1 ng•h/mL•kg. The elimination half-life ($t_{1/2\beta}$) of hydrastine was 4.8 ± 1.4 hours. Corresponding values for

berberine were 1.1 ± 1.2 ng/mL, 3.0 ± 3.3 hours and 0.15 ± 0.09 ng•h/mL•kg, respectively. Phase I metabolites of hydrastine underwent extensive glucuronidation, but not sulfation, while the phase I metabolites of berberine were primarily sulfated (Gupta $et\ al.$, 2010). The area under the curve of hydrastine in plasma is significantly higher than that of berberine, suggesting that the oral bioavailability of hydrastine is also higher. There was enterohepatic recycling of berberine, which also had a high volume of distribution (Gupta $et\ al.$, 2010).

In humans given berberine orally, plasma concentrations of berberine were very low and variable (Li $et\ al.$, 2000a; Hua $et\ al.$, 2007). For example, the plasma C_{max} of berberine was only 0.4 ng/mL after a single oral dose of 400 mg of berberine (Hua $et\ al.$, 2007). This suggested that berberine is poorly absorbed by the gastrointestinal wall. [The Working Group noted the discrepancy between pharmacokinetic parameters for purified berberine compared with those for goldenseal.]

The metabolites of berberine are mainly 1,3-dioxolane ring-opened, demethylated, demethylenated, glycosylated, and sulfonated products. Several clinical studies have been performed to identify these metabolites in the plasma and urine (Pan $et\ al.$, 2002; Qiu $et\ al.$, 2008).

In one study, five healthy male volunteers (aged 21–28 years) were given berberine chloride orally (900 mg/day; 100 mg tablets) for 3 days (Pan $et\ al.$, 2002). Urine samples were collected and the metabolites isolated and purified by polyporous resin column chromatography. Three metabolites were recovered and identified via electrospray ionization mass spectroscopy (ESI-MS) and proton nuclear magnetic resonance (^{1}H-NMR) spectroscopy: jatrorrhizine-3-sulfate, demethylene berberine-2-sulfate, and thalifendine-10-sulfate. The amounts of these purified metabolites in the urine were 250, 17, and 2 mg, respectively (Pan $et\ al.$, 2002).

In a later study with 12 healthy male volunteers (aged 22–26 years; body weight, 60–80 kg), additional metabolites were discovered (Qiu *et al.*, 2008). In this study, subjects were given an oral dose of berberine chloride of 300 mg, three times per day for 2 days, and urine samples were collected in the 72 hours after dosing. Using nuclear magnetic resonance spectroscopy in addition to liquid chromatography–mass spectrometry, the study identified the above three conjugated metabolites, plus previously unseen conjugates: demethyleneberberine-2-*O*-sulfate, jatrorrhizine-3-*O*-β-D-glucuronide, thalifendine-10-*O*-β-D-glucuronide, berberrubine-9-*O*-β-D-glucuronide, jatrorrhizine-3-*O*-sulfate, 3-10-demethylpalmatine-10-*O*-sulfate, and columbamin-2-*O*-β-D-glucuronide (40 mg, 6 mg, 4 mg, 6.1 mg, 2.2 mg, 1.2 mg, and 1 mg, per 16 L of urine, respectively) (Qiu *et al.*, 2008). In this study, both sulfates and glucuronides of berberine were observed.

Using the human intestinal Caco-2 model, Zhang *et al.* (2011) examined the intestinal absorption mechanisms of berberine. They found that the cellular uptake of berberine was 30.13 ± 0.57 μmol/g protein, at a substrate concentration of 10 μM, and that the apparent permeability (P_{app}) of berberine was 0.66 ± 0.04 (absorptive direction) and 15.91 ± 0.61 (secretory direction) × 10^{-6} cm/s, with an efflux ratio of 24.28 (Zhang *et al.*, 2011). Transport inhibition studies using cyclosporin A [ciclosporin] and verapamil [both potent inhibitors of P-glycoprotein 1 (P-gp/multidrug resistance protein 1)] indicated that berberine was a substrate of this transporter.

4.1.2 Experimental systems

The absorption of berberine in rats is very poor; in rats given berberine at an oral dose of 100 mg/kg bw, the plasma C_{max} of berberine was estimated to be only 4.0 ng/mL (Liu *et al.*, 2009, 2010).

The metabolism of berberine in vitro and in vivo has been well studied in rats (Qiu *et al.*, 2008; Liu *et al.*, 2009, 2010). In rat liver microsomes, or following intravenous administration, berberine was metabolized by several cytochromes P450 (CYPs) and UDP-glucuronosyltransferases. Oxidative demethylenation was the major metabolic pathway and the metabolite obtained can subsequently undergo glucuronidation (Liu *et al.*, 2009). In one study in vivo, male Wistar rats (age, 8–10 weeks) were given berberine at a dose of 100 mg/kg bw, and urine samples were collected for 48 hours; the five urinary metabolites of berberine isolated and identified included berberrubine-9-*O*-β-D-glucuronide, demethyleneberberine-2,3-di-*O*-β-D-glucuronide, demethyleneberberine-2-*O*-sulfate, 3,10-demethylpalmatine-10-*O*-sulfate, and thalifendine (Qiu *et al.*, 2008).

Berberine was found to undergo extensive first-pass metabolism in the rat intestine. After intragastric dosing, approximately half of the intact berberine passed through the gastrointestinal tract and another half was biotransformed by the small intestine, resulting in an extremely low absolute oral bioavailability in rats (0.36%) (Liu *et al.*, 2010).

[The above findings indicate that berberine is poorly absorbed in both rats and humans due to extensive first-pass disposition. Berberine is extensively metabolized by intestinal and hepatic phase I and II enzymes in rats and humans.]

4.1.3 Alterations in enzymes and metabolic capacity

Goldenseal strongly inhibits CYP2C9, CYP3A4, CYP2D6, and CYP2C19 in vitro (Budzinski *et al.*, 2000; Chatterjee & Franklin, 2003; Foster *et al.*, 2003). In one experiment, Etheridge *et al.* (2007) examined the effects of goldenseal on the activities of human CYPs in human liver microsomes, finding that goldenseal inhibited CYP2C8, CYP2D6, and CYP3A4 by ≥ 50% (Etheridge *et al.*, 2007).

In humans, goldenseal did not significantly affect the metabolism and pharmacokinetic of indinavir, a protease inhibitor, which is a substrate of CYP3A4, (Sandhu *et al.*, 2003). However, goldenseal has been shown to increase the plasma concentration of cyclosporine [ciclosporin] in healthy volunteers (Xin *et al.*, 2006) and in renal transplant patients (Wu *et al.*, 2005). In another study, single time-point phenotypic metabolic ratios of CYP probe drugs were administered to 12 healthy subjects (6 males and 6 females, all extensive metabolizers of CYP2D6) to determine whether a 28-day supplementation of goldenseal root extract (900 mg, three times per day, 2.70 g/day; no standardization claim) affected the activity of CYP1A2, CYP2D6, CYP2E1, or CYP3A4/5. The following probe cocktails were administered before and after supplementation: midazolam (CYP3A4) and caffeine (CYP1A2), followed 24 hours later by chlorzoxazone (CYP2E1) and debrisoquine (CYP2D6). The phenotypic traits of CYP3A4, CYP1A2, CYP2E1, and CYP2D6 activities were assessed using the 1-hydroxymidazolam/midazolam serum ratio at 1 hour, the paraxanthine/caffeine serum ratio at 6 hours, the 6-hydroxychlorzoxazone/chlorzoxazone serum ratio at 2 hours, and debrisoquine urinary recovery ratio after an 8-hour collection. Phenotypic ratios, taken before and after supplementation, show remarkable inhibition of CYP2D6 (~40%) and CYP3A4/5 (~40%) activities due to goldenseal supplementation. CYP1A2 and CYP2E1 activities were virtually unaffected (Gurley *et al.*, 2005). For CYP3A4/5, this clinical observation was confirmed by a more comprehensive study in which goldenseal caused a mean increase in midazolam $AUC_{0-\infty}$ and C_{max} by about 63% and 40%, respectively, while the $AUC_{0-\infty}$ and C_{max} of clarithromycin (an inhibitor of CYP3A4) increased about 5.5-fold and 2-fold, respectively (Gurley *et al.*, 2008a). However, goldenseal root extract is only a moderate inhibitor of CYP2D6 in humans (Gurley *et al.*, 2008b).

4.2 Genetic and related effects

4.2.1 Humans

No data were available to the Working Group.

4.2.2 Experimental systems

See also Table 4.1.

(a)   Mutagenicity

Goldenseal root powder (1000–10000 µg/plate) was not mutagenic in *Salmonella typhimurium* strains TA98 or TA100, or *Escherichia coli* strain WP2 *uvrA*/pKM101, with or without metabolic activation from rat liver S9 (NTP, 2010). Berberine was also not mutagenic in *S. typhimurium* strains TA97, TA98, TA100 and TA1535, with or without metabolic activation from rat or hamster liver S9. In three tests in TA98, berberine gave negative results in two tests and equivocal results in one.

(b)   Chromosomal damage

No increase in the frequency of micronucleated normochromatic erythrocytes or polychromatic erythrocytes was observed in blood from male or female mice exposed to diets containing goldenseal root powder at up to 50 000 ppm for 3 months. No increases in the frequency of micronucleated polychromatic erythrocytes were observed in bone marrow from male $B6C3F_1$ mice treated with berberine chloride at a dose of up to 658 mg/kg bw via three intraperitoneal injections at intervals of 24 hours (NTP, 2010).

(c)   Interaction with DNA

Data on the interaction of some goldenseal constituents with DNA are presented below (see Section 4.3.2).

Table 4.1 Genetic and related effects of goldenseal root and berberine

Test system	Results		Concentration or dose (LED or HID)	Reference
	Without exogenous metabolic system	With exogenous metabolic system		
Goldenseal root				
Salmonella typhimurium TA100, TA98 reverse mutation	–	–	10 000 µg/plate	NTP (2010)
Escherichia coli WP2 *uvrA*/pKM101 reverse mutation	–	–	10 000 µg/plate	NTP (2010)
Micronucleus formation in peripheral blood erythrocytes of male and female $B6C3F_1$ mice in vivo	–	NT	50 000 ppm [50 g/kg] in diet for 3 months	NTP (2010)
Berberine				
Salmonella typhimurium TA100, TA98, TA97, TA1535 reverse mutation	(–)[a]	–	1000 µg/plate	NTP (2010)
Inhibition of DNA repair activity, topoisomerase II inhibition, plasmid pUL402DNA	(+)[b]	NT	2.5 µM [0.9 µg/mL]	Kobayashi *et al.* (1995)
Inhibition of DNA repair activity, topoisomerase II inhibition,plasmid pBS DNA	(+)[b]	NT	50 µM [18 µg/mL]	Kim *et al.* (1998)
Micronucleus formation in bone-marrow polychromatic erythrocytes of male $B6C3F_1$ mice in vivo	–	NT	658 mg/kg bw, i.p. × 3	NTP (2010)

[a] One out of three tests in TA98 gave equivocal results.

[b] The test gave positive results with berberrubine, but weakly positive results with berberine.

+, positive; (+), weakly positive; –, negative; ?, inconclusive; HID, highest ineffective dose; i.p., intraperitoneal; LED, lowest effective dose; NR, not reported; NT, not tested

4.3 Other mechanistic data relevant to carcinogenicity

4.3.1 Humans

No data were available to the Working Group.

4.3.2 Experimental systems

Berberine alkaloids found in goldenseal root powder inhibited topoisomerases I (Topo I) and II (Topo II) (Krishnan & Bastow, 2000; Li *et al.*, 2000b; Kettmann *et al.*, 2004). The ability of berberine to disrupt Topo I and Topo II is related to its antitumour activity (Mazzini *et al.*, 2003). While the role of drug–DNA interactions in the inhibition of Topo I is unclear, the binding of berberine to DNA has been considered as the cause for inhibition.

It has been shown by nuclear magnetic resonance spectroscopy that berberine binds selectively to AT-rich sequences, interacting with several oligonucleotides (Mazzini *et al.*, 2003). Using a two-dimensional nuclear Overhauser effect assay, several contacts were detected between protons of the self-complementary oligomer d(AAGAATTCTT)$_2$ and the protons of berberine. Berberine was found on the convex side of the helix groove, the minor groove of the nucleotide (at the level of the A_4–T_7 and A_5–T_6 base pairs), presenting its positive nitrogen atom to the negative ionic surface of the oligonucleotide. The aromatic protons H-11 and H-12 are close to the ribose of cytidine C_8, while the methylenedioxy and ring A group are more external to the helix (Mazzini *et al.*, 2003).

Electrospray ionization-mass spectrometry (ESI-MS) has been used to study noncovalent complexes of protoberberine alkaloids, berberine, palmatine, jatrorrhizine, and coptisine with double-strand DNA oligonucleotides, showing that berberine has the lowest binding affinity and palmatine the highest (Chen *et al.*, 2004). These preliminary data suggested that berberine exhibited some sequence selectivities. Additional studies using ESI-MS to examine noncovalent complexes have produced new information (Chen *et al.*, 2005a, b). In one study, berberine exhibited different binding affinities to different nucleotides (Chen *et al.*, 2005b); however, ESI-MS and fluorescence titration experiments with these four alkaloids indicated that sequence selectivity was not significant and no specific AT- or GC-rich DNA binding preferences were observed, in contrast to the aforementioned reports (Mazzini *et al.*, 2003; Chen *et al.*, 2004).

Pang *et al.* (2005) suggested that berberine and its derivatives, especially those with a primary amino group, are able to bind strongly with calf-thymus DNA via an intercalation mechanism. Substitution at the C-9 position is an important determinant of the biological activity, as Park *et al.* (2004) demonstrated in these studies on the structure–activity relationships of the berberine analogues (Park *et al.*, 2004).

When berberine units are bridged at the C-9 position with different linker lengths (termed "bridged berberine derivatives"), they exhibit the highest binding affinity to DNA when they form a compound berberine dimer with a propyl chain (Chen *et al.*, 2005a; Qin *et al.*, 2006). DNA and RNA triplexes can be bound and stabilized better than their respective parent duplexes when they bind with the sanguinarine and berberine alkaloids (Das *et al.*, 2003).

4.4 Susceptibility

No data were available to the Working Group.

4.5 Mechanistic considerations

Goldenseal root powder gave negative results in several standard bacterial assays for mutation in the absence or presence of metabolic activation systems. The principal alkaloid in goldenseal root powder, berberine, also gave negative results in many of these assays. Goldenseal root powder gave negative results in the test for mouse peripheral blood micronucleated erythrocytes (normochromatic and polychromatic) after 3 months of dietary exposure. Berberine also gave negative results for induction of micronuclei in mouse bone-marrow polychromatic erythrocytes after three doses.

Goldenseal produced mostly negative results in assays for bacterial mutation (NTP, 2010). However, berberine, its metabolite, berberrubine, and several protoberberines have been shown to inhibit the activity of topoisomerases (Kobayashi *et al.*, 1995; Makhey *et al.*, 1995; Kim *et al.*, 1998; Li *et al.*, 2000b; Krishnan & Bastow, 2000). Etoposide, an inhibitor of topoisomerase II, was classified by the IARC *Monographs* as *carcinogenic to humans* (Group 1) (IARC, 2012).

5. Summary of Data Reported

5.1 Exposure data

Goldenseal (*Hydrastis canadensis* L.) is an endangered plant that is widely consumed in several countries. The root has been used traditionally in herbal medicine. Reported uses include the treatment of skin disorders, digestive disorders, anorexia, menstrual disorders, and mucosal inflammations. Currently, the main applications for this plant include the prevention and reduction of inflammation and related diseases. Goldenseal is available in the form of tea, capsules containing the crude drug or the extract, skin lotion, eyewash, and eardrops. In 2011, goldenseal ranked 37th among top-selling dietary supplements in the USA. Other countries that reported significant sales of goldenseal included Canada, France, and Germany.

5.2 Human carcinogenicity data

No data were available to the Working Group.

5.3 Animal carcinogenicity data

A well-characterized goldenseal root powder shown to contain all the major alkaloids characteristic of goldenseal was tested for carcinogenicity by oral administration in one study in mice and one study in rats.

In male mice fed a diet containing goldenseal root powder, there was a significant positive trend in the incidence of hepatoblastoma and of hepatocellular adenoma. There were no significant increases in the incidence of tumours in female mice.

In male and female rats fed a diet containing goldenseal root powder, there was an increased incidence of hepatocellular adenoma, which in F344/N rats is an uncommon tumour that is known to progress to malignancy. In addition, one rare hepatocellular carcinoma was observed in the group of males given the highest dose.

5.4 Mechanistic and other relevant data

The major alkaloid components of goldenseal, berberine and hydrastine, are absorbed from the gastrointestinal tract into the circulation and extensively metabolized in the liver after oral administration of goldenseal.

Goldenseal root powder gave negative results in several standard bacterial assays for mutation in the absence or presence of exogenous metabolic activation systems. Berberine also gave negative results in many of these assays. Likewise, goldenseal root powder gave negative results in the mouse peripheral blood micronucleated erythrocyte test (normochromatic and polychromatic erythrocytes) after dietary exposure. Berberine also gave negative results for the induction of micronuclei in mouse bone-marrow polychromatic erythrocytes.

Berberine and its metabolite, berberrubine, have been shown to inhibit DNA topoisomerases. Such inhibition may account for the carcinogenicity of goldenseal in experimental animals.

6. Evaluation

6.1 Cancer in humans

There is *inadequate evidence* in humans for the carcinogenicity of goldenseal.

6.2 Cancer in experimental animals

There is *sufficient evidence* in experimental animals for the carcinogenicity of goldenseal root powder.

6.3 Overall evaluation

Goldenseal root powder is *possibly carcinogenic to humans (Group 2B)*.

References

Abourashed EA & Khan IA (2001). High-performance liquid chromatography determination of hydrastine and berberine in dietary supplements containing goldenseal. *J Pharm Sci*, 90(7):817–22. doi:10.1002/jps.1035 PMID:11458331

AHP (2001). Golden root. In: Roy Upton, editor. American Herbal Pharmacopoeia and Therapeutic Compendium. Scotts Valley (CA), USA: AHP; pp. 1–36.

American Chemical Society (2014). SciFinder Database. Available from: https://scifinder.cas.org, accessed 10 September 2014.

BHMA; British Herbal Medicine Association (1983) British herbal pharmacopoeia. Bournemouth, UK: BHMA; pp 113–115.

BHMA; British Herbal Medicine Association (1992). British herbal compendium, volume I, Bournemouth, UK: BHMA; pp 119–120.

Borodina VM, Kirianova EE, Fedorova OV, Zelenin AV (1979). Cytochemical properties of interphase chromatin condensed as a result of treatment with caffeine. *Exp Cell Res*, 122(2):391–4. doi:10.1016/0014-4827(79)90316-1 PMID:92416

Brown PN & Roman MC (2008). Determination of hydrastine and berberine in goldenseal raw materials, extracts, and dietary supplements by high-performance liquid chromatography with UV: collaborative study. *J AOAC Int*, 91(4):694–701. PMID:18727526

Budzinski JW, Foster BC, Vandenhoek S, Arnason JT (2000). An in vitro evaluation of human cytochrome P450 3A4 inhibition by selected commercial herbal extracts and tinctures. *Phytomedicine*, 7(4):273–82. doi:10.1016/S0944-7113(00)80044-6 PMID:10969720

CDC (2013). National Health and Nutrition Examination Survey. Available from: http://www.cdc.gov/nchs/nhanes.htm, accessed 10 September 2014.

Chatterjee P & Franklin MR (2003). Human cytochrome p450 inhibition and metabolic-intermediate complex formation by goldenseal extract and its methylenedioxyphenyl components. *Drug Metab Dispos*, 31(11):1391–7. doi:10.1124/dmd.31.11.1391 PMID:14570772

Chen W-H, Chan C-L, Cai Z, Luo GA, Jiang ZH (2004). Study on noncovalent complexes of cytotoxic protoberberine alkaloids with double-stranded DNA by using electrospray ionization mass spectrometry. *Bioorg Med Chem Lett*, 14(19):4955–9. doi:10.1016/j.bmcl.2004.07.037 PMID:15341959

Chen W-H, Pang J-Y, Qin Y, Peng Q, Cai Z, Jiang ZH (2005a). Synthesis of linked berberine dimers and their remarkably enhanced DNA-binding affinities. *Bioorg Med Chem Lett*, 15(10):2689–92. doi:10.1016/j.bmcl.2004.10.098 PMID:15863343

Chen W-H, Qin Y, Cai Z, Chan CL, Luo GA, Jiang ZH (2005b). Spectrometric studies of cytotoxic protoberberine alkaloids binding to double-stranded DNA. *Bioorg Med Chem*, 13(5):1859–66. doi:10.1016/j.bmc.2004.10.049 PMID:15698803

Chi CW, Chang YF, Chao TW, Chiang SH, P'eng FK, Lui WY et al. (1994). Flowcytometric analysis of the effect of berberine on the expression of glucocorticoid receptors in human hepatoma HepG2 cells. *Life Sci*, 54(26):2099–107. doi:10.1016/0024-3205(94)00719-5 PMID:7516035

Choudhry VP, Sabir M, Bhide VN (1972). Berberine in giardiasis. *Indian Pediatr*, 9(3):143–6. PMID:4555485

CITES (2006). Convention on International Trade in Endangered Species of Wild Fauna and Flora. Fifty-fourth meeting of the Standing Committee, Geneva (Switzerland). SC54 Doc. 43.5. Available from: http://www.cites.org/eng/com/sc/54/E54-43-5.pdf, accessed 08 December 2014.

Creasey WA (1977). Plant Alkaloids. In: Becker FF, editor. Cancer, a Comprehensive Treatise: Chemotherapy. Vol. 5. New York and London: Plenum Press; pp. 379–425.

Creasey WA (1979). Biochemical effects of berberine. *Biochem Pharmacol*, 28(7):1081–4. doi:10.1016/0006-2952(79)90308-3 PMID:444265

Croom EM Jr & Walker L (1995). Botanicals in the pharmacy: new life for old remedies. *Drug Topics*, 139:84–93.

Das S, Kumar GS, Ray A, Maiti M (2003). Spectroscopic and thermodynamic studies on the binding of sanguinarine and berberine to triple and double helical DNA and RNA structures. *J Biomol Struct Dyn*, 20(5):703–14. doi:10.1080/07391102.2003.10506887 PMID:12643773

Duke JA, editor (2002). Handbook of medicinal herbs. 2nd ed. Boca Raton (FL): CRC Press; pp. 340–342.

Etheridge AS, Black SR, Patel PR, So J, Mathews JM (2007). An in vitro evaluation of cytochrome P450 inhibition and P-glycoprotein interaction with goldenseal, Ginkgo biloba, grape seed, milk thistle, and ginseng extracts and their constituents. *Planta Med*, 73(8):731–41. doi:10.1055/s-2007-981550 PMID:17611934

FDA (1994). Dietary Supplement Health and Education Act of 1994. Public Law 103-417, 103rd Congress., US Food and Drug Administration. Available from http://www.fda.gov/RegulatoryInformation/Legislation/FederalFoodDrugandCosmeticActFDCAct/SignificantAmendmentstotheFDCAct/ucm148003.htm, accessed 09 December 2014

Foster BC, Vandenhoek S, Hana J, Krantis A, Akhtar MH, Bryan M *et al.* (2003). In vitro inhibition of human cytochrome P450-mediated metabolism of marker substrates by natural products. *Phytomedicine*, 10(4):334–42. doi:10.1078/094471103322004839 PMID:12809364

Goldenseal Buccal (2010). Natural Health Products Ingredients Database. Health Canada. Available from: http://webprod.hc-sc.gc.ca/nhpid-bdipsn/monoReq.do?id=107&lang=eng, accessed 10 September 2014.

Govindan M & Govindan G (2000).A convenient method for the determination of the quality of goldensealA convenient method for the determination of the quality of goldenseal. *Fitoterapia*, 71(3):232–5. doi:10.1016/S0367-326X(99)00162-8 PMID:10844160

Gupta PK, Gurley BJ, Barone G, Hendrickson HP (2010). Clinical Pharmacokinetics and Metabolism of Berberine and Hydrastine Following an Oral Dose of Goldenseal Supplement. *Planta Med*, 76(05):110 doi:10.1055/s-0030-1251872

Gurley BJ, Gardner SF, Hubbard MA, Williams DK, Gentry WB, Khan IA *et al.* (2005). In vivo effects of goldenseal, kava kava, black cohosh, and valerian on human cytochrome P450 1A2, 2D6, 2E1, and 3A4/5 phenotypes. *Clin Pharmacol Ther*, 77(5):415–26. doi:10.1016/j.clpt.2005.01.009 PMID:15900287

Gurley BJ, Swain A, Hubbard MA, Hartsfield F, Thaden J, Williams DK *et al.* (2008a). Supplementation with goldenseal (Hydrastis canadensis), but not kava kava (Piper methysticum), inhibits human CYP3A activity in vivo. *Clin Pharmacol Ther*, 83(1):61–9. doi:10.1038/sj.clpt.6100222 PMID:17495878

Gurley BJ, Swain A, Hubbard MA, Williams DK, Barone G, Hartsfield F *et al.* (2008b). Clinical assessment of CYP2D6-mediated herb-drug interactions in humans: effects of milk thistle, black cohosh, goldenseal, kava kava, St. John's wort, and Echinacea. *Mol Nutr Food Res*, 52(7):755–63. doi:10.1002/mnfr.200600300 PMID:18214849

Hamon NW (1990). Herbal medicine: Goldenseal. *Can Pharm J*, 123:508–510.

Hobbs C (1990). Golden seal in early American medical botany. *Pharm Hist*, 32(2):79–82. PMID:11622733

HSDB (1997). The Hazardous Substance Data Bank. Berberine sulfate. Online database produced by the National Library of Medicine. Last Database Update: January 14, 2002.

Hua W, Ding L, Chen Y, Gong B, He J, Xu G (2007). Determination of berberine in human plasma by liquid chromatography-electrospray ionization-mass spectrometry. *J Pharm Biomed Anal*, 44(4):931–7. doi:10.1016/j.jpba.2007.03.022 PMID:17531424

Huang JH & Johnston GA (1990). (+)-Hydrastine, a potent competitive antagonist at mammalian GABAA receptors. *Br J Pharmacol*, 99(4):727–30. doi:10.1111/j.1476-5381.1990.tb12997.x PMID:2163278

Hwang BY, Roberts SK, Chadwick LR, Wu CD, Kinghorn AD (2003). Antimicrobial constituents from goldenseal (the Rhizomes of Hydrastis canadensis) against selected oral pathogens. *Planta Med*, 69(7):623–7. doi:10.1055/s-2003-41115 PMID:12898417

IARC (2012). Pharmaceuticals. Volume 100 A. A review of human carcinogens. *IARC Monogr Eval Carcinog Risks Hum*, 100:Pt A: 1–401. PMID:23189749

IMS Health (2012) Multinational Integrated Data Analysis (MIDAS). Plymouth Meeting, Pennsylvania: IMS Health, 2012.

Junio HA, Sy-Cordero AA, Ettefagh KA, Burns JT, Micko KT, Graf TN *et al.* (2011). Synergy-directed fractionation of botanical medicines: a case study with goldenseal (Hydrastis canadensis). *J Nat Prod*, 74(7):1621–9. doi:10.1021/np200336g PMID:21661731

Kettmann V, Kosfálová D, Jantová S, Cernáková M, Drímal J (2004). In vitro cytotoxicity of berberine against HeLa and L1210 cancer cell lines. *Pharmazie*, 59(7):548–51. PMID:15296093

Khin-Maung-U , Myo-Khin , Nyunt-Nyunt-Wai , Aye-Kyaw , Tin-U (1985). Clinical trial of berberine in acute watery diarrhoea. *Br Med J (Clin Res Ed)*, 291(6509):1601–5. doi:10.1136/bmj.291.6509.1601 PMID:3935203

Kim DI, Pedersen H, Chin CK (1990). Two stage cultures for the production of berberine in cell suspension cultures of Thalictrum rugosum. *J Biotechnol*, 16(3-4):297–303. doi:10.1016/0168-1656(90)90043-B PMID:1366939

Kim SA, Kwon Y, Kim JH, Muller MT, Chung IK (1998). Induction of topoisomerase II-mediated DNA cleavage by a protoberberine alkaloid, berberrubine. *Biochemistry*, 37(46):16316–24. doi:10.1021/bi9810961 PMID:9819224

Kobayashi Y, Yamashita Y, Fujii N, Takaboshi K, Kawakami T, Kawamura M *et al.* (1995). Inhibitors of DNA topoisomerase I and II isolated from the Coptis rhizomes. *Planta Med*, 61(5):414–8. doi:10.1055/s-2006-958127 PMID:7480201

Koehler's Medicinal-Plants (1887). Available from: http://pharm1.pharmazie.uni-greifswald.de/allgemei/koehler/koeh-eng.htm, accessed 10 September 2014.

Krishnan P & Bastow KF (2000). The 9-position in berberine analogs is an important determinant of DNA topoisomerase II inhibition. *Anticancer Drug Des*, 15(4):255–64. PMID:11200501

Kulkarni SK, Dandiya PC, Varandani NL (1972). Pharmacological investigations of berberine sulphate. *Jpn J Pharmacol*, 22(1):11–6. doi:10.1254/jjp.22.11 PMID:4260852

Li BX, Yang BF, Hao XM, Zhou H, Sun MZ (2000a). Study on the pharmacokinetics of berberine in single dosage and coadministration with oryzanol in rabbits and healthy volunteers. *Chin Pharm J*, 35:33–5.

Li TK, Bathory E, LaVoie EJ, Srinivasan AR, Olson WK, Sauers RR *et al.* (2000b). Human topoisomerase I poisoning by protoberberines: potential roles for both drug-DNA and drug-enzyme interactions. *Biochemistry*, 39(24):7107–16. doi:10.1021/bi000171g PMID:10852708

Li Y, Ren G, Wang YX, Kong WJ, Yang P, Wang YM *et al.* (2011). Bioactivities of berberine metabolites after transformation through CYP450 isoenzymes. *J Transl Med*, 9(1):62 doi:10.1186/1479-5876-9-62 PMID:21569619

Liu Y, Hao H, Xie H, Lv H, Liu C, Wang G (2009). Oxidative demethylenation and subsequent glucuronidation are the major metabolic pathways of berberine in rats. *J Pharm Sci*, 98(11):4391–401. doi:10.1002/jps.21721 PMID:19283771

Liu YT, Hao HP, Xie HG, Lai L, Wang Q, Liu CX *et al.* (2010). Extensive intestinal first-pass elimination and predominant hepatic distribution of berberine explain its low plasma levels in rats. *Drug Metab Dispos*, 38(10):1779–84. doi:10.1124/dmd.110.033936 PMID:20634337

Makhey D, Gatto B, Yu C *et al.* (1995). Protoberberine alkaloids and related compounds as dual inhibitors of mammalian topoisomerase I and II. *Med Chem Res*, 5:1–12.

Marin-Neto JA, Maciel BC, Secches AL, Gallo Júnior L (1988). Cardiovascular effects of berberine in patients with severe congestive heart failure. *Clin Cardiol*, 11(4):253–60. doi:10.1002/clc.4960110411 PMID:3365876

Martin EJ, Zell HC, Poon BT, editors (1978). Castor Oil to Chlorosulfuric Acid. In: Kirk-Othmer Encyclopedia of Chemical Technology. 3rd ed, Vol. 5. New York (NY): John Wiley and Sons; pp. 513–542.

Mazzini S, Bellucci MC, Mondelli R (2003). Mode of binding of the cytotoxic alkaloid berberine with the double helix oligonucleotide d(AAGAATTCTT)(2). *Bioorg Med Chem*, 11(4):505–14. doi:10.1016/S0968-0896(02)00466-2 PMID:12538015

McKenna DJ, Plotnikoff GA (2010). Goldenseal. In: Coates PM, Betz JM, editors. Encyclopedia of Dietary Supplements. 2nd ed. New York, USA: Informa Healthcare; pp. 379–390.

Mikeš V & Dadák V (1983). Berberine derivatives as cationic fluorescent probes for the investigation of the energized state of mitochondria. *Biochim Biophys Acta*, 723(2):231–9. doi:10.1016/0005-2728(83)90122-6 PMID:6849903

Mikeš V & Yaguzhinskij LS (1985). Interaction of fluorescent berberine alkyl derivatives with respiratory chain of rat liver mitochondria. *J Bioenerg Biomembr*, 17(1):23–32. doi:10.1007/BF00744986 PMID:3988724

Mikkelsen SL & Ash KO (1988). Adulterants causing false negatives in illicit drug testing. *Clin Chem*, 34(11):2333–6. PMID:3052928

Müller K, Ziereis K, Gawlik I (1995). The antipsoriatic Mahonia aquifolium and its active constituents; II. Antiproliferative activity against cell growth of human keratinocytes. *Planta Med*, 61(1):74–5. doi:10.1055/s-2006-958005 PMID:7700998

NBJ (2012a). Market Data and Overview. NBJ's Supplement Business Report. Nutrition Business Journal. 2009 Penton Media.

NBJ (2012b). NBJ's Supplement Business Report. An analysis of markets, trends, competition and strategy in the US dietary supplement industry. Penton Media, Inc., Neuw York, NY, USA.

NCCAM; National Center for Comprehensive and Alternative Medicine (2012). Goldenseal. In: Herbs at a glance. Available from: http://nccam.nih.gov/sites/nccam.nih.gov/files/Herbs_At_A_Glance_Goldenseal_071012_0.pdf?nav=gsa, accessed 10 September 2014.

Newall CA, Anderson LA, Phillipson JD (1996). Herbal Medicines. A guide for health-care professionals. 2nd ed, Pharmaceutical Press.

NMCD; Natural Medicines Comprehensive Database (2013). Goldenseal. Available from http://natural-database.therapeuticresearch.com/nd/Search.aspx?cs=&s=ND&pt=9&Product=Goldenseal&btnSearch.x=15&btnSearch.y=3, accessed 09 December 2014

NTP (2010). Toxicology and carcinogenesis studies of goldenseal root powder (Hydrastis Canadensis) in F344/N rats and B6C3F1 mice (feed studies). *Natl Toxicol Program Tech Rep Ser*, 562(562):1–188. PMID:21372858

O'NeilMJeditor. (2013). The Merck Index. 15th ed. Cambridge: The Royal Society of Chemistry; pp. 202–3, 301–2, 882–3.

Oldfield S (2005). IUCN/SSC Medicinal Plant Specialist Group PC 15 Inf. 3. Available from: http://www.cites.org/common/com/pc/15/X-PC15-03-Inf.pdf, accessed 10 September 2014.

Palmer EL (1975). Goldenseal, Orangeroot. Field book of Natural History. New York (NY): McGraw-Hill Book Co.; p. 173.

Pan J-F, Yu C, Zhu D-Y, Zhang H, Zeng JF, Jiang SH *et al.* (2002). Identification of three sulfate-conjugated metabolites of berberine chloride in healthy volunteers' urine after oral administration. *Acta Pharmacol Sin*, 23(1):77–82. PMID:11860742

Pang J-Y, Qin Y, Chen W-H, Luo GA, Jiang ZH (2005). Synthesis and DNA-binding affinities of monomodified berberines. *Bioorg Med Chem*, 13(20):5835–40. doi:10.1016/j.bmc.2005.05.048 PMID:15993616

Park H-S, Kim E-H, Kang M-R *et al.* (2004). Spectroscopic Studies on Interaction of Protoberberines with the Deoxyoligonucleotide d(GCCGTCGTTTTACA)2. *Bull Korean Chem Soc*, 25(10):1559–63. doi:10.5012/bkcs.2004.25.10.1559

Peng WH, Hsieh MT, Wu CR (1997). Effect of long-term administration of berberine on scopolamine-induced amnesia in rats. *Jpn J Pharmacol*, 74(3):261–6. doi:10.1254/jjp.74.261 PMID:9268086

Pengelly A, editor (2012) Goldenseal. *Hydrastis canadensis* L. In: Appalachian Plant Monographs. Frostburg (MD): Tai Sophia Institute for the Appalachian Center for Ethnobotanical Studies; pp. 1–41.

Qin Y, Pang J-Y, Chen W-H, Cai Z, Jiang ZH (2006). Synthesis, DNA-binding affinities, and binding mode of berberine dimers. *Bioorg Med Chem*, 14(1):25–32. doi:10.1016/j.bmc.2005.07.069 PMID:16169735

Qiu F, Zhu Z, Kang N, Piao S, Qin G, Yao X (2008). Isolation and identification of urinary metabolites of berberine in rats and humans. *Drug Metab Dispos*, 36(11):2159–65. doi:10.1124/dmd.108.021659 PMID:18703644

Ridler PJ & Jennings BR (1983). Electro-optical fluorescence studies on the DNA binding of medically active drugs. *Phys Med Biol*, 28(6):625–32. doi:10.1088/0031-9155/28/6/002 PMID:6308687

Sabir M, Akhter MH, Bhide NK (1978). Further studies on pharmacology of berberine. *Indian J Physiol Pharmacol*, 22(1):9–23. PMID:680944

Sabir M & Bhide NK (1971). Study of some pharmacological actions of berberine. *Indian J Physiol Pharmacol*, 15(3):111–32. PMID:4109503

Sandhu RS, Prescilla RP, Simonelli TM, Edwards DJ (2003). Influence of goldenseal root on the pharmacokinetics of indinavir. *J Clin Pharmacol*, 43(11):1283–8. doi:10.1177/0091270003258660 PMID:14551183

Schwarzhoff R & Cody JT (1993). The effects of adulterating agents on FPIA analysis of urine for drugs of abuse. *J Anal Toxicol*, 17(1):14–7. doi:10.1093/jat/17.1.14 PMID:8429620

Sinclair A & Catling PM (2000). Status of goldenseal, *Hydrastis canadensis* (Ranunculaceae), in Canada. *Can Field-Nat*, 114:111–120.

Sun Y, Xun K, Wang Y, Chen X (2009). A systematic review of the anticancer properties of berberine, a natural product from Chinese herbs. *Anticancer Drugs*, 20(9):757–69. doi:10.1097/CAD.0b013e328330d95b PMID:19704371

USP; United States Pharmacopeia (2013). 36th rev. and National Formulary. 31st ed. Rockville (MD): United States Pharmacopeial Convention, Inc.

Vennerstrom JL & Klayman DL (1988). Protoberberine alkaloids as antimalarials. *J Med Chem*, 31(6):1084–7. doi:10.1021/jm00401a006 PMID:3286870

Vennerstrom JL, Lovelace JK, Waits VB, Hanson WL, Klayman DL (1990). Berberine derivatives as antileishmanial drugs. *Antimicrob Agents Chemother*, 34(5):918–21. doi:10.1128/AAC.34.5.918 PMID:2360830

Wu X, Li Q, Xin H, Yu A, Zhong M (2005). Effects of berberine on the blood concentration of cyclosporin A in renal transplanted recipients: clinical and pharmacokinetic study. *Eur J Clin Pharmacol*, 61(8):567–72. doi:10.1007/s00228-005-0952-3 PMID:16133554

Xin HW, Wu XC, Li Q, Yu AR, Zhong MY, Liu YY (2006). The effects of berberine on the pharmacokinetics of cyclosporin A in healthy volunteers. *Methods Find Exp Clin Pharmacol*, 28(1):25–9. doi:10.1358/mf.2006.28.1.962774 PMID:16541194

Zeiger E and Tice R (1997). Goldenseal (*Hydrastis canadensis* L.) and two of its constituent alkaloids Berberine [2086-83-1] and hydrastine [118-08-1]. Integrated Laboratory Systems. Available from: http://ntp.niehs.nih.gov/ntp/htdocs/chem_background/exsumpdf/goldenseal_508.pdf. Accessed 08 December 2014.

Zhang X, Qiu F, Jiang J, Gao C, Tan Y (2011). Intestinal absorption mechanisms of berberine, palmatine, jateorhizine, and coptisine: involvement of P-glycoprotein. *Xenobiotica*, 41(4):290–6. doi:10.3109/00498254.2010.529180 PMID:21319959

Zieger E, Tice R (1997). Goldenseal (*Hydrastis canadensis* L.) and Two of Its Constituent Alkaloids. Integrated Laboratory Systems. pp. 1–52. Available from: http://ntp.niehs.nih.gov/ntp/htdocs/Chem_Background/ExSumPdf/GoldenSeal_508.pdf, accessed 10 September 2014.

GINKGO BILOBA

1. Exposure Data

Ginkgo biloba is one of the world's oldest living tree species. It has survived for more than 200 million years and has become popular as an ornamental tree in parks, gardens and city streets. Originating from China, *Ginkgo biloba* is now found all over the world (Gilman & Watson, 1993; ABC, 2000). Ginkgo seeds can be cooked and eaten as food. They have also been adopted in traditional Chinese medicine for many years. Some of the historical ethnomedical applications of ginkgo leaf extract include the treatment of a variety of ailments and conditions, such as asthma, bronchitis, and fatigue (Rai *et al.*, 1991). Nowadays, ginkgo leaf extracts are promoted for the improvement of memory, to treat or help prevent Alzheimer disease and other types of dementia, and to decrease intermittent claudication (Kleijnen & Knipschild, 1992; Kanowski *et al.*, 1996, 1997; Le Bars *et al.*, 1997; Morgenstern & Biermann, 1997; Nicolaï *et al.*, 2009; Snitz *et al.*, 2009; Herrschaft *et al.*, 2012; Vellas *et al.*, 2012). Some of these extracts are also used to treat multiple sclerosis, tinnitus, sexual dysfunction, and other health conditions (Oken *et al.*, 1998; Peters *et al.*, 1998; Lovera *et al.*, 2012; Herrschaft *et al.*, 2012; Evans, 2013; Nicolaï *et al.*, 2009; Hilton *et al.*, 2013).

1.1 Identification of the agent

1.1.1 Botanical data

(a) Nomenclature

Botanical name: *Ginkgo biloba* L.

Family: *Ginkgoaceae*

Genus: *Ginkgo*

Plant part: Leaf

Common names: Fossil tree; Kew tree; Japanese silver apricot; Maidenhair tree

From ABC (2000)

(b) Description

Ginkgo is a perennial plant with little invasive potential, which is resistant to insects and disease. Gingko grows slowly up to a height of about 40 m. The ginkgo plant is deciduous, with green leaves that turn golden in autumn. The leaves are simple, with alternate arrangement and lobed margins, fan-shaped with parallel venation, and a blade length of 2–4 inches [5–10 cm]. The female trees bear an inedible foul-smelling fruit containing a hard edible seed (Gilman & Watson, 1993; ABC, 2000).

1.1.2 Chemical constituents and their properties

The major bioactive constituents found in the leaves of ginkgo are reported to be flavonoids and terpene lactones, with the flavonoids present primarily as glycosides (Ding *et al.*, 2006; van Beek & Montoro, 2009). Major and minor flavonoids are described below. Standardized extracts of ginkgo leaves (CAS No. 122933-57-7; 123009-84-7; 401901-81-3) are frequently formulated to contain ~24% flavonoids and ~6% lactones (van Beek & Montoro, 2009). Other important constituents found in ginkgo include biflavonoids and traces of alkylphenols, such as ginkgolic acids (Wagner & Bladt, 1996; DeFeudis, 1991; Schötz, 2002; Siegers, 1999; van Beek & Montoro, 2009). Ginkgo also contains ginkgotoxin, which has been reported to be structurally related to vitamin B6 (Leistner & Drewke, 2010; Fig. 1.1).

CAS numbers and IUPAC names of the major components found in ginkgo are presented below (Chemical Abstracts Service, 2014).

(a)　Major flavonoids

(i)　Quercetin-3-β-D-glucoside

Chem. Abstr. Serv. Reg. No.: 482-35-9

IUPAC name: 2-(3,4-dihydroxyphenyl)-5,7-dihydroxy-3-[(2S,3R,4S,5S,6R)-3,4,5-trihydroxy-6-(hydroxymethyl)oxan-2-yl]oxychromen-4-one

(ii)　Quercitrin

Chem. Abstr. Serv. Reg. No.: 522-12-3

IUPAC name: 2-(3,4-dihydroxyphenyl)-5,7-dihydroxy-3-[(2S,3S,4R,5R,6S)-3,4,5-trihydroxy-6-methyloxan-2-yl]oxychromen-4-one

Description: Yellow crystalline substance (Ding *et al.*, 2006; van Beek & Montoro, 2009; O'Neil, 2013)

Melting-point: 174 °C

Solubility: Insoluble in cold water

(iii)　Rutin

Chem. Abstr. Serv. Reg. No.: 153-18-4

IUPAC name: 2-(3,4-dihydroxyphenyl)-5,7-dihydroxy-3-[α-L-rhamnopyranosyl-(1→6)-β-D-glucopyranosyloxy]-4H-chromen-4-one

Description: Yellow-brownish powder (Ding *et al.*, 2006; van Beek & Montoro, 2009; O'Neil, 2013)

Melting-point: 195 °C (O'Neil, 2013)

Solubility: Soluble in water (O'Neil, 2013)

(b)　Minor flavonoids

(i)　Quercetin

Chem. Abstr. Serv. Reg. No.: 117-39-5

IUPAC name: 2-(3,4-dihydroxyphenyl)-3,5,7-trihydroxy-4H-chromen-4-one

Description: Yellow crystalline substance (Ding *et al.*, 2006; van Beek & Montoro, 2009; O'Neil, 2013)

Melting-point: 316 °C

Solubility: Insoluble in water

Quercetin was previously evaluated by IARC (IARC, 1999) as *not classifiable as to its carcinogenicity to humans* (Group 3).

(ii)　Kaempferol

Chem. Abstr. Serv. Reg. No.: 520-18-3

IUPAC name: 3,5,7-trihydroxy-2-(4-hydroxyphenyl)-4H-chromen-4-one

Description: Yellow powder (Ding *et al.*, 2006; van Beek & Montoro, 2009; O'Neil, 2013)

Melting-point: 276 °C

Solubility: Slowly soluble in water

(iii)　Isorhamnetin

Chem. Abstr. Serv. Reg. No.: 480-19-3

IUPAC name: 3,5,7-trihydroxy-2-(4-hydroxy-3-methoxyphenyl)chromen-4-one

Description: Yellow powder (Ding *et al.*, 2006; van Beek & Montoro, 2009; O'Neil, 2013)

Melting-point: 307 °C

Fig. 1.1 Structural and molecular formulae and relative molecular mass of the major constituents found in *Ginkgo biloba*

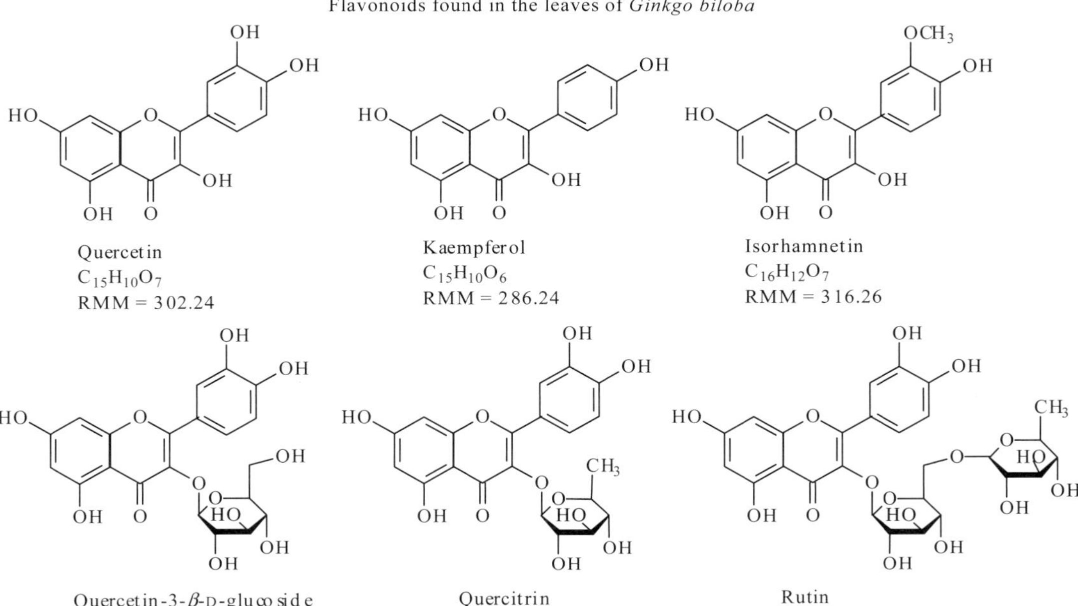

Ginkgolide A- RMM=408.40; $C_{20}H_{24}O_9$; Ginkgolide B- RMM=424.40; $C_{20}H_{24}O_{10}$
Ginkgolide C- RMM=440.40; $C_{20}H_{24}O_{11}$; Bilobalide - RMM=326.3; $C_{15}H_{18}O_8$

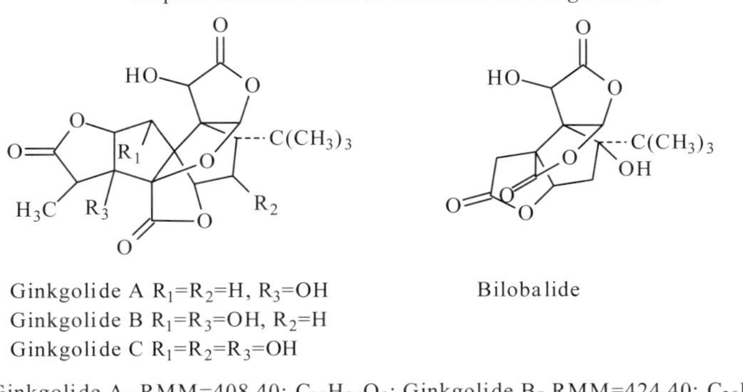

RMM, relative molecular mass
From Ding *et al.* (2006) and Leistner & Drewke (2010)

(c)   *Lactone components*

(i)   *Ginkgolide A*

Chem. Abstr. Serv. Reg. No.: 15291-75-5

IUPAC name: 9H-1,7a-(epoxymethano)-1H, 6aH-cyclopenta[c]furo[2,3-b]furo[3',2':3,4]-cyclopenta[1,2-days]furan-5,9,12(4H)-trione, 3-(1,1-dimethylethyl)hexahydro-4,7b-dihydroxy-8-methyl-, [1R-(1α,3β,3aS*,4β,6aα ,7aα,7bα,8α,10aα,11aS*)]-)

Description: White crystalline substance (Ding *et al.*, 2006; van Beek & Montoro, 2009; O'Neil, 2013)

Melting-point: 280 °C

(ii)   *Ginkgolide B*

Chem. Abstr. Serv. Reg. No.: 15291-77-7

IUPAC name: 9H-1,7a-(epoxymethano)-1H,6aH-cyclopenta[c]furo[2,3-b]furo[3',2':3,4]-cyclopenta[1,2-d]furan-5,9,12(4H)-trione, 3-(1,1-dimethylethyl)hexahydro-4,7b,11-trihydroxy-8-methyl-, [1R-(1α,3β,3aS *,4β,6aα,7aα,7bα,8α,10aα,11β,11aR*)]-)

Description: White crystalline substance (Ding *et al.*, 2006; van Beek & Montoro, 2009; O'Neil, 2013)

Melting-point: ~300 °C

(iii)   *Ginkgolide C*

Chem. Abstr. Serv. Reg. No.: 15291-76-6

IUPAC name: 9H-1,7a-(epoxymethano)-1H,6aH-cyclopenta[c]furo[2,3-b]furo[3',2':3,4]-cyclopenta[1,2-d]furan-5,9,12(4H)-trione, 3-(1,1-dimethylethyl)hexahydro-2,4,-7b,11-tetrahydroxy-8-methyl-, [1R-(1α,2α,3 β,3aS*,4β,6aα,7aα,7bα,8α,10aα,11α,11aR*)]-)

Description: White crystalline substance (Ding *et al.*, 2006; van Beek & Montoro, 2009; O'Neil, 2013)

Melting-point: ~300 °C

(iv)   *Bilobalide*

Chem. Abstr. Serv. Reg. No.: 33570-04-6

IUPAC name: (5aR-(3aS*,5aα,8b,8aS*,9a,10a-α))-9-(1,1-dimethylethyl)-10,10a-dihydro-8,9-dihydroxy-4H,5aH,9H-furo[2,3-b] furo[3',2':2,3]cyclopenta[1,2-c] furan-2,4,7(3H,8H)-trione

(v)   *Ginkgotoxin*

Chem. Abstr. Serv. Reg. No.: 1464-33-1

IUPAC name: 5-Hydroxy-3-(hydroxymethyl)-4-(methoxymethyl)-6-methylpyridine)

1.1.3 Technical and commercial products, and impurities

Products containing dried ginkgo leaf, dried ginkgo leaf extract, and standardized dried ginkgo leaf extract are sold worldwide as herbal medicinal products, dietary supplements, and food additives. Tablets and capsules containing between 40–60 mg of extract are sold in the USA as dietary supplements (Hänsel, 1991; Brestel & Van Dyke, 1991). In Europe, the extract has been sold primarily as a phytopharmaceutical in a variety of dosage forms such as tablets, liquids, and parenteral preparations (Hänsel, 1991; Brestel & Van Dyke, 1991), and is now available as a herbal medicinal product and food supplement (Lachenmeier *et al.*, 2012). Commercial products have been shown to contain variable amounts of the active constituents, and some also contain high amounts of ginkgolic acids (McKenna *et al.*, 2002; Consumer Council, 2000; Harnly *et al.*, 2012). The flavonoids present in ginkgo are primarily in the glycoside form (Ding *et al.*, 2006; van Beek & Montoro, 2009). The most widely used quality assurance assays (Association of Analytical Communities, AOAC; United States Pharmacopeia, USP, etc) are based on the measurement of free flavonoids obtained directly from the hydrolysis of the flavonoid glycosides. Addition of cheaper plant material containing large amounts of rutin or other flavonoids and flavonoid glycosides to boost the apparent content of flavonol glycosides has been reported, and more recent tests call for evaluation of flavonoid ratios to detect such adulteration (Harnly *et al.*, 2012).

Also, enzyme-assisted extraction has led to an increase in the amount of impurities in the extract (van Beek & Montoro, 2009). Commercial standardized *Ginkgo biloba* extracts are now prepared through a complex series of extractions and back-extractions using different solvents. The purpose is to purify the flavonol glycosides and to remove unwanted compounds (Harnly *et al.*, 2012).

Kressmann *et al.* (2002) investigated the pharmaceutical quality and phytochemical composition of several different brands of *Ginkgo biloba* sold as dietary supplements in the USA. In-vitro dissolution characteristics and phytochemical content varied between products, in some cases dramatically (as for the ginkgolic acid content). [This study highlighted the difficulty of estimating exposure to botanical products and their constituent phytochemicals, which may be marketed under the same name, but have very different compositions.]

1.2 Analysis

Identification tests for *Ginkgo biloba* in the USP are based on high-performance thin-layer chromatography (HPTLC). Botanical identity and composition are confirmed by HPTLC, as well as macroscopic and microscopic examination (USP, 2013). A standardized developing solvent system for flavonoids includes ethyl acetate, anhydrous formic acid, glacial acetic acid, and water (100:11:11:26). The spraying reagents include 5 mg/mL of 2-aminoethyl diphenylborinate in methanol and 50 mg/mL of polyethylene glycol 400 in alcohol. A standardized developing solvent system for terpene lactones includes toluene, ethyl acetate, acetone and methanol (20:10:10:1.2). Acetic anhydride is used as spraying reagent (USP, 2013).

The USP requires that a dry extract of *Ginkgo biloba* dried leaf is characterized by containing not less than 22% and not more than 27% of flavonoids calculated as flavonol glycosides via high-performance liquid chromatography (HPLC). The extract should also contains not less than 5.4% and not more than 12% of terpene lactones. *Ginkgo biloba* leaf extract is required to have a ratio of crude plant material to powdered extract between 35:1 and 67:1. A mobile phase composed of methanol, water, and phosphoric acid (100:100:1) is used for the content of flavonol glycosides. A gradient eluent mixture of methanol and water (25:75–90:10) is used for the content of terpene lactones (USP, 2013).

Validated HPLC methods for flavonoids and terpenes in ginkgo have been published (Gray *et al.*, 2007; Croom *et al.*, 2007). Quantitative determination of the major components of ginkgo have also been reported using combination methods including HPLC, gas chromatography (GC), nuclear magnetic resonance (NMR), and mass spectrometry (MS) (Ding *et al.*, 2006; van Beek & Montoro, 2009). Methods that have been recently standardized for the quantitation of the major components of ginkgo include reversed-phase HPLC/ESI-MS (high-performance liquid chromatography/electrospray ionization-mass spectrometry), HPLC/MS-MS, GC-MS, and ^{1}H-NMR (Ding *et al.*, 2006; van Beek & Montoro, 2009; Li *et al.*, 2004).

Pharmacopeial standards are mandatory in registered drug products, but not in dietary supplement or food products, so it is difficult to evaluate the composition of marketed non-drug products.

1.3 Uses

1.3.1 Indications

Ginkgo leaves and fruit are used medicinally for a variety of conditions. Among the uses reported for ginkgo are treatment of asthma, bronchitis, cardiovascular diseases, improvement of peripheral blood flow, and reduction of cerebral function (Perry, 1984; Mouren et al., 1994). Additional uses include allergies, bronchitis, tinnitus, dementia, and memory issues (Morgenstern & Biermann, 1997; Wang et al., 2010; Holgers et al., 1994). The World Health Organization and the German Commission E have included additional uses for peripheral arterial occlusive diseases (WHO, 1999).

Previous studies performed using standardized ginkgo extracts have also found therapeutic benefits for early stages of dementia, peripheral arterial occlusive diseases, cerebral insufficiency due to lack of adequate blood flow, and for other related ailments (Wesnes et al., 2000; Oken et al., 1998; Pittler & Ernst, 2000; Hopfenmüller, 1994). Lately, several clinical trials to evaluate cognitive performance for Alzheimer disease, multiple sclerosis, and for peripheral arterial diseases have been conducted with mixed results (Vellas et al., 2012; Schneider, 2012; Weinmann et al., 2010; Snitz et al., 2009; Herrschaft et al., 2012; Nicolaï et al., 2009; Hilton et al., 2013).

1.3.2 Dosage

According to the Commission E Monographs, 120–240 mg of standardized dry extract in liquid or solid pharmaceutical form for oral intake, is given in two or three daily doses for dementia syndromes, such as primary degenerative dementia, vascular dementia, and mixed forms of both. Doses of 120–160 mg of native dry extract is given in two or three daily doses for improvement of pain-free walking distance in peripheral arterial occlusive disease, and vertigo and tinnitus of vascular and involutional origin

(Blumenthal et al., 1998). These doses correspond to an estimate of 50 fresh ginkgo leaves to yield one standard dose of the extract. Dried extracts of leaves in the form of tablets, standardized to contain 24% flavone glycosides and 6% terpenes, are available commercially (Brestel & Van Dyke, 1991; McKenna et al., 2002; Hilton et al., 2013; Kleijnen & Knipschild, 1992).

1.3.3 Trends in use

According to USA National Health and Nutrition Survey (NHANES) data, there has been a steady decline in the prevalence of use in men and women from 1999–2002 (3.9%), and 2003–2006 (3.0%), to 2007–2010 (1.6%) (NHANES, 1999–2010). Barnes et al. (2008) reported that in a survey of users of complementary and alternative medicine that 11.3% of supplement-users had used ginkgo in the previous 30 days.

1.4 Production, sales, and consumption

1.4.1 Production

Ginkgo has been planted on a large scale in France and USA since the 1980s and plantations are found in the south eastern USA with a density of 10 million ginkgo trees per 1000 acres (Del Tredici, 1991, 2005). A large amount of the ginkgo sold in the USA comes from plantations in China (Schmid & Balz, 2005).

1.4.2 Sales

Ginkgo biloba is the most frequently prescribed herbal medicine in Germany and one of the most commonly used over-the-counter herbal preparations in the USA (Diamond et al., 2000). The use of dietary supplements in the USA has significantly increased in the past few years. According to the 2012 Nutrition Business Journal Annual report (Nutrition Business

Journal, 2012), ginkgo was the 37th best-selling herbal dietary supplement in the USA in 2011, and the 13th best-selling (by dollar volume) herbal dietary supplement at US$ 90 million. An estimated 3 million individuals in the USA used ginkgo in 2007, a relatively steady decline from approximately 7.7 million users, and sales of US$ 151 million in 2002 (Wu *et al.*, 2011). According to IMS Health MIDAS data (IMS Health, 2012), total worldwide sales of *Ginkgo biloba* products in 2012 were US$ 1.26 billion. China accounted for 46% of sales (US$ 578 million). Fifty-six individuals per 1000 reported using natural health products containing ginkgo in a Canadian survey in 2006 (Singh & Levine, 2006). Other countries with substantial sales included Germany (US$ 152 million), Australia (US$ 61 million), France (US$ 53 million), Brazil (US$ 48 million), Republic of Korea (US$ 40 million), and Viet Nam (US$ 37 million).

1.4.3 Consumption

Consumption of ginkgo occurs orally or topically in pharmaceutical or dietary-supplement formulations (Hänsel, 1991; Brestel & Van Dyke, 1991; Blumenthal *et al.*, 1998). Consumers may also be exposed through products containing ginkgo, such as teas, yogurts, and cosmetics that are sold over the internet. [The Working Group also noted that besides the use in medicinal products and supplements, ginkgo has also been used in Europe as ingredient in foods, as in the so-called "wellness" beverages.]

Ginkgo biloba extract is one of four herbal preparations refunded by health insurance in Germany, on prescription by a medical doctor (AMR, 2013).

1.5 Occupational exposure

No data were available to the Working Group. Workers on ginkgo plantations and in ginkgo-processing plants are probably exposed.

1.6 Regulations and guidelines

According to the 1994 Dietary Supplement Health and Education Act (DSHEA) in the USA, ginkgo is considered a dietary supplement under the general umbrella of "foods" (FDA, 1994). In the USA, dietary supplements put on the market before 15 October 1994 do not require proof of safety; however, the labelling recommendations for dietary supplements include warnings, dosage recommendations, and substantiated "structure or function" claims. The product label must declare prominently that the claims have not been evaluated by the Food and Drug Administration, and bear the statement "This product is not intended to diagnose, treat, cure, or prevent any disease" (Croom & Walker, 1995).

In Europe, ginkgo is available either as food supplement or as medicinal product. The Commission E approved different types of ginkgo preparations for human consumption (Diamond *et al.*, 2000) and published a monograph dedicated to standardized ginkgo leaf extract (Mills & Bone, 2005). In Europe, most herbal products, including ginkgo, were marketed as medicinal products. This changed when Directive 65/65/EEC (Council of the European Economic Community, 1965) was implemented, with the requirement of quality, efficacy, and safety data on medicinal products. Many medicinal products did not satisfy those requirements and were nevertheless marketed as food supplements, often just changing the label. This is currently the case for ginkgo, which is widely marketed as a food supplement in Europe (Lachenmeier *et al.*, 2012).

2. Cancer in Humans

2.1 Background

The available epidemiological studies on ginkgo and cancer consisted of one randomized controlled trial (the Ginko Evaluation of

Memory, GEM study), four nested case–control studies from the Vitamins and Lifestyle (VITAL) cohort, and one population based case–control study of cancer of the ovary.

2.2 Randomized controlled trial

See Table 2.1

The Ginkgo Evaluation of Memory (GEM) study is a randomized, double-blind, placebo-controlled clinical trial on *Ginkgo biloba* extract (EGb 761®) for the prevention of dementia (DeKosky *et al.*, 2008; Biggs *et al.*, 2010). Participants aged 75 years and older (*n* = 3069) from four clinical centres in the USA were enrolled between 2000 and 2002, and were randomized to either the placebo group, or the group receiving ginkgo as two daily doses of 120 mg of ginkgo extract. Participants were followed until 2008, with a median follow-up of 6.1 years. [The authors did not specify the period of treatment.] Invasive cancer (excluding non-melanoma cancer of the skin) was evaluated as a secondary outcome, and identified from hospital admission and discharge records. Analyses were performed with intention to treat beginning at randomization and at 1 year after randomization. Adherence to study protocol was 64% for the placebo group and 59% for the group receiving gingko.

Of the 310 hospitalizations for cancer, 162 occurred in the group receiving gingko, and 148 occurred in the group receiving placebo (adjusted hazard ratio, HR, 1.09; 95% CI, 0.87–1.36). For the observation period beginning at randomization, elevated hazard ratios were reported for cancers of the colon and rectum (HR, 1.62; 95% CI, 0.92–2.87), urinary bladder (HR, 1.21; 95% CI, 0.65–2.26) and breast (HR, 2.15; 95% CI, 0.97–4.80) and a decreased hazard ratio was found for cancer of the prostate (HR, 0.71; 95% CI, 0.43–1.17). The hazard ratios for cancer of the lung and combined leukaemia and lymphoma were close to unity (see Table 2.1 for values). In general, hazard ratios for the second observation period, beginning 1 year after randomization, were generally similar, but with a statistically significant increase in the risk of cancer of the breast (HR, 2.50; 95% CI, 1.03–6.07) and lower risk of cancer of the bladder (HR, 0.99; 95% CI, 0.52–2.61). The hazard ratios from a sensitivity analysis excluding participants who reported cancer 5 years before baseline were within 20%, with the exception of an increase for cancer of the colorectum reaching statistical significance (HR, 2.15; 95% CI, 1.11–4.15) and a attenuation of risk of cancer of the breast, losing statistical significance (HR, 1.55; 95% CI, 0.66–3.63). [The major strengths of the study were randomization of treatment groups and adequate follow-up procedures for identifying cancer cases hospitalized during follow-up; however, incident cancers not resulting in hospitalization may have been missed and the follow-up was short, so the statistical power for cancer was low, and long-term carcinogenic effects due to exposure could not be evaluated. The study findings were difficult to interpret since the sites with statistically significant associations were not consistent in different analyses. Furthermore, the generalizability of the findings was limited by the clinical trial design.]

2.3 Case–control studies

See Table 2.2

The VITAL cohort includes 77 738 men and women, aged 50–76 years, in Washington state, USA, who completed a postal questionnaire on supplement use, diet, health history, and risk factors between 2000 and 2002 (White *et al.*, 2004). The overall response rate was about 23%. Detailed data on use of vitamins, mineral supplements, herbal preparations and related products in the past 10 years were obtained via questions regarding brand, current and past use, frequency and duration of use. Dose information was not obtained because of lack of accurate information on potency. Cohort members were followed for 5–6 years, with incident cancer cases or deaths

Table 2.1 Randomized intervention trial on exposure to *Ginkgo biloba* extract

Reference, study location and period	Total subjects	Study design	Organ site	Exposure categories	Exposed cases	Hazard ratio (95% CI)	Covariates Comments
Biggs *et al.* (2010), USA 2000–8	3069	Randomized double-blind, placebo-controlled clinical trial	Any	Ginkgo extract: 120 mg, 2× per day; randomization observation period	162	1.09 (0.87–1.36)	Adjusted for clinical centre. GEM study, participants aged ≥ 75 yrs, intention to treat % compliance: placebo, 64%; ginkgo extract, 59% Sensitivity analysis performed excluding participants with a 5-yr history of cancer before enrolment. Median follow-up, 6.1 yr End-point assessment from hospital admissions and discharge records
			Prostate		27	0.71 (0.43–1.17)	
			Lung		26	0.90 (0.53–1.52)	
			Colorectal		31	1.62 (0.92–2.87)	
			Urinary bladder		22	1.21 (0.65–2.26)	
			Breast		18	2.15 (0.97–4.80)	
			Leukaemia and lymphoma		13	1.07 (0.49–2.34)	
			Any	1 yr post-randomization observation period	150	1.07 (0.85–1.35)	
			Prostate		25	0.68 (0.41–1.14)	
			Lung		27	1.00 (0.58–1.70)	
			Colorectal		22	1.27 (0.68–2.40)	
			Urinary bladder		18	0.99 (0.52–1.91)	
			Breast		16	2.50 (1.03–6.07)	
			Leukaemia and lymphoma		13	1.17 (0.52–2.61)	

GEM, Ginkgo Evaluation of Memory; yr, year

Table 2.2 Case–control studies of cancer and exposure to *Ginkgo biloba* extract

Reference, study location and period	Total No. cases Total No. controls	Control source (hospital, population)	Exposure assessment	Organ site	Exposure categories	Exposed cases	Relative risk (95% CI)	Covariates Comments
Satia *et al.* (2009), Washington State, USA	Lung cancer, 665 76 460 Colorectal cancer, 428 76 084	Nested case–control study: VITAL cohort	Mailed baseline questionnaire; supplement use 10 yrs before baseline	Lung cancer Colorectal cancer	Any pill per day – previous 10 yrs	80 49	1.04 (0.82–1.32) 0.83 (0.59–1.17)	Age, sex, education, smoking Age, sex, education, physical activity, fruit and vegetable consumption, BMI, NSAID use, and sigmoidoscopy Age 50–76 yr; low response rate (21.8%); cases identified by cancer registry (SEER); follow-up until 2006 (mean, 5 yr)
Hotaling *et al.* (2011) Washington State, USA	330 76 720	Nested case–control study: VITAL cohort	Same as Satia *et al.* (2009)	Urothelial carcinoma of the bladder	10 yr daily average	NR	NR (no statistical signficant association in multivariate analysis)	Age, sex, race, education, family history of bladder cancer, smoking, and fruit and vegetable intake Age 50–76 yr; cases identified by cancer registry (SEER); follow-up, 6 yr
Brasky *et al.* (2010), Washington State, USA	880 34 136	Nested case–control study: VITAL cohort	Same as Satia *et al.* (2009)	Breast cancer	Former	47	1.06 (0.77–1.45)	Adjusted for age, race, education, BMI, height, fruit & vegetable consumption, alcohol consumption, physical activity, reproductive history, history of hysterectomy, hormone therapy, family history of breast cancer and benign breast biopsy, mammography, use of aspirin, ibuprofen, naproxen and multivitamins. Postmenopausal women; excluded women with history of breast cancer or with in-situ breast cancer; participation rate, 23%; mean follow-up, 6 yr
					Current 10 yr daily average	56	0.85 (0.64–1.13)	
					low (< 4 days/wk or any use < 3 yr)	82	0.98 (0.77–1.25)	
					high (≥ 4 days/wk for ≥ 3 yr)	40	0.88 (0.63–1.24)	
					Trend		*P* = 0.51	

Table 2.2 (continued)

Reference, study location and period	Total No. cases Total No. controls	Control source (hospital, population)	Exposure assessment	Organ site	Exposure categories	Exposed cases	Relative risk (95% CI)	Covariates Comments
Brasky *et al.* (2011), Washington State, USA	1602 33 637	Cancer-registry study: VITAL cohort	Same as Satia *et al.* (2009)	Prostate cancer (invasive)	*Use* Average, 10 yr	165	1.03 (0.87–1.22)	Age, race, education, BMI, PSA test, history of prostate disease, family history of prostate cancer, multivitamin use, memory loss, diabetes. Males: age 50–76 yr.; low response rate (~22%); cases identified by cancer registry (SEER); follow-up; 6 yr
					Low (< 4 days/wk or any use < 3 yr)	127	1.08 (0.90–1.31)	
					High (≥ 4 days/ wk for ≥ 3 yr)	85	1.04 (0.82–1.31)	
					Trend		*P* = 0.52	
Ye *et al.* (2007) MA, NH, USA, 1998–2003	668 721	Population	In-person interviews and self-administered dietary questionnaires	Ovarian cancer (epithelial)	Weekly; at least 6 months	11	0.41 (0.20–0.84)	Age, study centre, oral contraceptive use, parity, and Jewish ethnic background RR similar for current versus no-longer-using, no association with exposure duration; however, small number of exposed cases. Participation rate: cases, 52%; controls, 39%
					Ginkgo alone (not other drugs)	6	0.36 (0.14–0.91)	
					Tumour type			
					Mucinous	3	1.17 (0.34–4.05)	
					Non-mucinous	8	0.33 (0.15–0.74)	

BMI, body mass index; NR, not reported; NSAID, nonsteroidal anti-inflammatory drugs; PSA, prostate-specific antigen; RR, relative risk; SEER, Surveillance, Epidemiology, and End Results programme of the National Cancer Institute; VITAL; VITamins and Lifestyle Cohort Study; wk, week; yr, year identified via linkage system to the SEER cancer registry, state death files, and other databases.

Associations between ginkgo intake and cancer were investigated in nested case–control studies with the large VITAL cohort for cancers of the lung and colorectum (Satia *et al.*, 2009), prostate (Brasky *et al.*, 2011), breast (Brasky *et al.*, 2010), and urothelial carcinoma of the bladder (Hotaling *et al.*, 2011) (see Table 2.2 for more information). No statistically significant increase or decrease in the occurrence of any of the cancers examined was observed in these studies. Hazard ratios were near unity for all associations reported, except cancer of the colorectum and any use of ginko (HR, 0.83; 95% CI, 0.59–1.17) and cancer of the breast and current use (HR, 0.85; 95% CI, 0.65–1.13) or high average use (HR, 0.88; 95% CI, 0.63–1.24). [The strengths of these studies were the prospective design, adequate case-ascertainment, broad age range of the study participants, and large size. The major limitations were use of self-reported exposure information, which was not updated after baseline; short follow-up time; low response rates, and inadequate evaluation of exposure–response and exposure–time relationships. These limitations would most likely bias the findings towards the null.]

Ye *et al.* (2007) conducted a population-based case–control study of 668 incident cases of cancer of the ovary (identified from state registries and tumour boards) and 721 age- and residence-matched general population controls. Approximately 53% of eligible cases and 39% of eligible controls participated. Intake of ginkgo and other herbal remedies, dietary information and other factors was assessed via in-person interview and self-administered questionnaire. Ginkgo intake at least weekly for 6 months or more was associated with a decreased risk of cancer of the ovary (adjusted odds ratio, OR, 0.41; 95% CI, 0.20–0.84). However, the reduced risk was restricted to women with non-mucinous ovarian tumours (OR, 0.33; 9%% CI, 0.15–0.74; eight exposed cases). This study also included

cell-culture analyses showing antiproliferative effects of *G. biloba* extract in serous (non-mucinous), but not in mucinous ovarian cancer cells. [The consistency of findings in cell culture and humans was a strength of this study. Limitations of the study were low statistical power, low participation rates, exposure assessment only for 1 year before diagnosis, and lack of information on dose.]

3. Cancer in Experimental Animals

3.1 Mouse

See Table 3.1

In one study of oral administration, groups of 50 male and 50 female $B6C3F_1$ mice (age, 6–7 weeks) were given *Ginkgo biloba* extract at a dose of 0 (corn oil vehicle, 5 mL/kg body weight, bw), 200, 600, or 2000 mg/kg bw by gavage, 5 days per week, for 104 weeks. The *G. biloba* extract contained 31.2% flavonol, 15.4% terpene lactones (bilobalide, 6.94%; ginkgolide A, 3.74%; ginkgolide B, 1.62%; ginkgolide C, 3.06%), and ginkgolic acid at 10.45 ppm. Survival of males at 600 and 2000 mg/kg bw was significantly less than that of controls; survival of females at 600 mg/kg bw was significantly greater than that of controls. Mean body weights of males at 600 and 2000 mg/kg bw were less (10% or more) than those of the controls after weeks 85 and 77, respectively; mean body weights of females at 2000 mg/kg bw were generally less (10% or more) than those of the controls between weeks 17 and 69, and after week 93.

In males, the incidence of hepatocellular carcinoma, hepatocellular adenoma or carcinoma (combined), and hepatoblastoma was significantly increased in the groups receiving the lowest, intermediate, and highest dose, and had a significant positive trend. Hepatocellular carcinoma and hepatoblastoma were observed in the same animal on multiple occasions. The

Table 3.1 Studies of carcinogenicity with *Ginkgo biloba* extracts in mice

Strain (sex) Duration Reference	Dosing regimen, Animals/group at start	Incidence of tumours	Significance[a]	Comments
B6C3F$_1$ (M, F) 104–105 wk NTP (2013), Hoenerhoff *et al.* (2013)	0 (control), 200, 600, 2000 mg/kg bw, by gavage in corn oil, 5 days/wk for 104–105 wk 50 M and 50 F/group (age, 6–7 wk)	Hepatocellular adenoma: 17/50*, 37/50**, 41/50**, 48/50** (F) Hepatocellular carcinoma: 22/50*, 31/50***, 41/50**, 47/50** (M) 9/50*, 10/50, 15/50, 44/50** (F) Hepatocellular adenoma or carcinoma (combined): 39/50*, 46/50****, 46/50****, 49/50** (M) 20/50*, 39/50**, 41/50**, 49/50** (F) Hepatoblastoma: 3/50*, 28/50**, 36/50**, 38/50** (M) 1/50*, 1/50, 8/50***, 11/50****(F) Thyroid gland follicular cell adenoma: 0/49, 0/49, 2/50, 2/50 (4%) (M)[b]	*$P < 0.001$ (trend) **$P \leq 0.001$ ***$P \leq 0.05$ ****$P \leq 0.01$	*Ginkgo biloba* study material contained: 31.2% flavonol, 15.4% terpene lactones (bilobalide, 6.94%; ginkgolide A, 3.74% ; ginkgolide B, 1.62%; ginkgolide C, 3.06%), ginkgolic acid, 10.45 ppm HPLC/UV profiles identified 37 components: quercetin, 34.08%; kaempferol, 27.7%; isorhamnetin, 5.43%. HPLC/ELS profiles identified 18 components: bilobalide, 17.31%; ginkgolide C, 3.25%; ginkgolide A, 9.06%; ginkgolide B, 2.05%; quercetin, 28.74%; kaempferol, 12.58%; isorhamnetin, 2.24%. Mean body weight of males at 600 and 2000 mg/kg bw were $\geq$ 10% less than the vehicle-control groups after wk 85 and 77, respectively. Mean body weight of females at 2000 mg/kg bw was $\geq$ 10% less than the vehicle-control group between wk 17 and 69 and after wk 93

[a] The Poly-3 test was used for all statistical analysis in this table.

[b] Historical incidence for 2-year gavage studies with corn oil vehicle-control groups (mean ± standard deviation): 1/349 (0.3% ± 0.8%), range, 0–2%; all routes: 7/1143 (0.6% ± 1.0%), range, 0–2%.

bw, body weight; ELS, evaporative light scattering; F, female; HPLC/UV, high-performance liquid chromatography/ultraviolet; M, male; wk, week

Table 3.2 Studies of carcinogenicity with *Ginkgo biloba* extracts in rats

Strain (sex) Duration Reference	Dosing regimen, Animals/group at start	Incidence of tumours	Significance[a]	Comments
F344/N (M, F) 104– 105 wk NTP (2013)	0 (control), 100, 300, 1000 mg/kg bw, by gavage in corn oil, 5 days/wk for 104–105 wk 50 M and 50 F/group (age, 6–7 wk)	Mononuclear cell leukaemia: 9/50*, 12/50, 22/50**, 21/45** (M) Thyroid follicular cell adenoma: 2/50***, 1/50, 3/50, 5/45 (M) 1/49, 0/50, 3/49, 1/49 (F)[b] Thyroid follicular cell carcinoma: 0/49, 0/50, 1/49, 1/49 (F)[c] Nose respiratory epithelium adenoma: 0/49, 0/49, 2/50, 0/46 (F)[d]	*P = 0.004 (trend) **P ≤ 0.01 ***P = 0.04	*Ginkgo biloba* study material contained: 31.2% flavonol, 15.4% terpene lactones (bilobalide, 6.94%, ginkgolide A, 3.74%; ginkgolide B, 1.62%; ginkgolide C, 3.06%), ginkgolic acid. 10.45 ppm HPLC/UV profiles identified 37 components: quercetin, 34.08%; kaempferol, 27.7%; isorhamnetin, 5.43% HPLC/ELS profiles identified 18 components: bilobalide, 17.31%; ginkgolide C, 3.25%; ginkgolide A, 9.06%; ginkgolide B, 2.05%; quercetin, 28.74%; kaempferol, 12.58%; isorhamnetin, 2.24% Mean body weight of males at 300 mg/kg bw, ≥ 10% less than the vehicle-control group after wk 93; at 1000 mg/kg bw, ≥ 10% less than the vehicle-control group after wk 89. Mean body weight of females: at 300 mg/kg bw: ≥ 10% less than the vehicle-control group after wk 93; at 1000 mg/kg bw, ≥ 10% less than the vehicle-control group after wk 89. Body-weight suppression at highest dose could have reduced tumour incidences.

[a] The Poly-3 test was used for all statistical analyses in this table.

[b] Historical incidence for 2-year gavage studies with corn-oil vehicle-control groups (mean ± standard deviation): 3/298 (1.0% ± 1.1%), range 0–2%; all routes: 8/1186 (0.7% ± 1.0%), range, 0–2%

[c] Historical incidence for 2-year gavage studies with corn-oil vehicle-control groups (mean ± standard deviation): 1/298 (0.3% ± 0.8%), range 0–2%; all routes: 5/1186 (0.4% ± 1.0%), range, 0–4%

[d] Historical incidence 2-year gavage studies with corn-oil vehicle-control groups (mean ± standard deviation): 0/299; all routes: 1/1196 (0.1% ± 0.4%), range, 0–2%

bw, body weight; ELS, evaporative light scattering; F, female; HPLC/UV, high-performance liquid chromatography/ultraviolet; M, male; wk, week incidence of thyroid follicular cell adenoma was higher in the group receiving the intermediate dose (2 out of 50; 4%) and highest dose (2 out of 50; 4%) groups than among the historical controls in the National Toxicology Program (NTP) Technical Report study series (historical incidence range, 0–2%; corn oil vehicle controls, 1 out of 349; all routes, 7 out of 1449).

In females, the incidence of hepatocellular adenoma was significantly higher in the groups receiving the lowest, intermediate, and highest dose, and had a significant positive trend. The incidence of hepatocellular carcinoma was significantly higher in the group receiving the highest dose, and had a significant positive trend. The incidence of hepatocellular adenoma or carcinoma (combined) was significantly higher in the groups receiving the lowest, intermediate, and highest dose, and had a significant positive trend. The incidence of hepatoblastoma was significantly higher at the intermediate and highest dose, and had a significant positive trend (Hoenerhoff *et al.*, 2013; NTP, 2013).

3.2 Rat

See Table 3.2

In one study of oral administration, groups of 50 male and 50 female F344/N rats (age, 6–7 weeks) were given *G. biloba* extract at a dose of 0 (corn oil vehicle, 2.5 mL/kg bw), 100, 300, or 1000 mg/kg bw by gavage, 5 days per week, for 104 weeks for males or 105 weeks for females. The *G. biloba* extract contained 31.2% flavonol, 15.4% terpene lactones (bilobalide, 6.94%; ginkgolide A, 3.74%; ginkgolide B, 1.62%; ginkgolide C, 3.06%), and ginkgolic acid at 10.45 ppm. Survival of males at 1000 mg/kg bw was significantly less than that of the controls. Mean body weights of males and females at 300 mg/kg bw were less (10% or more) than those of the controls after week 93, and those of males and females at 1000 mg/kg bw were less (10% or more) after week 89.

In males, the incidence of mononuclear cell leukaemia was significantly higher in groups at the intermediate and highest dose, and had a significant positive trend. The incidence of thyroid follicular cell adenoma (2 out of 50, 4%; 1 out of 50, 2%; 3 out of 50, 6%; and 5 out of 45, 10%) had a significant positive trend. In females, the incidences of thyroid follicular cell adenoma (1 out of 49, 0 out of 50, 3 out of 49, 1 out of 49), thyroid follicular cell carcinoma (0 out of 49, 0 out of 50, 1 out of 49, 1 out of 49), and nose respiratory epithelium adenoma (0 out of 49, 0 out of 49, 2 out of 50, 0 out of 46) in the dosed groups were higher than the ranges for historical controls (all routes: 8 out of 1186 [0–2%], 5 out of 1186 [0–4%] and 1 out of 1186 [0–2%], respectively) in the NTP Technical Report study series (NTP, 2013). [The Working Group noted that body-weight suppression at the highest dose could have reduced the tumour incidence, and that nose respiratory epithelium adenomas are rare spontaneous tumours in F344/N rats.]

4. Mechanistic and Other Relevant Data

4.1 Absorption, distribution, metabolism, and excretion

4.1.1 Humans

Several pharmacokinetics studies on the main active components of *Ginkgo biloba* in humans have been reported (Fourtillan *et al.*, 1995; Wójcicki *et al.*, 1995; Pietta *et al.*, 1997; Mauri *et al.*, 2001; Drago *et al.*, 2002; Wang *et al.*, 2003).

Wójcicki *et al.* (1995) investigated the pharmacokinetics of flavonoid glycosides in 18 healthy volunteers given one of three different formulations of *Ginkgo biloba* (capsules, drops, and tablets) by oral administration. The area-under-the-curve values were similar for all formulations. Drago *et al.* (2002) evaluated the pharmacokinetics of ginkgolide B, the main active ingredient in *G. biloba* extract, in 12 healthy volunteers given different doses (80 mg once daily, or 40 mg twice daily, for 7 days). The results indicated that the maximum concentration time (T_{max}) was 2.3 hours for both dosages, and the elimination half-life ($t_{1/2\beta}$) and mean residence time (MRT) were longer for the dose of 40 mg given twice daily than that for a single 80 mg dose, although the latter had a higher concentration peak (C_{max}) (Drago *et al.*, 2002). After oral administration of a tablet containing *G. biloba* extract in humans, two polyphenols, quercetin and kaempferol were found in urine mainly as glucuronides, and to a lesser extent, sulfates (Wang *et al.*, 2003).

As part of a clinical study to determine the metabolites of *G. biloba* after human oral consumption, an extract of *G. biloba* leaves was given to six healthy volunteers [sex, age, and weight not specified] as a single dose of 4.0 g per day (Pietta *et al.*, 1997). Urine samples were collected for 2 days, and blood samples were withdrawn every 30 minutes for 5 hours. The samples were purified through solid-phase extraction with C_{18} cartridges (SPE C_{18} cartridges) and analysed by reversed-phase liquid chromatography–diode array detection for the presence of metabolites. Only urine samples contained detectable amounts of substituted benzoic acids, i.e. 4-hydroxybenzoic acid conjugate, 4-hydroxyhippuric acid, 3-methoxy-4-hydroxyhippuric acid, 3,4-dihydroxybenzoic acid, 4-hydroxybenzoic acid, hippuric acid and 3-methoxy-4-hydroxybenzoic acid (vanillic acid). No metabolites were detected in the blood (Pietta *et al.*, 1997; see Fig. 4.1).

The pharmacokinetics of quercetin and its glycosides (components of *G. biloba*) have been extensively studied in humans (Prior, 2006). Quercetin glycoside was originally assumed to be absorbed from the small intestine after cleavage of the β-glycoside linkage by colonic microflora

(Griffiths & Smith, 1972). Excretion of quercetin or its conjugates in human urine ranged from 0.07% to 17.4% of intake. Only quercetin glucuronides, but not free quercetin, could be detected in the plasma (Prior, 2003).

4.1.2 Experimental systems

Several studies have addressed the issue of absorption and excretion of *Ginkgo biloba* in rats and mice (Moreau *et al.*, 1986; Chen *et al.*, 2007; Ude *et al.*, 2013). In one study in which ^{14}C-labelled *G. biloba* extract (360 mg/kg bw) was administered orally to rats, the amount expired as carbon dioxide only accounted for 16% of the original dose within the first 3 hours. About 38% of the administered dose was exhaled as carbon dioxide after 72 hours; 22% was excreted in the urine, and 29% was excreted in the faeces. Absorption reached at least 60%. A half-life of 4.5 hours and peak of 1.5 hours marked the pharmacokinetics of *G. biloba* in serum, with the characterization of a first-order phase kinetic model. After 48 hours of gradual uptake, radiolabel was primarily found in the plasma. The activity in the erythrocytes was similar to that in the plasma. It was also present in the neuronal, glandular, and ocular tissue, and it was suggested that the upper gastrointestinal tract plays a role in absorption (Moreau *et al.*, 1986). In rats but not in humans, phenylacetic acid or phenylpropionic acid derivatives were found in the urine after oral administration of *G. biloba* leaf extract (Pietta *et al.*, 1995). Recent studies in rats have shown that significant amounts of terpene trilactones (ginkgolides A and B, and bilobalide) and flavonoids (quercetin, kaempferol, and isorhamnetin) cross the blood–brain barrier and enter the central nervous system after intravenous and oral administration of *G. biloba* extract (Chen *et al.*, 2007; Rangel-Ordóñez *et al.*, 2010).

Fig. 4.1 Metabolites of *Ginkgo biloba* in humans

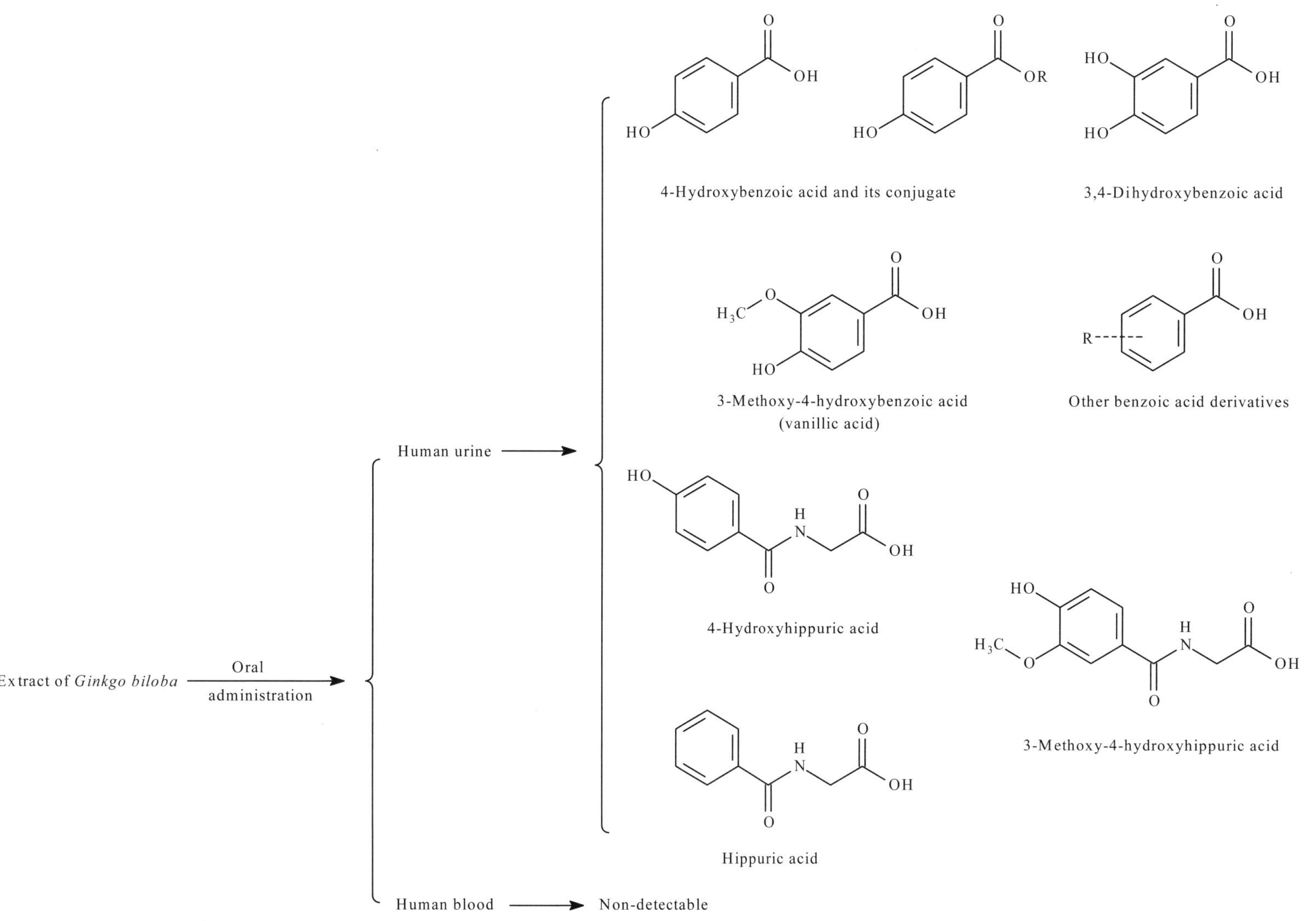

Subjects were given *Gingko biloba* extract orally. Urine samples contain detectable amounts of metabolites of *Ginkgo biloba*, but no metabolites were detected in the blood
Compiled by the Working Group from data in Pietta *et al.* (1997)

4.1.3 Herb–drug interactions

Despite potential therapeutic effects, the widespread use of *G. biloba* extract may also cause herb–drug interactions, altering drug efficiency or leading to undesired toxic effects of concurrent medications, especially for drugs with narrow therapeutic indices. A growing body of literature has shown that *G. biloba* extract and its constituents may influence the pharmacokinetics of coadministered drugs via altering the expression and activity of drug-metabolizing enzymes and transporters. However, the results from in-vitro studies were not always in agreement with those from in-vivo studies; and two similar clinical studies also showed disparities. For instance, in-vitro studies with human microsomes demonstrated that *G. biloba* extract inhibited cytochrome P450 (CYP) CYP2C9 (Mohutsky *et al.*, 2006; Etheridge *et al.*, 2007), while clinical studies showed that *G. biloba* extract had no significant effect on CYP2C9 (Greenblatt *et al.*, 2006; Mohutsky *et al.*, 2006; Uchida *et al.*, 2006). Robertson *et al.* (2008) reported that *G. biloba* extract induced the activity of CYP3A4 in a clinical study, while other studies reported that *G. biloba* extract did not alter CYP3A4 (Gurley *et al.*, 2002; Zadoyan *et al.*, 2012), or decreased CYP3A4 activity (Uchida *et al.*, 2006). [The discrepancy was probably due to multiple factors, for example, different approaches for assessing enzyme activity were applied, different formulations of herbal materials were used, some studies did not include a sufficient sample size to meet statistical requirements; and the sensitivity of detection methods was different; or the studies were conducted in different ethnic groups.]

Clinical studies and case reports have identified herb–drug interactions potentiated by the concurrent use of *G. biloba* extract and prescription drugs, many of which are substrates of CYPs and/or transport P-glycoprotein 1 (multidrug resistance protein 1); these studies are reviewed by Chen *et al.* (2011, 2012).

4.2 Genetic and related effects

4.2.1 Humans

No data were available to the Working Group.

4.2.2 Experimental systems

See Table 4.2

(a) Mutagenicity

Ginkgo biloba extract (up to 10 000 µg/plate) was mutagenic in *Salmonella typhimurium* strains TA98 and TA100 and *Escherichia coli* strain WP2 *uvrA* pKM101 with or without metabolic activation from rat liver S9 (NTP, 2013). Two components of *G. biloba* extract, quercetin and kaempferol, were also found to give positive results in these assays and in other assays for mutagenicity with and without metabolic activation (NTP, 1992, 2013). *G. biloba* constituents that induce mutagenicity include quercetin (Bjeldanes & Chang, 1977; Hardigree & Epler, 1978; Carver *et al.*, 1983; NTP, 1992; Zeiger *et al.*, 1992; Chan *et al.*, 2007), kaempferol (Silva *et al.*, 1997), and ginkgolic acids (Westendorf & Regan, 2000).

(b) Chromosomal damage

No increase in the frequency of micronucleus formation in peripheral blood erythrocytes was observed in male B6C3F$_1$ mice, but results were equivocal in female B6C3F$_1$ mice exposed to *G. biloba* extract at a dose of up to 2.0 g/kg bw per day by gavage for 3 months (NTP, 2013). Quercetin and kaempferol were also found to produce chromosomal alteration in various types of cells (NTP 1992, 2013; Gaspar *et al.*, 1994; Caria *et al.*, 1995; Silva *et al.*, 1997).

(c) DNA damage

A study has examined and compared the genotoxicity of flavonoids in human somatic cells and germ cells. Human somatic cells (human

Table 4.2 Genetic and related effects of *Ginkgo biloba* extract

Test system	Results		Concentration or dose (LED or HID)	Reference
	Without exogenous metabolic system	With exogenous metabolic system		
Salmonella typhimurium TA100 and TA98, reverse mutation	+	+	10 000 µg/plate	NTP (2013)
Escherichia coli WP2 *uvrA*/pKM101 reverse mutation	+	+	10 000 µg/plate	NTP (2013)
Micronucleus formation in peripheral blood erythrocytes of male and female B6C3F$_1$ mice in vivo	– (males), EQ (females)	NT	Up to 2.0 g/kg bw per day by gavage for 3 months	NTP (2013)

+, positive; (+), weakly positive; –, negative; bw, body weight; LED, lowest effective dose; NT, not tested; NR, not reported; EQ, equivocal

lymphocytes) and germ cells (human sperm cells) were treated with flavonoids (including quercetin, kaempferol, and rutin, which are present in *G. biloba* extract) at a concentration of 50–500 µM and their DNA damage potentials were examined using the comet assay (Anderson *et al.*, 1997). Results show that DNA damage was observed in lymphocytes and sperm cells over a similar dose range. [The Working Group noted that genotoxic responses occurred in somatic and germ cells in approximately a one-to-one ratio.] In another study Duthie *et al.* (1997) showed DNA strand breaks (as measured by comet assay) in human cell lines Caco-2 (colon), HepG2 (liver), HeLa (epithelium) and normal lymphocytes after treatment with quercetin.

4.3 Other mechanistic data relevant to carcinogenicity

4.3.1 Effects on cell physiology

Increased levels of thyroid stimulating hormone (TSH) were observed in rats after treatment with *G. biloba* extract for 14 weeks (NTP, 2013). In a 3-month study, follicular cell hypertrophy was observed in male and female rats (NTP, 2013).

G. biloba extract and its constituents including quercetin, kaempferol, and isorhamnetin, may exert estrogenic activity by directly binding both estrogen receptors α and β (Oh & Chung, 2004, 2006). The proliferation of MCF-7 cells in response to *G. biloba* extract was biphasic depending on the concentrations of extract and E2 (17β-estradiol) via estrogen receptor-dependent and independent pathways. In MCF-7 cells, *G. biloba* extract induced cell proliferation at low concentrations of E2, which has little or no estrogenic activity, but blocked the cell proliferation caused by higher concentrations of E2, which shows high estrogenic activity (Oh & Chung, 2006).

Most studies have focused on the pharmacological effects of *G. biloba*. *G. biloba* extract and its constituents have been shown to be involved in many cellular activities, such as anti-oxidant activity, anti-platelet activating factor, anti-inflammatory effect, inhibition of mitochondrial dysfunction, inhibition of amyloid β aggregation in neuroblastoma cells, and anti-apoptosis activity (Smith & Luo, 2004; Chan *et al.*, 2007; Shi *et al.*, 2010a, b).

4.3.2 Effects on cell function

No data were available to the Working Group.

4.4 Susceptibility

No data were available to the Working Group.

4.5 Mechanistic considerations

The genotoxicity of *G. biloba* extract could be one of the mechanisms responsible for its possible carcinogenicity. In addition, quercetin and kaempferol, the two flavonoid constituents that are present in high levels in *G. biloba* extract, are mutagenic as examined in several assays in vitro and may thus contribute to the genotoxicity of the *G. biloba* extract.

Quercetin and kaempferol have also been shown to suppress the activities of DNA topoisomerases (López-Lázaro *et al.*, 2010; Russo *et al.*, 2012). Although some topoisomerase suppressors have therapeutic efficacy in human cancer, the clinical use of topoisomerase inhibitors can also cause formation of secondary tumours, and increased maternal consumption of flavonoids (some are topoisomerase inhibitors) during pregnancy may be associated with infant acute leukaemia (Ross *et al.*, 1996; Strick *et al.*, 2000; Mistry *et al.*, 2005; Ezoe, 2012) by interfering with DNA repair processes and inducing chromosomal aberrations. It is possible that an inhibitory effect on topoisomerase is the underlying mechanism for quercetin- or kaempferol-associated chromosomal damage.

Genotoxicity or topoisomerase inhibition may be mechanisms of *G. biloba*-associated carcinogenicity.

5. Summary of Data Reported

5.1 Exposure data

Ginkgo biloba, also known as the "fossil tree," is the oldest living tree. Products containing ginkgo leaf extract have been widely consumed in Europe for many years, and are also popular in the USA and other parts of the world, including China. Major reported indications are for asthma, bronchitis, cardiovascular diseases, improvement of peripheral blood flow, and reduction of cerebral insufficiency, allergies, tinnitus, dementia, and memory issues. The main parts of the plant used for these applications are the leaves and the seeds. Ginkgo seeds are cooked and eaten as food. Various forms of processed and unprocessed ginkgo leaf are present in dietary supplements, herbal medicinal products and in foods. Considerable sales were reported from China, the USA, Germany, Australia, France, Brazil, the Republic of Korea, Viet Nam, and Canada.

5.2 Human carcinogenicity data

The potential carcinogenicity of *G. biloba* extract has been evaluated in few epidemiological studies: one randomized controlled trial (the Ginko Evaluation of Memory study, GEM), four nested case–control studies from the VITamins And Lifestyle (VITAL) cohort, and one population-based case–control study of cancer of the ovary.

The GEM study was considered to be informative because of its randomized design; however, the population was limited to people aged > 75 years and compliance in the placebo and ginkgo treatment groups was only about 60%. The strengths of the VITAL study were its prospective design, the large number of exposed cases, and the broad age range of the study participants; however, no information was available on use of ginkgo after enrolment.

The VITAL and GEM studies both reported risk estimates for cancers of the breast, colorectum, lung, prostate, and for urothelial cell carcinoma, and the GEM study also reported a risk estimate for leukaemia and lymphoma combined. Increased risk for cancers of the breast and colorectum was reported in the GEM random clinical trial. The findings for cancer of the colorectum were considered to be stronger in this study because, in a sensitivity analysis that excluded participants reporting a history of cancer 5 years before baseline, the relative risk increased and reached statistical significance, while the relative risk of cancer of the breast was attenuated and no longer statistically significant in the sensitivity analysis. The VITAL cohort did not corroborate the GEM findings for cancers of the colorectum or breast, finding somewhat decreased risk for both types of cancer and ginkgo intake. The differences in findings between the two studies could be due to differences in age or window of exposure. Risks for other types of cancers were either null or somewhat decreased in both studies. The population case–control study found a decreased risk of non-mucinous ovarian cancer, but not mucinous ovarian cancer, but the analysis was based on small numbers of exposed cases.

5.3 Animal carcinogenicity data

A *G. biloba* extract was tested for carcinogenicity in two studies of oral administration in mice and rats. In male and female mice treated by gavage, a *G. biloba* extract containing 31.2% flavonol, 15.4% terpene lactones (bilobalide, 6.94%; ginkgolide A, 3.74%; ginkgolide B, 1.62%; ginkgolide C, 3.06%), and ginkgolic acid at a concentration of 10.45 ppm, produced a significant increase in the incidences of hepatocellular adenoma or carcinoma (combined), hepatocellular carcinoma and hepatoblastoma. In male mice receiving the extract, the incidence of thyroid follicular cell adenoma exceeded the range for historical controls in the study series. In male rats given *G. biloba* extract by gavage, there was a significant positive trend in the incidence of thyroid follicular cell adenoma and a significant increase in the incidence of mononuclear cell leukaemia. In female rats, the incidences of thyroid follicular cell adenoma, thyroid follicular cell carcinoma, and nasal respiratory epithelium adenoma exceeded the range for historical controls in the study series.

5.4 Mechanistic and other relevant data

Components of *G. biloba* extract are extensively metabolized in rodents and humans after oral administration.

G. biloba extract gave positive results in standard bacterial assays for mutation in the absence or presence of exogenous metabolic activation. Two components of *G. biloba* extract, quercetin and kaempferol, also gave positive results in standard tests for genotoxicity. Quercetin, kaempferol, and rutin, a third component of *G. biloba* extract, produced chromosomal damage.

Quercetin and kaempferol are inhibitors of DNA topoisomerases.

Genotoxicity and/or topoisomerase inhibition may be mechanisms of carcinogenicity associated with *G. biloba* extract.

6. Evaluation

6.1 Cancer in humans

There is *inadequate evidence* in humans for the carcinogenicity of *Ginkgo biloba* extract.

6.2 Cancer in experimental animals

There is *sufficient evidence* in experimental animals for the carcinogenicity of *Ginkgo biloba* extract.

6.3 Overall evaluation

Ginkgo biloba extract is *possibly carcinogenic to humans (Group 2B).*

References

ABC; American Botanical Council (2000). Boston: Integrative Medicine Communications. American Botanical Counsel. Integrative Medicine Communications. Copyright.

AMR (2013). Guidelines of the Federal Committee of Physicians and Health Insurances on the prescription of medicines within the Statutory Health Care ("Arzneimittel-Richtlinien/AMR"). Available from: http://www.g-ba.de/downloads/83-691-314/AM-RL-I-OTC_2013-04-05.pdf, accessed 09 December 2014

Anderson D, Basaran N, Dobrzyńska MM, Basaran AA, Yu TW (1997). Modulating effects of flavonoids on food mutagens in human blood and sperm samples in the comet assay. *Teratog Carcinog Mutagen*, 17(2):45–58. doi:10.1002/(SICI)1520-6866(1997)17:2<45::AID-TCM1>3.0.CO;2-E PMID:9261919

Barnes PM, Bloom B, Nahin RL (2008). Complementary and alternative medicine use among adults and children: United States, 2007. *Natl Health Stat Report*, 12(12):1–23. PMID:19361005

Biggs ML, Sorkin BC, Nahin RL, Kuller LH, Fitzpatrick AL (2010). Ginkgo biloba and risk of cancer: secondary analysis of the Ginkgo Evaluation of Memory (GEM) Study. *Pharmacoepidemiol Drug Saf*, 19(7):694–8. doi:10.1002/pds.1979 PMID:20582906

Bjeldanes LF & Chang GW (1977). Mutagenic activity of quercetin and related compounds. *Science*, 197(4303):577–8. doi:10.1126/science.327550 PMID:327550

Blumenthal M, Busse WR, Goldberg A et al., editors Klein K, Rister RS (trans.). (1998). *The Complete German Commission E Monographs Therapeutic Guide to Herbal Medicines*. Austin.

Brasky TM, Kristal AR, Navarro SL, Lampe JW, Peters U, Patterson RE et al. (2011). Specialty supplements and prostate cancer risk in the VITamins and Lifestyle (VITAL) cohort. *Nutr Cancer*, 63(4):573–82. doi:10.1080/01635581.2011.553022 PMID:21598177

Brasky TM, Lampe JW, Potter JD, Patterson RE, White E (2010). Specialty supplements and breast cancer risk in the VITamins And Lifestyle (VITAL) Cohort. *Cancer Epidemiol Biomarkers Prev*, 19(7):1696–708. doi:10.1158/1055-9965.EPI-10-0318 PMID:20615886

Brestel EP, Van Dyke K (1991). "Chapter 42" in *Modern Pharmacology*, 3rd ed., C.R. Craig and R. E. Stitzel, eds., Little, Brown, Boston, pp. 567–569.

Caria H, Chaveca T, Laires A, Rueff J (1995). Genotoxicity of quercetin in the micronucleus assay in mouse bone marrow erythrocytes, human lymphocytes, V79 cell line and identification of kinetochore-containing (CREST staining) micronuclei in human lymphocytes. *Mutat Res*, 343(2–3):85–94. doi:10.1016/0165-1218(95)90075-6 PMID:7791812

Carver JH, Carrano AV, MacGregor JT (1983). Genetic effects of the flavonols quercetin, kaempferol, and galangin on Chinese hamster ovary cells in vitro. *Mutat Res*, 113(1):45–60. doi:10.1016/0165-1161(83)90240-6 PMID:6828043

Chan PC, Xia Q, Fu PP (2007). Ginkgo biloba leave extract: biological, medicinal, and toxicological effects. *J Environ Sci Health C Environ Carcinog Ecotoxicol Rev*, 25(3):211–44. doi:10.1080/10590500701569414 PMID:17763047

Chemical Abstracts Service (2014). Scifinder. Columbus, OH, USA. American Chemical Society. Available at: https://scifinder.cas.org:443/, accessed 09 December 2014

Chen WD, Liang Y, Xie L, Lu T, Liu XD, Wang GJ (2007). Pharmacokinetics of the ginkgo B following intravenous administration of ginkgo B emulsion in rats. *Biol Pharm Bull*, 30(1):1–5. doi:10.1248/bpb.30.1 PMID:17202649

Chen XW, Serag ES, Sneed KB, Liang J, Chew H, Pan SY et al. (2011). Clinical herbal interactions with conventional drugs: from molecules to maladies. *Curr Med Chem*, 18(31):4836–50. doi:10.2174/092986711797535317 PMID:21919844

Chen XW, Sneed KB, Pan SY, Cao C, Kanwar JR, Chew H et al. (2012). Herb-drug interactions and mechanistic and clinical considerations. *Curr Drug Metab*, 13(5):640–51. doi:10.2174/1389200211209050640 PMID:22292789

Consumer Council (2000). Test casts doubt on clinical benefits of Ginkgo leaf products with nonstandardized extract. Hong Kong, Choice No. 289 pp. 15.

Council of the European Economic Community (1965). Council Directive 65/65/EEC of 26 January 1965 on the approximation of provisions laid down by Law, Regulation or Administrative Action relating to proprietary medicinal products. Off. J. 022, 0369–0373.

Croom E, Pace R, Paletti A, Sardone N, Gray D (2007). Single-laboratory validation for the determination of terpene lactones in Ginkgo biloba dietary supplement crude materials and finished products by high-performance liquid chromatography with evaporative light-scattering detection. *J AOAC Int*, 90(3):647–58. PMID:17580616

Croom EM Jr & Walker L (1995). Botanicals in the pharmacy: New life for old remedies. *Drug Topics*, 139:84–93.

DeFeudis FV (1991). *Ginkgo biloba extract (EGb 761): pharmacological activities and clinical applications*. Amsterdam, Elsevier, pp 10–13.

DeKosky ST, Williamson JD, Fitzpatrick AL, Kronmal RA, Ives DG, Saxton JA et al.; Ginkgo Evaluation of Memory (GEM) Study Investigators (2008). Ginkgo biloba for prevention of dementia: a randomized controlled trial. *JAMA*, 300(19):2253–62. doi:10.1001/jama.2008.683 PMID:19017911

Del Tredici P (1991). Ginkgos and people —A thousand years of interaction. *Arnoldia*, 51:2–15.

Del Tredici P (2005). The evolution, ecology, and cultivation of *Ginkgo biloba*. In: *Ginkgo biloba*. Van Beek TA, Harwood Academic Publishers, p. 20. Available from: http://books.google.com/books?id=g_MPcQ1gu3MC&dq=ginkgo+plantations&lr=&source=gbs_navlinks_s, accessed 09 December 2014

Diamond BJ, Shiflett SC, Feiwel N, Matheis RJ, Noskin O, Richards JA *et al.* (2000). Ginkgo biloba extract: mechanisms and clinical indications. *Arch Phys Med Rehabil*, 81(5):668–78. PMID:10807109

Ding S, Dudley E, Plummer S, Tang J, Newton RP, Brenton AG (2006). Quantitative determination of major active components in Ginkgo biloba dietary supplements by liquid chromatography/mass spectrometry. *Rapid Commun Mass Spectrom*, 20(18):2753–60. doi:10.1002/rcm.2646 PMID:16921563

Drago F, Floriddia ML, Cro M, Giuffrida S (2002). Pharmacokinetics and bioavailability of a Ginkgo biloba extract. *J Ocul Pharmacol Ther*, 18(2):197–202. doi:10.1089/108076802317373941 PMID:12002672

Duthie SJ, Johnson W, Dobson VL (1997). The effect of dietary flavonoids on DNA damage (strand breaks and oxidised pyrimdines) and growth in human cells. *Mutat Res*, 390(1–2):141–51. doi:10.1016/S0165-1218(97)00010-4 PMID:9150762

Etheridge AS, Black SR, Patel PR, So J, Mathews JM (2007). An in vitro evaluation of cytochrome P450 inhibition and P-glycoprotein interaction with goldenseal, Ginkgo biloba, grape seed, milk thistle, and ginseng extracts and their constituents. *Planta Med*, 73(8):731–41. doi:10.1055/s-2007-981550 PMID:17611934

Evans JR (2013). Ginkgo biloba extract for age-related macular degeneration. *Cochrane Database Syst Rev*, 1:CD001775 PMID:23440785

Ezoe S (2012). Secondary leukemia associated with the anti-cancer agent, etoposide, a topoisomerase II inhibitor. *Int J Environ Res Public Health*, 9(7):2444–53. doi:10.3390/ijerph9072444 PMID:22851953

FDA (1994). Dietary Supplement Health and Education Act of 1994. Public Law 103–417, 103rd Congress. Available from: http://www.fda.gov/opacom/laws/dshea.html, accessed 09 December 2009.

Fourtillan JB, Brisson AM, Girault J, Ingrand I, Decourt JP, Drieu K *et al.* (1995). [Pharmacokinetic properties of Bilobalide and Ginkgolides A and B in healthy subjects after intravenous and oral administration of Ginkgo biloba extract (EGb 761)] *Therapie*, 50(2):137–44. PMID:7631288

Gaspar J, Rodrigues A, Laires A, Silva F, Costa S, Monteiro MJ *et al.* (1994). On the mechanisms of genotoxicity and metabolism of quercetin. *Mutagenesis*, 9(5):445–9. doi:10.1093/mutage/9.5.445 PMID:7837978

Gilman EF & Watson DG (1993). *Ginkgo biloba* Maidenhair Tree. *Fact Sheet,*, ST-273:1–3.

Gray D, LeVanseler K, Meide P, Waysek EH (2007). Evaluation of a method to determine flavonol aglycones in Ginkgo biloba dietary supplement crude materials and finished products by high-performance liquid chromatography: collaborative study. *J AOAC Int*, 90(1):43–53. PMID:17373435

Greenblatt DJ, von Moltke LL, Luo Y, Perloff ES, Horan KA, Bruce A *et al.* (2006). Ginkgo biloba does not alter clearance of flurbiprofen, a cytochrome P450–2C9 substrate. *J Clin Pharmacol*, 46(2):214–21. doi:10.1177/0091270005283465 PMID:16432273

Griffiths LA & Smith GE (1972). Metabolism of myricetin and related compounds in the rat. Metabolite formation in vivo and by the intestinal microflora in vitro. *Biochem J*, 130(1):141–51. PMID:4655415

Gurley BJ, Gardner SF, Hubbard MA, Williams DK, Gentry WB, Cui Y *et al.* (2002). Cytochrome P450 phenotypic ratios for predicting herb-drug interactions in humans. *Clin Pharmacol Ther*, 72(3):276–87. doi:10.1067/mcp.2002.126913 PMID:12235448

Hänsel R. (1991). *Phytopharmaka*, 2nd ed., Berlin, Springer-Verlag, pp. 59–72.

Hardigree AA & Epler JL (1978). Comparative mutagenesis of plant flavonoids in microbial systems. *Mutat Res*, 58(2–3):231–9. doi:10.1016/0165-1218(78)90014-9 PMID:370575

Harnly JM, Luthria D, Chen P (2012). Detection of adulterated Ginkgo biloba supplements using chromatographic and spectral fingerprints. *J AOAC Int*, 95(6):1579–87. doi:10.5740/jaoacint.12-096 PMID:23451372

Health IMS (2012). Multinational Integrated Data Analysis (MIDAS). Plymouth Meeting, Pennsylvania: IMS Health.

Herrschaft H, Nacu A, Likhachev S, Sholomov I, Hoerr R, Schlaefke S (2012). Ginkgo biloba extract EGb 761® in dementia with neuropsychiatric features: a randomised, placebo-controlled trial to confirm the efficacy and safety of a daily dose of 240 mg. *J Psychiatr Res*, 46(6):716–23. doi:10.1016/j.jpsychires.2012.03.003 PMID:22459264

Hilton MP, Zimmermann EF, Hunt WT (2013). Ginkgo biloba for tinnitus. *Cochrane Database Syst Rev*, 3:CD003852 PMID:23543524

Hoenerhoff MJ, Pandiri AR, Snyder SA, Hong HH, Ton TV, Peddada S *et al.* (2013). Hepatocellular carcinomas in B6C3F1 mice treated with Ginkgo biloba extract for two years differ from spontaneous liver tumors in cancer gene mutations and genomic pathways. *Toxicol Pathol*, 41(6):826–41. doi:10.1177/0192623312467520 PMID:23262642

Holgers KM, Axelsson A, Pringle I (1994). Ginkgo biloba extract for the treatment of tinnitus. *Audiology*, 33(2):85–92. doi:10.3109/00206099409071870 PMID:8179518

Hopfenmüller W (1994). [Evidence for a therapeutic effect of Ginkgo biloba special extract. Meta-analysis of 11 clinical studies in patients with cerebrovascular insufficiency in old age] *Arzneimittelforschung*, 44(9):1005–13. PMID:7986236

Hotaling JM, Wright JL, Pocobelli G, Bhatti P, Porter MP, White E (2011). Long-term use of supplemental vitamins and minerals does not reduce the risk of urothelial cell carcinoma of the bladder in the VITamins And Lifestyle study. *J Urol*, 185(4):1210–5. doi:10.1016/j.juro.2010.11.081 PMID:21334017

IARC (1999). Some chemicals that cause tumours of the kidney or urinary bladder in rodents and some other substances. *IARC Monogr Eval Carcinog Risks Hum*, 73:1–674.

Kanowski S, Hermann WM, Stephan K *et al.* (1997). Proof of the efficacy of the *Ginkgo biloba* special extract EGb 761 in outpatients suffering from mild to moderate dementia of the Alzheimer's type or multi-infarct dementia. *Phytomedicine*, 4:3–13. doi:10.1016/S0944-7113(97)80021-9 PMID:23195239

Kanowski S, Herrmann WM, Stephan K, Wierich W, Hörr R (1996). Proof of efficacy of the ginkgo biloba special extract EGb 761 in outpatients suffering from mild to moderate primary degenerative dementia of the Alzheimer type or multi-infarct dementia. *Pharmacopsychiatry*, 29(2):47–56. doi:10.1055/s-2007-979544 PMID:8741021

Kleijnen J & Knipschild P (1992). Ginkgo biloba for cerebral insufficiency. *Br J Clin Pharmacol*, 34(4):352–8. doi:10.1111/j.1365-2125.1992.tb05642.x PMID:1457269

Kressmann S, Müller WE, Blume HH (2002). Pharmaceutical quality of different Ginkgo biloba brands. *J Pharm Pharmacol*, 54(5):661–9. doi:10.1211/0022357021778970 PMID:12005361

Lachenmeier DW, Steffen C, el-Atma O, Maixner S, Löbell-Behrends S, Kohl-Himmelseher M (2012). What is a food and what is a medicinal product in the European Union? Use of the benchmark dose (BMD) methodology to define a threshold for "pharmacological action". *Regul Toxicol Pharmacol*, 64(2):286–95. doi:10.1016/j.yrtph.2012.08.017 PMID:22960033

Le Bars PL, Katz MM, Berman N, Itil TM, Freedman AM, Schatzberg AF (1997). A placebo-controlled, double-blind, randomized trial of an extract of Ginkgo biloba for dementia. North American EGb Study Group. *JAMA*, 278(16):1327–32. doi:10.1001/jama.1997.03550160047037 PMID:9343463

Leistner E & Drewke C (2010). Ginkgo biloba and ginkgotoxin. *J Nat Prod*, 73(1):86–92. doi:10.1021/np9005019 PMID:20041670

Li CY, Lin CH, Wu CC, Lee KH, Wu TS (2004). Efficient 1H nuclear magnetic resonance method for improved quality control analyses of Ginkgo constituents. *J Agric Food Chem*, 52(12):3721–5. doi:10.1021/jf049920h PMID:15186088

López-Lázaro M, Willmore E, Austin CA (2010). The dietary flavonoids myricetin and fisetin act as dual inhibitors of DNA topoisomerases I and II in cells. *Mutat Res*, 696(1):41–7. doi:10.1016/j.mrgentox.2009.12.010 PMID:20025993

Lovera JF, Kim E, Heriza E, Fitzpatrick M, Hunziker J, Turner AP *et al.* (2012). Ginkgo biloba does not improve cognitive function in MS: a randomized placebo-controlled trial. *Neurology*, 79(12):1278–84. doi:10.1212/WNL.0b013e31826aac60 PMID:22955125

Mauri P, Simonetti P, Gardana C, Minoggio M, Morazzoni P, Bombardelli E *et al.* (2001). Liquid chromatography/atmospheric pressure chemical ionization mass spectrometry of terpene lactones in plasma of volunteers dosed with Ginkgo biloba L. extracts. *Rapid Commun Mass Spectrom*, 15(12):929–34. doi:10.1002/rcm.316 PMID:11400198

McKenna OJ Jones K Hughes K Tyler VM 2002). Botanical medicines: the desk reference for major herbal supplements. 2nd ed. New York: The Haworth Herbal Press; pp. 480-8.

Mills S Bone K 2005). Ginkgo. In: Mills S Bone K editors. Safety Monographs. Part II. The essential guide to herbal safety. Elsevier; pp. 425-32.

Mistry AR, Felix CA, Whitmarsh RJ, Mason A, Reiter A, Cassinat B *et al.* (2005). DNA topoisomerase II in therapy-related acute promyelocytic leukemia. *N Engl J Med*, 352(15):1529–38. doi:10.1056/NEJMoa042715 PMID:15829534

Mohutsky MA, Anderson GD, Miller JW, Elmer GW (2006). Ginkgo biloba: evaluation of CYP2C9 drug interactions in vitro and in vivo. *Am J Ther*, 13(1):24–31. doi:10.1097/01.mjt.0000143695.68285.31 PMID:16428919

Moreau JP, Eck CR, McCabe J, Skinner S (1986). [Absorption, distribution and elimination of a labelled extract of Ginkgo biloba leaves in the rat] *Presse Med*, 15(31):1458–61. PMID:2947082

Morgenstern C & Biermann E (1997). *Ginkgo biloba* special extract EGb 761 in the treatment of tinnitus aurium: Results of a randomized, double-blind, placebo-controlled study. *Fortschr Med*, 115:711

Mouren X, Caillard P, Schwartz F (1994). Study of the antiischemic action of EGb 761 in the treatment of peripheral arterial occlusive disease by TcPo2 determination. *Angiology*, 45(6):413–7. doi:10.1177/000331979404500601 PMID:8203766

Nicolaï SP, Kruidenier LM, Bendermacher BL, Prins MH, Teijink JA (2009). Ginkgo biloba for intermittent claudication. *Cochrane Database Syst Rev*, 2(2):CD006888 PMID:19370657

NTP (1992). Toxicology and carcinogenesis studies of quercetin (CAS No. 117-39-5) in F344/N rats (feed studies). *Natl Toxicol Program Tech Rep Ser*, 409:

NTP (2013). Toxicology and carcinogenesis studies of *Ginkgo biloba* extract (CAS No. 90045-36-6) in F344/N rats and B6C3F1/N mice (gavage studies). *Natl Toxicol Program Tech Rep Ser*, 578(578):1–183. PMID:23652021

Nutrition Business Journal (2012). Nutrition Business Journal Annual Report. Available from: http://nutritionbusinessjournal.com/, accessed 09 December 2014

O'Neil MJ (2013). *An Encyclopedia of Chemicals, Drugs, and Biologicals*. 15th Ed., Merck Sharp & Dohme Corp. Whitehouse, NJ, 2013, RSC Publishing.

Oh SM & Chung KH (2004). Estrogenic activities of Ginkgo biloba extracts. *Life Sci*, 74(11):1325–35. doi:10.1016/j.lfs.2003.06.045 PMID:14706564

Oh SM & Chung KH (2006). Antiestrogenic activities of Ginkgo biloba extracts. *J Steroid Biochem Mol Biol*, 100(4–5):167–76. doi:10.1016/j.jsbmb.2006.04.007 PMID:16842996

Oken BS, Storzbach DM, Kaye JA (1998). The efficacy of Ginkgo biloba on cognitive function in Alzheimer disease. *Arch Neurol*, 55(11):1409–15. doi:10.1001/archneur.55.11.1409 PMID:9823823

Perry LM (1984). Medicinal Plants of East and Southeast Asia: Attributed Properties and Uses, MIT Press: Cambridge, MA.

Peters H, Kieser M, Hölscher U (1998). Demonstration of the efficacy of ginkgo biloba special extract EGb 761 on intermittent claudication–a placebo-controlled, double-blind multicenter trial. *Vasa*, 27(2):106–10. PMID:9612115

Pietta PG, Gardana C, Mauri PL (1997). Identification of Gingko biloba flavonol metabolites after oral administration to humans. *J Chromatogr B Biomed Sci Appl*, 693(1):249–55. doi:10.1016/S0378-4347(96)00513-0 PMID:9200545

Pietta PG, Gardana C, Mauri PL, Maffei-Facino R, Carini M (1995). Identification of flavonoid metabolites after oral administration to rats of a Ginkgo biloba extract. *J Chromatogr B Biomed Appl*, 673(1):75–80. doi:10.1016/0378-4347(95)00252-E PMID:8925077

Pittler MH & Ernst E (2000). Ginkgo biloba extract for the treatment of intermittent claudication: a meta-analysis of randomized trials. *Am J Med*, 108(4):276–81. doi:10.1016/S0002-9343(99)00454-4 PMID:11014719

Prior RL (2003). Fruits and vegetables in the prevention of cellular oxidative damage. *Am J Clin Nutr*, 78(3):Suppl: 570S–8S. PMID:12936951

Prior RL (2006). Phytochemicals. In: Shils ME, Shike M, Ross AC, Caballero B Cousins RJ (eds) 10th ed. Modern Nutrition in Health and Disease. Philadelphia: Lippincott, Williams and Wilkins, 582–593.

Rai GS, Shovlin C, Wesnes KA (1991). A double-blind, placebo controlled study of Ginkgo biloba extract ('tanakan') in elderly outpatients with mild to moderate memory impairment. *Curr Med Res Opin*, 12(6):350–5. doi:10.1185/03007999109111504 PMID:2044394

Rangel-Ordóñez L, Nöldner M, Schubert-Zsilavecz M, Wurglics M (2010). Plasma levels and distribution of flavonoids in rat brain after single and repeated doses of standardized Ginkgo biloba extract EGb 761®. *Planta Med*, 76(15):1683–90. doi:10.1055/s-0030-1249962 PMID:20486074

Robertson SM, Davey RT, Voell J, Formentini E, Alfaro RM, Penzak SR (2008). Effect of Ginkgo biloba extract on lopinavir, midazolam and fexofenadine pharmacokinetics in healthy subjects. *Curr Med Res Opin*, 24(2):591–9. doi:10.1185/030079908X260871 PMID:18205997

Ross JA, Potter JD, Reaman GH, Pendergrass TW, Robison LL (1996). Maternal exposure to potential inhibitors of DNA topoisomerase II and infant leukemia (United States): a report from the Children's Cancer Group. *Cancer Causes Control*, 7(6):581–90. doi:10.1007/BF00051700 PMID:8932918

Russo P, Del Bufalo A, Cesario A (2012). Flavonoids acting on DNA topoisomerases: recent advances and future perspectives in cancer therapy. *Curr Med Chem*, 19(31):5287–93. doi:10.2174/092986712803833272 PMID:22998568

Satia JA, Littman A, Slatore CG, Galanko JA, White E (2009). Associations of herbal and specialty supplements with lung and colorectal cancer risk in the VITamins and Lifestyle study. *Cancer Epidemiol Biomarkers Prev*, 18(5):1419–28. doi:10.1158/1055-9965.EPI-09-0038 PMID:19423520

Schmid W & Balz JP (2005). Cultivation of *Ginkgo biloba* L. on three continents. [ISHS]*Acta Hortic*, 676:177–180.Available fromhttp://www.actahort.org/books/676/676_23.htmaccessed 09 December 2014

Schneider LS (2012). Ginkgo and AD: key negatives and lessons from GuidAge. *Lancet Neurol*, 11(10):836–7. doi:10.1016/S1474-4422(12)70212-0 PMID:22959218

Schötz K (2002). Detection of allergenic urushiols in Ginkgo biloba leaves. *Pharmazie*, 57(7):508–10. PMID:12168544

Shi C, Liu J, Wu F, Yew DT (2010a). Ginkgo biloba extract in Alzheimer's disease: from action mechanisms to medical practice. *Int J Mol Sci*, 11(1):107–23. doi:10.3390/ijms11010107 PMID:20162004

Shi C, Wu F, Yew DT, Xu J, Zhu Y (2010b). Bilobalide prevents apoptosis through activation of the PI3K/Akt pathway in SH-SY5Y cells. *Apoptosis*, 15(6):715–27. doi:10.1007/s10495-010-0492-x PMID:20333467

Siegers CP (1999). Cytotoxicity of alkylphenols from Ginkgo biloba. *Phytomedicine*, 6(4):281–3. doi:10.1016/S0944-7113(99)80021-X PMID:10589448

Silva ID, Rodrigues AS, Gaspar J, Maia R, Laires A, Rueff J (1997). Involvement of rat cytochrome 1A1 in the biotransformation of kaempferol to quercetin: relevance to the genotoxicity of kaempferol. *Mutagenesis*, 12(5):383–90. doi:10.1093/mutage/12.5.383 PMID:9379919

Singh SR & Levine MAH (2006). Natural health product use in Canada: analysis of the National Population Health Survey. *Can J Clin Pharmacol*, 13(2):e240–50. PMID:16921199

Smith JV & Luo Y (2004). Studies on molecular mechanisms of Ginkgo biloba extract. *Appl Microbiol Biotechnol*, 64(4):465–72. doi:10.1007/s00253-003-1527-9 PMID:14740187

Snitz BE, O'Meara ES, Carlson MC, Arnold AM, Ives DG, Rapp SR *et al.*; Ginkgo Evaluation of Memory (GEM) Study Investigators (2009). Ginkgo biloba for preventing cognitive decline in older adults: a randomized trial. *JAMA*, 302(24):2663–70. doi:10.1001/jama.2009.1913 PMID:20040554

Strick R, Strissel PL, Borgers S, Smith SL, Rowley JD (2000). Dietary bioflavonoids induce cleavage in the MLL gene and may contribute to infant leukemia. *Proc Natl Acad Sci USA*, 97(9):4790–5. doi:10.1073/pnas.070061297 PMID:10758153

Uchida S, Yamada H, Li XD, Maruyama S, Ohmori Y, Oki T *et al.* (2006). Effects of Ginkgo biloba extract on pharmacokinetics and pharmacodynamics of tolbutamide and midazolam in healthy volunteers. *J Clin Pharmacol*, 46(11):1290–8. doi:10.1177/0091270006292628 PMID:17050793

Ude C, Schubert-Zsilavecz M, Wurglics M (2013). Ginkgo biloba extracts: a review of the pharmacokinetics of the active ingredients. *Clin Pharmacokinet*, 52(9):727–49. doi:10.1007/s40262-013-0074-5 PMID:23703577

USP; United States Pharmacopeia (2013). 36th rev. and *National Formulary*, 31th ed., Rockville, MD: United States Pharmacopeial Convention, Inc.

van Beek TA & Montoro P (2009). Chemical analysis and quality control of Ginkgo biloba leaves, extracts, and phytopharmaceuticals. *J Chromatogr A*, 1216(11):2002–32. doi:10.1016/j.chroma.2009.01.013 PMID:19195661

Vellas B, Coley N, Ousset PJ, Berrut G, Dartigues JF, Dubois B *et al.*; GuidAge Study Group (2012). Long-term use of standardised Ginkgo biloba extract for the prevention of Alzheimer's disease (GuidAge): a randomised placebo-controlled trial. *Lancet Neurol*, 11(10):851–9. doi:10.1016/S1474-4422(12)70206-5 PMID:22959217

Wagner H, Bladt S (1996). *Plant drug analysis: a thin layer chromatography atlas*, 2nd Ed., Berlin, SpringerVerlag, p 237.

Wang BS, Wang H, Song YY, Qi H, Rong ZX, Wang BS *et al.* (2010). Effectiveness of standardized ginkgo biloba extract on cognitive symptoms of dementia with a six-month treatment: a bivariate random effect meta-analysis. *Pharmacopsychiatry*, 43(3):86–91. doi:10.1055/s-0029-1242817 PMID:20104449

Wang FM, Yao TW, Zeng S (2003). Determination of quercetin and kaempferol in human urine after orally administrated tablet of ginkgo biloba extract by HPLC. *J Pharm Biomed Anal*, 33(2):317–21. doi:10.1016/S0731-7085(03)00255-3 PMID:12972097

Weinmann S, Roll S, Schwarzbach C, Vauth C, Willich SN (2010). Effects of Ginkgo biloba in dementia: systematic review and meta-analysis. *BMC Geriatr*, 10(1):14 doi:10.1186/1471-2318-10-14 PMID:20236541

Wesnes KA, Ward T, McGinty A, Petrini O (2000). The memory enhancing effects of a Ginkgo biloba/Panax ginseng combination in healthy middle-aged volunteers. *Psychopharmacology (Berl)*, 152(4):353–61. doi:10.1007/s002130000533 PMID:11140327

Westendorf J & Regan J (2000). Induction of DNA strand-breaks in primary rat hepatocytes by ginkgolic acids. *Pharmazie*, 55(11):864–5. PMID:11126011

White E, Patterson RE, Kristal AR, Thornquist M, King I, Shattuck AL *et al.* (2004). VITamins And Lifestyle cohort study: study design and characteristics of supplement users. *Am J Epidemiol*, 159(1):83–93. doi:10.1093/aje/kwh010 PMID:14693663

WHO; World Health Organization (1999). Ginkgo folium. *WHO Monographs on Selected Medicinal Plants*, Vol. 1. Geneva: World Health Organization.

Wójcicki J, Gawrońska-Szklarz B, Bieganowski W, Patalan M, Smulski HK, Samochowiec L *et al.* (1995). Comparative pharmacokinetics and bioavailability of flavonoid glycosides of Ginkgo biloba after a single oral administration of three formulations to healthy volunteers. *Mater Med Pol*, 27(4):141–6. PMID:9000837

Wu C-H, Wang C-C, Kennedy J (2011). Changes in herb and dietary supplement use in the U.S. adult population: a comparison of the 2002 and 2007 National Health Interview Surveys. *Clin Ther*, 33(11):1749–58. doi:10.1016/j.clinthera.2011.09.024 PMID:22030445

Ye B, Aponte M, Dai Y, Li L, Ho MC, Vitonis A *et al.* (2007). Ginkgo biloba and ovarian cancer prevention: epidemiological and biological evidence. *Cancer Lett*, 251(1):43–52. doi:10.1016/j.canlet.2006.10.025 PMID:17194528

Zadoyan G, Rokitta D, Klement S, Dienel A, Hoerr R, Gramatté T *et al.* (2012). Effect of Ginkgo biloba special extract EGb 761® on human cytochrome P450 activity: a cocktail interaction study in healthy volunteers. *Eur J Clin Pharmacol*, 68(5):553–60. doi:10.1007/s00228-011-1174-5 PMID:22189672

Zeiger E, Anderson B, Haworth S, Lawlor T, Mortelmans K (1992). Salmonella mutagenicity tests: V. Results from the testing of 311 chemicals. *Environ Mol Mutagen*, 19(S21):Suppl 21: 2–141. doi:10.1002/em.2850190603 PMID:1541260

KAVA

1. Exposure Data

The kava plant is indigenous to Oceania (Lebot *et al.*, 1997; Ramzan & Tran, 2004) and has been used both ceremonially and recreationally in certain cultures of the South Pacific for at least 1500 years. Europeans documented its use when they travelled to Polynesia in the 18th century (WHO, 2007). The cultural history of the use of kava has been reviewed by Singh (1992).

In the past, traditional use of kava was widespread, but, in certain cultures, custom determined who could use kava and for what purposes. In recent years, as part of the processes of modernization, major changes have occurred with regard to who uses kava, and where and how it is consumed. In some places, kava is now being consumed much like alcohol in western countries, as a beverage that is drunk socially (McDonald & Jowitt, 2000).

1.1 Identification of the agent

1.1.1 Botanical data

(a) Nomenclature

Chem. Abstr. Serv. Reg. No.: 9000-38-8
Chem. Abstr. Name: Kava-kava resin (8Cl)
Botanical name: *Piper methysticum* G. Forst
Family: *Piperaceae*
Genus: *Piper*
Plant part: Rhizome

(WHO, 2004; O'Neil *et al.*, 2006; NTP, 2012; and SciFinder, 2013)

According to WHO (2007), some other species such as *Piper wichmanni*, *Piper aduncum* and *Piper auritum* have also been marketed as "kava."

Common names: Kava; Kava-kava; Ava-ava; Antares; Ava; Ava pepper; Ava pepper shrub; Ava root; Awa; Fijian kava; Gea; Gi; Grog; Intoxicating long pepper; Intoxicating pepper; Kao; Kava kava rhizome; Kava root; Kavapiper; Kavapyrones; Kavarod; Kavasporal forte; Kavekave; Kawa; Kawa kawa; Kawa pepper; Kawa Pfeffer; Kew; Long pepper; *Macropiper latifolium*; Malohu; Maluk; Maori kava; Meruk; Milik; Pepe kava; Piperis methystici rhizome; Rhizoma piperis methystici; Sakaua; Sakau; Tonga; Yagona; Yangona; Yaqona; Yongona

(b) Description

See Fig. 1.1

The tropical shrub *Piper methysticum* is a hardy, fairly succulent, slow-growing perennial that is widely cultivated in Oceania. The species is sterile and reproduces asexually. Due to its traditional use as a ritual beverage known for promoting relaxation and a sense of well-being, the kava plant spread widely throughout Oceania, in Polynesia, Melanesia, and the Federated States of Micronesia (Norton & Ruze, 1994; NTP, 2012).

The leaves are heart-shaped, pointed, 8–25 cm in length, and smooth and green on both sides. Kava is cultivated for its rootstock (rhizome), also

Fig. 1.1 *Piper methysticum* G. Forst

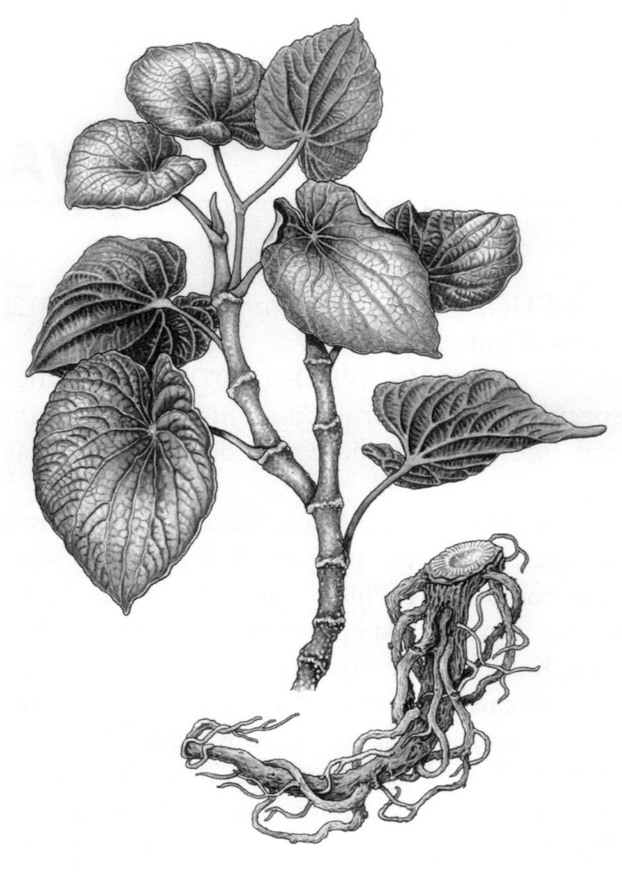

From Spohn (2013)
© Roland Spohn

referred to as the stump. The stump is knotty, thick, and sometimes tuberous and often contains holes or cracks created by partial destruction of the parenchyma. A fringe of lateral roots up to 2–3 m in length extends from the pithy rhizome. The roots comprise a multitude of ligneous fibres and consist of > 60% starch. Rhizome colour varies from white to dark yellow, depending upon the amount of kavalactones contained in the lemon-yellow resin. The plant is usually harvested when it is about 2–2.5 m in height (Singh, 1992; Lebot *et al.*, 1997; NTP, 2012).

The cultivation and selection of kava has produced numerous varieties or cultivars recognized by differences in the internodes (space between stem joints), colour of stems, intensity of leaf colour, and quality of the root. Different varieties are classified, named, and used for different purposes by the indigenous people (NTP, 2012).

The dried rhizome consists of irregular, transverse and longitudinal pieces, varying considerably in size and shape: 3–20 cm in length and 1–5 cm in diameter. The outer surface is light yellowish or greyish-brown, longitudinally wrinkled, with large, whitish, circular root scars. The fracture is coarsely fibrous, the inner surface is yellow-white, with thin bark, radiate xylem, and large pith (WHO, 2004).

1.1.2 Chemical constituents and their properties

Analysis of the composition of kava rhizome indicates that the fresh material is on average 80% water. When dried, the rhizome consists of approximately 43% starch, 20% fibres, 12% water, 3.2% sugars, 3.6% proteins, 3.2% minerals, and 15% kavalactones, although the kavalactone component can vary between 3% and 20% of the dry weight of the rhizome, depending on the age of the plant and the cultivar. The bioactive principles of kava rhizome are mostly, if not entirely, contained in the lipid-soluble resin. The compounds of greatest pharmacological interest are the substituted α-pyrones or kavapyrones, commonly known as kavalactones. At least 15 lactones have been isolated from kava rhizome. The following six compounds are present in the highest concentrations and account for approximately 96% of the lipid resin: kavain, dihydrokavain, yangonin, desmethoxyyangonin, methysticin, and dihydromethysticin (see Fig. 1.2). Other constituents of kava include chalcones and other flavanones, and conjugated diene ketones (Shulgin, 1973; Dentali, 1997; WHO, 2004; NTP, 2012).

In the past, "kavain" has been used to indicate a racemic mixture resulting from chemical synthesis, and "kawain" for the naturally

Fig. 1.2 Structures of the major kavalactones occurring in kava rhizome

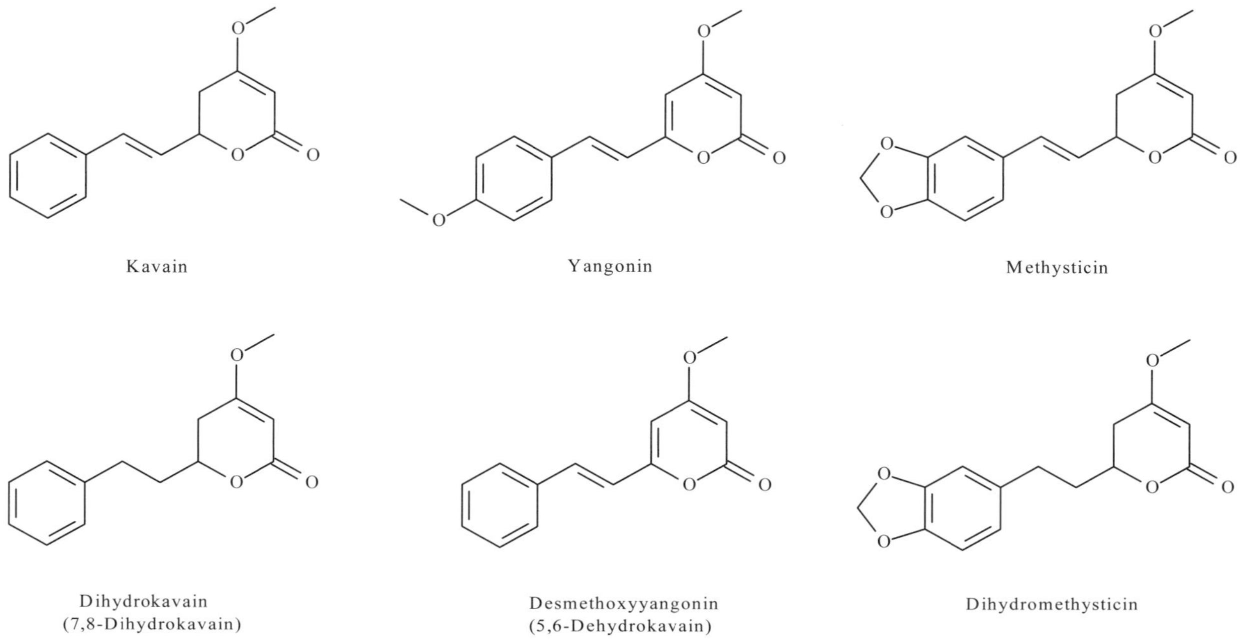

Kavain

Yangonin

Methysticin

Dihydrokavain
(7,8-Dihydrokavain)

Desmethoxyyangonin
(5,6-Dehydrokavain)

Dihydromethysticin

Compiled by the Working Group

occurring compound, which is a dextro-isomer. Currently, the two terms, kavain and kawain, are frequently used interchangeably in the scientific literature, but the term kavain has started to supersede kawain (Singh, 2004a).

The chemistry of kava and kavalactones has been reviewed in detail by Ramzan & Tran (2004).

1.1.3 Technical and commercial products

Kava biomass is normally sold as the rhizome, with the periderm and roots removed. The peeled rhizome is also the desired material for solvent extraction to produce kava extracts. Kava may also be sold as an unpeeled rhizome covered with the cork or with the roots attached. Peelings from the root and stump have also been used in commerce (Morgan *et al.*, 2005). Powdered forms of rhizome are available in commercial markets in Fiji and have been described to be adulterated

to the extent that they only contain 71–78% of the expected active constituents (Clough *et al.*, 2000). Singh (2004a) mentioned adulteration with sawdust, flour, or soil. Adulteration of kava with plants resembling the genuine kava, but lacking the kavalactones and the distinct kava odour has also been reported. The main "false kava" species are *P. auritum* and *P. aduncum* (Singh, 2004b).

Very few data exist on kava contamination by bacteria or with mycotoxins (Teschke *et al.*, 2011). A study on ochratoxin A contamination found concentrations of 3.0 ng/g in one sample of kava root (Trucksess *et al.*, 2006). The level of contamination with aflatoxin B_1 in four samples of ground kava was 0.5 ng/g (Weaver & Trucksess, 2010).

The part of the plant used, processing techniques, and specifically the extraction solvent and the ratio between solvent/plant material in the case of kava extracts, may have considerable influence on the chemical composition of the end product. For example, the alkaloid pipermethystine was not detectable in some commercial kava extracts (Teschke *et al.*, 2011).

[The Working Group noted that the influences on composition mentioned above may hinder the comparison of studies, especially if the applied kava material was not specified exactly.]

1.2 Analysis

The chemical analysis and quality control of both kava and its extracts obtained by aqueous acetone or aqueous methanol, and supercritical fluid extraction – typically with carbon dioxide modified with methanol as solvent – were reviewed by Bilia *et al.* (2004). Both gas chromatography (GC) and high-performance liquid chromatography (HPLC) can be used for the analysis of kavalactones with some advantages and disadvantages for each method. Using GC analysis, methysticin and yangonin, which are two of the major components, are generally not separated. In addition, the high temperature of the injection port causes the decomposition of methysticin. Concerning HPLC analyses, reversed-phase separation is generally better because it is highly reproducible with a very low detection limit for all compounds even if the quantitative analysis of the kavalactones by HPLC needs to be carried out in the absence of light to prevent the *cis/trans* isomerization of yangonin (Bilia *et al.*, 2004). Besides various chromatographic approaches reviewed by Bilia *et al.* (2004), near infrared spectroscopy and nuclear magnetic resonance spectroscopy have been suggested to directly determine kavalactones without the need for separation (Table 1.1).

1.3 Use

1.3.1 Indications

(a) Medicinal use

According to WHO (2004), the medicinal uses supported by clinical data are short-term symptomatic treatment of mild states of anxiety or insomnia due to nervousness, stress or tension; the medicinal uses described in pharmacopoeias and in traditional systems of medicine are to induce relaxation, reduce weight, and treat fungal infections. Uses described in traditional medicine, but not supported by experimental or clinical data, are treatment of asthma, common cold, cystis, gonorrhoea, headaches, menstrual irregularities, urinary infections, and warts.

The German Commission E has approved kava for use in conditions of nervous anxiety, stress, and restlessness (Anonymous, 2000).

(b) Traditional food and recreational use

A local traditional drink, also known under the name kava, is obtained from the root or rhizome of the kava plant. The kava drink is made from water extracts, with water-insoluble substances made available to the drinker by emulsification, which may be accomplished by pounding or chewing of the rhizome (WHO, 2007).

On some islands in the South Pacific, fresh kava root or rhizome is used to prepare the traditional drink, while on others it is the dried and ground roots or rhizomes that are used. For fresh preparations, the root is chewed by young women, who spit the juice into the kava bowl without swallowing it themselves. The juice is then mixed with water or coconut milk and further processed. Most people drink only the water extracts of kava. This is obtained by adding water to kava roots which are finely ground and then filtered using cheese-cloth (WHO, 2007).

The kava drink has been described to have a psychoactive activity, and potency can vary

Table 1.1 Selected methods of analysis of constituents of kava in various matrices

Sample matrix	Analyte/purpose of analysis	Sample preparation	Assay method	Detection limit	Reference
Serum and urine	Kavain and metabolites/metabolism	Glucuronidase treatment, extraction with dichloromethane:diethylether (7:3, v:v)	HPLC-DAD and LC-MS	1 ng/mL	Tarbah *et al.* (2003)
Urine	Kavalactones/metabolism	Chloroform extraction	GC-MS, HPLC	NA	Duffield *et al.* (1989)
Kava root from botanical supplier	Ochratoxin A/contamination	Immunoaffinity column cleanup	HPLC-FD	NA	Trucksess *et al.* (2006)
Dried kava roots	Kavain and other major kavalactones/isolation	Ethanol extraction	HSCCC	NA	Schäfer & Winterhalter (2005)
Commercial kava extract, and kava finely powdered	Kavalactones and a range of other compounds/quality assessment	Solution with DMSO-d_6	NMR	NA	Bilia *et al.* (2002)
Kava root extract	Kavalactones/structural elucidation	Extraction with methylene chloride	NMR	NA	Dharmaratne *et al.* (2002)
Kava dry extracts	Kavain and total kavalactones/routine quality control	None	NIRS	NA	Gaub *et al.* (2004)
Food supplements containing kava	Total kavalactones/regulatory control	Solution in ethanol, buffer addition	NMR	NA	Monakhova *et al.* (2013)

DMSO, dimethyl sulfoxide; GC, gas chromatography; HPLC, high-performance liquid chromatography; HPLC-DAD, high-performance liquid chromatography with diode-array detection; HPLC-FD, high performance liquid chromatography with fluorescence detection; HSCCC, high-speed counter-current chromatography; LC, liquid chromatography; MS, mass spectrometry; NA, not applicable; NIRS, near infrared spectroscopy; NMR, nuclear magnetic resonance spectroscopy; v:v, volume:volume considerably. Kava drinking initially produces a slight numbing of the tongue. Delayed effects have been described as relief of fatigue, reduction of anxiety, and production of a pleasant, cheerful, and sociable attitude in the drinker (WHO, 2007).

The consumption of kava is part of everyday life on islands such as Fiji, Tonga, and Vanuatu, and occurs during important events or social gatherings (Singh, 1992).

It is difficult to compare the psychopharmacological effects of kava between published studies as methods of preparation, means of ingestion, and the potency and quantity of dosages actually consumed vary considerably (Cairney et al., 2002).

Kava bars, at which prepared kava can be purchased to drink on the spot or to take away, are an increasingly common feature throughout Oceania (McDonald & Jowitt, 2000).

(c) Non-traditional food use

Non-traditional kava products are marketed in Europe and North America typically as food or dietary supplements in tablet form (Morris & Avorn, 2003; Teschke & Lebot, 2011). Interestingly, these food supplements are often marketed over the internet (Morris & Avorn, 2003). In some countries this may be due to difficulties with regulatory acceptance. For example, in Europe this practice is illegal, but kava products are nevertheless available (Monakhova et al., 2013).

(d) Cosmetic use

Kava extracts from various parts of the plant may be used as skin-conditioning agents in cosmetics. However, the USA Cosmetic Ingredient Review expert panel concluded that the available data were insufficient to support the safety of kava extracts for cosmetic use (Robinson et al., 2009).

1.3.2 Dosage

(a) Medicinal use

The comminuted crude drug and extracts are used for oral use. Daily dosage for crude drug and extracts is equivalent to 60–210 mg of kavalactones (WHO, 2004). The recommended oral dose for use of commercial kava extracts as an anxiolytic is 50–70 mg of kavalactones, two to four times per day and, as a hypnotic, 150–210 mg in a single oral dose before bedtime (Bilia et al., 2002b).

The pharmaceutical industry was primarily interested in the organic solvent (such as 95% ethanol or acetone) extracts of kava containing the organic compounds of commercial interest. Some marketed products, referred to as "synthetic," consist of a single kavalactone, l-kavain (WHO, 2007).

A review of standardized kava brands in the USA found an approximate equivalence of actual [measured] and labelled amounts of kavalactones in 13 products that listed amounts of constituents. Kavalactones per tablet or capsule ranged from 50 to 110 mg. Two brands that did not label amounts of constituents contained 10–15 mg per tablet or capsule (Ulbricht et al., 2005).

Typical usage has ranged from 70 to 280 mg of kavalactones per day as a single bedtime dose or divided doses (60–120 mg of kavalactones per day). Many practitioners allegedly start at a lower dose and titrate up as needed (Ulbricht et al., 2005).

(b) Traditional food and recreational use

Only rough estimations exist on the dosage of traditional food and in recreational use of kava. Heavy consumers may drink the equivalent of at least 610 g/week of kava powder, which, with an estimated kavalactone content of 12.5%, may equate to approximately 76 g of lactones per week or more than 50 times the recommended therapeutic dose (Cairney et al., 2002).

In Arnhem Land, Australia, weekly per capita consumption was estimated as 145 g of powder for 1989–90 and 368 g of powder for 1990–91. When seven cups of 100 mL are consumed in 1 hour, about 3.8 g of lactones may be consumed. In a detailed review of the literature on weekly consumption levels and possible lactone contents, the estimations encompassed a wide variation from 39 to 1840 g of kava powder consumed, and from 4.1 g to 188.6 g of lactones consumed per week (Clough *et al.*, 2000).

Typical dosage of dried root or by decoction was reported to be 6–12 g per day (Morgan *et al.*, 2005).

(c)   Non-traditional food use

The Dietary Supplements Label Database lists 11 products that contain kava as active ingredient in amounts of 60–1000 mg. Of the 11 products, 4 are listed as discontinued (NLM, 2012).

Kava food supplements, illegally sold over the internet in Germany, contained 8–10 mg of kava-lactones per capsule (Monakhova *et al.*, 2013).

(d)   Cosmetic use

The Cosmetic, Toiletry, and Fragrance Association (CTFA) provided a use concentration of 0.0001–0.01% for leaf/root/stem extract, and of 0.1% for root extract (Robinson *et al.*, 2009).

1.4 Production, sales, and consumption

1.4.1 Production

(a)   Production process

Kava production including cultivation, diseases and pests, harvesting and processing has been reviewed by Singh (2004b).

(b)   Production volume

Kava was one of the most extensively used herbal products in the USA in the 1990s (NTP, 2012). According to Morris & Avorn (2003), sales of kava were US$ 69 million in 2000. In 2003, 62 retail sites were identified that sold kava over the internet (Morris & Avorn, 2003).

In Australia, trade in kava rhizome in Arnhem Land was approximately 28 tonnes in 1992, and between 27 and 36 tonnes in 1997. At the end of 1999, by which time trade in kava was illegal, trade was estimated to be 20 tonnes, while in 2000 the trade was approximately 15 tonnes (Clough, 2003).

1.4.2 Sales

By the mid-1990s, North Americans, Europeans, and Australians had begun using kava products as an alternative medicine and herbal relaxant. Commercial kava bars promoted recreational kava drinking, which can often occur for extended periods. Drug stores and supermarkets offered a variety of kava products in pill, capsule, tea, and liquid form. In addition, powdered kava root was available by mail order from several internet sites. Most of this exported kava derived from Fiji and Vanuatu, and to a lesser extent, Samoa and Tonga (Lindstrom, 2004). Kava abuse has been reported, especially in Pacific Island nations, leading to significant health and social problems (McDonald & Jowitt, 2000; Rychetnik & Madronio, 2011).

Current use in North America, Europe, and Australia may have been influenced by regulatory measures (see Section 1.6) and reports of adverse events in the popular press.

According to the 2012 Nutrition Business Journal Annual Report, kava was the 36th best-selling dietary supplement in the USA in 2011. There has been a considerable decline in kava sales in the USA from US$ 52 million in 2000 to US$ 17 million in 2004. Sales remained at a similar level between US$ 18 and 22 million

Fig. 1.3 Sales of kava as a dietary supplement in the USA

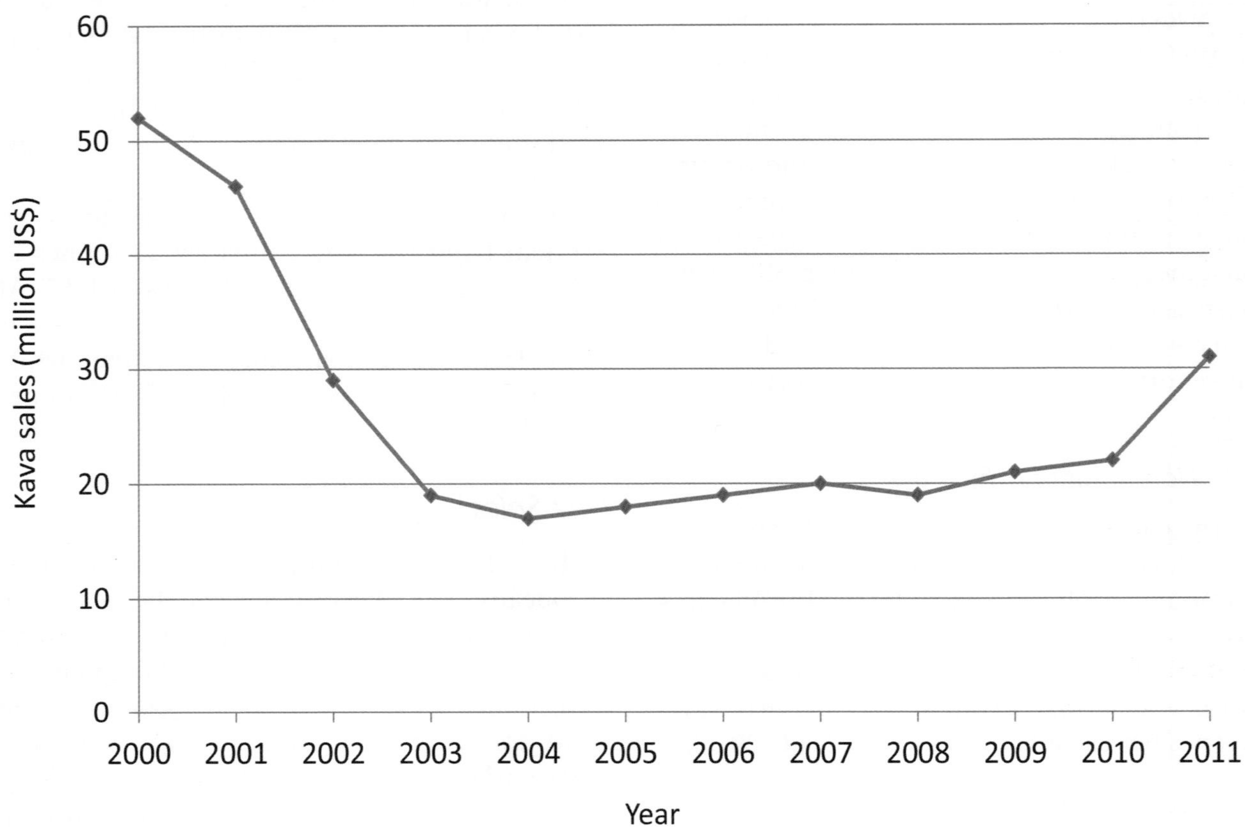

Compiled by the Working Group from data from Nutrition Business Journal (2010, 2012).

during 2005–2011, and then increased to US$ 31 million in 2011 (Fig. 1.3; Nutrition Business Journal, 2010, 2012). Total global sales of kava (*Piper methysticum*) as an herbal supplement were US$ 8 million in 2012, and appreciable sales volumes occurred in the USA (US $3 million), Brazil (US$ 2 million), and Hungary (US$1 million) (IMS Health, 2012).

[The Working Group suggested that prohibition in some countries may have resulted in increases in unrecorded sales of kava, e.g. unrecorded individual imports, or illegal sales.]

1.4.3 Consumption

Consumers of products specified in Section 1.3 are exposed to kava. No literature about the degree of population-based exposure to kava was available to the Working Group. [The Working Group estimated that current exposure to kava was expected to be a fraction of what it was in the previous decade due to withdrawal of marketing authorization in many countries (see Section 1.6).]

Table 1.2 Guidelines for dried kava rhizome

Characteristic	Guideline
Content	Not less than 3.5% kavapyrones [kavalactones], as determined by IR spectroscopy
Identity tests	Macroscopic, microscopic and microchemical examinations, and TLC for the presence of characteristic unsaturated α-pyrones known as kavapyrones [kavalactones]
Microbiological purity, heavy metals, radioactive residues	Limits according to WHO guidelines on quality control methods for medicinal plants
Foreign organic matter	Not more than 2%
Total ash	Not more than 8%
Acid-insoluble ash	Not more than 1.5%
Water-soluble extractive	Not less than 5%
Loss on drying	Not more than 12%
Pesticide residues	Aldrin and dieldrin not more than 0.05 mg/kg. For other pesticides, general guidelines apply.

IR, infrared; TLC, thin-layer chromatography
From WHO (2004)

1.5 Occupational exposure

No specific studies on occupational exposure were available to the Working Group. It can be assumed that workers in kava production for food, cosmetic, or medicinal use may be exposed.

1.6 Regulations and guidelines

Several cases of liver damage have been associated with exposure to kava in Europe, and have led to withdrawal of the product license (NTP, 2012). Reviews on the cases of adverse effects potentially caused by exposure to kava have been compiled by Schmidt *et al.* (2005) (detailed analysis of 83 cases), as by WHO (2007) (analysis of 93 cases). Speculations about the causes of the adverse effects included the use of less expensive stem peelings in commercial materials instead of the usual peeled rhizomes (Teschke *et al.*, 2011).

Sales of kava have been suspended or withdrawn in several countries, including Australia, Canada, France, Germany, Spain, and Switzerland, and due to reported association with hepatotoxicity in humans (Russmann *et al.*, 2001, 2003; Campo *et al.*, 2002; De Smet, 2002; Parkman, 2002; Clough *et al.*, 2003; Humberston

et al., 2003; Teschke *et al.*, 2003; Ulbricht *et al.*, 2005; NTP, 2012).

Although sales of kava were not regulated or controlled in the USA in 2012 (NTP, 2012), the Food and Drug Administration (FDA) had issued a public warning in 2001 that kava might be be associated with serious liver damage, including hepatitis, cirrhosis, and liver failure (FDA, 2002). The regulatory action taken by various countries around the world from the year 2000 after concerns about hepatotoxicity is summarized in WHO (2007). Current regulatory status was summarized by Teschke & Lebot (2011), and included suggested chemical standards and agricultural standardizations. WHO (2004) provided some guidelines for the quality control of kava (see Table 1.2).

2. Cancer in Humans

Steiner (2000) investigated the association between cancer incidence and consumption of kava in an ecological study of six countries in the South Pacific. Exposure was estimated by a surrogate measure of consumption based on the number of kava plants under cultivation in each country. Exposure estimates and data on cancer incidence for men in the 1980s were used in the analysis on the assumption that all kava produced before 1990 was consumed locally, and primarily by men. An inverse correlation was observed between the incidence of all cancers in men and estimated exposure, but no test of statistical significance or confidence intervals, was reported. [The Working Group considered this study as uninformative because of its ecological design, the use of crude measures of exposure and outcome, and inadequate assessment of the role of chance.]

3. Cancer in Experimental Animals

3.1 Mouse

See Table 3.1

In one study of oral administration, groups of 50 male and 50 female B6C3F$_1$ mice (age, 5–6 weeks) were given kava extract at a dose of 0 (corn oil vehicle, 10 mL/kg body weight, bw), 0.25, 0.5, or 1.0 g/kg bw per day by gavage, 5 days per week, for 105 weeks. The purity of the kava extract was 98.04% by high-performance liquid chromatography/ultraviolet (HPLC/UV) profiles. The extract contained 27% kavalactones identified as kavain, dihydrokavain, methysticin, dihydromethysticin, yangonin, and desmethoxyyangonin. In males, the mean body weight of the dosed groups was similar to that in the control group. In females, the mean body weight of the group at 1.0 g/kg bw was 11% less than that in the control group after week 21. The mean survival time of male and female mice in the dosed groups was similar to that of the controls.

In males, the incidence of hepatoblastoma was significantly higher in the groups receiving the intermediate and highest dose, and had a significant positive trend. The incidence of hepatocellular carcinoma and hepatoblastoma (combined) was significantly higher in the group receiving the intermediate dose. The incidence of eosinophilic hepatocyte foci, a preneoplastic hepatocyte lesion, was significantly higher in the groups receiving the intermediate or highest dose.

In females, the incidence of hepatocellular carcinoma was significantly higher in the group receiving the lowest dose. The incidence of hepatocellular adenoma or carcinoma (combined) was significantly higher in the groups receiving the lowest and intermediate doses. The incidence of hepatocellular carcinoma and hepatoblastoma (combined) was significantly higher in the group receiving the lowest dose. [The Working Group noted that reduced body weight may have reduced one tumour response in females at the highest dose.] The incidence of eosinophilic hepatocyte foci was significantly higher in the group receiving the highest dose. The incidence of squamous cell hyperplasia of the forestomach was significantly higher in the groups receiving the lowest or intermediate doses (Behl *et al.*, 2011; NTP, 2012).

3.2 Rat

See Table 3.1

In one study of oral administration, groups of 49 or 50 male and 50 female F344/N rats (age, 6–7 weeks) were given kava extract at 0 (corn-oil vehicle, 5 mL/kg bw), 0.1, 0.3, or 1.0 g/kg bw per day by gavage, 5 days per week, for 104 (male rats) or 105 (female rats) weeks. The purity of the kava extract was 98.04% by HPLC/UV profiles. The extract contained 27% kavalactones identified as kavain, dihydrokavain, methysticin, dihydromethysticin, yangonin, and desmethoxyyangonin. The mean body weight of the groups at 1.0 g/kg bw was 10% less than that of the control group after week 65 in males and after week 41 in females. The mean survival time for rats in the dosed groups was similar to that of controls for both sexes.

Table 3.1 Studies of carcinogenicity with kava extracts in mice and rats

Species, strain (sex) Duration Reference	Dosing regimen, Animals/group at start	Incidence of tumours	Significance[a]	Comments
Mouse, B6C3F$_1$ (M, F) 105 wk NTP (2012), Behl *et al.* (2011)	0 (control), 0.25, 0.5, or 1.0 g/kg bw by gavage in corn oil, 5 days/wk for 105 wk 50 M and 50 F/group (age, 5–6 wk)	Hepatocellular carcinoma: 3/50, 13/50*, 8/50, 8/50 (F) Hepatocellular adenoma or carcinoma (combined): 38/50, 39/50, 39/50, 40/50 (M); 10/50, 21/50*, 20/50**, 13/50 (F) Hepatoblastoma: 0/50*, 4/50, 9/50**, 12/50*** (M); 0/50, 0/50, 1/50, 0/50 (F) Hepatocellular carcinoma or hepatoblastoma (combined): 20/50, 21/50, 30/50*, 25/50 (M); 3/50, 13/50**, 9/50, 8/50 (F)	*P = 0.007 *P = 0.015 **P = 0.036 *P < 0.001 (trend) **P = 0.002 ***P < 0.001 *P < 0.05 **P = 0.007	Extract purity, 98.04% (HPLC/UV profiles), containing 27% kavalactones Mean body weight of females at 1.0 g/kg bw was 11% less than that in the vehicle-control group after wk 21
Rat, F344 (M, F) 104– 105 wk NTP (2012), Behl *et al.* (2011)	0 (control), 0.1, 0.3, or 1.0 g/kg bw by gavage in corn oil, 5 days/wk for 104 (M) or 105 (F) wk 49 or 50 M, and 50 F (age, 6–7 wk)	Testis interstitial (Leydig) cell adenoma[b]: 37/49 (76%)*, 44/50 (88%), 49/50 (98%)**, 46/50 (92%)***(M)	*P = 0.003 (trend) **P = 0.002 ***P < 0.001	Extract purity, 98.04% (HPLC/UV profiles), containing 27% kavalactones Mean body weight of group at 1.0 g/kg bw was 10% less than that of the vehicle-control group after wk 65 (M) and wk 41 (F) No significant increase in the incidence of any neoplasm in females

[a] Poly-3 test

[b] Historical incidence in 2-year studies with administration by gavage with corn oil vehicle-control group (mean ± standard deviation): 176/199 (88.4% ± 8.6%), range 76–94%; all routes: 1053/1298 (81.1% ± 13.4%), range 54–98%

bw, body weight; F, female; HPLC/UV, high-performance liquid chromatography/ultraviolet; M, male; wk, week

In males, the incidence of testis interstitial (Leydig) cell adenoma was significantly higher in the groups at the intermediate or highest dose, and had a significant positive trend. [The incidence of this tumour in controls was low (76%) compared with that in historical controls (corn oil vehicle controls: range, 76–94%; all routes: range, 54–98%).] The incidence of renal pelvis transitional cell hyperplasia was significantly higher in the group receiving the highest dose. In females, the incidence of renal pelvis transitional cell hyperplasia was significantly higher in the groups at the highest or intermediate dose. There was no significant increase in the incidence of any neoplasm in females (Behl *et al.*, 2011; NTP, 2012).

4. Mechanistic and Other Relevant Data

4.1 Absorption, distribution, metabolism, and excretion

4.1.1 Humans

The metabolism of kava and individual kava-lactones has been studied in humans (Duffield *et al.*, 1989; Köppel & Tenczer, 1991; Johnson *et al.*, 2003; Zou *et al.*, 2005). Demethylation and hydroxylation products were found in human urine after ingestion of kava extract (Duffield *et al.*, 1989), or its constituent kavain. The metabolites were mainly excreted as conjugates (Köppel & Tenczer, 1991).

Ten urinary metabolites were identified when kavain was given as a therapeutic oral dose of 200 mg to five healthy volunteers. The structures of kavain and its metabolites are shown in Fig. 4.1. The major metabolite was a hydroxydihydrokavain. Hydroxylation of the phenyl ring, reduction of the 7,8 double bond, hydroxylation of the lactone ring with subsequent dehydration, and opening of the lactone ring appeared to be the main metabolic pathways (Köppel & Tenczer, 1991).

Zou *et al.* (2005) identified a pyrone ring-opened product, 6-phenyl-3-hexen-2-one, a proposed metabolite of kava, as its mercapturic acid adduct, in urinary samples from two kava drinkers. This metabolite was possibly formed from enzymatic demethylation of 7,8-dihydromethysticin, followed by ring opening of the α-pyrone ring, and rearrangement (Zou *et al.*, 2005).

11,12-Dihydroxy-7,8-dihydrokavain-*o*-quinone and 11,12-dihydroxykavain-*o*-quinone, two electrophilic metabolites, were identified as glutathione conjugates when kava extract was incubated with human liver microsomes. The glucuronic acid and sulfate conjugates of these two urinary metabolites were detected in a human volunteer who ingested a single dose of a dietary supplement containing kava extract (about 90 mg of kavalactones) (Johnson *et al.*, 2003).

4.1.2 Experimental systems

(a) Absorption, distribution, and excretion

Few studies have been published on the absorption, distribution, and excretion of the constituents of kava (kavain, dihydrokavain, methysticin, dihydromethysticin, yangonin, desmethoxyyangonin, and dihydroyangonin).

Kavain is rapidly absorbed from the gastrointestinal tract, distributed to tissues, and eliminated.

In male F344 rats given kavain at a single oral dose of 100 mg/kg bw, the maximum blood concentration of kavain was measured at 0.88 hours, after which plasma concentrations declined with a mean terminal half-life of 1.3 hours. The mean oral bioavailability of kavain in F344 rats was about 50% (Mathews *et al.*, 2005).

In male F344 rats given kavain orally for 7 days, kavain was primarily excreted in the urine, with about 77% recovered during the

Fig. 4.1 Structures of kavain and its eight identified metabolites

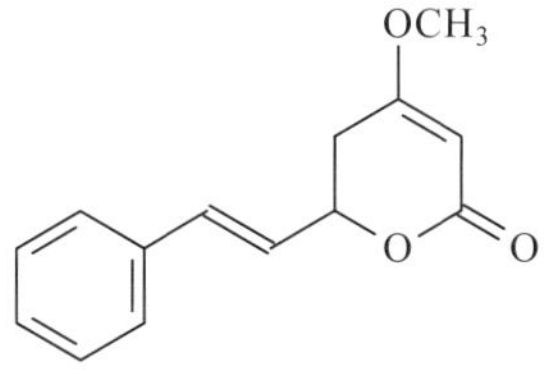

Kavain

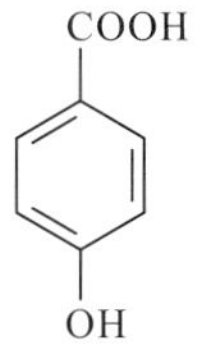

m-Hydroxybenzoic acid

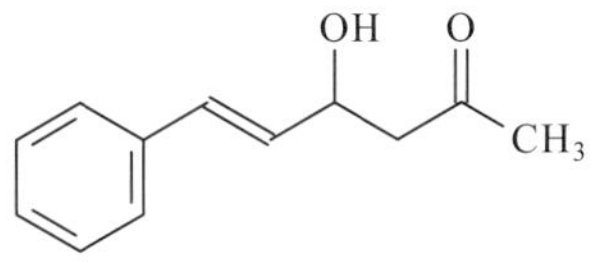

4-Hydroxy-6-phenyl-5-hexen-2-one

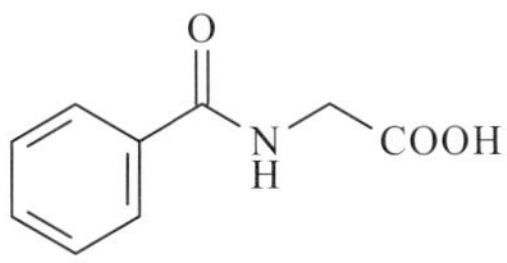

Hippuric acid

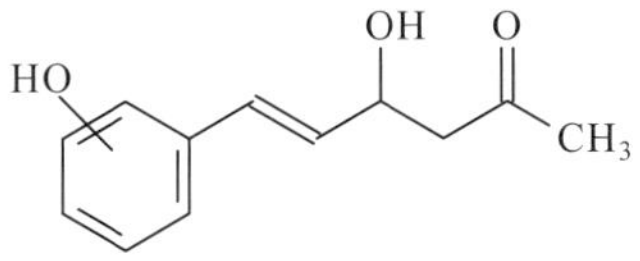

4-Hydroxy-6-hydroxyphenyl-5-hexen-2-one

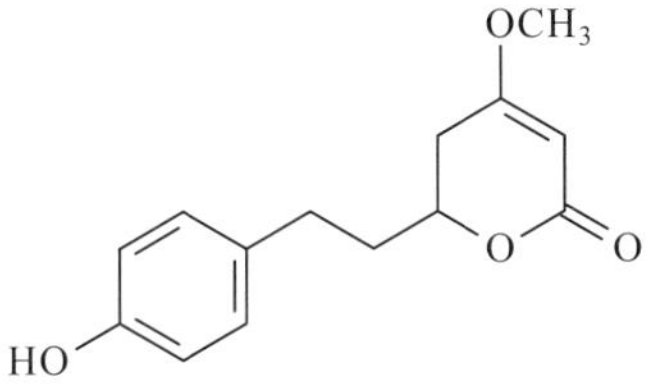

12-Hydroxydihydrokavain

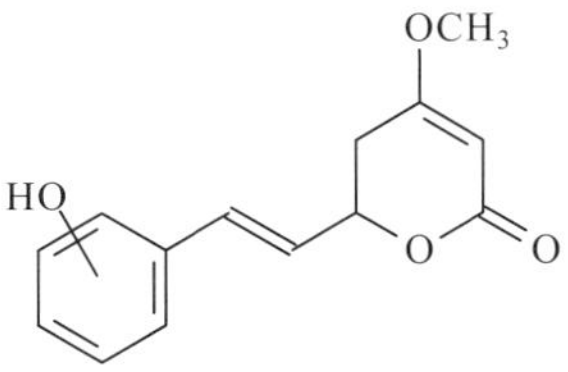

x-Hydroxykavain

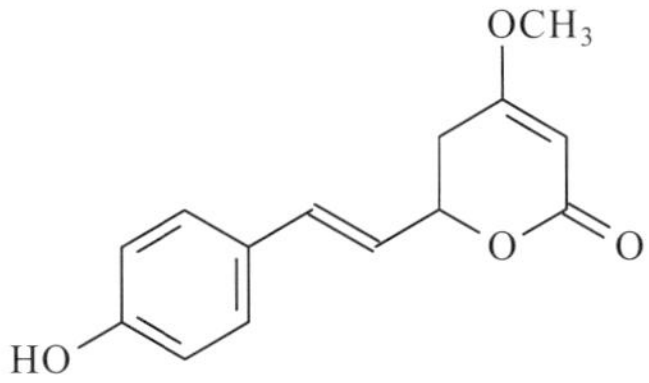

12-Hydroxykavain

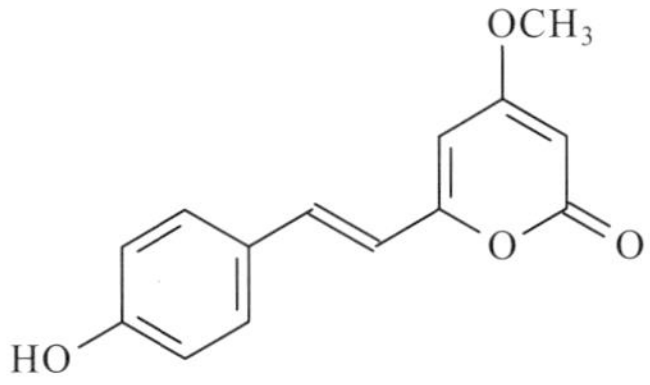

12-Hydroxy-5,6-dehydrokavain

Compiled by the Working Group

72 hours after the last dose. Faecal excretion accounted for about 14% of the administered dose. Only 0.4% of the kavain was retained in the tissues, and kavain did not accumulate preferentially in any particular tissue. In addition, there were no differences in the pharmacokinetics of kavain when administered as a single dose or as repeated doses (Mathews *et al.*, 2005).

Oral absorption of kavain, dihydrokavain, methysticin, dihydromethysticin, yangonin, and desmethoxyyangonin was investigated in mice (Meyer, 1967). Kavain and dihydrokavain were rapidly absorbed from the gastrointestinal tract (with a peak at 10 minutes), followed by methysticin and dihydromethysticin (30–45 minutes). Yangonin and desmethoxyyangonin were poorly absorbed, and rapid elimination occurred (Meyer, 1967; Robinson *et al.*, 2009).

In male F344 rats given an intravenous injection of kavain at a dose of 7 mg/kg bw, kavain was rapidly eliminated from the systemic circulation, with a terminal half-life of 0.63 hours. Systemic clearance and volume of distribution were 89 mL/minutes per kg and 2.70 L/kg, respectively, indicating that a significant amount of kavain was rapidly distributed out of the plasma into tissues and quickly cleared from the body (Mathews *et al.*, 2005).

Keledjian *et al.* (1988) observed a peak concentration at 5 minutes in brain for kavain and 7,8-dihydrokavain; the compounds were rapidly eliminated after intraperitoneal administration (100 mg/kg bw) of individual kava constituents in male Balb/c mice. The maximum concentrations of kavain and 7,8-dihydrokavain were 64.7 and 29.3 ng/mg wet brain tissue, respectively. The maximum concentrations of desmethoxyyangonin and yangonin were 10.4 and 1.2 ng/mg wet brain tissue, lower than those of kavain or 7,8-dihydrokavain. When kava extract was given intraperitoneally to male Balb/c mice, the maximum concentrations of kavain and yangonin increased in the brain, while the concentrations of 7,8-dihydrokavain and desmethoxyyangonin were similar to those measured after they were injected separately (Keledjian *et al.*, 1988).

(b) Metabolism

Rasmussen *et al.* (1979) investigated the metabolism of five kavalactones (kavain, dihydrokavain, methysticin, yangonin, and dihydroyangonin) in male albino rats. The individual kavalactones were administered orally (400 mg/kg bw) or intraperitoneally (100 mg/kg bw), the metabolites and the recovered parent substrate in the urine were then identified. Kavalactones were metabolized to several products via demethylation, mono- and dihydroxylation, and reduction and pyrone ring-opening (Rasmussen *et al.*, 1979; NTP, 2012).

With 7,8-dihydrokavain, large amounts of the parental compound were found in the urine. Nine metabolites were identified, with 12-hydroxydihydrokavain being the most abundant. About two thirds of the metabolites were hydroxylated forms, and one third of the metabolites were formed by scission of the 5,6-dihydro-α-pyrone ring (Fig. 4.2). The proposed metabolic pathways for 7,8-dihydrokavain are depicted in Fig. 4.2 (adapted from NTP (2012).

With kavain, a total of 10 metabolites were formed in very small amounts. Eight were determined structurally and two remained unidentified. Both hydroxylated and ring-opened products were formed (Fig. 4.1).

With methysticin, only small amounts of two metabolites (11,12-dihydroxykavain and 11,12-dihydroxydihydrokavain) were formed by demethylenation of the methylenedioxyphenyl moiety (Fig. 4.3).

Metabolites of yangonin and dihydroyangonin were formed via *O*-demethylation. No ring-opened products were detected (Fig. 4.4 and Fig. 4.5).

4.1.3 Effects on drug-metabolizing enzymes

Studies *in vivo* and *in vitro* have shown that kava extract and its constituents altered drug-metabolizing enzymes. Table 4.1 lists the major enzymes affected by kava.

4.2 Genetic and related effects

4.2.1 Humans

No data were available to the Working Group.

4.2.2 Experimental systems

See Table 4.2

(a) Mutagenicity

Kava extract (up to 10 000 µg/plate) was not mutagenic in *Salmonella typhimurium* strains TA97, TA98, TA1535 or TA100, or *Escherichia coli* strain WP2 *uvr*A pKM101 with or without metabolic activation (rat liver S9) (NTP, 2012). In one trial out of three of which two of the results were negative, kava extract tested equivocal in TA97 with metabolic activation (NTP, 2012). Kava extracts were not mutagenic in an assay in L5178Y mouse lymphoma cells (Whittaker *et al.*, 2008).

Fig. 4.2 The proposed metabolic pathways for 7,8-dihydrokavain

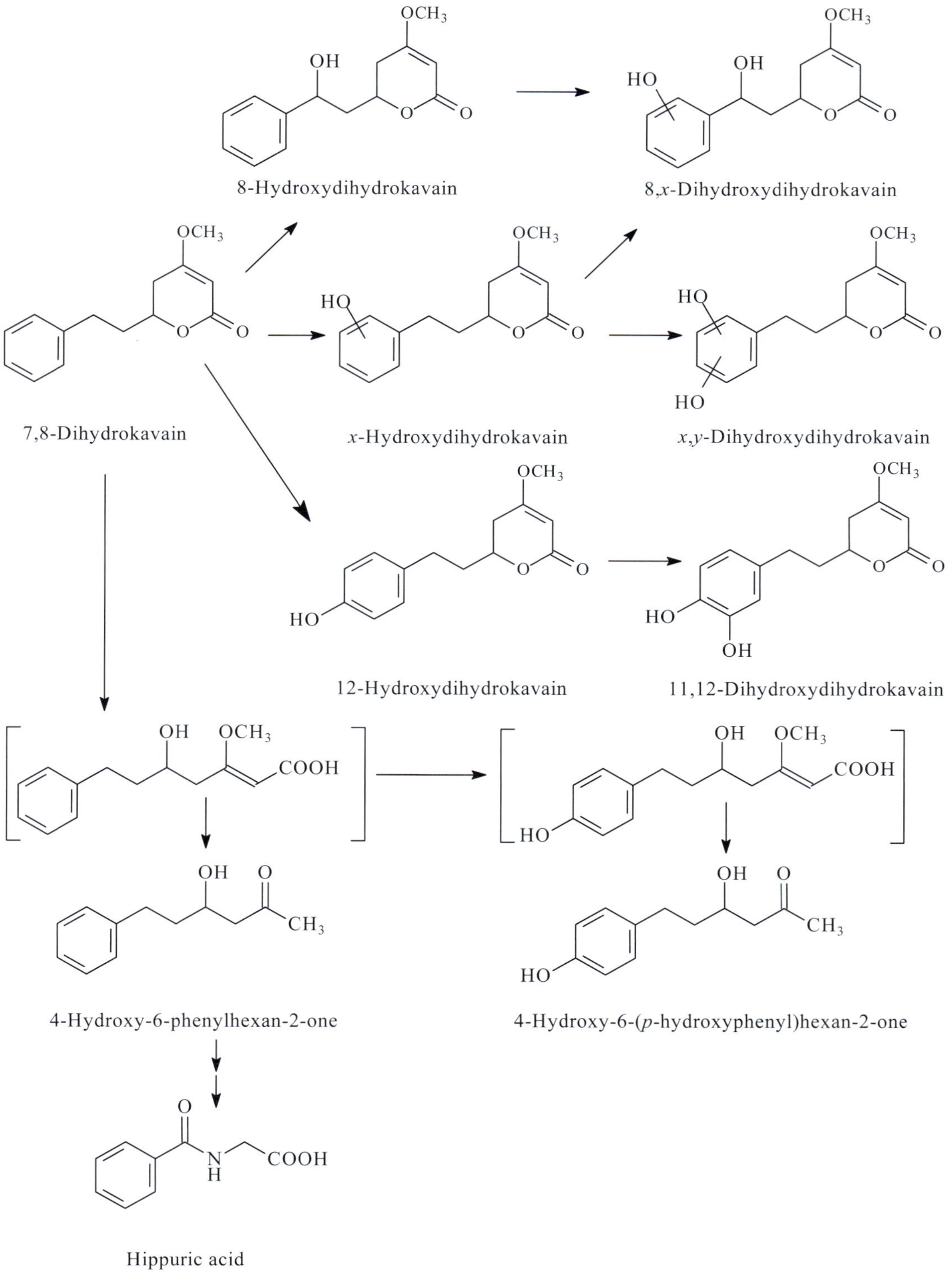

Compiled by the Working Group using data from NTP (2012).

Fig. 4.3 Structures of methysticin and its two metabolites

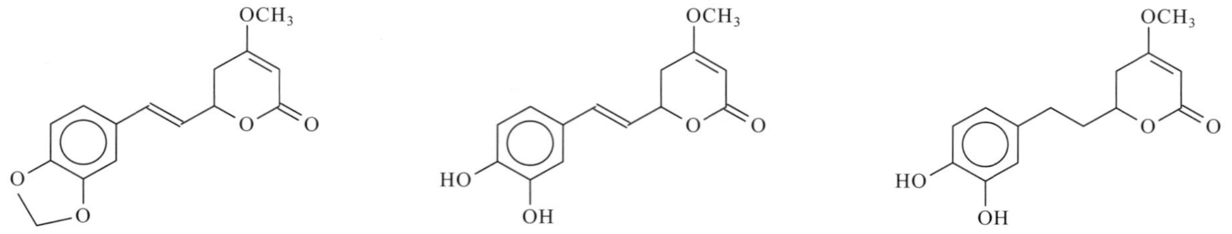

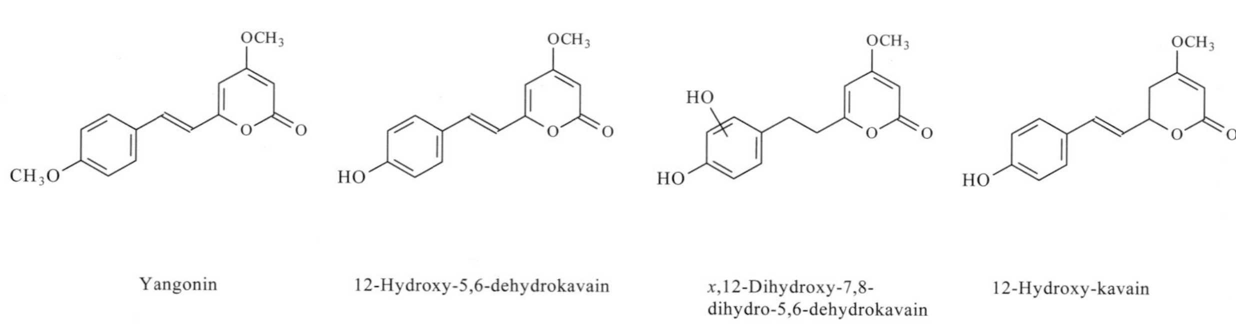

| Methysticin | 11,12-Dihydroxykavain | 11,12-Dihydroxydihydrokavain |

Compiled by the Working Group using data from Fu *et al.* (2008)

Fig. 4.4 Structures of 7,8-dihydroyangonin and its three metabolites

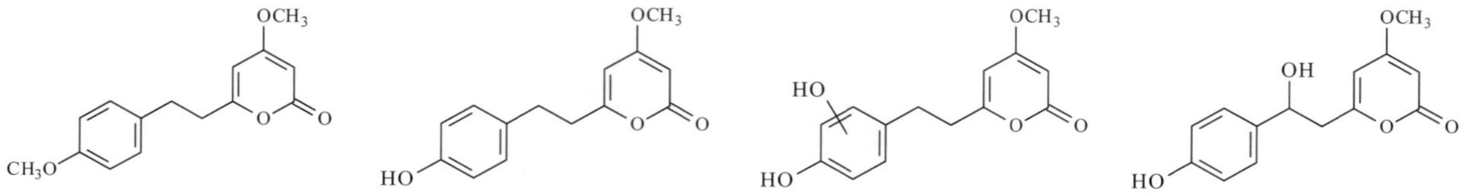

7,8-Dihydroyangonin   12-Hydroxy-5,6-dehydro-7,8-dihydrokavain I   Dihydroxy-5,6-dehydro-7,8-dihydrokavain I II   Dihydroxy-5,6-dehydro-7,8-dihydrokavain II III

For the metabolites II and III the positioning of the second hydroxyl group (m, o or at C8) are uncertain.
Compiled by the Working Group using data from Fu *et al.* (2008)

Fig. 4.5 Structures of yangonin and its three metabolites

Yangonin   12-Hydroxy-5,6-dehydrokavain   x,12-Dihydroxy-7,8-dihydro-5,6-dehydrokavain   12-Hydroxy-kavain

Compiled by the Working Group using data from Fu *et al.* (2008)

Table 4.1 Effects of kava extract and kavalactones on metabolizing enzymes

Reference	Species or cell type	Kava preparation	Dose	Duration of treatment	Detection method	Result
In vivo						
Russmann *et al.* (2005)	Human	Aqueous extract	7–27 g of kavalactones per wk, oral	6 yr	Substrate turnover	CYP1A2 (inhibition)
Guo *et al.* (2010)	Mouse	Methanolic and aqueous extracts	0.125–2.0 g/kg bw per day, 5 days/wk, gavage	98 days	Gene expression	CYP4A10 (inhibition); CYP2A5, CYP2B20, CYP2C55, GSTA1, GSTA2 (induction)
Guo *et al.* (2009)	Rat	Methanolic and aqueous extracts	0.125–2.0 g/kg bw per day, 5 days/wk, gavage	98 days	Gene expression	CYP3A13, CYP17A1, ABCB9 (inhibition); CYP1A1, CYP1A2, CYP3A1, CYP3A3, ABCC3, NQO1, UGT1A6 (induction)
Yamazaki *et al.* (2008)	Rat	Kava extracts (not specified)	Kava extract (kavalactones, 380 mg/kg bw per day), gavage	8 days	Rat liver microsomes/ enzyme assay, gene expression, protein expression	CYP1A1, CYP1A2 (induction)
Lim *et al.* (2007)	Rat	Acetone kava leave extract	100 mg/kg/ bw per day, gavage	14 days	Protein expression	CYP1A2, CYP2E1 (induction)
Clayton *et al.* (2007)	Rat	Methanolic and aqueous extracts	0.125–2.0 g/kg bw per day, 5 days/wk, gavage	90 days	Protein expression	CYP2D1 (inhibition); CYP1A2, CYP2B1, CYP3A1 (induction)
Mathews *et al.* (2005)	Rat	Methanol or acetone kava extract	256 mg/kg bw, 1 g/kg bw, gavage	7 days	Rat liver microsomes/ enzyme assay	CYP2D1, 2C11 (inhibition); CYP1A2, 2B1, 2C6, 2D1, 3A1/2 (induction)
In vitro						
Li *et al.* (2011)	Hepa1c1c7	Methanolic and aqueous extracts, methysticin, 7,8-dihydromethysticin	Various concentrations to 25 µM of kava constituents or 6.25 µg/mL of kava extract	24 h	Cell-based enzymatic assay/enzyme assay, gene expression, protein expression	CYP1A1 (induction)
Mathews *et al.* (2005)	Human liver microsomes	Methanol or acetone kava extract, yangonin, dihydrokavain, methysticin, dihydromethysticin, composite kavalactones	1, 10, 100 µM	10 min	Recombinant protein/ enzyme assay	CYP2C9, 2C19, 2D6, 3A4 (inhibition); P-glycoprotein ATPase (inhibition)

Table 4.1 (continued)

Reference	Species or cell type	Kava preparation	Dose	Duration of treatment	Detection method	Result
Weiss et al. (2005)	P388 and P388/dx cell lines	Methanol aqueous kava extracts, kavain, dihydrokavain, methysticin, dihydromethysticin, yangonin, and desmethoxyyangonin	Various concentrations (to the highest soluble concentration)	NR	Calcein uptake	ABCB1 (inhibition)
Zou et al. (2004)	Baculovirus/ insect cell system and cryopreserved human hepatocytes	Ethanol extract, methysticin, desmethoxyyangonin, yangonin	Various concentrations up to 100 μM	15–45 min	Recombinant enzyme/ enzyme assay	CYP1A2, 2C9, 2C19, 2E1, 3A4 (inhibition)
Côté et al. (2004)	Human liver microsomes/	Methanol, acetone, ethanol or aqueous kava extracts	Various concentrations up to 200 μg/mL	5 min	Enzyme assay	CYP3A4, CYP1A2, CYP2C9, CYP2C19 (inhibition)
Raucy (2003)	Primary human hepatocytes and HepG2	Kava extract (not specified)	100 μg/mL	48 h	Gene expression, report gene assay	CYP3A4 (induction)
Mathews et al. (2002)	Human liver microsomes/	Methanol or acetone extract, desmethoxyyangonin, methysticin, dihydromethysticin	Kava extract normalized to 100 μM kavalactones	15 min	Enzyme assay	CYP1A2, CYP2C9, CYP2C19, CYP2D6, CYP3A4, CYP4A9/11 (induction)
Unger et al. (2002)	Baculovirus/ insect cell system	Methanol, acetone and ethyl acetate extracts	1–100 mg/mL	30 min	Recombinant enzyme/ enzyme assay	CYP3A4 (inhibition)
Zou et al. (2002)	cDNA human CYP isoforms	Methysticin, desmethoxyyangonin, dihydromethysticin, kavain, dihydrokavain	Various concentrations up to ~200 μM	30–45 min	Recombinant enzyme/ enzyme assay	CYP1A2, CYP2C9, CYP2C19, CYP2D6, CYP3A4 (inhibition)

ABC, ATP-binding cassette; CYP, cytochrome; GST, glutathione-S-transferase; min, minute; NR, not reported; NQO, NAD(P)H quinone oxidoreductase; UGT, UDP glycosyltransferase; wk, week; yr, year

Table 4.2 Genetic and related effects of kava extract

Test system	Results[a]		Concentration or dose (LED or HID)	Reference
	Without exogenous metabolic system	With exogenous metabolic system		
Salmonella typhimurium TA100, TA98, TA1535, reverse mutation	–	–	10 000 µg/plate	NTP (2012)
Salmonella typhimurium TA97, reverse mutation	–	Equivocal in 1 out of 3 tests	10 000 µg/plate	NTP (2012)
L5178Y mouse lymphoma mutation assay	–	NR	300 µg/mL	Whittaker et al. (2008)
umu point mutation assay	+[a]	+[a]	2330 µg/mL extract 300 µM pure kavalactones	Jhoo et al. (2007)
Escherichia coli WP2 *uvrA*/pKM101, reverse mutation	–	–	10 000 µg/plate	NTP (2012)
Micronucleus induction in peripheral blood erythrocytes of male and female B6C3F$_1$ mice in vivo	–	NT	Up to 2.0 g/kg bw per day by gavage for 3 months	NTP (2012)

+, positive; (+), weakly positive; –, negative; HID, highest ineffective dose; LED, lowest effective dose; NT, not tested; NR, not reported

[a] These data were not analysed statistically.

The only report of positive mutagenic activity with kava extracts (two positive results, but six negative results) involved the *umu* point mutation assay (Jhoo *et al.*, 2007). [The Working Group noted that these data were not analysed statistically.]

(b) Chromosomal damage

In male or female mice given kava extract at a dose of up to 2.0 g/kg bw per day by gavage for 3 months, there was no increase in the frequency of micronucleated normochromatic or polychromatic erythrocytes in blood (NTP, 2012).

4.3 Other mechanistic data relevant to carcinogenesis

Effects on hepatic cell physiology

Case reports of liver injury associated with kava intake have been described. The types of liver damage reported include fulminant hepatitis, necrosis, cirrhosis, and liver failure requiring liver transplantation or causing death (Russmann *et al.*, 2001; Bujanda *et al.*, 2002; Campo *et al.*, 2002; Brauer *et al.*, 2003; Gow *et al.*, 2003; Humberston *et al.*, 2003; Stickel *et al.*, 2003; Teschke *et al.*, 2003, 2008; Thomsen *et al.*, 2004).

4.4 Susceptibility

Genetic polymorphisms

Deficiency in CYP2D6, the major kavalactone-metabolizing enzyme, was detected in two patients with liver failure (Russmann *et al.*, 2001). Genetic polymorphism of CYP2D6 has a prevalence of 7–9% in Caucasian populations, but < 1% in Polynesian populations (Wanwimolruk *et al.*, 1998; Ingelman-Sundberg, 2005). Severe liver failure has not been observed in people using kava in the traditional way in islands in the South Pacific (Moulds & Malani, 2003; Anke & Ramzan, 2004).

4.5 Mechanistic considerations

Kava extract is not mutagenic based on the results of numerous studies of genotoxicity, including tests for mutagenicity in bacteria, induction of micronuclei *in vivo* (NTP, 2012), and the mouse lymphoma assay (Whittaker *et al.*, 2008). The reported carcinogenicity in mice is most probably mediated through nongenotoxic mechanisms.

5. Summary of Data Reported

5.1 Exposure data

The kava (or kava kava) plant *Piper methysticum* is a perennial tropical shrub that is widely cultivated in Oceania. The rhizome of the plant was originally used as an ingredient in local traditional drinks with psychopharmacological properties, and as traditional folk medicine. More recently, rhizome extracts have been used in medicinal products, food or dietary supplements, and cosmetics. Important chemical constituents of the resin contained in the kava rhizome are kavalactones, kavain being the major compound. The medicinal uses of kava supported by clinical data are short-term symptomatic treatment of mild states of anxiety or insomnia due to nervousness, stress, or tension. Use of kava was popular worldwide, but several case reports of liver damage associated with exposure to kava reduced sales, and caused kava to be banned in several countries.

5.2 Human carcinogenicity data

The Working Group was able to identify only one epidemiological study of cancer and kava consumption. This ecological study found an inverse correlation between all cancers in men and a proxy measure of kava consumption, but no confidence intervals or test of statistical significance were reported. The Working Group regarded the study as uninformative because the ecological design provided only weak support for causal inference at the individual level, the measures of exposure and outcome were crude, and the role of chance was not evaluated.

5.3 Animal carcinogenicity data

A kava extract was tested for carcinogenicity in one study in mice and one study in rats treated by gavage. In mice, the extract caused a significant increase in the incidence of hepatoblastoma in males, and of hepatocellular adenoma or carcinoma (combined), and hepatocellular carcinoma, in females. In male rats, the same extract caused a significant increase in the incidence of testis interstitial (Leydig) cell adenoma; however, the incidence in controls was low compared with that in historical controls. There was no significant increase in the incidence of any neoplasm in female rats.

5.4 Mechanistic and other relevant data

The major components of kava extract, kavalactones, are extensively metabolized in humans and experimental animals. Among the numerous metabolites are products from demethylation, hydroxylation, and ring-opening.

Kava extract gave negative results in several standard bacterial assays for mutation in the absence or presence of exogenous metabolic activation. Kavalactones gave negative results in most of these assays.

The reported carcinogenicity of kava in mice is most likely to be mediated through a nongenotoxic mechanism.

6. Evaluation

6.1 Cancer in humans

There is *inadequate evidence* in humans for the carcinogenicity of kava extract.

6.2 Cancer in experimental animals

There is *sufficient evidence* in experimental animals for the carcinogenicity of kava extract.

6.3 Overall evaluation

Kava extract is *possibly carcinogenic to humans (Group 2B)*.

References

Anke J & Ramzan I (2004). Kava hepatotoxicity: Are we any closer to the truth? *Planta Med*, 70(3):193–6. doi:10.1055/s-2004-815533 PMID:15114493

Anonymous (2000). Kava kava rhizome (root). In: Blumenthal M, Goldberg A, Brinckmann J, editors. Expanded Commission E Monographs. Herb Monographs, based on those created by a special expert committee of the German Federal Institute for Drugs and Medicinal Devices. Newton (MA), USA: Integrative Medicine Communications

Behl M, Nyska A, Chhabra RS, Travlos GS, Fomby LM, Sparrow BR *et al.* (2011). Liver toxicity and carcinogenicity in F344/N rats and B6C3F$_1$ mice exposed to Kava Kava. *Food Chem Toxicol*, 49(11):2820–9. doi:10.1016/j.fct.2011.07.067 PMID:21871523

Bilia AR, Bergonzi MC, Lazari D, Vincieri FF (2002). Characterization of commercial kava-kava herbal drug and herbal drug preparations by means of nuclear magnetic resonance spectroscopy. *J Agric Food Chem*, 50(18):5016–25. doi:10.1021/jf020049j PMID:12188601

Bilia AR, Gallon S, Vincieri FF (2002b). Kava-kava and anxiety: growing knowledge about the efficacy and safety. *Life Sci*, 70(22):2581–97. doi:10.1016/S0024-3205(02)01555-2 PMID:12269386

Bilia AR, Scalise L, Bergonzi MC, Vincieri FF (2004). Analysis of kavalactones from *Piper methysticum* (kava-kava). *J Chromatogr B Analyt Technol Biomed Life Sci*, 812(1-2):203–14. doi:10.1016/j.jchromb.2004.07.038 PMID:15556499

Brauer RB, Stangl M, Stewart JR, Pfab R, Becker K (2003). Acute liver failure after administration of herbal tranquilizer kava-kava (*Piper methysticum*). *J Clin Psychiatry*, 64(2):216–8. doi:10.4088/JCP.v64n0215c PMID:12633134

Bujanda L, Palacios A, Silvariño R, Sánchez A, Muñoz C (2002). [Kava-induced acute icteric hepatitis] *Gastroenterol Hepatol*, 25(6):434–5. doi:10.1016/S0210-5705(02)70281-1 PMID:12069710

Cairney S, Maruff P, Clough AR (2002). The neurobehavioural effects of kava. *Aust N Z J Psychiatry*, 36(5):657–62. doi:10.1046/j.1440-1614.2002.01027.x PMID:12225450

Campo JV, McNabb J, Perel JM, Mazariegos GV, Hasegawa SL, Reyes J (2002). Kava-induced fulminant hepatic failure. *J Am Acad Child Adolesc Psychiatry*, 41(6):631–2. doi:10.1097/00004583-200206000-00001 PMID:12049436

Clayton NP, Yoshizawa K, Kissling GE, Burka LT, Chan PC, Nyska A (2007). Immunohistochemical analysis of expressions of hepatic cytochrome P450 in F344 rats following oral treatment with kava extract. *Exp Toxicol Pathol*, 58(4):223–36. doi:10.1016/j.etp.2006.08.002 PMID:17059882

Clough A (2003). Enough! or too much. What is 'excessive' kava use in Arnhem Land? *Drug Alcohol Rev*, 22(1):43–51. doi:10.1080/0959523021000059820 PMID:12745358

Clough AR, Bailie RS, Currie B (2003). Liver function test abnormalities in users of aqueous kava extracts. *J Toxicol Clin Toxicol*, 41(6):821–9. doi:10.1081/CLT-120025347 PMID:14677792

Clough AR, Burns CB, Mununggurr N (2000). Kava in Arnhem Land: a review of consumption and its social correlates. *Drug Alcohol Rev*, 19(3):319–28. doi:10.1080/713659370

Côté CS, Kor C, Cohen J, Auclair K (2004). Composition and biological activity of traditional and commercial kava extracts. *Biochem Biophys Res Commun*, 322(1):147–52. doi:10.1016/j.bbrc.2004.07.093 PMID:15313185

De Smet PA (2002). Safety concerns about kava not unique. *Lancet*, 360(9342):1336 doi:10.1016/S0140-6736(02)11347-X PMID:12414243

Dentali SJ (1997). Herb safety review: Kava: *Piper methysticum* Forster F. (Piperaceae). Boulder (CO), USA: Herb Research Foundation.

Dharmaratne HR, Nanayakkara NP, Khan IA (2002). Kavalactones from Piper methysticum, and their 13C NMR spectroscopic analyses. *Phytochemistry*, 59(4):429–33. doi:10.1016/S0031-9422(01)00443-5 PMID:11830162

Duffield AM, Jamieson DD, Lidgard RO, Duffield PH, Bourne DJ (1989). Identification of some human urinary metabolites of the intoxicating beverage kava. *J Chromatogr A*, 475(2):273–81. doi:10.1016/S0021-9673(01)89682-5 PMID:2777959

FDA (2002). Kava-containing dietary supplements may be associated with severe liver injury. US Food and Drug

Administration. Available at: http://www.fda.gov/food/resourcesforyou/consumers/ucm085482.htm, accessed 18/04/2012.

Fu PP, Xia Q, Guo L, Yu H, Chan PC (2008). Toxicity of kava kava. *J Environ Sci Health C Environ Carcinog Ecotoxicol Rev*, 26(1):89–112. doi:10.1080/10590500801907407 PMID:18322868

Gaub M, Roeseler Ch, Roos G, Kovar KA (2004). Analysis of plant extracts by NIRS: simultaneous determination of kavapyrones and water in dry extracts of Piper methysticum Forst. *J Pharm Biomed Anal*, 36(4):859–64. doi:10.1016/j.jpba.2004.06.030 PMID:15533680

Gow PJ, Connelly NJ, Hill RL, Crowley P, Angus PW (2003). Fatal fulminant hepatic failure induced by a natural therapy containing kava. *Med J Aust*, 178(9):442–3. PMID:12720510

Guo L, Li Q, Xia Q, Dial S, Chan PC, Fu P (2009). Analysis of gene expression changes of drug metabolizing enzymes in the livers of F344 rats following oral treatment with kava extract. *Food Chem Toxicol*, 47(2):433–42. doi:10.1016/j.fct.2008.11.037 PMID:19100306

Guo L, Shi Q, Dial S, Xia Q, Mei N, Li QZ *et al.* (2010). Gene expression profiling in male B6C3F1 mouse livers exposed to kava identifies–changes in drug metabolizing genes and potential mechanisms linked to kava toxicity. *Food Chem Toxicol*, 48(2):686–96. doi:10.1016/j.fct.2009.11.050 PMID:19948201

IMS Health (2012) Multinational Integrated Data Analysis (MIDAS). Plymouth Meeting, 2012, Pennsylvania: IMS Health.

Humberston CL, Akhtar J, Krenzelok EP (2003). Acute hepatitis induced by kava kava. *J Toxicol Clin Toxicol*, 41(2):109–13. doi:10.1081/CLT-120019123 PMID:12733846

Ingelman-Sundberg M (2005). Genetic polymorphisms of cytochrome P450 2D6 (CYP2D6): clinical consequences, evolutionary aspects and functional diversity. *Pharmacogenomics J*, 5(1):6–13. doi:10.1038/sj.tpj.6500285 PMID:15492763

Jhoo JW, Ang CY, Heinze TM, Deck J, Schnackenberg LK, Beger RD *et al.* (2007). Identification of C-glycoside flavonoids as potential mutagenic compounds in kava. *J Food Sci*, 72(2):C120–5. doi:10.1111/j.1750-3841.2007.00278.x PMID:17995826

Johnson BM, Qiu SX, Zhang S, Zhang F, Burdette JE, Yu L *et al.* (2003). Identification of novel electrophilic metabolites of *Piper methysticum* Forst (kava). *Chem Res Toxicol*, 16(6):733–40. doi:10.1021/tx020113r PMID:12807356

Keledjian J, Duffield PH, Jamieson DD, Lidgard RO, Duffield AM (1988). Uptake into mouse brain of four compounds present in the psychoactive beverage kava. *J Pharm Sci*, 77(12):1003–6. doi:10.1002/jps.2600771203 PMID:3244102

Köppel C & Tenczer J (1991). Mass spectral characterization of urinary metabolites of D,L-kawain. *J Chromatogr A*, 562(1-2):207–11. doi:10.1016/0378-4347(91)80578-Z PMID:2026693

Lebot V, Merlin M, Lindstrom L (1997). Kava-the Pacific elixir: the definitive guide to its ethnobotany, history, and chemistry. Rochester (VT), USA: Healing Arts Press.

Li Y, Mei H, Wu Q, Zhang S, Fang JL, Shi L *et al.* (2011). Methysticin and 7,8-dihydromethysticin are two major kavalactones in kava extract to induce CYP1A1. *Toxicol Sci*, 124(2):388–99. doi:10.1093/toxsci/kfr235 PMID:21908763

Lim ST, Dragull K, Tang CS, Bittenbender HC, Efird JT, Nerurkar PV (2007). Effects of kava alkaloid, piper-methystine, and kavalactones on oxidative stress and cytochrome P450 in F-344 rats. *Toxicol Sci*, 97(1):214–21. doi:10.1093/toxsci/kfm035 PMID:17329236

Lindstrom L (2004). History, folklore, traditional and current uses of kava. In: Singh YN, editor. Kava: from ethnology to pharmacology. Boca Raton (FL), USA: CRC Press; pp. 10–28.

Mathews JM, Etheridge AS, Black SR (2002). Inhibition of human cytochrome P450 activities by kava extract and kavalactones. *Drug Metab Dispos*, 30(11):1153–7. doi:10.1124/dmd.30.11.1153 PMID:12386118

Mathews JM, Etheridge AS, Valentine JL, Black SR, Coleman DP, Patel P *et al.* (2005). Pharmacokinetics and disposition of the kavalactone kawain: interaction with kava extract and kavalactones in vivo and in vitro. *Drug Metab Dispos*, 33(10):1555–63. doi:10.1124/dmd.105.004317 PMID:16033948

McDonald D & Jowitt A (2000). Kava in the Pacific Islands: a contemporary drug of abuse? *Drug Alcohol Rev*, 19(2):217–27. doi:10.1080/713659319

Meyer HJ (1967). Pharmacology of kava. 1. *Psychopharmacol Bull*, 4(3):10–1. PMID:5616309

Monakhova YB, Kuballa T, Löbell-Behrends S, Maixner S, Kohl-Himmelseher M, Ruge W *et al.* (2013). Standardless 1H NMR determination of pharmacologically active substances in dietary supplements and medicines that have been illegally traded over the internet. *Drug Test Anal*, 5(6):400–11. doi:10.1002/dta.1367 PMID:22550015

Morgan M, Bone K, Mills S et al. (2005). Kava. Safety monograph. In: Mills S, Bone K, editors. The essential guide to herbal safety. St. Louis (MO), USA: Elsevier Churchill Livingstone; pp. 484–492.

Morris CA & Avorn J (2003). Internet marketing of herbal products. *JAMA*, 290(11):1505–9. doi:10.1001/jama.290.11.1505 PMID:13129992

Moulds RF & Malani J (2003). Kava: herbal panacea or liver poison? *Med J Aust*, 178(9):451–3. PMID:12720513

NTP (2012). Toxicology and carcinogenesis studies of kava kava extract (CAS No. 9000–38–8) in F344/N rats and B6C3F1 mice (gavage studies). *Natl Toxicol Program Tech Rep Ser*, 571(571):1–186. PMID:22441424

NLM (2012). Products that contain active ingredient - Kava Kava. Dietary supplements labels database. United States National Library of Medicine. Available from: http://www.dsld.nlm.nih.gov/dsld/rptQSearch.jsp?item=Kava+Kava&db=adsld, accessed 7 July 2014.

Norton SA & Ruze P (1994). Kava dermopathy. *J Am Acad Dermatol*, 31(1):89–97. doi:10.1016/S0190-9622(94)70142-3 PMID:8021378

Nutrition Business Journal (2010). NBJ's Supplement Business Report. An analysis of markets, trends, competition and strategy in the U.S. dietary supplement industry. New York (NY), USA: Penton Media, Inc.

Nutrition Business Journal (2012). NBJ's Supplement Business Report. An analysis of markets, trends, competition and strategy in the U.S. dietary supplement industry. . New York (NY), USA: Penton Media, Inc. Available from: http://newhope360.com/2012-supplement-business-report; accessed 4 September 2014.

O'Neil MJ, Heckelman PE, Koch CB et al. (2006). The Merck Index - An Encyclopedia of Chemicals, Drugs, and Biologicals. 14th ed. Version 14.6. Whitehouse Station (NJ), USA: Merck & Co., Inc.

Parkman CA (2002). Another FDA warning: Kava supplements. *Case Manager*, 13(4):26–8. doi:10.1067/mcm.2002.126437 PMID:12131903

Ramzan I, Tran VH (2004). Chemistry of kava and kavalactones. In: Singh YN, editor. Kava: from ethnology to pharmacology. Boca Raton (FL), USA: CRC Press; pp. 76–103.

Rasmussen AK, Scheline RR, Solheim E, Hänsel R (1979). Metabolism of some kava pyrones in the rat. *Xenobiotica*, 9(1):1–16. doi:10.3109/00498257909034699 PMID:760318

Raucy JL (2003). Regulation of CYP3A4 expression in human hepatocytes by pharmaceuticals and natural products. *Drug Metab Dispos*, 31(5):533–9. doi:10.1124/dmd.31.5.533 PMID:12695340

Robinson V, Bergfeld WF, Belsito DV, Klaassen CD, Marks JG Jr, Shank RC *et al.*; Cosmetic Ingredient Review Expert Panel (2009). Final report on the safety assessment of *Piper methysticum* leaf/root/stem extract and *Piper methysticum* root extract. *Int J Toxicol*, 28(6):Suppl: 175S–88S. doi:10.1177/1091581809350934 PMID:19966149

Russmann S, Barguil Y, Cabalion P, Kritsanida M, Duhet D, Lauterburg BH (2003). Hepatic injury due to traditional aqueous extracts of kava root in New Caledonia. *Eur J Gastroenterol Hepatol*, 15(9):1033–6. doi:10.1097/00042737-200309000-00015 PMID:12923378

Russmann S, Lauterburg BH, Barguil Y, Choblet E, Cabalion P, Rentsch K *et al.* (2005). Traditional aqueous kava extracts inhibit cytochrome P450 1A2 in humans: Protective effect against environmental carcinogens? *Clin Pharmacol Ther*, 77(5):453–4. doi:10.1016/j.clpt.2005.01.021 PMID:15900292

Russmann S, Lauterburg BH, Helbling A (2001). Kava hepatotoxicity. *Ann Intern Med*, 135(1):68–9. doi:10.7326/0003-4819-135-1-200107030-00036 PMID:11434754

Rychetnik L & Madronio CM (2011). The health and social effects of drinking water-based infusions of kava: a review of the evidence. *Drug Alcohol Rev*, 30(1):74–83. doi:10.1111/j.1465-3362.2010.00184.x PMID:21219501

Schäfer K & Winterhalter P (2005). Application of high speed countercurrent chromatography (HSCCC) to the isolation of kavalactones. *J Liquid Chromatogr Relat Technol*, 28(11):1703–16. doi:10.1081/JLC-200060451

Schmidt M, Morgan M, Bone K et al. (2005). Kava: a risk-benefit assessment. In: Mills S, Bone K, editors. The essential guide to herbal safety. St. Louis (MO), USA: Elsevier Churchill Livingstone; pp. 155–221.

SciFinder (2013). *CAS Registry Number 9000-38-8 (accessed: 15/01/2013)*. Columbus, Ohio, USA: Chemical Abstracts Service, American Chemical Society.

Shulgin AT (1973). The narcotic pepper - the chemistry and pharmacology of *Piper methysticum* and related species. *Bull Narc*, 25:59–74.

Singh YN (1992). Kava: an overview. *J Ethnopharmacol*, 37(1):13–45. doi:10.1016/0378-8741(92)90003-A PMID:1453702

Singh YN (2004a). An introduction to Kava *Piper methysticum*. In: Singh YN, editor. Kava: from ethnology to pharmacology. Boca Raton (FL), USA: CRC Press; pp. 1–9.

Singh YN (2004b). Kava: production, marketing and quality assurance. In: Singh YN, editor. Kava: from ethnology to pharmacology. Boca Raton (FL), USA: CRC Press; pp. 29–49.

Spohn R (2013). Water colour of *Piper methysticum*. Available from: http://www.spohns.de/heilpflanze-nillus/pipermethysticum.html, accessed 13 March 2013.

Steiner GG (2000). The correlation between cancer incidence and kava consumption. *Hawaii Med J*, 59(11):420–2. PMID:11149250

Stickel F, Baumüller HM, Seitz K, Vasilakis D, Seitz G, Seitz HK *et al.* (2003). Hepatitis induced by Kava (Piper methysticum rhizoma). *J Hepatol*, 39(1):62–7. doi:10.1016/S0168-8278(03)00175-2 PMID:12821045

Tarbah F, Mahler H, Kardel B, Weinmann W, Hafner D, Daldrup T (2003). Kinetics of kavain and its metabolites after oral application. *J Chromatogr B Analyt Technol Biomed Life Sci*, 789(1):115–30. doi:10.1016/S1570-0232(03)00046-1 PMID:12726850

Teschke R, Gaus W, Loew D (2003). Kava extracts: safety and risks including rare hepatotoxicity. *Phytomedicine*, 10(5):440–6. doi:10.1078/0944-7113-00314 PMID:12834011

Teschke R & Lebot V (2011). Proposal for a kava quality standardization code. *Food Chem Toxicol*, 49(10):2503–16. doi:10.1016/j.fct.2011.06.075 PMID:21756963

Teschke R, Qiu SX, Lebot V (2011). Herbal hepatotoxicity by kava: update on pipermethystine, flavokavain B, and mould hepatotoxins as primarily assumed culprits. *Dig Liver Dis*, 43(9):676–81. doi:10.1016/j.dld.2011.01.018 PMID:21377431

Teschke R, Schwarzenboeck A, Hennermann KH (2008). Kava hepatotoxicity: a clinical survey and critical analysis of 26 suspected cases. *Eur J Gastroenterol Hepatol*, 20(12):1182–93. doi:10.1097/MEG.0b013e3283036768 PMID:18989142

Thomsen M, Vitetta L, Schmidt M, Sali A (2004). Fatal fulminant hepatic failure induced by a natural therapy containing kava. *Med J Aust*, 180(4):198–9, author reply 199. PMID:14960147

Trucksess M, Weaver C, Oles C, D'Ovidio K, Rader J (2006). Determination of aflatoxins and ochratoxin A in ginseng and other botanical roots by immuno-affinity column cleanup and liquid chromatography with fluorescence detection. *J AOAC Int*, 89(3):624–30. PMID:16792061

Ulbricht C, Basch E, Boon H, Ernst E, Hammerness P, Sollars D *et al.* (2005). Safety review of kava (*Piper methysticum*) by the Natural Standard Research Collaboration. *Expert Opin Drug Saf*, 4(4):779–94. doi:10.1517/14740338.4.4.779 PMID:16011454

Unger M, Holzgrabe U, Jacobsen W, Cummins C, Benet LZ (2002). Inhibition of cytochrome P450 3A4 by extracts and kavalactones of Piper methysticum (Kava-Kava). *Planta Med*, 68(12):1055–8. doi:10.1055/s-2002-36360 PMID:12494328

Wanwimolruk S, Bhawan S, Coville PF, Chalcroft SC (1998). Genetic polymorphism of debrisoquine (CYP2D6) and proguanil (CYP2C19) in South Pacific Polynesian populations. *Eur J Clin Pharmacol*, 54(5):431–5. doi:10.1007/s002280050488 PMID:9754989

Weaver CM & Trucksess MW (2010). Determination of aflatoxins in botanical roots by a modification of AOAC Official Method 991.31: single-laboratory validation. *J AOAC Int*, 93(1):184–9. PMID:20334179

Weiss J, Sauer A, Frank A, Unger M (2005). Extracts and kavalactones of *Piper methysticum* G. Forst (kava-kava) inhibit P-glycoprotein in vitro. *Drug Metab Dispos*, 33(11):1580–3. doi:10.1124/dmd.105.005892 PMID:16051732

Whittaker P, Clarke JJ, San RH, Betz JM, Seifried HE, de Jager LS *et al.* (2008). Evaluation of commercial kava extracts and kavalactone standards for mutagenicity and toxicity using the mammalian cell gene mutation assay in L5178Y mouse lymphoma cells. *Food Chem Toxicol*, 46(1):168–74. doi:10.1016/j.fct.2007.07.013 PMID:17822821

WHO (2004). Rhizoma Piperis Methystici. In: WHO monographs on selected medicinal plants. Vol. 2, Geneva, Switzerland: World Health Organization. Available at http://apps.who.int/medicinedocs/en/d/Js4927e/23.html.

WHO (2007). Assessment of the risk of hepatotoxicity with kava products. Geneva, Switzerland: World Health Organization.

Yamazaki Y, Hashida H, Arita A, Hamaguchi K, Shimura F (2008). High dose of commercial products of kava (Piper methysticum) markedly enhanced hepatic cytochrome P450 1A1 mRNA expression with liver enlargement in rats. *Food Chem Toxicol*, 46(12):3732–8. doi:10.1016/j.fct.2008.09.052 PMID:18930106

Zou L, Harkey MR, Henderson GL (2002). Effects of herbal components on cDNA-expressed cytochrome P450 enzyme catalytic activity. *Life Sci*, 71(13):1579–89. doi:10.1016/S0024-3205(02)01913-6 PMID:12127912

Zou L, Harkey MR, Henderson GL (2005). Synthesis, in vitro, reactivity, and identification of 6-phenyl-3-hexen-2-one in human urine after kava-kava (Piper methysticum) ingestion. *Planta Med*, 71(2):142–6. doi:10.1055/s-2005-837781 PMID:15729622

Zou L, Henderson GL, Harkey MR, Sakai Y, Li A (2004). Effects of kava (Kava-kava, 'Awa, Yaqona, Piper methysticum) on c-DNA-expressed cytochrome P450 enzymes and human cryopreserved hepatocytes. *Phytomedicine*, 11(4):285–94. doi:10.1078/0944711041495263 PMID:15185840

1. Exposure Data

Pulegone is a monoterpene ketone present in the leaves and flowering tops of several members of the mint family *Lamiaceae*. Two enantiomeric forms occur in nature, the *R*-(+)-enantiomer being the most abundant in the essential oils (Hayes *et al.*, 2007; Barceloux, 2008).

1.1 Identification of the agent

1.1.1 Classification

(a) Nomenclature

Chem. Abstr. Serv. Reg. No: 89-82-7

IUPAC systematic name: (*R*)-5-Methyl-2-(1-methylethylidine) cyclohexanone

From Scifinder (2014).

(b) Description of origin

Pulegone is a major constituent of the volatile oils of European pennyroyal (*Mentha pulegium* L.) and American pennyroyal (*Hedeoma pulegioides* L.), where it comprises 85–97% (w/v) and about 30% (w/v) of the respective oil (Guenther, 1949; Smith & Levi, 1961; Smith *et al.*, 1963; Von Hefendehl & Ziegler, 1975; Farley & Howland, 1980). The compound is also a minor component of several other edible mint (*Mentha*) species and their derived volatile oils, including peppermint (*Mentha piperita*) and spearmint (*Mentha spicata*) (Virmani & Datta, 1968; Turner &

Croteau, 2004). It is found in different varieties of *M. piperita* oils at a range of 0.5% to 4.6%, and in *M. arvensis* oils at a range of 0.2% to 4.9%; oils in natural form contain lower concentrations of pulegone than those that have been partially dementholized (Smith & Levi, 1961). Pulegone is also found in various concentrations in Buchu leaf oils (*Barosma betulina* and *B. crenulata* with 3% and 50%, respectively) (Kaiser *et al.*, 1975).

1.1.2 Structural and molecular formulae and relative molecular mass

$C_{10}H_{16}O$

Relative molecular mass: 152.23

From Farley & Howland (1980), Thomassen *et al.* (1988), and Da Rocha *et al.* (2012).

1.1.3 Chemical and physical properties of the pure substance

Description: Colourless oil with a strong pungent aromatic mint smell.

Boiling point: 224 °C

Density: 0.9346 g/mL at 25 °C

Optical activity ($[\alpha]^{20}_{D}$): +22°

Solubility: Insoluble in water (Farley & Howland, 1980; O'Neil, 2013; Sigma Aldrich, 2013).

1.1.4 Analysis

Physical properties such as density and optical rotation are used to characterize essential oils. Gas chromatography with flame-ionization detection has been the standard method of analysis for essential oil composition. Petrakis *et al.* (2009) have developed a direct and rapid method to quantify pulegone using Fourier transform mid-infrared spectroscopy, which showed equivalent results to those obtained when using gas chromatography.

1.2 Production and use

1.2.1 Production

According to the United Nations Commodity Trade Statistics Database (United Nations Comtrade, 2013), 3.4–3.7 tonnes of essential oils of mint other than peppermint were imported by the China, Germany, Japan, Singapore, and USA and in recent years. No separate data were available for spearmint, peppermint, or pennyroyal oil from this source.

1.2.2 Use

Aerial parts [leaves and flowering tops] of plant species containing pulegone have been used as a traditional remedy, as flavouring, as spice, and for brewing teas. Pennyroyal oil has been used as a traditional medicine. It is also used to flavour alcoholic beverages, baked goods, candies, ice creams, as a fragrance component of detergents, cosmetics and oral hygiene products, and as an insect repellent (Karousou *et al.*, 2007; Da Rocha *et al.*, 2012).

(a) Medicinal indications

The aerial parts of both American and European pennyroyal plants have traditionally been used internally as a tea for non-ulcer dyspepsia, primary dysmenorrhoea, secondary amenorrhoea and oligomenorrhoea, as abortifacient, and as a diaphoretic. Pennyroyal oils have been used for these same medicinal indications (Hoppe, 1975; List & Hörhammer, 1976; Foster & Duke, 1990; Skenderi, 2003). Today, recorded uses for *Mentha piperita* and *Mentha pulegium* L. are for common cold, headache, and as diuretic, spasmolytic, anti-convulsive, anti-emetic, heart stimulant, and sedative (Karousou *et al.*, 2007). Peppermint oil is used for the treatment of the symptoms of inflammatory bowel syndrome (Cappello *et al.*, 2007).

(b) Dosage

No typical dose was found in the literature for pulegone. According to literature reports on levels of pulegone present in *M. piperita* oils, two capsules of 225 mg of oil taken twice per day could contain an amount of pulegone of between 4.5 and 41.4 mg (0.5–4.6%) (Smith & Levi, 1961). According to the European Union, the highest recommended daily dose is 1.2 mL of peppermint oil; 1080 mg of peppermint oil contains a maximum of 140 mg of pulegone, a daily intake of 2.3 mg/kg body weight (bw) for a person of 60 kg (EMEA, 2005).

1.3 Occurrence and exposure

1.3.1 Occurrence

Pulegone is naturally found in plants of the *Lamiaceae* (or *Labiatae*) family. The amount of pulegone in the various oils varies depending on several factors such as origin of the plant, yearly weather conditions, harvest date, plant age, fertilization, location and planting time (Farley & Howland, 1980; Weglarz & Zalecki, 1985; Murray *et al.*, 1988; Voirin *et al.*, 1990;

Marotti *et al.*, 1994; Kumar *et al.*, 2000; Misra & Srivastava, 2000; Dolzhenko *et al.*, 2010).

1.3.2 Consumer exposure

In addition to the use in medication, humans are exposed to pulegone as a constituent of the essential oil in flavourings, confectionery, and cosmetics (Karousou *et al.*, 2007; Barceloux, 2008). According to the Joint FAO/WHO Expert Committee on Food Additives (JECFA), the estimated intake of pulegone per capita is 2 µg per day and 0.04 µg/kg bw per day for Europe, and 12 µg per day and 0.03 µg/kg bw per day for the USA (IPCS, 2001).

1.3.3 Occupational exposure

No data were available to the Working Group. Workers from the flavouring, confectionary, and cosmetic industries are probably exposed to pulegone.

1.4 Regulations and guidelines

Limits in the use of pulegone in food products have been issued for different applications. According to regulation (EC) 1334/2008, the use of pulegone in food and beverages has limits of: 100 mg/kg for mint/peppermint containing alcoholic beverages; 20 mg/kg for mint/peppermint containing non-alcoholic beverages; 2000 mg/kg for "micro breath freshening confectionery"; 350 mg/kg for chewing gum; and 250 mg/kg for mint/peppermint containing confectionery, except the "micro breath." As a pure ingredient, pulegone may not be added to foodstuffs. According to the Committee of Experts on Flavoring Substances (CEFS), provisional consumption limits were established for pulegone at 20 mg/kg in food and beverages (European Commission, 2002, 2008).

In the USA, pulegone is not authorized as a synthetic flavouring substance (DHHS-FDA,

2012). According to the Cosmetic Ingredient Review Expert Panel, the concentration of pulegone in cosmetic formulations should not exceed 1% (Nair, 2001).

2. Cancer in Humans

No data were available to the Working Group.

3. Cancer in Experimental Animals

3.1 Mouse

See Table 3.1

In one study of oral administration, groups of 50 male and 50 female B6C3F$_1$ mice (age, 6–7 weeks) were given pulegone at a dose of 0 (corn oil only, 10 mL/kg bw), 37.5, 75, or 150 mg/kg body weight (bw) by gavage, 5 days per week for 105 weeks. The purity of pulegone was approximately 96%. Survival in all dosed groups was similar to that in the vehicle-control group. Mean body weights of males and females at 150 mg/kg bw were lower than those in the vehicle-control group after weeks 25 and 33, respectively.

In males, the incidence of hepatoblastoma was significantly higher in the group at the intermediate dose. The incidences of hepatocellular adenoma, and hepatocellular adenoma or carcinoma (combined) were also significantly higher in the group at the intermediate dose. The incidences of hepatocellular adenoma, hepatocellular carcinoma, or hepatoblastoma (combined) showed a significant positive trend. [The Working Group noted that the lower average body weight in the group at the highest dose may have reduced the incidences of liver tumours (Haseman *et al.*, 1997).] The incidence of liver clear cell foci was significantly higher in all dosed groups; the incidence of eosinophilic liver

Table 3.1 Studies of carcinogenicity with pulegone in mice and rats

Species, strain (sex) Duration Reference	Dosing regimen Animals/group at start	Incidence of tumours	Significance[a]	Comments
Mouse, B6C3F$_1$ (M, F) 105 wk NTP (2011)	0 (control), 37.5, 75, 150 mg/kg bw, by gavage in corn oil, 5 days per wk, for 105 wk 50 M and 50 F/group (age, 5–6 wk)	Hepatoblastoma: 1/50, 3/50, 7/50*, 2/50 (M); 0/50, 1/50, 2/50, 2/50 (F) Hepatocellular adenoma: 22/50, 31/50, 35/50*, 28/50 (M); 13/49**, 15/50, 13/50, 27/50*** (F) Hepatocellular carcinoma: 13/50, 11/50, 18/50, 15/50 (M); 5/50, 1/50, 4/50, 8/50 (F) Hepatocellular adenoma or carcinoma (combined): 29/50, 36/50, 42/50*, 35/50 (M); 17/49**, 15/50, 15/50, 32/50*** (F) Hepatocellular adenoma or carcinoma or hepatoblastoma (combined): 29/50*, 37/50, 42/50**, 36/50 (M); 17/49***, 15/50, 15/50, 33/50**** (F) Osteoma or osteosarcoma (combined[b]): 0/49, 0/50, 3/50#, 1/50 (F)	*P = 0.040 *P = 0.008 **P < 0.001 (trend) ***P < 0.002 *P = 0.004 **P = 0.001 (trend) ***P = 0.002 *P = 0.038 (trend) **P = 0.004 ***P < 0.001 (trend) ****P < 0.001 # Greater than historical controls	Purity, 96% (approximate) Body weight of group at 150 mg/kg bw was 10% less than that of the vehicle-control group after week 25 for males and after week 33 for females
Rat, F344 (M, F) 104 wk NTP (2011)	0 (control), 18.75 (M only), 37.5, 75 or 150 (F only) mg/kg bw, by gavage in corn oil, 5 days per wk, for 104 wk Dosing of males at the highest dose (75 mg/kg bw) and females at the highest dose (150 mg/kg bw) was stopped after wk 60 because of high morbidity and mortality. Surviving animals at these doses were treated with corn oil only from wk 60 to end of study. 50 M and 50 F/group (age, 6–7 wk)	Urinary bladder papilloma: 0/50, 0/49, 1/50 (2%), 3/47* (F) Urinary bladder carcinoma: 0/50, 0/49, 0/50, 2/47 (F) Urinary bladder papilloma or carcinoma (combined)[c]: 0/50, 0/49, 1/50, 5/47** (F)	*P = 0.044 **P = 0.005	Purity, 96% (approximate) Mean body weight of males and females at 75 mg/kg bw was 10% less than that of the vehicle-control group after week 13 and 21 respectively; and mean body weight in females at 150 mg/kg bw was 12% less than that in the vehicle-control group after week 9. No treatment-related increases in tumour incidences were found in males.

[a] Poly-3 test was used for all the statistical analyses in this table

[b] Historical incidence for 2-year gavage studies with corn oil vehicle-control groups: 1/248 (0.4% ± 0.9%); range 0–2%; for all routes: 8/1498 (0.5% ± 1.0%), range 0–4%

[c] Historical incidence for 2-year gavage studies with corn oil vehicle-control groups: 0/200; for all routes, 0/1347

bw, body weight; F, female; M, male; wk, week

cell foci was significantly higher in the groups receiving the intermediate and highest doses; and the incidence of mixed liver cell foci was significantly higher in the group at the highest dose. The incidence of forestomach squamous cell hyperplasia was significantly higher in the group at the highest dose.

In females, the incidence of hepatocellular adenoma was significantly higher in the group at the highest dose. The incidence of hepatocellular adenoma or carcinoma (combined) was significantly higher in the group at the highest dose and had a significant positive trend. The incidence of hepatocellular adenoma, hepatocellular carcinoma, or hepatoblastoma (combined) was significantly higher in the group at the highest dose and had a significant positive trend. The incidence of liver clear cell foci was significantly higher in all dosed groups; the incidence of eosinophilic liver cell foci was significantly higher in the high-dose group; and the incidence of mixed liver cell foci was significantly higher in the groups receiving the intermediate and highest doses. The incidence of osteoma or osteosarcoma (combined) was increased in the group at the intermediate dose (3 out of 50) compared with historical controls (historical incidence for gavage studies was 1 out of 248 (0.4% ± 0.9%); range, 0–2%). The incidence of forestomach squamous cell hyperplasia was significantly higher in the groups receiving the intermediate and highest doses (NTP, 2011).

3.2 Rat

See Table 3.1

In one study of oral administration, groups of 50 male and 50 female F344/N rats (age, 6–7 weeks) were given pulegone at 0 (corn oil only, 5 mL/kg bw), 18.75 (males only), 37.5, 75, or 150 (females only) mg/kg bw by gavage, 5 days per week for up to 104 weeks. Due to excessive morbidity and mortality, males at 75 mg/kg bw and females at 150 mg/kg bw were not given pulegone after week 60 (stop-exposure); these groups were given the corn-oil vehicle until the end of the study. Survival of males at 37.5 mg/kg bw was significantly lower than that of the vehicle controls; only two males in the group receiving 75 mg/kg bw and stop-exposure survived to the end of the study, and no females in the group receiving 150 mg/kg bw and stop-exposure. Compared with those of the rats in the vehicle-control group, mean body weights of males in the group receiving 75 mg/kg bw and stop-exposure, and of females in the group receiving 75 mg/kg bw, and of females receiving 150 mg/kg bw and stop-exposure were lower after weeks 13, 21 and 9, respectively.

In females, the incidence of urinary bladder papilloma was significantly higher in the group at the highest dose. The incidence of urinary bladder papilloma or carcinoma (combined) was significantly higher in the group at the highest dose (150 mg/kg bw with stop-exposure). [The Working Group noted that no urinary bladder papillomas or carcinoma were observed in 1347 control animals from previous studies (all routes of exposure) by the National Toxicology Program (NTP).] In males, no treatment-related increases in tumour incidences were found (NTP, 2011).

4. Mechanistic and Other Relevant Data

4.1 Absorption, distribution, metabolism, and excretion

Fig. 4.1 describes the metabolism of pulegone in humans and rodents.

4.1.1 Humans

A haematological post-mortem examination of a woman who ingested pennyroyal extract used as an abortifacient, indicated that both serum concentrations of pulegone at 18 ng/mL and menthofuran at 1 ng/mL possibly resulted

Fig. 4.1 Metabolism of pulegone in humans and rodents

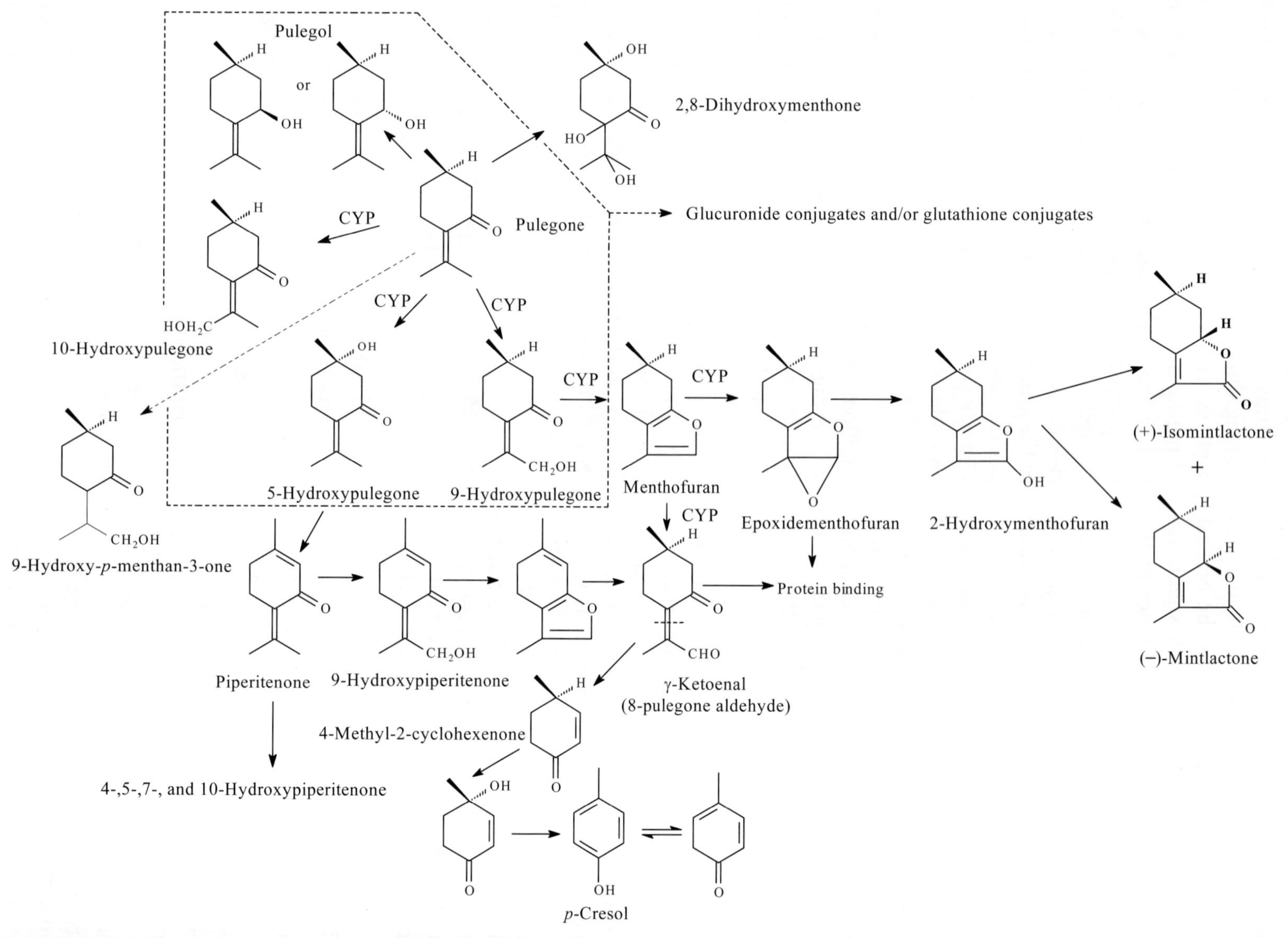

Most of the metabolites of pulegone are derived from menthofuran and piperitenone. A γ-ketoenal is generated as a major electrophilic metabolite from both pulegone and menthofuran.
CYP, cytochrome P450
Adapted from Chen et al. (2011) with permission from Elsevier

in fatal poisoning. Serum samples were analysed for both metabolites at 26 hours post mortem, 72 hours after ingestion (Anderson *et al.*, 1996). In another case, serum was found to contain menthofuran at 40 ng/mL, with no detectable pulegone, 10 hours after ingestion (Anderson *et al.*, 1996). Menthofuran is considered the major proximate toxic metabolite; however, pulegone oxidation produces other metabolites that may also be toxic (see Fig. 4.1; Anderson *et al.*, 1996).

Pulegone is metabolized by multiple human liver CYPs to menthofuran, a toxic metabolite of pulegone (Khojasteh-Bakht *et al.*, 1999). In a study by Khojasteh-Bakht *et al.* (1999), pulegone (200 µM) was separately incubated with individual human CYPs, namely CYP1A2, CYP2A6, CYP2C9, CYP2C19, CYP2D6, CYP2E1, or CYP3A4. It was found that CYP2E1, CYP1A2, and CYP2C19 metabolized the oxidation of pulegone to menthofuran with the following K_m and V_{max}: CYP2E: K_m, 29 µM; V_{max}, 8.4 nmol/min per nmol protein; CYP1A2: K_m, 94 mM; V_{max}, 2.4 nmol/min per nmol protein; and for CYP2C19: K_m, 31 µM; and V_{max}, 1.5 nmol/min per nmol protein.

Menthofuran was metabolized by the same human liver CYPs involved in the metabolism of pulegone except for the addition of CYP2A6 (Khojasteh-Bakht *et al.*, 1999).

After oral administration of (*R*)-(+)-pulegone at 0.5 mg/kg bw or (*S*)-(–)-pulegone at 1 mg/kg bw to six volunteers, six metabolites were identified in the urine. The major metabolite of (*R*)-(+)-pulegone was 10-hydroxypulegone (Engel, 2003). Although 10-hydroxypulegone was shown to convert to menthofuran *in vitro*, menthofuran and its metabolites were found in relative small amounts in the urine. Alternatively, pulegone may be reduced to menthone, a product that is detected in small amounts in the urine. It might be possible that pulegone is also reduced at carbonyl group first; however, no trace of pulegol was found in the urine. Consequently, it was also proposed that pulegol can be reduced to menthol

or rearranged under conditions found in the human body, forming α,α,4-trimethyl-1-cyclohexene-1-methanol (3-*p*-menthen-8-ol) as a minor metabolite (Engel, 2003). It was also deduced that the reduction of the carbonyl group in menthone leads to the formation of menthol, while oxidation at C-5 also yields the menthone metabolite. The formation of α,α,4-trimethyl-1-cyclohexene-1-methanol from pulegol occurs at a body pH of 6.5. However, the formation of the same metabolite from pulegol as an artefact during enzymatic hydrolysis with sulfatase and glucuronidase cannot be totally excluded (Engel, 2003). The major metabolite, 9-hydroxy-*p*-menthan-3-one, is formed through the oxidation of 10-hydroxypulegone via the reduction of the exocyclic double bond (Engel, 2003). Although the results of this study suggested that menthofuran is not a relevant metabolite in humans, menthofuran was found to be present in the serum of two individuals, hours after ingestion of a large amount of pennyroyal oil in a study by Anderson *et al.* (1996). Additionally, it should be noted that toxicity seems to be stereospecific, in that for (*R*)-(+)-pulegone both reduction steps (to menthone and from 10-hydroxypulegone to 9-hydroxy-*p*-menthan-3-one) are much less favoured by the conformation of the terpene, as opposed to the (*S*)-(–)-pulegone enantiomer (Engel, 2003). Subsequently, 10-hydroxypulegone is accumulated and further oxidation at the hydroxyl group leads to pulegon-10 aldehyde, a toxic metabolite.

In summary, from a general perspective, minimal data existed on the excretion of pulegone in humans.

4.1.2 Experimental systems

The majority of experimental studies used the toxic stereoisomer (*R*)-(+)-pulegone, which is the natural component of pennyroyal oil, but the (*S*)-(–)-isomer is also metabolized in the same manner (Speijers, 2001). A total of approximately

14 phase I metabolites exist in rats *in vivo*, with approximately 10 identified phase II metabolites (Thomassen *et al.*, 1991; Chen *et al.*, 2001; Zhou *et al.*, 2005). Observed metabolites account for only 3% of total radiolabel typically excreted in bile, with glucuronide conjugates and minimal glutathione conjugates being found in highest quantities (Speijers, 2001). The most common biliary metabolites observed were the glucuronide conjugates of hydroxylated pulegone and pulegol (Speijers, 2001).

The metabolism of pulegone involves three major metabolic pathways: (i) hydroxylation to give monohydroxylated pulegones at C-5 or methyl (9- or 10-), followed by conjugation with glucuronic acid or with glutathione; the conjugates being further metabolized; (ii) reduction of the carbon–carbon double bond that leads to the formation of menthofuran; and (iii) the formation of piperitenone after 5-hydroxylation, followed by dehydration (see Fig. 4.1) (Thomassen *et al.*, 1990; Speijers, 2001; Chen *et al.*, 2011). Most of the metabolites of pulegone are derived from menthofuran and piperitenone, and 4-methyl-2-cyclohexenone is one of these metabolites. A γ-ketoenal is generated as a major electrophilic metabolite from both pulegone and menthofuran (Thomassen *et al.*, 1992; Speijers, 2001). This reactive enonal may be derived directly from incipient oxycarbonium ions formed in the oxidation of menthofuran by cytochrome P450 (CYP), or from an epoxyfuran intermediate (Thomassen *et al.*, 1992). Mintlactones are formed as stable products of the γ-ketoenal, but also may be formed by direct proton loss from an incipient oxycarbonium ion (Chen *et al.*, 2011).

As shown experimentally, pulegone is specifically metabolized to menthofuran and *para*-mentha-1,4(8)-dien-3-one, commonly known as piperitenone (Speijers, 2001). In subsequent reactions, the tertiary ring carbon (C-5) is hydroxylated to obtain 5-hydroxypulegone (Speijers, 2001). This product is then dehydrated to piperitenone, which is further metabolized in terms of ring- and side-chain oxidation to obtain numerous hydroxylated by-products (Speijers, 2001). For the predominant pathway, the isopropylidene substituent of pulegone is subjected to regiospecific allylic oxidation to yield 9-hydroxypulegone, which forms menthofuran cyclically (Gordon *et al.*, 1987; Madyastha & Raj, 1993). As a minor pathway, it is presumed that the exocyclic alkene of pulegone is oxidized (with the assumption of an epoxide intermediate) to yield 2,8-dihydroxymenthone, (Speijers, 2001). Additionally, pulegone is reduced to pulegol which is then rearranged to isopulegone with the aid of a supposed free-radical intermediate (Gordon *et al.*, 1987; Speijers, 2001).

When pulegone is converted to menthofuran, it undergoes a reaction where an oxycarbonium ion is created via CYP-mediated oxidation of menthofuran, generating an intermediate, γ-ketoenal (one of the primary reactive metabolites), but also another intermediate epoxyfuran (Chen *et al.*, 2011). Additionally, *p*-cresol is also generated via pulegone metabolism and also depletes glutathione with minor hepatotoxic effects (Chen *et al.*, 2011).

In addition to cyclizing to obtain menthofuran, 9-hydroxypulegone can also be oxidized in a secondary detoxication pathway to 9-carboxy-pulegone, also called 5-methyl-2-(1-methyl-1-carboxyethylidene) cyclohexanone (Speijers, 2001). This product is then partially cyclized to hydroxylactone or is assumed to be oxidized and hydrated to hydroxyacids that are eliminated through urine (Speijers, 2001). Studies of oral administration in rats have shown piperitenone is hydroxylated: metabolites found in the urine were isolated and found to be hydroxylated at the 4, 5, 7, 9, and 10 positions (Speijers, 2001). 9-Piperitenone can be further converted to an analogous furan metabolite and to the γ-ketoenal (Chen *et al.*, 2011).

According to studies in experimental animals treated orally, gastrointestinally absorbed pulegone is excreted in the urine within 24 hours.

Additional studies have demonstrated that pulegone is excreted and eliminated at 6–24% in faecal matter, and a small amount in expired air (NTP, 2011).

4.2 Genetic and related effects

4.2.1 Humans

No data were available to the Working Group.

4.2.2 Experimental systems

A limited number of studies of genotoxicity have been conducted with pulegone (Table 4.1).

(a) Mutation

(i) Bacteria

Pulegone was not mutagenic in *Salmonella typhimurium* strains TA97, TA98, TA100, TA1535, or TA1537, with or without metabolic activation (Andersen & Jensen, 1984).

Three additional assays for gene mutation in bacteria were conducted and results were mixed (NTP, 2011). In the first two studies, pulegone was not mutagenic with or without metabolic activation. Bacterial strains tested in the first study included *S. typhimurium* TA97, TA98, TA100, and TA1535, with and without metabolic activation (10% or 30% S9 from Syrian hamster or Sprague-Dawley rat liver). Strains tested in the second study included *S. typhimurium* strains TA98 and TA100, and *Escherichia coli* strain WP2 *uvrA*/pKM101, with and without metabolic activation (10% S9 from rat liver S9). The third study also tested pulegone in *S. typhimurium* and *E. coli*; results were positive in *S. typhimurium* strain TA98 and *E. coli* strain WP2 *uvrA*/pKM101 in the presence of metabolic activation. [There was no explanation for the discrepancy between the multiple assays for mutagenicity.]

(ii) Drosophila melanogaster

Pulegone was reported to be weakly mutagenic in the *Drosophila melanogaster* somatic mutation and recombination test. However, a sample of pennyroyal oil that was reported to contain pulegone at 75.7% was not mutagenic in this assay (Franzios *et al.*, 1997).

(b) Cytogenetic effects

In B6C3F$_1$ mice given pulegone at doses up to 150 mg/kg bw per day by gavage for 3 months, there was no increase in the frequency of micronucleus formation in peripheral blood erythrocytes (NTP, 2011).

4.3 Other mechanistic data

4.3.1 Humans

In a review of published reports, excessive consumption of pennyroyal oil has been shown to induce moderate to severe toxicity (Anderson *et al.*, 1996; Speijers, 2001; NTP, 2011). Consumption of amounts greater than 15 mL or approximately 250 mg/kg bw may result in death (Anderson *et al.*, 1996; Speijers, 2001; NTP, 2011). Adverse physiological reactions following excessive consumption lead to massive centrilobular hepatic necrosis, pulmonary oedema, internal bleeding, and body weight loss (Anderson *et al.*, 1996; Speijers, 2001).

Eighteen cases of hepatotoxicity were described in people who had ingested 10 mL or more of pennyroyal oil (Anderson *et al.*, 1996; NTP, 2011). Symptoms of toxicity included coma, seizures, liver, and kidney effects, while consumption of less than 10 mL of pennyroyal oil resulted in gastritis and mild toxicity of the central nervous system (Anderson *et al.*, 1996; NTP, 2011). There was no clear correlation between dose and toxicological effect (NTP, 2011).

Functionally, reactive metabolites of pulegone and menthofuran bind to cellular proteins.

Table 4.1 Genetic and related effects of pulegone

Test system	Results[a]		Dose or concentration (LED or HID)	Reference
	Without exogenous metabolic system	With exogenous metabolic system		
Salmonella typhimurium TA100, TA1535, TA1537, TA98, TA97, reverse mutation	–	–	800 µg/plate	Andersen & Jensen (1984)
Salmonella typhimurium TA100, TA1535, TA98, TA97, reverse mutation	–	–[b]	2167 µg/plate	NTP (2011)
Salmonella typhimurium TA100, TA98, *Escherichia coli* WP2, *uvrA* pKM101	–	–[b]	3500 µg/plate	NTP (2011)
Salmonella typhimurium TA98, *Escherichia coli* WP2, *uvrA* pKM101	–	+[c]	500 µg/plate	NTP (2011)
Salmonella typhimurium TA100	–	–[c]	1500 µg/plate	NTP (2011)
Drosophila melanogaster, somatic mutation (and recombination)	–	NT	2.1 µL, applied to filter paper[d]	Franzios *et al.* (1997)
Drosophila melanogaster, somatic mutation (and recombination)	+	NT	0.2 µL, applied to filter paper[d]	Franzios *et al.* (1997)
Micronucleus formation in peripheral blood lymphocytes, B6C3F$_1$ male and female mice in vivo	–	NT	150 mg/kg bw per day by gavage, for 3 months	NTP (2011)

[a] +, positive; –, negative
[b] 10% or 30% S9 from Syrian hamster or Sprague-Dawley rat liver
[c] 10% S9 from Sprague-Dawley rat liver
[d] Larval feeding for 18 hours
HID, highest ineffective dose; LED, lowest effective dose; NT, not tested

Reactive metabolites of pulegone deplete hepatic glutathione concentrations, whereas mentho-furan, only slightly diminishes these concentrations. On a molecular level, diminished concentrations of pulegone-induced glutathione result from the generation of electrophili-cally metabolites that form covalent adducts with glutathione (Anderson *et al.*, 1996). Thus, *N*-acetylcysteine serves as a protectant against pennyroyal oil poisoning within the first few hours after ingestion and may also protect cells from further damage in late-stage injuries (Anderson *et al.*, 1996).

Bakerink *et al.* (1996) have reported two cases of infant death following the ingestion of mint tea containing pulegone. The male patient (aged 6 months) was given mint tea rich in pule-gone along with two crushed aspirin tablets. Presentation of this case indicated hepatic fulmi-nation with cerebral oedema and necrosis, and the patient died with a serum concentration of menthofuran of 10 ng/mL. Most importantly, characteristic hepatotoxicity findings included hepatomegaly, poor perfusion, and dark blood from the nasogastric tube and rectum. The second case presented with hepatic dysfunction and severe epileptic encephalopathy and had serum concentrations of pulegone at 25 ng/mL, and menthofuran at 41 ng/mL. Overall, find-ings were similar for both cases, suggesting that pulegone intake is associated with marked hepa-totoxicity (Bakerink *et al.*, 1996).

4.3.2 Experimental systems

Many studies in experimental animal have observed that *p*-cresol, a pulegone metabolite, induces diminished hepatic function, increased liver and kidney weight, gastrointestinal and nasal epithelial irritation, and atrophy of female reproductive organs (Chen *et al.*, 2011).

Female Fischer rats (age, 6 weeks) were given pulegone orally at a dose of 0, 75, or 150 mg/kg bw per day, 5 days per week, for 4 or 6 weeks.

Urinary bladders from treated rats showed super-ficial cell layer necrosis and exfoliation in both treated groups, and a significant increase in the incidence of cellular proliferation in the group at the highest dose (150 mg/kg bw) (Da Rocha *et al.*, 2012). Examination of urine collected during week 6 of treatment revealed the pres-ence of pulegone, piperitone, piperitenone, and menthofuran. Piperitenone was concentrated in the urine at cytotoxic levels in rats treated with pulegone at the highest dose.

4.4 Susceptibility

No relevant data were available to the Working Group.

4.5 Mechanistic considerations

Studies in humans and rodents indicated that the metabolism of pulegone to menthofuran generates electrophilic species that can bind to proteins. This may result in chronic regenera-tive cell proliferation that may be related to the carcinogenicity in the liver and urinary bladder that is observed in experimental animals (see Section 3).

5. Summary of Data Reported

5.1 Exposure data

Pulegone is present as a major constituent in pennyroyal oils, and to a minor extent in the oil of several other species of mint. Pulegone is also found in Buchu leaf oils. Pennyroyal oil has been used as flavouring in confectionery, as a spice, and in brewing teas. Pennyroyal leaves and oil are used in traditional medicine applications, for the treatment of dyspepsia and menstrual disorders, and as a diaphoretic. Pennyroyal oil has also been used as a fragrance in foods and in cosmetics, and as a flea repellent. Given the wide range of uses of mint, there is a possibility of exposure to pulegone on a daily basis. Limits to the use of pulegone have been issued for foods and beverages. Synthetic pulegone is not authorized as a flavouring substance in the USA or Europe.

5.2 Human carcinogenicity data

No data were available to the Working Group.

5.3 Animal carcinogenicity data

Pulegone was tested for carcinogenicity after oral administration in one study in mice and one study in rats.

In male and female mice given pulegone by gavage, there was a significant increase in the incidences of hepatocellular adenoma, and hepatocellular adenoma and carcinoma (combined) in males and females, and of hepatoblastoma in males. In female mice, the incidence of osteoma or osteosarcoma (combined) was higher than that in historical controls.

In female rats given pulegone by gavage, there was an increase in the incidence of urinary bladder papilloma and of urinary bladder papilloma or carcinoma (combined). In males, there were no treatment-related increases in tumour incidences.

5.4 Mechanistic and other relevant data

Pulegone is readily absorbed in humans. It is metabolized in humans and rodents to isomers of hydroxypulegone, predominantly by hepatic oxidation at the 5-, 9-, and 10-positions. In rodents, 9-hydroxypulegone is further oxidized to menthofuran, which is converted to a reactive epoxide and a reactive aldehyde (γ-ketoenal). 5-Hydroxypulegone is converted to piperitenone,

which is then hydroxylated at the 9-position and further converted to an analogous furan metabolite and to the γ-ketoenal. Further metabolism of the γ-ketoenal produces 4-methyl-2-cyclohexenone and *p*-cresol.

Pulegone was not mutagenic in standard bacterial assays, either with or without exogenous metabolic activation.

Studies in humans and rodents indicated that some of the pulegone metabolites deplete hepatic levels of glutathione and can bind to cellular proteins. This may result in chronic regenerative cell proliferation, which may be related to the carcinogenicity observed in the liver and urinary bladder in experimental animals.

6. Evaluation

6.1 Cancer in humans

There is *inadequate evidence* in humans for the carcinogenicity of pulegone.

6.2 Cancer in experimental animals

There is *sufficient evidence* in experimental animals for the carcinogenicity of pulegone.

6.3 Overall evaluation

Pulegone is *possibly carcinogenic to humans (Group 2B)*.

References

Andersen PH & Jensen NJ (1984). Mutagenic investigation of peppermint oil in the Salmonella/mammalian-microsome test. *Mutat Res*, 138:17–20. doi:10.1016/0165-1218(84)90080-6 PMID:6387476

Anderson IB, Mullen WH, Meeker JE *et al.* (1996). Pennyroyal toxicity: measurement of toxic metabolite levels in two cases and review of the literature. *Ann Intern Med*, 124:726–734. doi:10.7326/0003-4819-124-8-199604150-00004 PMID:8633832

Bakerink JA, Gospe SM Jr, Dimand RJ, Eldridge MW (1996). Multiple organ failure after ingestion of pennyroyal oil from herbal tea in two infants. *Pediatrics*, 98:944–947. PMID:8909490

Barceloux DG (2008). Pennyroyal and Pulegone (Mentha pulegium L.). In: Medical Toxicology of Natural Substances: Foods, Fungi, Medicinal Herbs, Plants and Venomous Animals. Hoboken, NJ: John Wiley & Sons, Inc.; pp. 563–567.

Cappello G, Spezzaferro M, Grossi L, Manzoli L, Marzio L (2007). Peppermint oil (Mintoil) in the treatment of irritable bowel syndrome: a prospective double blind placebo-controlled randomized trial. *Dig Liver Dis*, 39(6):530–6. doi:10.1016/j.dld.2007.02.006 PMID:17420159

Chen LJ, Lebetkin EH, Burka LT (2001). Metabolism of (R)-(+)-pulegone in F344 rats. *Drug Metab Dispos*, 29:1567–1577. PMID:11717176

Chen XW, Serag ES, Sneed KB, Zhou SF (2011). Herbal bioactivation, molecular targets and the toxicity relevance. *Chem Biol Interact*, 192:161–176. doi:10.1016/j.cbi.2011.03.016 PMID:21459083

Da Rocha MS, Dodmane PR, Arnold LL, Pennington KL, Anwar MM, Adams BR et al. (2012). Mode of action of pulegone on the urinary bladder of F344 rats. *Toxicol Sci*, 128(1):1–8. doi:10.1093/toxsci/kfs135 PMID:22499580

DHHS-FDA (2012). Synthetic flavouring substances and adjuvants. 21CFR182.60. Department of Health and Human Services, Food and Drug Administration. Available from: http://www.gpo.gov/fdsys/granule/CFR-2011-title21-vol3/CFR-2011-title21-vol3-sec182-60/content-detail.html. Accessed 18 June 2014.

Dolzhenko Y, Bertea CM, Occhipinti A, Bossi S, Maffei ME (2010). UV-B modulates the interplay between terpenoids and flavonoids in peppermint (Mentha x piperita L.). *J Photochem Photobiol B*, 100(2):67–75. doi:10.1016/j.jphotobiol.2010.05.003 PMID:20627615

EMEA; European Medicines Agency (2005). Public Statement on the use of herbal medicinal products containing pulegone and menthofuran. EMEA/HMPC/138386/2005. London, United Kingdom: Committee on Herbal Medicinal products (HMPC). Available from: http://www.ema.europa.eu/docs/en_GB/document_library/Scientific_guideline/2010/04/WC500089958.pdf. Accessed 18 June 2014.

Engel W (2003). *In vivo* studies on the metabolism of the monoterpene pulegone in humans using the metabolism of ingestion-correlated amounts (MICA) approach: explanation for the toxicity differences between (S)-(-)- and (R)-(+)-pulegone. *J Agric Food Chem*, 51:6589–6597. doi:10.1021/jf034702u PMID:14558782

European Commission (2002). Opinion of the Scientific Committee on Food on pulegone and menthofuran. Brussels, Belgium: Scientific Committee on Food. Available from: http://ec.europa.eu/food/fs/sc/scf/out133_en.pdf. Accessed 18 June 2014.

European Commission (2008). Regulation (EC) No 1334/2008 of the European Parliament and of the Council of 16 December 2008 on flavourings and certain food ingredients with flavouring properties for use in and on foods and amending Council Regulation (EEC) No 1601/91, Regulations (EC) No 2232/96 and (EC) No 110/2008 and Directive 2000/13/EC. *Off J Eur Union L*, 354:34

Farley DR & Howland V (1980). The natural variation of the pulegone content in various oils of peppermint. *J Sci Food Agric*, 31(11):1143–51. doi:10.1002/jsfa.2740311104

Foster S, Duke J (1990). A field guide to medicinal plants. Boston (MA): Houghton Mifflin Co.; p. 190.

Franzios G, Mirotsou M, Hatziapostolou E et al. (1997). Insecticidal and Genotoxic activities of mint essential oils. *J Agric Food Chem*, 45:2690–2694. doi:10.1021/jf960685f

Gordon WP, Huitric AC, Seth CL et al. (1987). The metabolism of the abortifacient terpene, (R)-(+)-pulegone, to a proximate toxin, menthofuran. *Drug Metab Dispos*, 15:589–594. PMID:2891472

Guenther E (1949). The Essential Oils. New York (NY): D Van Nostrand Company Inc.

Haseman JK, Young E, Eustis SL, Hailey JR (1997). Body weight-tumor incidence correlations in long-term rodent carcinogenicity studies. *Toxicol Pathol*, 25:256–263. doi:10.1177/019262339702500302 PMID:9210256

Hayes JR, Stavanja MS, Lawrence BM (2007). Biological and toxicological properties of mint oils and their major isolates: Safety assessment. In: Lawrence BM, editor. Mint: The Genus *Mentha*. CRC Press, Taylor & Francis Group; pp. 462–477.

Hoppe HA (1975). Drogenkunde, 8th Ed. Berlin: Walter de Gruyter; Vol 1, p. 764.

IPCS (2001).WHO food additives series 46: Pulegone and related substances. Available from: http://www.inchem.org/documents/jecfa/jecmono/v46je10.htm#_46101200. Accessed 19 June 2014.

Kaiser R, Lamparsky D, Schudel P (1975). Analysis of buchu leaf oil. *J Agric Food Chem*, 23(5):943–50. doi:10.1021/jf60201a021

Karousou R, Balta M, Hanlidou E, Kokkini S (2007). "Mints", smells and traditional uses in Thessaloniki (Greece) and other Mediterranean countries. *J Ethnopharmacol*, 109(2):248–57. doi:10.1016/j.jep.2006.07.022 PMID:16962274

Khojasteh-Bakht SC, Chen W, Koenigs LL et al. (1999). Metabolism of (R)-(+)-pulegone and (R)-(+)-menthofuran by human liver cytochrome P-450s: evidence for formation of a furan epoxide. *Drug Metab Dispos*, 27:574–580. PMID:10220485

Kumar S, Bahl JR, Bansal RP, Kukreja AK, Garg SN, Naqvi AA (2000). Profits of Indian menthol mint Mentha arvensis cultivars at different stages of crop growth in northern plains *J Med Arom Plant Sci*, 22:774–786.

List PH, Hörhammer L, editors (1976). Hagers handbook of pharmaceutical practice. 4th Ed. Berlin: Springer-Verlag; Vol 5, p. 20.

Madyastha KM & Raj CP (1993). Studies on the metabolism of a monoterpene ketone, R-(+)-pulegone–a hepatotoxin in rat: isolation and characterization of new metabolites. *Xenobiotica*, 23(5):509–18. doi:10.3109/00498259309059391 PMID:8342298

Marotti M, Piccaglia R, Giovanelli E, Deans SG, Eaglesham E (1994). Effects of planting time and mineral fertilization on peppermint (*Mentha piperita* L.) essential oil composition and its biological activity. *Flavour Fragrance J*, 9(3):125–9. doi:10.1002/ffj.2730090307

Misra A & Srivastava NK (2000). Influence of water stress on Japanese mint. *J Herbs Spices Med Plants*, 7(1):51–8. doi:10.1300/J044v07n01_07

Murray MJ, Marble P, Lincoln D, Hefendehl FW (1988). Peppermint oil quality differences and the reason for them. In: Lawrence BM, Mookherjee BD, Willis BJ, editors. Flavor and Fragrances: A World Perspective. Amsterdam, the Netherlands: Elsevier Press; pp. 189–210.

Nair B (2001). Final report on the safety assessment of Mentha Piperita (Peppermint) Oil, Mentha Piperita (Peppermint) Leaf Extract, Mentha Piperita (Peppermint) Leaf, and Mentha Piperita (Peppermint) Leaf Water. *Int J Toxicol*, 20(4):Suppl 3: 61–73. doi:10.1080/10915810152630747 PMID:11766133

NTP; National Toxicology Program (2011). Toxicology and carcinogenesis studies of pulegone (CAS No. 89–82–7) in F344/N rats and B6C3F1 mice (gavage studies). *Natl Toxicol Program Tech Rep Ser*, 563:1–201. PMID:21921962

O'Neil MJ (2013). An Encyclopedia of Chemicals, Drugs, and Biologicals. 15th Ed. Whitehouse (NJ): Merck Sharp & Dohme Corp., RSC Publishing.

Petrakis EA, Kimbaris AC, Pappas CS, Tarantilis PA, Polissiou MG (2009). Quantitative determination of pulegone in pennyroyal oil by FT-IR spectroscopy. *J Agric Food Chem*, 57(21):10044–8. doi:10.1021/jf9026052 PMID:19817373

Scifinder (2014). CAS Database: Pulegone. American Chemical Society. Available from: https://scifinder.cas.org

Sigma Aldrich (2013). Pulegone. MSDS Analytical Standard. Available from: http://www.sigmaaldrich.com/catalog/product/aldrich/w296309?lang=en®ion=US. Accessed 19 June 2014.

Skenderi G (2003). Herbal Vade Mecum. Rutherford (NJ): Herbacy Press; p. 287.

Smith DM & Levi L (1961). Essential oils, treatment of compositional data for the characterization of essential oils. Determination of geographical origins of peppermint oils by gas chromatographic analysis. *J Agric Food Chem*, 9(3):230–44. doi:10.1021/jf60115a017

Smith DM, Skakum W, Levi L (1963). Determination of botanical and geographical origin of spearmint oils by gas chromatographic and ultraviolet analysis. *J Agric Food Chem*, 11(3):268–76. doi:10.1021/jf60127a010

Speijers GJA (2001). WHO Food Additives Series 46: Pulegone and related substances. Bilthoven, the Netherlands: National Institute of Public Health and the Environment, Section on Public Health, Centre for Substances and Risk Assessment. Available from: http://www.inchem.org/documents/jecfa/jecmono/v46je10.htm. Accessed 22 July 2014.

Thomassen D, Knebel N, Slattery JT *et al.* (1992). Reactive intermediates in the oxidation of menthofuran by cytochromes P-450. *Chem Res Toxicol*, 5:123–130. doi:10.1021/tx00025a021 PMID:1581528

Thomassen D, Pearson PG, Slattery JT, Nelson SD (1991). Partial characterization of biliary metabolites of pulegone by tandem mass spectrometry. Detection of glucuronide, glutathione, and glutathionyl glucuronide conjugates. *Drug Metab Dispos*, 19(5):997–1003. PMID:1686249

Thomassen D, Slattery JT, Nelson SD (1988). Contribution of menthofuran to the hepatotoxicity of pulegone: assessment based on matched area under the curve and on matched time course. *J Pharmacol Exp Ther*, 244(3):825–9. PMID:3252034

Thomassen D, Slattery JT, Nelson SD (1990). Menthofuran-dependent and independent aspects of pulegone hepatotoxicity: roles of glutathione. *J Pharmacol Exp Ther*, 253:567–572. PMID:2338648

Turner GW & Croteau R (2004). Organization of monoterpene biosynthesis in Mentha. Immunocytochemical localizations of geranyl diphosphate synthase, limonene-6-hydroxylase, isopiperitenol dehydrogenase, and pulegone reductase. *Plant Physiol*, 136(4):4215–27. doi:10.1104/pp.104.050229 PMID:15542490

United Nations Comtrade (2013). United Nations Comtrade Database. Available from: http://comtrade.un.org/, accessed 17 December 2014.

Virmani OP & Datta SC (1968). Oil of spearmint *Perfume Essential Oil Rec*, 59:351–362.

Voirin B, Brun N, Bayet C (1990). Effects of day length on the monoterpene. composition of leaves of Mentha × piperita. *Phytochemistry*, 29(3):749–55. doi:10.1016/0031-9422(90)80012-6

Von Hefendehl FW & Ziegler E (1975). Analysis of peppermint oil. *Deut Lebens-Ritnds*, 8:287–290.

Weglarz Z & Zalecki R (1985). Investigations of dependence of the crop season of peppermint (*Mentha piperita* L.) herb upon the crop itself and the quality of the raw material. *Herba Pol*, 31:175–180.

Zhou S, Chan E, Duan W *et al.* (2005). Drug bioactivation, covalent binding to target proteins and toxicity relevance. *Drug Metab Rev*, 37:41–213. PMID:15747500

METHYLENE BLUE

1. Exposure Data

Methylene blue was originally synthesized in 1876 as an aniline-based dye for the textile industry (Berneth, 2008), but scientists such as Robert Koch and Paul Ehrlich were quick to realize its potential for use in microscopy stains (Ehrlich, 1881; Oz *et al.*, 2011). The observation of selective staining and inactivation of microbial species led to the testing of aniline-based dyes against tropical diseases (Oz *et al.*, 2011). Methylene blue was the first such compound to be administered to humans, and was shown to be effective in the treatment of malaria (Guttmann & Ehrlich, 1891; Oz *et al.*, 2011). Methylene blue was also the first synthetic compound ever used as an antiseptic in clinical therapy, and the first antiseptic dye to be used therapeutically. In fact, the use of methylene blue and its derivatives was widespread before the advent of sulfonamides and penicillin (Oz *et al.*, 2011).

1.1 Chemical and physical data

1.1.1 Nomenclature

Chem. Abstr. Serv. Reg. No.: 61-73-4 (anhydrous); 7220-79-3 (methylene blue trihydrate)

According to recent research, methylene blue occurs in the form of several different hydrates, but not as trihydrate (Rager *et al.*, 2012). [The Working Group noted that most of the scientific literature refers only to "methylene blue" independent of hydration state. Due to its hygroscopic nature, commercial methylene blue is typically sold as the hydrate, but is sometimes incorrectly presented as the trihydrate.]

Chem. Abstr. Serv. Name: Phenothiazin-5-ium, 3,7-bis(dimethylamino)-, chloride (O'Neil *et al.*, 2006)

IUPAC Systematic Name: [7-(Dimethylamino)phenothiazin-3-ylidene]-dimethylazanium chloride (PubChem, 2013)

Synonyms: Aizen methylene blue; Basic blue 9 (8CI); Calcozine blue ZF; Chromosmon; C.I. 52 015; Methylthionine chloride; Methylthioninium chloride; Phenothiazine-5-ium,3,7-bis, (dimethylamino)-, chloride; Swiss blue; Tetramethylene blue; Tetramethyl thionine chloride (NTP, 2008; PubChem, 2013).

1.1.2 Structural and molecular formulae and relative molecular mass

$C_{16}H_{18}ClN_3S$

Relative molecular mass (anhydrous form): 319.85 (PubChem, 2013)

1.1.3 Chemical and physical properties of the pure substance

Description: Dark green crystals or crystalline powder with bronze lustre, odourless, stable in air, deep blue solution in water or alcohol, forms double salts (PubChem, 2013)

Melting point: 100–110 °C (decomposition) (PubChem, 2013)

Density: 1.0 g/mL at 20 °C (ChemNet, 2013)

Solubility: 43.6 g/L in water at 25 °C; also soluble in ethanol (PubChem, 2013)

Vapour pressure: 1.30×10^{-7} mm Hg at 25 °C (estimated) (PubChem, 2013).

1.1.4 Technical products and impurities

(a) Trade names

Desmoid piller; desmoidpillen; panatone; urolene blue; vitableu (NTP, 2008)

(b) Impurities

- 3-Amino-7-(dimethylamino)phenothiazin-5-ium chloride (azure A) (PubChem, 2013)

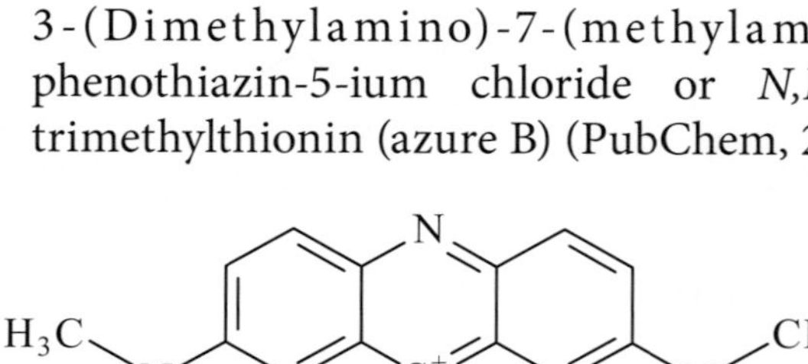

- 3-(Dimethylamino)-7-(methylamino)phenothiazin-5-ium chloride or N,N,N'-trimethylthionin (azure B) (PubChem, 2013)

- 3-(Amino)-7-(methylamino)phenothiazin-5-ium chloride (azure C) (PubChem, 2013)

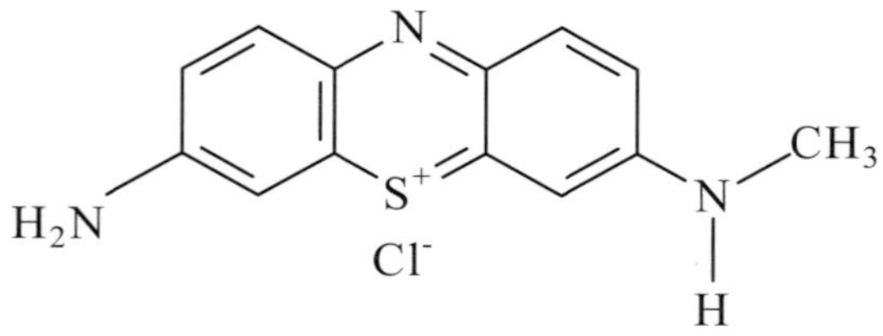

1.2 Analysis

There are several compendial and non-compendial methods for the analysis of methylene blue (Table 1.1). To quantify methylene blue in formulations, ultraviolet-visible spectroscopy can be conducted. For the quantification of methylene blue in biological specimens, liquid chromatography coupled with different detectors seems to be the method of choice.

1.3 Production and use

1.3.1 Production

Methylene blue is synthesized commercially by oxidation of N,N-dimethyl-phenylenediamine with sodium dichromate ($Na_2Cr_2O_7$) in the presence of sodium thiosulfate ($Na_2S_2O_3$), followed by further oxidation in the presence of N,N-dimethylaniline (NTP, 2008). Methylene blue hydrochloride is isolated by addition of 30% hydrochloric acid and of a saturated common salt solution to the dye solution; after filtration, the product is washed with a 2% common salt solution. Instead of sodium dichromate, manganese dioxide, and catalytic amounts of copper sulfate can be used for the oxidation (Berneth, 2008).

Methylene blue of high purity can be obtained by chloroform extraction of impurities from solutions of raw dye in borate buffer at pH 9.5–10, followed by acidification of the aqueous solution and isolation of the dye (Berneth, 2008).

Table 1.1 Some compendial and non-compendial methods for the analysis of methylene blue

Matrix	Sample preparation	Assay method	Detection limit	Reference
Compendial methods				
Assay	–	UV-visible spectroscopy Wavelength: 663 nm	–	US Pharmacopeial Convention (2013)
Assay	–	Iodimetric titration Titration with sodium thiosulfate using starch solution as indicator	–	British Pharmacopoeia Commission (2005)
Related substance test	–	LC-UV Column: C_{18} Mobile phase: acetonitrile and phosphoric acid (3.4 mL in 1000 mL of water) (27 : 73, v/v) Flow rate: 1 mL/min Wavelength: 246 nm	–	British Pharmacopoeia Commission (2005)
Non-compendial methods				
Human blood	Addition of NaCl and dichloroethane, centrifugation, analysis of dichloroethane layer	UV-visible spectroscopy Wavelength: 660 nm	0.02 µg/mL (LOD)	DiSanto & Wagner (1972)
Human urine	Addition of NaCl and dichloroethane, centrifugation, analysis of dichloroethane layer	UV-visible spectroscopy Wavelength: 660 nm	0.02 µg/mL (LOD)	DiSanto & Wagner (1972)
Rat tissue	Blotting on filter paper, addition of 0.1 N hydrochloric acid, homogenization, addition of NaCl and dichloroethane, centrifugation, analysis of dichloroethane layer	UV-visible spectroscopy Wavelength: 660 nm	0.02 µg/mL (LOD)	DiSanto & Wagner (1972)
Human blood	Haemolysis, addition of sodium hexanesulfonate, extraction (dichloroethane), centrifugation, analysis of organic layer	UV-visible spectroscopy Wavelength: 657 nm	0.1 µg/mL (LOQ)	Belaz-David *et al.* (1997)
Human plasma	Addition of sodium hexanesulfonate, extraction (dichloroethane), centrifugation, analysis of organic layer	UV-visible spectroscopy Wavelength: 657 nm	0.1 µg/mL (LOQ)	Belaz-David *et al.* (1997)
Human urine	Reduction of leucomethylene blue into methylene blue, addition of sodium hexanesulfonate, extraction (dichloroethane), centrifugation, analysis of organic layer	UV-visible spectroscopy Wavelength: 657 nm	3 µg/mL (LOQ)	Belaz-David *et al.* (1997)

Table 1.1   (continued)

Matrix	Sample preparation	Assay method	Detection limit	Reference
Human blood	Mixing with sodium hexanesulfonate, extraction (dichloroethane), centrifugation, evaporation	LC-UV Column: cyano Mobile phase: ammonium dihydrogen phosphate, acetonitrile and methanol pH 2.75 Flow rate: 0.7 mL/min Wavelength: 660 nm	9 nmol/L (LOQ)	Peter *et al.* (2000)
Human urine	Reduction of leucomethylene blue into methylene blue, mixing with sodium hexanesulfonate, extraction (dichloroethane), centrifugation, evaporation	LC-UV Column: cyano Mobile phase: ammonium dihydrogen phosphate, acetonitrile and methanol pH 2.75 Flow rate: 0.7 mL/min Wavelength: 660 nm	9 nmol/L (LOQ)	Peter *et al.* (2000)
Human blood and plasma	Precipitation with acetonitrile, centrifugation, and analysis of clear supernatant	LC-ESI-MS Column: C_{18} Mobile phase: 0.1% acetic acid in 5 mM acetate buffer and acetonitrile Flow rate: 0.35 mL/min	0.5 ng/mL (LOQ)	Rengelshausen *et al.* (2004)
Human blood and plasma	Acidic protein precipitation, centrifugation, analysis of clear supernatant	IEX-MS Column: uptisphere mixed mode Mobile phase: 0.1% acetic acid including 100 mM ammonium acetate (solvent A) and 2.5% formic acid/acetonitrile (1 : 1, v/v) including 500 mM ammonium acetate (solvent B) Flow rate: 0.45 mL/min	75 ng/mL (LOQ)	Burhenne *et al.* (2008)
Dried blood	Cutting of paper sheet, soaking in demineralized water, ultrasonication, protein precipitation, and analysis of clear supernatant	IEX-MS Column: uptisphere mixed mode Mobile phase: 0.1% acetic acid including 100 mM ammonium acetate (solvent A) and 2.5% formic acid/acetonitrile (1 : 1, v/v) including 500 mM ammonium acetate (solvent B) Flow rate: 0.45 mL/min	75 ng/mL (LOQ)	Burhenne *et al.* (2008)
Human urine	Dilution of urine	FIA-PIF Wavelength: λ_{ex} at 345 nm and λ_{em} at 485 nm pH 13 Flow rate: 2 mL/min	16 ng/mL (LOD) 0.06 µg/mL (LOQ)	Laassis *et al.* (1994)

Table 1.1 (continued)

Matrix	Sample preparation	Assay method	Detection limit	Reference
Human urine	Addition of sodium hexanesulfonate, extraction (dichloromethane), evaporation, reconstitution in water	CE-UV Extended light path(bubble) capillary Mobile phase: 100 mM phosphate buffer with 25% acetonitrile pH 2.5 Wavelength: 292 and 592 nm	1 µg/mL (LOQ)	Borwitzky et al. (2005)
Rat urine and mouse urine	Addition of 1 M sodium chloride solution, mixing, addition of dichloroethane, centrifugation, collection of dichloroethane layer, evaporation, reconstitution in 0.1% trifluoroacetic acid and acetonitrile	LC-UV Column: C_{18} Mobile phase: acetonitrile and 0.1% trifluoroacetic acid in water pH adjusted to ~2.74 with triethylamine Flow rate: 1 mL/min Wavelength: 660 nm	3.9 ng/mL (LOD) 13 ng/mL (LOQ)	Gaudette & Lodge (2005)
Rat blood	Addition of p-toluene sulfonic acid, buffering at pH 3 with ammonium acetate buffer, addition of acetonitrile and ultrasonic extraction, defatting of liquid phase with hexane, addition of dichloromethane, centrifugation, evaporation, reconstitution in water	CE-ESI-MS Fused silica capillary Electrolyte: 2 mol/L acetic acid Sheath liquid: methanol : water (80 : 20, v/v)	0.22 µg/mL (LOD) 0.5 µg/mL (LOQ)	Yang et al. (2011)
Cows' milk	Addition of acetonitrile, centrifugation, transferring of liquid into separating funnel, addition of NaCl, extraction with chloroform twice, collection of lower layer, evaporation, dissolve in acetonitrile, column clean-up with CBA column, evaporation of eluent, reconstitution in methanol	LC-UV Column: cyano Mobile phase: acetonitrile and acetate buffer pH 4.5 Flow rate: 1 mL/min Wavelength: 627 nm	2.5 ppb [ng/mL] (LOD) 5 ppb [ng/mL] (LOQ)	Munns et al. (1992)
Muscle of fish (rainbow trout)	Addition of McIlvaine buffer (pH 3.0), homogenization, addition of acetonitrile, centrifugation, washing of supernatant with n-hexane twice, addition of 10% NaCl solution and dichloromethane, addition of sodium sulfate to dichloromethane layer, filtration, evaporation, reconstitution with methanol	LC-UV Column: C_{18} Mobile phase: 0.1 M citrate buffer, acetonitrile pH 3.0 Flow rate: 0.8 mL/min Wavelength: 636 nm	3 µg/kg (LOD)	Kasuga et al. (1991)

Table 1.1   (continued)

Matrix	Sample preparation	Assay method	Detection limit	Reference
Fish tissue	Homogenization with ammonium acetate (pH 4.5) and acetonitrile, addition of basic aluminium oxide, centrifugation, transferring of supernatant into separating funnel, re-extraction of solid residue in the same manner, further extraction (dichloromethane), addition of DDQ and formic acid to dichloromethane layer, clean-up with isolute strong cation-exchange cartridge	LC-ESI-MS Column: C_{18} Mobile phase: ammonium acetate and acetonitrile pH 4.5 Flow rate: 0.3 mL/min	23.8 µg/kg (LOD)	Tarbin *et al.* (2008)
Edible aquatic products (eel, shrimp)	Addition of *p*-toluene sulfonic acid, buffering at pH 4.5 with sodium acetate buffer, extraction (acetonitrile, dichloromethane and diglycol), centrifugation, evaporation, reconstitution in acetonitrile, clean-up with neutral alumina and weak cation-exchange cartridges, evaporation, reconstitution in 3 : 7 (v/v) methanol : water solution	LC-ESI-MS Column: C_{18} Mobile phase: methanol, 0.1% formic acid pH 4.5 Flow rate: 250 µL/mL	0.1 µg/kg (LOD) 0.5 µg/kg (LOQ)	Xu *et al.* (2009)
Formulation	–	LC-ED Column: cyano Mobile phase: methanol, 0.1 M sodium acetate pH 4.5 Flow rate: 0.8 mL/min	3 pmol (LOD)	Roybal *et al.* (1989)
Formulation	–	First derivative UV spectroscopy Wavelength: 273 nm	6 µg/mL (LOQ)	Onur & Acar (1992)
Formulation	–	HPLC-PO-CL Colum: C_{18} Mobile phase: acetonitrile and 25 mM imidazole buffer containing 10 mM sodium 1-propanesulfonate pH 6.5 CL reaction solution: 0.25 mM TDPO and 25 mM H_2O_2 in acetonitrile Flow rate: for eluent, 1 mL/min; and for CL solution, 1.3 mL/min	120 fmol (LOD)	Kimoto *et al.* (1996)

λ_{ex}, λ excitation; λ_{em}, λ emission; CBA, carboxylic acid; CE-ESI-MS, capillary electrophoresis/electrospray ionization mass spectrometry; CE-UV, capillary electrophoresis ultraviolet spectroscopy; CL, chemiluminescence; DDQ, 2,3-dichloro-5,6-dicyano-1,4-benzoquinone; FIA-PIF, flow injection analysis photochemically induced fluorescence; HPLC-PO-CL, high-performance liquid chromatography peroxyoxalate chemiluminescence; IEX-MS, ion exchange chromatography mass spectrometry; LC-ED, liquid chromatography electrochemical detection; LC-ESI-MS, liquid chromatography electrospray ionization mass spectrometry; LC-UV, liquid chromatography ultraviolet spectroscopy; LOD, limit of detection; LOQ, limit of quantitation; ppb, parts per billion; NaCl, sodium chloride; TDPO, bis(4-nitro-2-(3,6,9-trioxadecyloxycarbonyl)phenyloxalate

1.3.2 Medical use

(a)   Indications

Methylene blue is used in human and veterinary medicine for several therapeutic and diagnostic procedures, including as a stain in bacteriology, as a redox colorimetric agent, as a targeting agent for melanoma, as an antihaemoglobinaemic, as an antidote, and as an antiseptic and disinfectant (O'Neil *et al.*, 2006; NTP, 2008).

Methylene blue is used clinically in a wide range of indications, including the emergency treatment of methaemoglobinemia, ifosfamid-induced encephalopathy or poisoning by cyanide, nitrate or carbon monoxide, and for intraoperative tissue staining (Oz *et al.*, 2011; Schirmer *et al.*, 2011).

One of the most common clinical applications of methylene blue is for the treatment of methaemoglobinaemia induced by overexposure to drugs, to industrial chemicals such as nitrophenols (ATSDR, 1992), or to environmental poisons such as excessive nitrate in well-water, or cyanide compounds (Sills & Zinkham, 1994; Christensen *et al.*, 1996).

Methylene blue is used in the treatment of some psychiatric disorders because of the anxiolytic and antidepressant properties attributed to its ability to block activation of guanyl cyclase by nitric oxide (Naylor *et al.*, 1986; Eroğlu & Cağlayan, 1997). In 2011, however, the Food and Drug Administration of the United States issued a safety warning concerning the risk of serotonin syndrome when methylene blue is given concurrently with serotonergic psychiatric medications (FDA, 2011).

Recent studies suggested that methylene blue may have beneficial effects in the treatment of Alzheimer disease and memory improvement (Oz *et al.*, 2011).

The use of methylene blue as a candidate antimalarial drug was revived in 1995, with the major goal to develop an affordable, available, and accessible therapy for uncomplicated falciparum malaria in children in Africa. In malaria combination therapy, methylene blue is also advantageous because the blue colour of the urine can be used as an indicator that the drug combination containing methylene blue has not been counterfeited, which is a serious problem in developing countries (Schirmer *et al.*, 2011). Some phase II trials have shown promising results, especially when methylene blue is combined with a more rapidly acting partner drug (Zoungrana *et al.*, 2008; Coulibaly *et al.*, 2009; Bountogo *et al.*, 2010).

(b)   Dosage

In clinical use, methylene blue is either dissolved in sterile water to a concentration of 10 mg/mL (1%) injectable solution or administered orally in gelatin capsules to avoid staining of the oral mucous membranes and to ensure complete gastrointestinal delivery (Oz *et al.*, 2011). The dosage depends on the therapeutic indication (Schirmer *et al.*, 2011). For inherited methaemoglobinaemia, the suggested oral dosage was 1×50–250 mg/day (for a lifetime), while for acute methaemoglobinaemia the suggested dosage was 1–2×1.3 mg/kg body weight (bw), given intravenously over 20 minutes. In ifosfamid-induced neurotoxicity, oral or intravenous doses of 4×50 mg/day were used. For prevention of urinary-tract infections in elderly patients, a dose of 3×65 mg/day was given orally. In Alzheimer disease, the dosage was 3×60 mg/day, and for paediatric malaria it was 2×12 mg/kg bw orally for 3 days (Schirmer *et al.*, 2011). In a controlled trial in semi-immune adults with uncomplicated falciparum malaria, the oral dosage was 390 mg twice per day (Bountogo *et al.*, 2010). According to Medscape (2013), a solution (10 mg/mL) may be injected at the following intravenous dosages: 1–2 mg/kg bw over 5–10 minutes for methaemoglobinaemia, and 50 mg every 6 to 8 hours until symptoms resolve for prevention of ifosfamid-induced encephalopathy.

(c) Sales volume

Worldwide sales of methylene blue totalled US$ 44 million in 2012, with 59% occurring in the USA. The only other nation to report substantial sales volumes was Brazil (US$ 11 million) (IMS Health, 2012).

1.3.3 Other uses

Methylene blue is used as a disinfectant and biological stain (NTP, 2008; Oz *et al.*, 2011). As a disinfectant, methylene blue is sold to end-consumers as an aquarium fungicide (Schirmer *et al.*, 2011). Most recently, methylene blue has been used as an optical probe in biophysical systems, as an intercalator in nanoporous materials, as a redox mediator, and in photoelectrochromic imaging (NTP, 2008).

Methylene blue is used to dye paper and office supplies, but also to tone up silk colours (Berneth, 2008). In analytical chemistry, methylene blue is applied to determine anionic surfactants, which are termed "methylene blue active substances" (Kosswig, 2000). Methylene blue is also used in pH and redox indicator reagents (Sabnis *et al.*, 2009).

1.4 Occurrence and exposure

1.4.1 Natural occurrence

Methylene blue is a synthetic substance and does not occur naturally.

1.4.2 Occupational exposure

A National Occupational Exposure Survey in the USA indicated that an estimated 69 563 workers were potentially exposed to methylene blue in the workplace between 1981 and 1983 (NTP, 2008).

1.4.3 General population and consumers

In 20 paediatric patients in Burkina Faso who were treated for malaria with methylene blue at an oral dose of 20 mg/kg bw, the concentrations in samples of dried whole blood on paper spots ranged between 531 and 2645 ng/mL within 1 hour after administration (Burhenne *et al.*, 2008). In a phase 1 study of malaria treatment, mean plasma concentrations after a single dose of methylene blue in healthy adults were 748 ng/mL (50 mg, intravenous injection; $n = 16$) and 3905 ng/mL (500 mg, oral administration; $n = 16$) (Walter-Sack *et al.*, 2009).

No systematic data on other exposures, e.g. environmental contamination, were available to the Working Group. While methylene blue may hypothetically enter the food chain after application in veterinary medicine (which would be illegal in most jurisdictions), or as a contaminant in drinking-water, no systematic data on residue levels in food or water were available. In the few available studies, it was found that metabolites rather than methylene blue itself were detectable, e.g. in milk from dairy cattle treated with methylene blue (Roybal *et al.*, 1996).

1.5 Regulations and guidelines

No permissible exposure limits for methylene blue have been established in the USA by the Occupational Safety and Health Administration, the National Institute for Occupational Safety and Health, or the American Conference of Governmental Industrial Hygienists (NTP, 2008). In the European Union, the use of methylene blue in food-producing animals is not allowed. According to Xu *et al.* (2009), Japan has established a maximum residue limit of 10 µg/kg for methylene blue in aquatic products, because it is used as a replacement for other antifungal dyes in aquaculture.

Table 1.2 Specifications for methylene blue

Parameter	WHO International Pharmacopoeia, 4th edition	United States Pharmacopoeia 36	European Pharmacopoeia 7.0
Content $C_{16}H_{18}ClN_3S$ (dried substance)	97.0–101.0%	98.0–103.0%	95.0–101.0%
Identity tests	A. IR B. Colour reaction with hydrochloric acid and zinc powder C. General identification test as characteristic of chlorides	IR	A. UV/VIS B. TLC C. Colour reaction with glacial acetic acid and zinc powder D. Reaction of chlorides
Copper or zinc	Absence of zinc; copper, max. 0.20 mg/g	Absence of zinc; copper max. 0.02%	Zinc, max. 100 ppm; copper, max. 300 ppm
Metals besides copper and zinc	Iron, max. 0.10 mg/g	Arsenic, max. 8 ppm	Max. contents: aluminium, 300 ppm; cadmium, 1 ppm; chromium, 100 ppm; tin, 10 ppm; iron, 200 ppm; manganese, 10 ppm; mercury, 1 ppm; molybdenum, 10 ppm; nickel, 10 ppm; lead, 10 ppm
Sulfated ash	Max. 10 mg/g		Max. 0.25%
Loss on drying	80–220 mg/g	8.0–18.0%	8.0–22.0%
Foreign substances/chromatographic purity/related substances	TLC: no spots besides the characteristic spots	TLC: max. four spots	HPLC: detailed specification of max. peak areas of impurities
Residue on ignition		Max. 1.2%	
Organic volatile impurities		Meets the requirements	
Bacterial endotoxins	Max. 2.5 IU of endotoxin per mg		
Methanol-insoluble substances			Max. 10.0 mg (1.0%)

HPLC, high-performance liquid chromatography; IR, infrared; IU, international unit; max., maximum; TLC, thin-layer chromatography; UV/VIS, ultraviolet and visible absorption spectrophotometry

From EDQM (2008), WHO (2011), US Pharmacopeial Convention (2013)

Specifications for methylene blue are published in several official pharmacopoeias (Table 1.2).

2. Cancer in Humans

No data were available to the Working Group.

3. Cancer in Experimental Animals

3.1 Mouse

In a study of oral administration, groups of 50 male and female B6C3F$_1$ (age, 6 weeks) received methylene blue (in a 0.5% aqueous methylcellulose solution) at a dose of 0 (control), 2.5, 12.5, or 25 mg/kg bw per day by gavage on 5 days per week for up to 106 weeks. There was an increase in mean body weight in females at the intermediate and highest doses compared with controls. Survival of treated groups was similar to that of controls.

In males, there was a significant positive increase in the trend in the incidence of carcinoma ($P = 0.027$, poly-3 trend test) and of adenoma or carcinoma (combined) of the small intestine ($P = 0.029$, poly-3 trend test). The incidences of carcinoma were: 0/50 (0%), 1/50 (2%), 2/50 (4%), 4/50 (8%); and the incidences of adenoma or carcinoma (combined) were: 1/50 (2%), 2/50 (4%), 4/50 (8%), 6/50 (12%). The incidences in the dosed groups were not significant by pairwise comparison. The incidence of adenoma or carcinoma (combined) in the group receiving the highest dose (12%) exceeded the range for historical controls (39/1508; range, 0–10%); while the incidence in controls (2%) was consistent with the range for historical controls.

In males, the incidence of bronchiolo-alveolar carcinoma of the lung occurred with a significant positive trend: 1/50 (2%), 4/50 (8%), 5/50 (10%), 7/50 (14%); $P = 0.043$, poly-3 trend test); and the incidence was significantly increased in the group at the highest dose ($P = 0.039$; poly-3 test). The incidence in males receiving methylene blue were within the range for historical controls for all routes of administration (151/1507; range, 4–24%) and the incidence in controls in the current study was below the range for historical controls. [The Working Group considered that the significantly increased incidence and significant positive trend in the incidence of bronchiolo-alveolar carcinoma was therefore not related to treatment with methylene blue.] In females, the incidences of bronchiolo-alveolar carcinoma were decreased in all groups of treated mice (5/50, 0/50, 0/50, 1/50), and the decreases were significant ($P \leq 0.05$, poly-3 test) in the groups receiving the lowest and intermediate dose.

The incidence of malignant lymphoma in females occurred with a significant positive trend: 6/50 (12%), 4/50 (8%), 9/50 (18%), 12/50 (24%); $P = 0.025$, poly-3 trend test. However, the incidence in females at the highest dose (24%) was well within the range for historical controls (308/1508; range, 6–58%) for this neoplasm with a highly variable incidence. In males, the incidences were 2/50 (4%), 2/50 (4%), 2/50 (4%), 5/50 (10%). While the incidence in the group at the highest dose was higher than in controls, it was not significantly increased, and barely exceeded the range for historical controls (70/1508; range, 0–8%) (NTP, 2008; Auerbach *et al.*, 2010).

3.2 Rat

In a study of oral administration, groups of 50 male and 50 female F344/N rats (age, 6 weeks) received methylene blue in a 0.5% aqueous methylcellulose solution at a dose of 0 (control), 5, 25, or 50 mg/kg bw, by gavage once per day on 5 days per week for up to 106 weeks. The mean body weights of males and females in groups at the intermediate and highest dose were decreased compared with controls at the end of the study.

There was no effect on body weight in groups at the lowest dose. Survival of treated groups was similar to that of the controls.

In males, the trend in the incidence of pancreatic islet cell adenoma and of adenoma or carcinoma (combined) were non-significantly increased. The incidences of adenoma were: 4/50 (8%), 9/50 (18%), 12/50 (24%), and 8/50 (16%); and the incidences of adenoma or carcinoma (combined) were: 4/50 (8%), 9/50 (18%), 14/50 (28%), and 8/50 (16%). The incidences were significantly increased only in the group receiving the intermediate dose (adenoma, $P = 0.037$; adenoma or carcinoma (combined), $P = 0.013$; poly 3-test), and the incidence of islet cell carcinoma of the pancreas (2/50; 4%) in the group receiving the intermediate dose was within the range for historical controls (26/1448; range, 0–8%). [Although the incidence of pancreatic islet cell hyperplasia was significantly increased in the group at the highest dose versus controls (26/50 versus 13/50; $P \leq 0.01$), and in view of the fact that islet cell hyperplasia, adenoma, and carcinoma are thought to constitute a morphological and biological continuum in the progression of islet cell proliferation, the Working Group considered that the positive trend in the incidence of adenoma or carcinoma (combined) was mainly the result of the increased trend in the incidence of adenoma].

There was no increase in the incidence of any neoplasm in exposed females (NTP, 2008; Auerbach *et al.*, 2010).

4. Mechanistic and Other Relevant Data

4.1 Absorption, distribution, metabolism, and excretion

4.1.1 Humans

After an intravenous bolus injection of 100 mg, the mean plasma concentration of methylene blue was reported to be 5 µM in healthy volunteers [number not specified] (Aeschlimann *et al.*, 1996).

Methylene blue is well absorbed, reduced, and excreted largely in the urine as the reduced leucomethylene blue (colourless) form (DiSanto & Wagner, 1972a; Fig. 4.1). The *N*-demethylated metabolites azure A (minor), azure B, and azure C (minor), which have the potential to undergo deprotonation to a neutral quinone imine, have been reported (Munns *et al.*, 1992; Schirmer *et al.*, 2011; Fig. 4.2), but their pharmacokinetic characteristics do not appear to have been investigated. One study mentioned the presence of azure B in autopsied peripheral organs from a patient who had received 200 mg of methylene blue intravenously, at levels (475–2943 ng/g) higher than those (74–208 ng/g) of methylene blue in the same tissues (Warth *et al.*, 2009). [The Working Group noted that the metabolites of methylene blue are anticipated to have greater lipophilicity than the parent compound and may accumulate in tissues.]

When administered orally to seven healthy human subjects at a dose of 10 mg in capsule form, the total urinary recovery ranged from 53% to 97% of the administered dose, with an average of 74%. Of the material recovered, an average of 78% was excreted as leucomethylene blue and the remainder as methylene blue. Excretion rate–time plots for methylene blue and leucomethylene blue suggested a circadian rhythm (DiSanto & Wagner, 1972a).

Fig. 4.1 Structures of methylene blue and leucomethylene blue

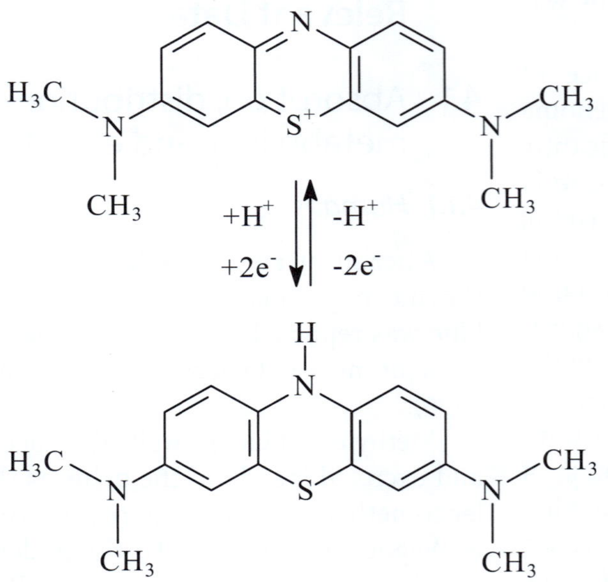

Compiled by the Working Group

In another study, the concentration of methylene blue in whole blood was measured in healthy individuals, before and after oxidation, following intravenous ($n = 7$) or oral ($n = 7$) administration of 100 mg of methylene blue. The concentration of methylene blue in whole blood after intravenous administration showed a multiphasic time course with an estimated terminal half-life of 5.25 hours. The area under the curve (AUC) was 0.134 ± 0.025 μmol/mL.min and the systemic clearance was 3.0 ± 0.7 L/min. After oral administration (in capsule form), maximum concentrations were reached within 1–2 hours; the AUC (0.01 ± 0.004 μmol/mL.min) was one order of magnitude lower than upon intravenous administration. The urinary excretion of total methylene blue (methylene blue and leucomethylene blue), between 4 and 14 hours, was significantly ($P < 0.01$) higher after intravenous administration than after oral administration ($28.6 \pm 3.0\%$ and $18.4 \pm 2.4\%$ of the administered dose, respectively). In this study, approximately one third of the methylene blue

excreted in the urine was in the leuco form (Peter *et al.*, 2000).

Another study compared the administration of single doses of methylene blue: 50 mg intravenously ($n = 16$) versus 500 mg orally ($n = 16$). The mean plasma AUCs were estimated to be 7.6 ± 3.4 μg/mL.h and 51.2 ± 17.1 μg/mL.h after intravenous and oral administration, respectively. The absolute bioavailability was $72.3 \pm 23.9\%$ (Walter-Sack *et al.*, 2009).

The pharmacokinetics of methylene blue were investigated in the setting of lymphatic mapping of cancer of the breast. A subareolar injection of 4 mL of a methylene blue solution at 1.25 mg/mL (total dose, 5 mg) resulted in rapid absorption (time to peak, 23 minutes) and an average peak serum concentration of 71.3 ng/mL. The elimination was slow ($t_{1/2} = 11.1$ hours), and 32% of the initial dose was recovered within 48 hours. The highest serum concentration was 280 ng/mL (Pruthi *et al.*, 2011). Of note, methylene blue concentrations have been found to be four- to fivefold higher in whole blood than in plasma (Peter *et al.*, 2000; Rengelshausen *et al.*, 2004).

Fig. 4.2 Structures of the methylene blue metabolites azure B, azure A, and azure C

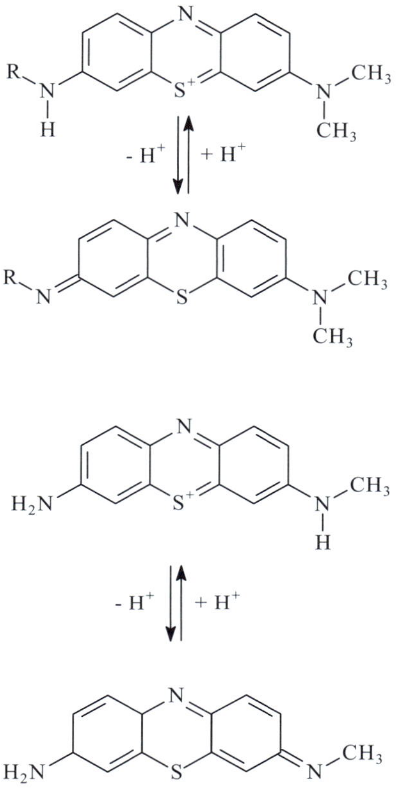

Compiled by the Working Group

[The Working Group noted that leuco-methylene blue is readily oxidized in air and forms stable complexes in the urine, but not blood (DiSanto & Wagner, 1972b, c). It is not clear whether or not discrepancies in the relative proportions of methylene blue and the leuco form between studies may be due to different aeration conditions during sample processing.]

4.1.2 Experimental animals

In one male and one female dog given methylene blue orally at a dose of 15 mg/kg bw, methylene blue was not detectable in the blood. The female was catheterized and urine was collected for 10 hours after dosing; the recovery was 2.4% of the administered dose. When the female was given methylene blue orally at a dose of 10 mg/kg bw, 3.8% of the administered dose was recovered in the urine within 14 hours (DiSanto & Wagner, 1972a). In comparison with the data obtained for humans in the same study (see Section 4.1.1), this low recovery indicated that methylene blue is well absorbed in humans and poorly absorbed in dogs after oral administration.

In another study, male Sprague-Dawley rats were treated intravenously with methylene blue at a dose of 2–25 mg/kg bw and killed 3 minutes after dosing; lungs, liver, kidneys, and heart were removed and assayed for methylene blue. An average of 29.8% of the administered dose (range, 25.2–35.8%) was recovered in the four tissues, which is consistent with very rapid and extensive uptake of methylene blue by tissues; the uptake was best described by a nonlinear model (DiSanto & Wagner, 1972c).

The distribution of total methylene blue in different tissues of male Wistar rats was measured after intravenous or intraduodenal administration of a single dose at 10 mg/kg bw. The rats were killed after 1 hour and samples from several different tissues were collected. The concentrations of the drug in the blood and brain were significantly higher ($P < 0.05$) after intravenous than after intraduodenal administration. In contrast, the concentrations in the intestinal wall and in the liver were significantly ($P < 0.05$) higher after intraduodenal administration, while concentrations in bile, and biliary excretion, were not affected by the route of administration. Less than 3% of the administered dose was found in the intestinal lumen 1 hour after intraduodenal administration (Peter *et al.*, 2000).

When a 10% solution of methylene blue was administered by intramammary infusion to lactating goats, the drug passed quickly into systemic circulation, peaked at 3 hours, and was still detectable in the blood 12 hours after infusion (Ziv & Heavner, 1984).

Azure B, together with methylene blue and leucomethylene blue, was reported to be present in the urine of male and female Fischer 344 rats ($n = 5$) given methylene blue as a single intravenous dose of 2.5 mg/kg bw, or a single oral dose of either 2.5 or 50 mg/kg bw. The methylene blue used in the experiment was contaminated with azure B at approximately 15%; metabolism of methylene blue through *N*-demethylation was inferred from a time-dependent increase in the amount of azure B present in the urine, but quantification of azure B was not provided (Gaudette & Lodge, 2005).

Methylene blue was reported to bind strongly to rabbit plasma (71–77% of bound drug). Extensive tissue and protein binding was proposed to account for the high apparent volume of distribution (21 L/kg) in rabbits (Kozaki & Watanabe, 1981).

4.2 Genetic and related effects

See Table 4.1

4.2.1 Humans

In mucosal cells from Barrett oeosophagus in humans undergoing endoscopy, methylene blue dye (0.5% solution) (which was used to identify specific areas of interest for biopsy) induced DNA damage as detected by the alkaline comet assay and the modified comet assay using the enzyme formamide pyrimidine-DNA glycosylase (FPG) to detect damage associated with reactive oxygen species (Olliver *et al.*, 2003). Fifteen patients undergoing endoscopy were biopsied at oesophageal mucosal sites that were treated with methylene blue, and at adjacent sites not treated with methylene blue. Comet assays revealed that elevated levels of DNA damage were observed in oesophageal mucosal cells exposed to methylene blue in all 15 patients, while samples adjacent to the methylene blue-exposed sites had significantly lower levels of DNA damage, despite photosensitization with white light from the endoscope (Olliver *et al.*, 2003). Exposure in vitro of normal oesophageal tissue, obtained by biopsy, to methylene blue (0.5% for 1 minute) in the absence of light did not result in an increase in DNA damage (Olliver *et al.*, 2003), confirming the role of white light-activated methylene blue in the induction of DNA damage. Similarly, an increase in DNA damage (alkali-labile sites and FPG-sensitive sites) was seen in biopsied colonic epithelium sprayed with methylene blue dye (0.1%) during colonoscopy (which used illumination with white light) compared with colonic epithelial cells sampled in the same region before spraying with methylene blue (Davies *et al.*, 2007).

Table 4.1 Genetic and related effects of methylene blue and its metabolites

Test system	Results[a]		Dose (LED or HID)	Reference
	Without exogenous metabolic system	With exogenous metabolic system[b]		
Methylene blue				
Bacteriophage PM2 cell-free, DNA damage, in the presence of white-light activation	+	NT	10 µg/mL	Epe *et al.* (1988)
Bacteriophage pAQ1 in *Salmonella typhimurium* TA1535 and TA1978, DNA damage, in the presence of white-light activation	+[c]	NT	10 µM	Epe *et al.* (1989)
Bacteriophage PM2 cell-free, DNA damage, in the presence of white-light activation	+[c]	NT	27 µM	Epe *et al.* (1993)
Bacteriophage pAQ1 in *Salmonella typhimurium* TA1978, DNA damage in PM2 with white-light activation	+[c]	NT	27 µM	Epe *et al.* (1993)
Single-stranded M13mp2 bacteriophage, DNA damage with photoactivation[d]	+	NT	2.5 µM	McBride *et al.* (1992)
Calf thymus DNA, intercalation, with photoactivation	+	NT	1.83 µM	Lee *et al.* (1973)
Calf thymus DNA, intercalation, with photoactivation	+	NT	NR[e]	Nordén & Tjerneld (1982)
DNA–protein crosslinks, calf thymus DNA, calf thymus histone type II, with photoactivation	+	NT	5 µM	Villanueva *et al.* (1993)
Salmonella typhimurium TA100, TA1535, TA1537, TA1538, TA98, reverse mutation	+ (TA98)	+ (TA98)	5 µg/plate	Chung *et al.* (1981)
Salmonella typhimurium TA100, reverse mutation	+	+	20 µg/plate	Yamaguchi (1981)
Salmonella typhimurium TA100, TA1530, TA1535, TA98, reverse mutation	+ (TA1530, TA98)	+ (TA98)	1000 µg/plate	Lunn & Sansone (1991)
Salmonella typhimurium TA100, reverse mutation	(±)	+[f]	33 µg/plate	NTP (2008)
Salmonella typhimurium TA98, reverse mutation	+	+[f]	33 µg/plate, –S9 3.3 µg/plate, +S9	NTP (2008)
Salmonella typhimurium TA100, reverse mutation	+	+	0.25 µg/plate, –S9 10 µg/plate, +S9	NTP (2008)
Salmonella typhimurium TA98, reverse mutation	+	+	1 µg/plate, –S9 10 µg/plate, +S9	NTP (2008)
Salmonella typhimurium TA1535, TA1538, reverse mutation, with and without photoactivation	+ (TA1535)[g]	NT	20 µg/plate	Gutter *et al.* (1977)
Salmonella typhimurium TA1535, TA2638, TA100, TA104, reverse mutation, with photoactivation	+	NT	10 µg/mL	Epe *et al.* (1989)

Table 4.1 (continued)

Test system	Results[a]		Dose (LED or HID)	Reference
	Without exogenous metabolic system	With exogenous metabolic system[b]		
Escherichia coli WP2, WP2 *uvrA*⁻, WP67 *uvrA*⁻ *polA*⁻, CM611 *uvrA*⁻ *lexA*⁻, WP100 *uvrA*⁻ *recA*⁻, W3110 *polA*⁺, p3478 *polA*⁻, DNA damage	+ (CM611, WP100, p3478)	NT	160 µg/well (p3478 *polA*⁻)	McCarroll *et al.* (1981)
Escherichia coli AB1157, B/r, WP2, WP2s,WP10, WP6 (*polA1*), resistance to bacteriophage T5	+ (AB1157, WP2s, WP10)	NT	2 µM	Webb & Hass (1984)
Escherichia coli K-12/343/113, reverse mutation to *Arg*+, with white-light activation	+	NT	10–40 µM (LED, NR)	Mohn *et al.* (1984)
Escherichia coli WP2 *uvrA* pKM101, reverse mutation	+	+	0.5 µg/plate, –S9 25 µg/plate, +S9	NTP (2008)
Saccharomyces cerevisiae, gene conversion, with white light photoactivation (λmax 664 nm)	–	NT	0.95 (OD$_{\lambda max}$)[h]	Ito & Kobayashi (1977)
Saccharomyces cerevisiae 507.4/2b, MT182/8d, CM106/5a, gene mutations, no photoactivation	–	NT	20 µg/mL	Tuite *et al.* (1981)
Bacteriophage *Serratia* phage *kappa*, mutagenicity, with photoactivation	+	NT	NR	Brendel (1973)
DNA damage (alkali-labile sites) (comet assay), male Sprague-Dawley rat, primary hepatocytes, with visible light activation in vitro	+	NT	0.31 µM × 2 min	Lábaj *et al.* (2007)
DNA damage (FPG-sensitive sites) (comet assay), male Sprague-Dawley rat, primary hepatocytes, with visible light activation in vitro	+	NT	0.31 µM × 2 min	Lábaj *et al.* (2007)
DNA damage (alkali-labile sites; FPG-sensitive sites) (comet assay), male Sprague Dawley rat, primary hepatocytes, in vitro	–	NT	0.31 µM × 3 min	Lábaj *et al.* (2007)
DNA damage (alkali-labile sites; FPG-sensitive sites) (comet assay), male Sprague-Dawley rat, primary hepatocytes, in vitro	+	NT	0.31 µM × 3 min	Horváthová *et al.* (2012)
DNA damage (alkali-labile sites) (comet assay), male Sprague Dawley rat, primary hepatocytes, with visible light activation in vitro	+	NT	0.31 µM × 3 min	Horváthová *et al.* (2012)
DNA damage (FPG-sensitive sites) (comet assay), male Sprague-Dawley rat, primary hepatocytes, with visible light activation in vitro	+	NT	0.31 µM × 3 min	Horváthová *et al.* (2012)
DNA damage (alkali-labile sites) (comet assay), MCF-7 cells, with visible light activation in vitro	+	NT	0.1% × 5 min	Masannat *et al.* (2009)
DNA damage (FPG-sensitive sites) (comet assay), MCF-7 cells, with visible light activation in vitro	–	NT	1.0% × 5 min	Masannat *et al.* (2009)
DNA damage (alkali-labile sites) (comet assay), HB-2 cells, with visible light activation in vitro	+	NT	1.0% × 5 min	Masannat *et al.* (2009)
DNA damage (FPG-sensitive sites) (comet assay), HB-2 cells, with visible light activation in vitro	–	NT	1.0% × 5 min	Masannat *et al.* (2009)
DNA damage (comet assay), CaCo-2 cells, in vitro	–	NT	0.1% × 2 min	Davies *et al.* (2007)

Table 4.1 (continued)

Test system	Results[a]		Dose (LED or HID)	Reference
	Without exogenous metabolic system	With exogenous metabolic system[b]		
DNA damage (alkali-labile sites) (comet assay), CaCo-2 cells, with visible light activation in vitro	+	NT	0.1% × 2 min	Davies *et al.* (2007)
DNA damage (FPG-sensitive sites) (comet assay), CaCo-2 cells, with visible light activation in vitro	+	NT	0.1% × 2 min	Davies *et al.* (2007)
DNA damage (alkali-labile sites) (comet assay), human colonic mucosa cells, with visible light activation during colonoscopy in vivo	+		0.1%	Davies *et al.* (2007)
DNA damage (FPG-sensitive sites) (comet assay), human colonic mucosa cells, with visible light activation during colonoscopy in vivo	+		0.1%	Davies *et al.* (2007)
DNA damage (comet assay), human Barrett oesophagus cells (biopsy), in vitro	–	NT	0.5% × 1 min	Olliver *et al.* (2003)
DNA damage (alkali-labile sites) (comet assay), human Barrett oesophagus cells, with visible light activation during endoscopy in vivo	+		0.5%	Olliver *et al.* (2003)
DNA damage (FPG-sensitive sites) (comet assay), human Barrett oesophagus cells, with visible light activation during endoscopy in vivo	+		0.5%	Olliver *et al.* (2003)
DNA damage (alkali-labile sites) (comet assay), human OE33 cells, with white-light activation in vitro	+	NT	15 mM (0.5%) × 5 min	Sturmey *et al.* (2009)
DNA damage (alkali-labile sites) (comet assay), human OE33 cells, with red light activation in vitro	+	NT	15 mM (0.5%) × 5 min	Sturmey *et al.* (2009)
DNA damage (FPG-sensitive sites) (comet assay), human OE33 cells, with red light activation in vitro	+	NT	1.5 mM × 5 min	Sturmey *et al.* (2009)
DNA damage (alkali-labile sites) (comet assay), human OE33 cells, with green light activation in vitro	–	NT	15 mM (0.5%) × 3 min	Sturmey *et al.* (2009)
DNA damage (alkali-labile sites) (comet assay), human OE33 cells, with blue light activation in vitro	–	NT	15 mM (0.5%) × 3 min	Sturmey *et al.* (2009)
DNA damage (alkali-labile sites) (comet assay), human OE33 cells, with filtered white light (to remove 580–800 nm red spectrum) activation in vitro	–	NT	15 mM (0.5%) × 3 min	Sturmey *et al.* (2009)
Drosophila melanogaster, sex-linked recessive lethal mutation, in germ cells, larval feeding	–		0.1% in feed	Clark (1953)
Drosophila melanogaster, somatic mutation and recombination test (SMART), with photoactivation	+		0.01 mM in feed	Smijs *et al.* (2004)
Sister-chromatid exchange, Chinese hamster V79 cells, in vitro	–	NT	1.0 µg/mL	Popescu *et al.* (1977)

Table 4.1 (continued)

Test system	Results[a]		Dose (LED or HID)	Reference
	Without exogenous metabolic system	With exogenous metabolic system[b]		
Sister-chromatid exchange, Chinese hamster V79 cells, in vitro, no photoactivation	+	NT	0.1 µg/mL	Speit & Vogel (1979)
Sister-chromatid exchange, Chinese hamster V79 cells, in vitro, with photoactivation	–	NT	1.0 µg/mL	Speit & Vogel (1979)
Sister-chromatid exchange, Syrian hamster BHK-1 cells, with/without photoactivation in vitro	–	NT	27 µg/mL	MacRae *et al.* (1980)
Sister-chromatid exchange, Chinese hamster ovary cells, in vitro	+	+	0.63 µg/mL (–S9) 4.7 µg/mL (+S9)	NTP (2008)
Chromosomal aberrations, Chinese hamster ovary cells, in vitro	–	NT	20 µM[i]	Au & Hsu (1979)
Chromosomal aberrations, Chinese hamster V79 cells, in vitro	–		1.0 µg/mL	Popescu *et al.* (1977)
Chromosomal aberrations, Chinese hamster ovary cells, in vitro	+	+	7.5 µg/mL (–S9) 4.7 µg/mL (+S9)	NTP (2008)
Sister chromatid exchanges, Chinese hamster bone-marrow cells, in vivo	–		12 mg/kg bw, ip × 1	Speit (1982)
Micronucleus formation, male B6C3F$_1$ mice, bone-marrow cells or peripheral blood erythrocytes, in vivo	–		150 mg/kg bw, ip × 1	NTP (2008)
Micronucleus formation, male and female B6C3F$_1$ mice, peripheral blood erythrocytes, in vivo	–		200 mg/kg bw per day, gavage × 14 wk	NTP (2008)
Azure A				
Salmonella typhimurium TA100, reverse mutation	+	+	10 µg/plate, –S9 50 µg/plate, +S9	NTP (2008)
Salmonella typhimurium TA98, reverse mutation	+	+	10 µg/plate, –S9 100 µg/plate, +S9	NTP (2008)
Escherichia coli WP2 *uvrA* pKM101, reverse mutation	+	+	50 µg/plate, –S9 250 µg/plate, +S9	NTP (2008)
Chromosomal aberrations, Chinese hamster ovary cells, in vitro	+	NT	10 µM[j]	Au & Hsu (1979)
Azure B				
Salmonella typhimurium TA100, TA98, reverse mutation	+	+	10 µg/plate	NTP (2008)
Escherichia coli WP2 *uvrA* pKM101, reverse mutation	+	+	10 µg/plate, –S9 100 µg/plate, +S9	NTP (2008)
Chromosomal aberrations, Chinese hamster ovary cells, in vitro	+	NT	20 µM[j]	Au & Hsu (1979)

Table 4.1 (continued)

Test system	Results[a]		Dose (LED or HID)	Reference
	Without exogenous metabolic system	With exogenous metabolic system[b]		
Azure C				
Salmonella typhimurium TA100, reverse mutation	+	+	25 µg/plate, –S9 100 µg/plate, +S9	NTP (2008)
Salmonella typhimurium TA98, reverse mutation	+	+	10 µg/plate, –S9 250 µg/plate, +S9	NTP (2008)
Escherichia coli WP2 *uvrA* pKM101, reverse mutation	+	+	25 µg/plate, –S9 100 µg/plate, +S9	NTP (2008)
Chromosomal aberrations, Chinese hamster ovary cells, in vitro	+	NT	20 µM[j]	Au & Hsu (1979)

[a] +, positive; –, negative; (±), equivocal
[b] S9 from Aroclor 1254-treated Sprague-Dawley rats, unless otherwise noted
[c] DNA damage was in the form of base modifications consistent with singlet oxygen generation
[d] 8-hydroxydeoxyguanosine and SOS-induced mutations implicating generation of lesions (ionic) other than 8-hydroxydeoxyguanosine in methylene blue plus white light oxidative DNA damage
[e] Intercalation orientation is changed by ionic strength; at low ionic strength, methylene blue is oriented co-planar with the DNA bases and at higher ionic strength, orientation changes
[f] S9 from Aroclor 1254-treated Sprague-Dawley rats or Syrian hamsters
[g] Photoactivation required; no increase in mutations in the absence of photoactivation with white light. Dose–response observed in the presence of white light (2-hour exposure) over a range of 10–100 µg/plate
[h] Concentrated stock solution was diluted with 0.067 M phosphate buffer to give a final concentration of OD ≥ 1 at its absorption peak
[i] Not possible to accurately interpret the data; duration of exposure was only 5 hours, only 50 cells were evaluated for aberrations per concentration tested, gaps were included in the overall assessment of chromosomal damage, and data were presented as total aberrations rather than percentage of aberrant cells
[j] Not possible to accurately interpret the data; high levels of cytotoxicity were noted at ≥ 10 µM for azure A. For azure B and C, only the cytotoxic concentration (20 µM) was tested
bw, body weight; HID, highest ineffective dose; ip, intraperitoneal; LED, lowest effective dose; min, minute; NR, not reported; NT, not tested; po, oral; wk, week

4.2.2 Experimental systems

(a) Mutation

(i) Assays in bacteria or yeast

Methylene blue was shown to be mutagenic without photoactivation in a variety of *Salmonella typhimurium* tester strains, inducing both base-substitution and frameshift mutations, with and without metabolic activation (Chung *et al.*, 1981; Yamaguchi, 1981; Lunn & Sansone, 1991; NTP, 2008); mutagenic activity or induction of DNA damage was also reported in several strains of *Escherichia coli* (McCarroll *et al.*, 1981; Mohn *et al.*, 1984; Webb & Hass, 1984; NTP, 2008). In contrast, photoactivated (664 nm) methylene blue did not induce gene conversion in the yeast *Saccharomyces cerevisiae* (Ito & Kobayashi, 1977), and no induction of gene mutation was seen in *S. cerevisiae* treated with methylene blue at a single concentration of 20 μg/mL in the absence of photoactivation (Tuite *et al.*, 1981). It was suggested that the negative results in the yeast assays resulted from the inability of methylene blue to penetrate the yeast cell wall (Ito & Kobayashi, 1977).

(ii) Drosophila melanogaster

No increase in the frequency of sex-linked recessive lethal mutation was detected in germ cells of male *Drosophila melanogaster* given methylene blue via a larval feeding regimen (Clark, 1953). However, when photoactivated with white light, methylene blue induced high levels of homologous mitotic recombination in a somatic mutation and recombination test (SMART) in *D. melanogaster* (Smijs *et al.*, 2004).

(b) DNA damage

Positive results were reported in several in-vitro tests for mutagenicity or DNA damage induction with photoactivated methylene blue, presumably the result of singlet oxygen production (Brendel, 1973; Gutter *et al.*, 1977; Epe *et al.*, 1988, 1989, 1993; McBride *et al.*, 1992).

Methylene blue was shown to intercalate into calf thymus DNA (Lee *et al.*, 1973), and to bind to calf thymus DNA in an orientation perpendicular to the helix axis, coplanar with the bases, at low methylene blue : DNA binding ratios and low ionic strengths (Nordén & Tjerneld, 1982). Villanueva *et al.* (1993) reported that methylene blue induced light-dose-dependent increases in DNA–protein crosslinks (calf thymus DNA, calf thymus histone type II), which was attributed to the production of singlet oxygen.

Several studies of DNA damage using the comet assay have been conducted with the majority demonstrating a requirement for methylene blue activation by visible (white) light to induce both alkali-labile and FPG-sensitive (oxidized guanine) sites. Studies were conducted in male Sprague-Dawley rat primary hepatocytes (Lábaj *et al.*, 2007; Horváthová *et al.*, 2012), MCF-7 breast cancer cells (Masannat *et al.*, 2009), HB-2 normal human breast cells (Masannat *et al.*, 2009), cultured colonic adenocarcinoma CaCo-2 cells (Davies *et al.*, 2007), and Barrett-associated adenocarcinoma OE33 cells (Sturmey *et al.*, 2009). Masannat *et al.* (2009) reported no increase in the number of FPG-sensitive sites in MCF-7 cells treated with 1% methylene blue for 5 minutes in the presence of white light, but alkali-labile sites were significantly increased by this treatment, as was total DNA damage. Similar results were reported by Sturmey *et al.* (2009) with OE33 cells treated with methylene blue and white light (significant increase in alkali-labile sites, but not FPG-sensitive sites). In all other cell lines, DNA damage in the form of both alkali-labile sites and FPG-sensitive sites) was observed after treatment with methylene blue in the presence of white light. To determine if one particular portion of the spectrum was involved in the photoactivation of methylene blue, Sturmey *et al.* (2009) conducted a series of experiments using white light and filtered light to activate methylene blue and assess DNA damage levels in OE33 cells. The concentrations of methylene blue ranged from 0.015 to 15 mM (0.0005–0.5%), with the highest concentration equal to the clinically relevant concentration used in colonoscopies to visualize suspicious areas for biopsy. Only the highest concentration of methylene blue induced significant increases in DNA damage in OE33 cells with white-light activation. However, red light (580–700 nm) induced DNA damage at a lower concentration of methylene blue (1.5 mM or 0.05%) and increased the frequency of both alkali-labile sites and FPG-sensitive sites; no increases in DNA damage were seen when light was filtered to allow only the blue or the green portions of the spectrum to interact with methylene blue. Lowering the concentration of methylene blue used in the clinic, and/or eliminating the red portion of the white-light spectrum used to illuminate colonic epithelium during colonoscopy might thus result in reduction of DNA damage in sensitive tissues during these medical procedures.

(c) Chromosomal damage

(i) In vitro

The results of tests measuring induction of sister-chromatid exchange in cultured Chinese hamster lung V79 cells (Popescu *et al.*, 1977), and Syrian hamster fibroblast (baby hamster kidney) BHK-1 cells (MacRae *et al.*, 1980) treated with methylene blue in the absence of photoactivation were generally negative. One exception was reported, where Chinese hamster V79 cells showed significant increases in the frequency of sister-chromatid exchange in the absence, but not in the presence, of photoactivation (Speit & Vogel, 1979). No induction of chromosomal aberration was seen in Chinese hamster V79 cells treated with methylene blue in the absence of photo-activation (Popescu *et al.*, 1977). Negative results were also reported in another test for chromosomal aberration in Chinese hamster ovary cells (Au & Hsu, 1979). [The Working Group noted that caution should be used in interpreting the results of Au & Hsu (1979) due to the inadequate description of the protocol and other deficiencies, including the brief exposure time and the small number of cells scored.] In a study by the National Toxicology Program (NTP, 2008), induction of sister-chromatid exchange and of chromosomal aberration with and without metabolic activation was observed in Chinese hamster ovary cells treated with methylene blue.

(ii) In vivo

Despite extensive evidence for mutagenicity and induction of DNA damage by methylene blue in vitro, particularly with white-light activation, no evidence for genotoxicity has been observed in a limited number of standard tests in vivo, all of which investigated some aspect of chromosomal damage. No significant increase in the frequency of sister-chromatid exchange was seen in bone-marrow cells of adult Chinese hamsters given a single intraperitoneal injection of methylene blue at 12 mg/kg bw (Speit, 1982). Similarly, no increases in the frequency of micronucleated erythrocytes were observed in bone-marrow cells or peripheral blood erythrocytes of male $B6C3F_1$ mice given a single intraperitoneal dose of methylene blue, or in peripheral blood erythrocytes of male $B6C3F_1$ mice treated by gavage with methylene blue for 5 days per week for 3 months (NTP, 2008).

4.2.3 Metabolites of methylene blue

(a) Azure A

Azure A was mutagenic in *Salmonella typhimurium* strains TA98 and TA100, and *Escherichia coli* strain WP2 *uvrA* pKM101, with and without exogenous metabolic activation (NTP, 2008). Azure A also induced chromosomal damage in cultured Chinese hamster ovary cells in the absence of exogenous metabolic activation at doses (10 and 20 µM) that produced marked cytotoxicity (Au & Hsu, 1979).

(b)   Azure B

Azure B was mutagenic in *Salmonella typhimurium* strains TA98 and TA100, and *Escherichia coli* strain WP2 *uvrA* pKM101, with and without exogenous metabolic activation (NTP, 2008). Azure B also induced chromosomal damage in cultured Chinese hamster ovary cells in the absence of exogenous metabolic activation at a dose (20 µM) that produced marked cytotoxicity (Au & Hsu, 1979).

(c)   Azure C

Azure C was mutagenic in *Salmonella typhimurium* strains TA98 and TA100, and *Escherichia coli* strain WP2 *uvrA* pKM101, with and without exogenous metabolic activation (NTP, 2008). Azure C also induced chromosomal damage in cultured Chinese hamster ovary cells in the absence of exogenous metabolic activation at a dose (20 µM) that produced marked cytotoxicity (Au & Hsu, 1979).

4.3   Other relevant mechanisms

4.3.1 General adverse effects

In humans, large intravenous doses of methylene blue (~500 mg) have been reported to cause nausea, abdominal and chest pain, cyanosis, methaemoglobinaemia, sweating, dizziness, headache, and confusion (Clifton & Leikin, 2003; Oz *et al.*, 2011). Toxicity in infants exposed to methylene blue during prenatal or perinatal diagnostic or therapeutic procedures is well documented: hyperbilirubinaemia, haemolytic anaemia, formation of Heinz bodies, erythrocytic blister cells, skin discoloration, and photosensitization are the most commonly reported adverse effects (Sills & Zinkham, 1994; Porat *et al.*, 1996; Cragan, 1999).

A series of acute toxic effects have been described in animals exposed to methylene blue, including haemoconcentration, hypothermia, acidosis, hypercapnia, hypoxia, increases in blood pressure, changes in respiratory frequency and amplitude, corneal injury, conjunctival damage, and formation of Heinz bodies (Auerbach *et al.*, 2010).

4.3.2 Haematological toxicity

Severe toxic methaemoglobinaemia can be treated by intravenous administration of methylene blue (1–2 mg/kg bw). In the presence of reduced nicotinamide adenine dinucleotide phosphate (NADPH), the dye is converted by methaemoglobin reductases in erythrocytes to leucomethylene blue, which then reduces methaemoglobin nonenzymatically, restoring functional haemoglobin and methylene blue. This redox cycle is sustained by regeneration of NADPH via the hexose monophosphate shunt (pentose phosphate pathway). However, at higher concentrations, methylene blue oxidizes ferrous iron in haemoglobin to the ferric state, producing methaemoglobin (Bradberry *et al.*, 2001).

Given that glucose-6-phosphate dehydrogenase is required for the enzymatic pentose phosphate pathway that produces NADPH, patients with glucose-6-phosphate dehydrogenase deficiency have depleted NADPH levels. In these patients, methylene blue may exacerbate haemolytic anaemia, and haemolysis favours the formation of methylene blue-induced methaemoglobin (Smith & Thron, 1972; Bilgin *et al.*, 1998).

A study compared the responses of several species to a single intraperitoneal injection of methylene blue (20–100 mg/kg bw in cats, dogs, and guinea-pigs; 20–200 mg/kg bw in mice, rabbits, and rats). Although the tolerance for methylene blue varied considerably, most species had a decrease in erythrocytes and haemoglobin, and an increase in reticulocytes within a few days after treatment. Cats and dogs were the most sensitive species, with Heinz bodies detected 4 and 6 hours, respectively, after administration of methylene blue. Heinz bodies were also detected in mice (100% incidence, at 200 mg/kg bw after

24 hours), rats (12% incidence, at 200 mg/kg bw after 96 hours), rabbits (70% incidence, at 200 mg/kg bw after 96 hours), and guinea-pigs (incidence was 4%, at 100 mg/kg bw, after 72 hours) (Rentsch & Wittekind, 1967).

In a 90-day study of toxicity by the NTP, methylene blue was administered at doses of 0, 25, 50, 100, and 200 mg/kg bw by gavage to F344/N rats and B6C3F$_1$ mice. The treatment resulted in methaemoglobin formation, oxidative damage to erythrocytes, and dose-related regenerative Heinz-body anaemia in rats and mice. Splenomegaly and an increase in splenic haematopoiesis occurred in treated rats and mice. Splenic congestion and bone-marrow hyperplasia were also observed in treated rats. Mice showed increased liver haematopoiesis (100 mg/kg bw and above) and an accumulation of haemosiderin in Kupffer cells (50 mg/kg bw and above). These observations suggested the development of haemolytic anaemia. There was also a dose-related increase in the reticulocyte count in treated rats and mice, suggesting a compensatory response to anaemia (Hejtmancik *et al.*, 2002; NTP, 2008).

The haematological toxicity documented in the 90-day study by the NTP (see above) served as the basis for selecting the doses of methylene blue for a long-term bioassay (0, 5, 25, and 50 mg/kg bw per day for rats; 0, 2.5, 12.5, and 25 mg/kg bw per day for mice; 5 days per week for 2 years). Similarly to the 90-day study, development of methaemoglobinemia, formation of Heinz bodies, and macrocytic responsive anaemia were observed in treated rats, while methaemoglobinaemia and formation of Heinz bodies also occurred in treated mice (NTP, 2008; Auerbach *et al.*, 2010).

4.3.3 Additional mechanisms

Amino acids can undergo photo-oxidation by methylene blue and methylene blue derivatives (Knowles & Gurnani, 1972); multiple studies have been conducted on the photoinactivation of a variety of enzymes by methylene blue (reviewed in Moura & Cordeiro, 2003).

In pharmacological studies, methylene blue (1–10 μM) is used routinely to inhibit soluble guanylate cyclase for the analysis of cyclic guanosine monophosphate (cGMP)-mediated processes. Methylene blue also inhibits constitutive and inducible forms of nitric oxide synthase by oxidation of ferrous iron bound to the enzyme, and inactivates nitric oxide by generation of superoxide anions (reviewed in Oz *et al.*, 2011).

Methylene blue penetrates cellular and mitochondrial membranes, accumulates within mitochondria, and improves mitochondrial respiration at low concentrations (0.5–2 μM) by shuttling electrons to oxygen in the electron transport chain. When acting as an alternative electron acceptor in mitochondria, methylene blue also inhibits the production of superoxide by competing with molecular oxygen. Methylene blue has been described to increase the enzymatic activity of cytochrome oxidase in the brain (reviewed in Oz *et al.*, 2009).

Methylene blue and its metabolite, azure B, are reversible inhibitors of monoamine oxidase. This inhibition may underlie adverse effects, but also psycho- and neuromodulatory actions associated with methylene blue taken as a drug (Ramsay *et al.*, 2007; Petzer *et al.*, 2012).

4.4 Susceptibility

No data were available to the Working Group.

4.5 Mechanistic considerations

Methylene blue absorbs energy directly from a light source and then transfers this energy to molecular oxygen, generating singlet oxygen ($^1O_2$). Singlet oxygen is electrophilic and can oxidize electron-rich double bonds in bio(macro)molecules (Tardivo *et al.*, 2005).

Two mechanisms of action, involving photo-activation, can also be envisaged. Excitation of methylene blue can produce both a singlet and a triplet species; the excess triplet energy can be transferred through electrons (type I mechanism) or energy (type II mechanism) (Tardivo *et al.*, 2005). Both mechanisms can damage bio(macro) molecules. Energy transfer can cause strand breaks in nucleic acids, thereby leading to DNA damage. Electron transfer can produce reactive oxygen species, including hydroxyl radicals and hydroperoxides, which can be detrimental to the integrity of nucleic acids, proteins, and lipids.

Although the carcinogenicity of methylene blue may partly arise via photoactivation, the rodent biossays were conducted without light activation. Therefore other mechanisms are likely to operate. It is currently unclear whether the effects of methylene blue upon enzyme-mediated processes, such as inhibition of nitric oxide synthase, with possible generation of superoxide anions, are a factor in the process.

5. Summary of Data Reported

5.1 Exposure data

Methylene blue is a synthetic chemical dye. Methylene blue has a variety of medical uses, including use as an antidote to methaemoglobin-aemia induced by environmental poisons such as excessive nitrate in well-water or cyanide compounds. Other indications include treatment of psychiatric disorders. Recent studies have investigated its use in Alzheimer disease and therapy for malaria. Other uses include staining in bacteriology, and uses as a redox colorimetric agent, as a contrast agent in medical procedures, as a dye, or as a disinfectant. Occupational exposure has been documented. Overall, data on exposure are limited, but substantial sales have been reported in the USA and Brazil.

5.2 Human carcinogenicity data

No data were available to the Working Group.

5.3 Animal carcinogenicity data

Methylene blue was tested for carcinogenicity in one study in mice treated by gavage for 2 years, and one study in rats treated by gavage for 2 years.

In the study in mice, methylene blue caused a significant positive trend in the incidence of carcinoma, and of adenoma or carcinoma (combined), of the small intestine in males. In males, a significant positive trend and a significant increase in the incidence of bronchiolo-alveolar carcinoma of the lung at the highest dose were considered not to be related to treatment. Treatment with methylene blue caused the incidence of malignant lymphoma in females to increase with a significant positive trend, but all incidences were well within the range for historical controls.

In the study in rats treated by gavage, methylene blue caused a significant increase in the incidence of pancreatic islet cell adenoma in males at the intermediate dose. The incidence of pancreatic islet cell adenoma or carcinoma (combined) in males at the intermediate dose was significantly increased only as the result of the increased incidence of adenoma; the incidence of carcinoma was within the range for historical controls. No significant increase in the incidence of any neoplasm was observed in females.

5.4 Mechanistic and other relevant data

Methylene blue is well absorbed, reduced, and is excreted largely in the urine as the reduced form, leucomethylene blue.

Methylene blue and its *N*-demethylated metabolites, azure A, azure B, and azure C, have given positive results in an extensive series of standard in-vitro assays for genotoxicity, both in the absence and presence of exogenous metabolic activation.

At high doses, methylene blue oxidizes ferrous iron in haemoglobin to the ferric state, producing methaemoglobin. Exposure to methylene blue results in haematological toxicity, including formation of Heinz bodies and haemolytic anaemia, in several species.

Photoactivation of methylene blue produces high-energy species that have the potential to damage DNA, proteins, and lipids, either directly or through the production of reactive oxygen species. In the absence of light activation, the carcinogenicity of methylene blue is likely to arise from other mechanisms. A potential mechanism is the inhibition of nitric oxide synthase, with possible generation of superoxide anions.

6. Evaluation

6.1 Cancer in humans

No data were available to the Working Group.

6.2 Cancer in experimental animals

There is *limited evidence* for the carcinogenicity of methylene blue in experimental animals.

6.3 Overall evaluation

Methylene blue is *not classifiable as to its carcinogenicity in humans (Group 3)*.

References

Aeschlimann C, Cerny T, Küpfer A (1996). Inhibition of (mono)amine oxidase activity and prevention of ifosfamide encephalopathy by methylene blue. *Drug Metab Dispos*, 24:1336–1339. PMID:8971139

ATSDR (1992). Toxicological profile for nitrophenols. Atlanta (GA): Agency for Toxic Substances and Disease Registry, United States Public Health Service.

Au W, Hsu TC (1979). Studies on the clastogenic effects of biologic stains and dyes. *Environ Mutagen*, 1:27–35. doi:10.1002/em.2860010109 PMID:95447

Auerbach SS, Bristol DW, Peckham JC *et al.* (2010). Toxicity and carcinogenicity studies of methylene blue trihydrate in F344N rats and B6C3F1 mice. *Food Chem Toxicol*, 48:169–177. doi:10.1016/j.fct.2009.09.034 PMID:19804809

Belaz-David N, Decosterd LA, Appenzeller M *et al.* (1997). Spectrophotometric determination of methylene blue in biological fluids after ion-pair extraction and evidence of its adsorption on plastic polymers. *Eur J Pharm Sci*, 5:335–345. doi:10.1016/S0928-0987(97)00061-4

Berneth H (2008). Azine dyes. In: Ullmann's Encyclopedia of Industrial Chemistry. Weinheim, Germany: Wiley-VCH Verlag GmbH & Co. KGaA, pp. 475–514. doi:10.1002/14356007.a03_213.pub3.

Bilgin H, Özcan B, Bilgin T (1998). Methemoglobinemia induced by methylene blue pertubation during laparoscopy. *Acta Anaesthesiol Scand*, 42:594–595. doi:10.1111/j.1399-6576.1998.tb05173.x PMID:9605379

Borwitzky H, Haefeli WE, Burhenne J (2005). Analysis of methylene blue in human urine by capillary electrophoresis. *J Chromatogr B Analyt Technol Biomed Life Sci*, 826:244–251. doi:10.1016/j.jchromb.2005.09.013 PMID:16182616

Bountogo M, Zoungrana A, Coulibaly B *et al.* (2010). Efficacy of methylene blue monotherapy in semi-immune adults with uncomplicated falciparum malaria: a controlled trial in Burkina Faso. *Trop Med Int Health*, 15:713–717. doi:10.1111/j.1365-3156.2010.02526.x PMID:20374561

Bradberry SM, Aw T-C, Williams NR, Vale JA (2001). Occupational methaemoglobinaemia. *Occup Environ Med*, 58:611–615, quiz 616. doi:10.1136/oem.58.9.611 PMID:11511749

Brendel M (1973). Different photodynamic action of proflavine and methylene blue on bacteriophage. II. Mutation induction in extracellularly treated *Serratia* phage kappa. *Mol Gen Genet*, 120:171–180. doi:10.1007/BF00267245 PMID:4568530

British Pharmacopoeia Commission (2005). British Pharmacopoeia 2005. London: Medicines and Healthcare products Regulatory Agency.

Burhenne J, Riedel KD, Rengelshausen J *et al.* (2008). Quantification of cationic anti-malaria agent methylene blue in different human biological matrices using cation exchange chromatography coupled to tandem mass spectrometry. *J Chromatogr B Analyt Technol Biomed Life Sci*, 863:273–282. doi:10.1016/j.jchromb.2008.01.028 PMID:18258499

ChemNet (2013). Methylene blue. Royal Society of Chemistry. Available from: http://chemnet.rsc.org.

Christensen CM, Farrar HC, Kearns GL (1996). Protracted methemoglobinemia after phenazopyridine overdose in an infant. *J Clin Pharmacol*, 36:112–116. doi:10.1002/j.1552-4604.1996.tb04175.x PMID:8852386

Chung KT, Fulk GE, Andrews AW (1981). Mutagenicity testing of some commonly used dyes. *Appl Environ Microbiol*, 42:641–648. PMID:7039509

Clark AM (1953). Mutagenic activity of dyes in *Drosophila melanogaster*. *Am Nat*, 87:295–305. doi:10.1086/281787

Clifton J 2nd, Leikin JB (2003). Methylene blue. *Am J Ther*, 10:289–291. doi:10.1097/00045391-200307000-00009 PMID:12845393

Coulibaly B, Zoungrana A, Mockenhaupt FP *et al.* (2009). Strong gametocytocidal effect of methylene blue-based combination therapy against falciparum malaria: a randomised controlled trial. *PLoS ONE*, 4:e5318 doi:10.1371/journal.pone.0005318 PMID:19415120

Cragan JD (1999). Teratogen update: methylene blue. *Teratology*, 60:42–48. doi:10.1002/(SICI)1096-9926(199907)60:1<42::AID-TERA12>3.0.CO;2-Z PMID:10413340

Davies J, Burke D, Olliver JR *et al.* (2007). Methylene blue but not indigo carmine causes DNA damage to colonocytes *in vitro* and *in vivo* at concentrations used in clinical chromoendoscopy. *Gut*, 56:155–156. doi:10.1136/gut.2006.107300 PMID:17172595

DiSanto AR, Wagner JG (1972). Pharmacokinetics of highly ionized drugs. I. Methylene blue–whole blood, urine, and tissue assays. *J Pharm Sci*, 61(4):598–602. doi:10.1002/jps.2600610422 PMID:5014319

DiSanto AR, Wagner JG (1972a). Pharmacokinetics of highly ionized drugs. II. Methylene blue–absorption, metabolism, and excretion in man and dog after oral administration. *J Pharm Sci*, 61:1086–1090. doi:10.1002/jps.2600610710 PMID:5044807

DiSanto AR, Wagner JG (1972b). Pharmacokinetics of highly ionized drugs. I. Methylene blue–whole blood, urine, and tissue assays. *J Pharm Sci*, 61:598–602. doi:10.1002/jps.2600610422 PMID:5014319

DiSanto AR, Wagner JG (1972c). Pharmacokinetics of highly ionized drugs. III. Methylene blue–blood levels in the dog and tissue levels in the rat following intravenous administration. *J Pharm Sci*, 61:1090–1094. doi:10.1002/jps.2600610711 PMID:5044808

EDQM (2008). Methylthionimium chloride. In: European Pharmacopoeia. Strasbourg, France: European Directorate for the Quality of Medicines & HealthCare.

Ehrlich P (1881). Ueber das Methylenblau und seine klinisch-bakterioskopische Verwerthung. *Z Klin Med*, 2:710–713. [German]

Epe B, Hegler J, Wild D (1989). Singlet oxygen as an ultimately reactive species in *Salmonella typhimurium* DNA damage induced by methylene blue/visible light. *Carcinogenesis*, 10:2019–2024. doi:10.1093/carcin/10.11.2019 PMID:2680144

Epe B, Mützel P, Adam W (1988). DNA damage by oxygen radicals and excited state species: a comparative study using enzymatic probes *in vitro*. *Chem Biol Interact*, 67:149–165. doi:10.1016/0009-2797(88)90094-4 PMID:2844422

Epe B, Pflaum M, Boiteux S (1993). DNA damage induced by photosensitizers in cellular and cell-free systems. *Mutat Res*, 299:135–145. doi:10.1016/0165-1218(93)90091-Q PMID:7683082

Eroğlu L, Cağlayan B (1997). Anxiolytic and antidepressant properties of methylene blue in animal models. *Pharmacol Res*, 36:381–385. doi:10.1006/phrs.1997.0245 PMID:9441729

FDA (2011). Drug Safety Communication: Serious CNS reactions possible when methylene blue is given to patients taking certain psychiatric medications. Safety announcement dated 26 July 2011. Silver Spring (MD): United States Food and Drug Administration. Available from: http://www.fda.gov/Drugs/DrugSafety/ucm263190.htm, accessed 1 October 2014.

Gaudette NF, Lodge JW (2005). Determination of methylene blue and leucomethylene blue in male and female Fischer 344 rat urine and B6C3F$_1$ mouse urine. *J Anal Toxicol*, 29:28–33. doi:10.1093/jat/29.1.28 PMID:15808010

Gutter B, Speck WT, Rosenkranz HS (1977). A study of the photoinduced mutagenicity of methylene blue. *Mutat Res*, 44:177–181. doi:10.1016/0027-5107(77)90075-6 PMID:331101

Guttmann P, Ehrlich P (1891). Ueber die Wirkung des Methylenblau bei Malaria. *Berl Klin Wochenschr*, 28:953–956. [German]

Hejtmancik MR, Ryan MJ, Toft JD *et al.* (2002). Hematological effects in F344 rats and B6C3F$_1$ mice during the 13-week gavage toxicity study of methylene blue trihydrate. *Toxicol Sci*, 65:126–134. doi:10.1093/toxsci/65.1.126 PMID:11752692

Horváthová E, Kozics K, Srančíková A *et al.* (2012). Borneol administration protects primary rat hepatocytes against exogenous oxidative DNA damage. *Mutagenesis*, 27:581–588. doi:10.1093/mutage/ges023 PMID:22544524

IMS Health (2012). Multinational Integrated Data Analysis (MIDAS). IMS Health, Plymouth Meeting, 2012, Pennsylvania, USA.

Ito T, Kobayashi K (1977). A survey of *in vivo* photodynamic activity of xanthenes, thiazines, and acridines in yeast cells. *Photochem Photobiol*, 26:581–587. doi:10.1111/j.1751-1097.1977.tb07536.x

Kasuga Y, Hishida M, Tanahashi N (1991). Simultaneous determination of malachite green and methylene blue in cultured fishes by high performance liquid chromatography. *Shokuhin Eiseigaku Zasshi*, 32:137–141. doi:10.3358/shokueishi.32.137

Kimoto K, Gohda R, Murayama K *et al.* (1996). Sensitive detection of near-infrared fluorescent dyes using high-performance liquid chromatography with peroxyoxalate chemiluminescence detection system. *Biomed Chromatogr*, 10:189–190. doi:10.1002/(SICI)1099-0801(199607)10:4<189::AID-BMC585>3.0.CO;2-P PMID:8831965

Knowles A, Gurnani S (1972). A study of the methylene blue-sensitized oxidation of amino acids. *Photochem Photobiol*, 16:95–108. doi:10.1111/j.1751-1097.1972.tb07341.x PMID:5052681

Kosswig K (2000). Surfactants. In: Ullmann's Encyclopedia of Industrial Chemistry. Weinheim, Germany: Wiley-VCH Verlag GmbH & Co. KGaA, pp. 487–505. doi:10.1002/14356007.a25_747

Kozaki A, Watanabe J (1981). Dose dependency of apparent volumes of distribution for methylene blue in rabbits. *J Pharmacobiodyn*, 4:49–57. doi:10.1248/bpb1978.4.49 PMID:7277192

Laassis B, Aaron J-J, Mahedero MC (1994). Fluorimetric determination of phenothiazine derivatives by photooxidation in a flow-injection system. *Talanta*, 41:1985–1989. doi:10.1016/0039-9140(94)00162-6 PMID:18966160

Lábaj J, Slamenová D, Lazarová M, Kosíková B (2007). Induction of DNA-lesions in freshly isolated rat hepatocytes by different genotoxins and their reduction by lignin given either as a dietary component or in *in vitro* conditions. *Nutr Cancer*, 57:209–215. doi:10.1080/01635580701277643 PMID:17571955

Lee CH, Chang CT, Wetmur JG (1973). Induced circular dichroism of DNA-dye complexes. *Biopolymers*, 12:1099–1122. doi:10.1002/bip.1973.360120514 PMID:4710250

Lunn G, Sansone EB (1991). Decontamination of aqueous solutions of biological stains. *Biotech Histochem*, 66:307–315. doi:10.3109/10520299109109992 PMID:1725856

MacRae WD, Chan GF, Wat CK *et al.* (1980). Examination of naturally occurring polyacetylenes and alpha-terthienyl for their ability to induce cytogenetic damage. *Experientia*, 36:1096–1097. doi:10.1007/BF01965990 PMID:7418849

Masannat YA, Hanby A, Horgan K, Hardie LJ (2009). DNA damaging effects of the dyes used in sentinel node biopsy: possible implications for clinical practice. *J Surg Res*, 154:234–238. doi:10.1016/j.jss.2008.07.039 PMID:19181339

McBride TJ, Schneider JE, Floyd RA, Loeb LA (1992). Mutations induced by methylene blue plus light in single-stranded M13mp2. *Proc Natl Acad Sci USA*, 89:6866–6870. doi:10.1073/pnas.89.15.6866 PMID:1495976

McCarroll NE, Piper CE, Keech BH (1981). An E. coli microsuspension assay for the detection of DNA damage induced by direct-acting agents and promutagens. *Environ Mutagen*, 3:429–444. doi:10.1002/em.2860030404 PMID:7021147

Medscape (2013). Methylene blue (Rx). Dosing and uses. Available from: http://reference.medscape.com/drug/methylene-blue-343739, accessed 5 June 2013.

Mohn GR, Kerklaan PR, van Zeeland AA *et al.* (1984). Methodologies for the determination of various genetic effects in permeable strains of *E. coli* K-12 differing in DNA repair capacity. Quantification of DNA adduct formation, experiments with organ homogenates and hepatocytes, and animal-mediated assays. *Mutat Res*, 125:153–184. doi:10.1016/0027-5107(84)90067-8 PMID:6230533

Moura JC, Cordeiro N (2003). 3,7-*Bis*(dialkylamino) phenothiazin-5-ium derivatives: biomedical applications and biological activity. *Curr Drug Targets*, 4:133–141. doi:10.2174/1389450033346902 PMID:12558066

Munns RK, Holland DC, Roybal JE *et al.* (1992). Liquid chromatographic determination of methylene blue and its metabolites in milk. *J AOAC Int*, 75:796–800.

Naylor GJ, Martin B, Hopwood SE, Watson Y (1986). A two-year double-blind crossover trial of the prophylactic effect of methylene blue in manic-depressive psychosis. *Biol Psychiatry*, 21:915–920. doi:10.1016/0006-3223(86)90265-9 PMID:3091097

Nordén B, Tjerneld F (1982). Structure of methylene blue-DNA complexes studied by linear and circular dichroism spectroscopy. *Biopolymers*, 21:1713–1734. doi:10.1002/bip.360210904 PMID:7126754

NTP (2008). Toxicology and carcinogenesis studies of methylene blue trihydrate (Cas No. 7220–79–3) in F344/N rats and B6C3F1 mice (gavage studies). *Natl Toxicol Program Tech Rep Ser*, 540:1–224. PMID:18685714

O'Neil MJ, Heckelman PE, Koch CB et al. (2006). The Merck Index: an encyclopedia of chemicals, drugs, and biologicals, 14th Edition (Version 14.6). Whitehouse Station (NJ): Merck & Co., Inc.

Olliver JR, Wild CP, Sahay P *et al.* (2003). Chromoendoscopy with methylene blue and associated DNA damage in Barrett's oesophagus. *Lancet*, 362:373–374. doi:10.1016/S0140-6736(03)14026-3 PMID:12907012

Onur F, Acar N (1992). Simultaneous determination of methylene blue, hexamethylene tetramine and resorcinol in pharmaceutical formulations by first-derivative UV spectrophotometry. *Int J Pharm*, 78:89–91. doi:10.1016/0378-5173(92)90359-A

Oz M, Lorke DE, Hasan M, Petroianu GA (2011). Cellular and molecular actions of Methylene Blue in the nervous system. *Med Res Rev*, 31:93–117. doi:10.1002/med.20177 PMID:19760660

Oz M, Lorke DE, Petroianu GA (2009). Methylene blue and Alzheimer's disease. *Biochem Pharmacol*, 78:927–932. doi:10.1016/j.bcp.2009.04.034 PMID:19433072

Peter C, Hongwan D, Küpfer A, Lauterburg BH (2000). Pharmacokinetics and organ distribution of intravenous and oral methylene blue. *Eur J Clin*

Pharmacol, 56:247–250. doi:10.1007/s002280000124 PMID:10952480

Petzer A, Harvey BH, Wegener G, Petzer JP (2012). Azure B, a metabolite of methylene blue, is a high-potency, reversible inhibitor of monoamine oxidase. *Toxicol Appl Pharmacol*, 258:403–409. doi:10.1016/j.taap.2011.12.005 PMID:22197611

Popescu NC, Turnbull D, DiPaolo JA (1977). Sister chromatid exchange and chromosome aberration analysis with the use of several carcinogens and noncarcinogens. *J Natl Cancer Inst*, 59:289–293. PMID:406414

Porat R, Gilbert S, Magilner D (1996). Methylene blue-induced phototoxicity: an unrecognized complication. *Pediatrics*, 97:717–721. PMID:8628613

Pruthi S, Haakenson C, Brost BC *et al.* (2011). Pharmacokinetics of methylene blue dye for lymphatic mapping in breast cancer-implications for use in pregnancy. *Am J Surg*, 201:70–75. doi:10.1016/j.amjsurg.2009.03.013 PMID:21167367

PubChem (2013). Methylene blue. Pubchem database. National Center for Biotechnology Information. Available from: https://pubchem.ncbi.nlm.nih.gov/ [online database].

Rager T, Geoffroy A´, Hilfiker R, Storey JMD (2012). The crystalline state of methylene blue: a zoo of hydrates. *Phys Chem Chem Phys*, 14:8074–8082. doi:10.1039/c2cp40128b PMID:22481217

Ramsay RR, Dunford C, Gillman PK (2007). Methylene blue and serotonin toxicity: inhibition of monoamine oxidase A (MAO A) confirms a theoretical prediction. *Br J Pharmacol*, 152:946–951. doi:10.1038/sj.bjp.0707430 PMID:17721552

Rengelshausen J, Burhenne J, Fröhlich M *et al.* (2004). Pharmacokinetic interaction of chloroquine and methylene blue combination against malaria. *Eur J Clin Pharmacol*, 60:709–715. doi:10.1007/s00228-004-0818-0 PMID:15619134

Rentsch G, Wittekind D (1967). Methylene blue and erythrocytes in the living animal. Contribution to the toxicology of methylene blue and formation of Heinz bodies. *Toxicol Appl Pharmacol*, 11:81–87. doi:10.1016/0041-008X(67)90029-4 PMID:6056158

Roybal JE, Munns RK, Hurlbut JA, Shimoda W (1989). High-performance liquid chromatography of gentian violet, its demethylated metabolites, leucogentian violet and methylene blue with electrochemical detection. *J Chromatogr*, 467:259–266. doi:10.1016/S0021-9673(01)93970-6 PMID:2753937

Roybal JE, Pfenning AP, Turnipseed SB et al. (1996). Dye residues in foods of animal origin. ACS Symposium Series, 636: 169–184. doi:10.1021/bk-1996-0636-ch018

Sabnis RW, Ross E, Köthe J et al. (2009). Indicator reagents. In: Ullmann's Encyclopedia of Industrial Chemistry. Weinheim, Germany: Wiley-VCH Verlag GmbH & Co. KGaA, pp. 9–53. doi:10.1002/14356007.a14_127.pub2

Schirmer RH, Adler H, Pickhardt M, Mandelkow E (2011). "Lest we forget you - methylene blue…" *Neurobiol Aging*, 32:2325.e7–2325.e16. doi:10.1016/j.neurobiolaging.2010.12.012 PMID:21316815

Sills MR, Zinkham WH (1994). Methylene blue-induced Heinz body hemolytic anemia *Arch Pediatr Adolesc Med*, 148:306–310. doi:10.1001/archpedi.1994.02170030076017 PMID:8130867

Smijs TG, Nivard MJ, Schuitmaker HJ (2004). Development of a test system for mutagenicity of photosensitizers using *Drosophila melanogaster*. *Photochem Photobiol*, 79:332–338. doi:10.1562/2003-12-03-RA.1 PMID:15137509

Smith RP, Thron CD (1972). Hemoglobin, methylene blue and oxygen interactions in human red cells. *J Pharmacol Exp Ther*, 183:549–558. PMID:4636392

Speit G (1982). Intercalating substances do not induce sister-chromatid exchanges (SCEs) *in vivo*. *Mutat Res*, 104:261–266. doi:10.1016/0165-7992(82)90154-3 PMID:7110164

Speit G, Vogel W (1979). The effect on sister-chromatid exchanges of drugs and dyes by intercalation and photoactivation. *Mutat Res*, 59:223–229. doi:10.1016/0027-5107(79)90161-1 PMID:35743

Sturmey RG, Wild CP, Hardie LJ (2009). Removal of red light minimizes methylene blue-stimulated DNA damage in oesophageal cells: implications for chromoendoscopy. *Mutagenesis*, 24:253–258. doi:10.1093/mutage/gep004 PMID:19218330

Tarbin JA, Chan D, Stubbings G, Sharman M (2008). Multiresidue determination of triarylmethane and phenothiazine dyes in fish tissues by LC-MS/MS. *Anal Chim Acta*, 625:188–194. doi:10.1016/j.aca.2008.07.018 PMID:18724993

Tardivo JP, Del Giglio A, de Oliveira CS, Gabrielli DS, Junqueira HC, Tada DB *et al.* (2005). Methylene blue in photodynamic therapy: From basic mechanisms to clinical applications. *Photodiagn Photodyn Ther*, 2(3):175–91. doi:10.1016/S1572-1000(05)00097-9 PMID:25048768

Tuite MF, Mundy CR, Cox BS (1981). Agents that cause a high frequency of genetic change from [*psi*+] to [*psi*-] in Saccharomyces cerevisiae. *Genetics*, 98:691–711. PMID:7037537

US Pharmacopeial Convention (2013). *Methylene blue. United States* Pharmacopeia,*USP36*. Rockville (MD): The United States Pharmacopeial Convention.

Villanueva A, Cañete M, Trigueros C *et al.* (1993). Photodynamic induction of DNA-protein cross-linking in solution by several sensitizers and visible light. *Biopolymers*, 33:239–244. doi:10.1002/bip.360330206 PMID:8485298

Walter-Sack I, Rengelshausen J, Oberwittler H, Burhenne J, Mueller O, Meissner P *et al.* (2009). High absolute bioavailability of methylene blue given as an aqueous oral formulation. *Eur J Clin Pharmacol*, 65(2):179–89. doi:10.1007/s00228-008-0563-x PMID:18810398

Warth A, Goeppert B, Bopp C *et al.* (2009). Turquoise to dark green organs at autopsy. *Virchows Arch*, 454:341–344. doi:10.1007/s00428-009-0734-x PMID:19189125

Webb RB, Hass BS (1984). Biological effects of dyes on bacteria. VI. Mutation induction by acridine orange and methylene blue in the dark with special reference to *Escherichia coli* WP6 (*polA1*). *Mutat Res*, 137:1–6. doi:10.1016/0165-1218(84)90105-8 PMID:6379434

WHO (2011). The International Pharmacopoeia, Fourth Edition. Geneva, Switzerland: World Health Organization. Available from: http://apps.who.int/phint/en/p/about/.

Xu JZ, Dai L, Wu B *et al.* (2009). Determination of methylene blue residues in aquatic products by liquid chromatography-tandem mass spectrometry. *J Sep Sci*, 32::4193–4199. doi:10.1002/jssc.200900364 PMID:20066681

Yamaguchi T (1981). Mutagenicity of low Molecular substances in various superoxide generating systems. *Agric Biol Chem*, 45:327–330. doi:10.1271/bbb1961.45.327

Yang F, Xia S, Liu Z *et al.* (2011). Analysis of methylene blue and its metabolites in blood by capillary electrophoresis/electrospray ionization mass spectrometry. *Electrophoresis*, 32:659–664. doi:10.1002/elps.201000514 PMID:21328395

Ziv G, Heavner JE (1984). Permeability of the blood-milk barrier to methylene blue in cows and goats. *J Vet Pharmacol Ther*, 7:55–59. doi:10.1111/j.1365-2885.1984.tb00879.x PMID:6708167

Zoungrana A, Coulibaly B, Sié A *et al.* (2008). Safety and efficacy of methylene blue combined with artesunate or amodiaquine for uncomplicated falciparum malaria: a randomized controlled trial from Burkina Faso. *PLoS ONE*, 3:e1630 doi:10.1371/journal.pone.0001630 PMID:18286187

PRIMIDONE

1. Exposure Data

1.1 Identification of the agent

1.1.1 Nomenclature

Chem. Abstr. Serv. Reg. No.: 125-33-7 (O'Neil, 2006)

Chem. Abstr. Serv. Name: 4,6(1*H*,5*H*)-Pyrimidinedione, 5-ethyldihydro-5-phenyl- (O'Neil, 2006; US Pharmacopeia, 2007)

IUPAC Systematic Name: 5-Ethyl-5-phenyl-1,3-diazinane-4,6-dione (DrugBank, 2013)

Synonym: 2-Deoxyphenobarbital

See WHO (2007) for names in other languages.

1.1.2 Structural and molecular formulae and relative molecular mass

$C_{12}H_{14}N_2O_2$
Relative molecular mass: 218.25

1.1.3 Chemical and physical properties of the pure substance

Description: White or almost white, crystalline powder (European Pharmacopoeia, 2008); white crystalline powder, odourless, very slight bitter taste, with no acidic properties (Japanese Pharmacopoeia, 2007; US Pharmacopeia, 2009)

Density: 1.138 ± 0.06 g/cm³ (predicted) (SciFinder, 2013)

Melting-point: 279–284 °C (Japanese Pharmacopoeia, 2007; US Pharmacopeia, 2007); 281–282 °C (O'Neil, 2006)

Spectroscopy Data: Data from infrared spectroscopy have been reported (Daley, 1973)

Solubility: Very slightly soluble in water, slightly soluble in ethanol (96%). It dissolves in alkaline solution (O'Neil, 2006; European Pharmacopoeia, 2008; US Pharmacopeia, 2009); soluble to 100 mM in dimethylsulfoxide (Tocris, 2013); soluble in dimethylformamide, sparingly soluble in pyridine, and practically insoluble in diethyl ether (Japanese Pharmacopoeia, 2007)

Stability data: Stable; finished product has shelf-life of 5 years (US Pharmacopeia, 2009; MHRA, 2013)

Octanol/water partition coefficient (log P): 0.91 (US Pharmacopeia, 2009)

1.1.4 Technical products and impurities

(a)   Trade names

Mysoline; Cyral; Liskantin; Majsolin; Midone; Mylepsinum; Mysedon; Primoline; Primron; Prysoline; Resimatil; Sertan (NTP, 2000; O'Neil, 2006)

(b)   Specified impurities and enantiomer

Several impurities have been detected in the technical product (European Pharmacopoeia, 2008), including:

- R1 = NH$_2$, R2 = CO-NH$_2$: 2-ethyl-2-phenyl-propanediamide (ethylphenylmalonamide)
- R1 = NH$_2$, R2 = H: (2RS)-2-phenylbutanamide
- R1 = NH$_2$, R2 = CN: (2RS)-2-cyano-2-phenylbutanamide
- R1 = OH, R2 = H: (2RS)-2-phenylbutanoic acid
- Phenobarbital
- 5-Ethyl-5-phenyl-2-[(1RS)-1-phenylpropyl] dihydropyrimidine-4,6(1H,5H)-dione

1.2   Analysis

Selected compendial and noncompendial methods are presented in Table 1.1. Primidone can be quantitatively determined using ultraviolet spectroscopy, liquid chromatography using ultraviolet detection, and gas chromatography using flame ionization detection.

Primidone can be analysed in human plasma by extraction followed by protein precipitation, centrifugation and finally subjecting to ultra-performance liquid chromatography with electrospray ionization mass spectrometry, with a limit of detection of < 0.05 mg/mL (Kuhn & Knabbe, 2013).

The physical properties of the substance (spectroscopy, melting point) are used for the identification of the substance.

1.3   Production and use

1.3.1 Production and consumption volume

The synthetic dug primidone is not used frequently, with around 250 000 uses in the USA per year in 2005–2012 mentioned by office-based physicians in visits with patients. Based on the same source, approximately 80 000 patients in the USA were exposed to primidone in 2012 (IMS Health, 2012a). According to the National Prescription Audit Plus (IMS Health, 2012b), there were a total of 1.5 million prescriptions for primidone dispensed in the USA in 2012, similar to the 1.4 million prescriptions dispensed in 2008. [The Working Group recognized that these prescription figures were larger than expected based on the drug uses reported by office-based physicians.]

Total worldwide sales of primidone in 2012 were US$ 41 million (IMS Health, 2012c), with 60% occurring in the USA. The only other country with appreciable use was Germany, with sales of US$ 3 million.

1.3.2 Use

(a)   Indications

Primidone is an anticonvulsant that metabolizes to phenobarbital and phenylethylmalonamide. All three compounds are thought to be biologically active. Primidone is used in the treatment of a range of conditions, including seizure disorders, tremor, neuropathic pain, trigeminal neuralgia, tinnitus, and migraine headache. Its use for seizure disorders has declined substantially with a shift to newer medications with

Table 1.1 Analytical methods for primidone

Sample matrix	Sample preparation	Assay method	Detection limit	Reference
Compendial methods				
Assay	–	UV-visible Wavelength: 257 nm	–	European Pharmacopoeia (2008)
Assay	–	UV-visible Wavelength: minima 254 nm, 261 nm, and maxima 257 nm	–	US Pharmacopeia (2013)
Assay (tablet and suspension)	–	GC Column: glass column packed with acid-washed, silanized diatomaceous support coated with phenyl methyl silicone fluid	–	British Pharmacopoeia (2013)
Assay (tablet and suspension)	–	GC Column: 10% liquid phase G3 on support S1AB Flow rate: 40 mL/min	–	US Pharmacopeia (2013)
Non-compendial methods				
Human plasma or serum	Protein precipitation, vortex-mixing, centrifugation, analysis of clear organic supernatant	UPLC-ESI-MS-MS Column: C_{18} Mobile phase: solvent A, 0.1% formic acid in water containing 2 mmol/L ammonium acetate; and solvent B, 0.1% formic acid in methanol containing 2 mmol/L ammonium acetate Flow rate: 0.5 mL/min MRM: 219.0 *m/z* reducing to 162.0 *m/z*	< 0.05 mg/L	Kuhn & Knabbe (2013)
Human serum	Centrifugation, supernatant injected onto the anti-primidone column, washing with methanol and water, elution with methanol and acetic acid, evaporation, sonication	MIP-ESI-MS Needle voltage: 11.40 kV Target electrode voltage: 9.00 kV Liquid flow rate: 6 µL/min Drift field: 600 V/cm Desolvation field: 600 V/cm Drift gas flow (N_2): 500 mL/min Desolvation gas flow (N_2): 900 mL/min Drift tube length: 11 cm Shutter grid pulse: 0.3 ms	0.0051 µg/mL	Rezaei *et al.* (2009)
Human plasma	Extraction by a liquid-liquid extraction system, vortex mixing and centrifugation, organic layer evaporated, reconstituted with methanol in water for injection on to the MECC system	MECC Capillary: fused-silica Wavelength: 210 and 285 nm Buffer: 10 mM monobasic sodium phosphate, with 6 mM tetraborate, and 75 mM SDS pH 9.0	0.7 µg/mL	Lanças *et al.* (2003)

Table 1.1 (continued)

Sample matrix	Sample preparation	Assay method	Detection limit	Reference
Tablet	Nitration of primidone with sulfuric-nitric acid mixture to form 3-nitrophenyl derivative	Polarography Electrode: dropping mercury electrode	Observed half-wave potential was −0.17 V vs the saturated calomel electrode	Daley (1973)
Human serum	Acidified and extracted with $CHCl_3$ and isopropanol (70 : 30)	LC-UV Column: C_{18} Mobile phase: acetonitrile and water (12 : 88)	50–1000 ng/mL (LOQ)	Sato *et al.* (1986)
Tablet	Dissolved in DMSO-d_6 using maleic acid as internal standard	Proton NMR	Chemical shift value: primidone, 7.53 ppm; and maleic acid, 6.50 ppm	Özden *et al.* (1989)
Serum or plasma	Serum or plasma + anticoagulants, centrifugation	Immunoassay The enzyme activity is determined spectrophotometrically at 340 nm	0.5 µg/mL	Thermoscientific (2004)
Rat urine	Extraction by LRC column	LC-UV Column: C_{18} Mobile phase: 0.01 M potassium phosphate buffer, methanol and acetonitrile (270 : 30 : 30) pH: 4.0 Flow rate: 1.0 mL/min Wavelength: 227 nm	0.5 mg/mL	Ferranti *et al.* (1998)
Rat plasma	Solid phase extraction Bond-Elut C-18 cartridge column	LC-UV Column: C_{18} Mobile phase: acetonitrile and 0.01 M KH_2PO_4 (25 : 75) Flow rate: 0.8 mL/min Wavelength: 210 nm	0.1 µg/mL	Moriyama *et al.* (1994)

DMSO, dimethylsulfoxide; GC, gas chromatography; LC, liquid chromatography; LOQ, limit of quantitation; LRC, large reserve capacity; MECC, micellar electrokinetic capillary chromatography; MIP-ESI-IMS, molecular imprinted polymer electrospray ionization ion mobility spectrometry; MRM, multiple reaction monitoring; NMR, nuclear magnetic resonance; SDS, sodium dodecyl sulfate; UPLC-ESI-MS-MS, ultra-performance liquid chromatography with electrospray ionization and tandem mass spectrometry; UV, ultraviolet spectroscopy; vs, versus

Table 1.2 Most commonly reported clinical indications for primidone in the USA, 2011–2012

Diagnosis	ICD-9 code[a]	Drug uses (in thousands)	Percentage of total
Benign essential tremor	333.101	263	52.5
Tremor, NOS	781.005	139	27.8
Convulsion, NOS	780.301	39	7.8
Familial tremor	333.102	14	2.8
Parkinson disease	332.005	9	1.7
Migraine, NOS	346.903	7	1.5
All other diagnoses	–	28	5.8
Total with reported diagnoses	–	502	100.0

[a] The ICD-9 code listed is a more detailed, proprietary version developed by IMS Health

NOS, not otherwise specified

From IMS Health (2012a)

fewer adverse effects, fewer drug interactions, and less potential for addiction and abuse. Once a key medication in the management of seizure disorders, primidone is now considered at best a third-line medication for partial and tonic-clonic seizures (MicroMedex, 2013).

In the USA, primidone is currently labelled for use as a treatment for epilepsy in children and adults, either alone or as an adjunct to other anticonvulsants (FDA, 2013; MicroMedex, 2013). Most prescriptions in the USA are for off-label indications (Table 1.2).

Primidone is used relatively infrequently as anticonvulsant, accounting for 0.4% of all medications reported as therapies for seizure disorders (whether alone or in combination with other agents) (IMS Health, 2012a). There are numerous other anticonvulsants with overlapping clinical indications that have largely replaced primidone, even in cases of non-responsiveness to multiple medications. In contrast, there are few comparatively effective treatments for essential tremor (Zesiewicz *et al.*, 2011). As a result, primidone comprises the largest fraction (35%) of all medications reported as therapies for essential tremor (IMS Health, 2012a).

In the European Union, primidone is indicated for essential tremor, and in the management of grand mal and psychomotor (temporal lobe) epilepsy (eMC, 2013).

[Given its use for chronic conditions, primidone therapy would be expected to be long-term in the absence of short- or long-term adverse effects.]

(b) Dosage

Primidone is available in tablets of 50 mg and 250 mg, with a tablet of 125 mg and an oral suspension formulation being available in some countries (MicroMedex, 2013; eMC, 2013). Therapy is initiated at lower doses and then increased, although lower doses may be taken when primidone is employed as an adjunct (MicroMedex, 2013). There is a wide range of dosing regimens, varying from 50 mg once per day to 500 mg twice per day; 50 mg once or twice daily are the most common regimens, each representing 21% of all uses. The mean daily dosage for primidone is 183 mg per day (IMS Health, 2012a).

1.4 Occurrence and exposure

Primidone has been reported in groundwater, spring water and well-water (Morasch, 2013). Primidone, and its metabolite phenobarbital, were detected in groundwater within the catchment area of a drinking-water treatment plant located downstream of a former sewage farm in Berlin, Germany. The age of shallow groundwater samples ranged from years to a decade, whereas the age of groundwater was up to four decades. Concentrations of the compounds in groundwater increased with age. This indicated a strong persistence of these compounds in the environment under anoxic aquifer conditions (Hass *et al.*, 2012).

Human exposure is largely limited to use as a medication. Workers in pharmaceutical manufacturing plants may be exposed, but no specific data were available to the Working Group.

1.5 Regulations and guidelines

Primidone has been widely approved by drug regulatory agencies. Primidone was approved by the United States Food and Drug Administration in 1954 (FDA, 2013).

There were no extraordinary regulatory restrictions on use. Primidone was listed in 1999 as a "chemical known to the State to cause cancer" by the Office of Environmental Health Hazard Assessment of the State of California, requiring public notice of potential environmental exposures (OEHHA, 2013). The basis of this listing was an evaluation by the United States National Toxicology Program (NTP, 2000).

2. Cancer in Humans

Primidone has been used to treat grand seizures in epilepsy patients. Elevated risks of several types of cancers, mainly tumours of the brain and central nervous system, lymphoma, myeloma, and cancers of the lung, liver, pancreas, and gastrointestinal tract have been seen in some but not all studies of epilepsy patients, suggesting that epilepsy and long-term use of anti-epileptic drugs may be risk factors for cancer (Lamminpää *et al.*, 2002; Olsen *et al.*, 1989). The evaluation of causality was complicated because epileptic seizures can be early symptoms of tumours of the brain, or can prompt clinical examinations, thus

the observed associations between anti-epileptic drugs and cancer may be attributable to detection bias (Adelöw *et al.*, 2006).

Few studies have conducted analysis specific for individual anti-epileptic drugs such as primidone. The epidemiological studies available for evaluating exposure to primidone were limited to two case–control studies nested in a cohort of epileptic patients conducted by Olsen and colleagues in Denmark (Olsen *et al.*, 1993, 1995). The cohort study (Olsen *et al.*, 1989) provided information on the source population for the case–control studies; several anti-epileptic drugs were used in this cohort. A cohort study of offspring of mothers from the Danish cohort, which provided limited information on exposure to primidone, is also briefly discussed (Olsen *et al.*, 1990).

2.1 Cohort studies

A cohort study of patients at the Filadelfia epilepsy treatment community, in Dianalund, Denmark, was the only cohort study to report on incidence of cancer after treatment with primidone (Olsen *et al.*, 1989). The cohort consisted of 8004 patients admitted between 1933 and 1962, who had not died before 1943, and who had hospital stays of 4 weeks or greater and traceable records. Patients were treated primarily with phenobarbital, phenytoin, and primidone (500–1500 mg per day starting in mid-1950). Newer drugs became more common in the 1960s. The cohort was followed for cancer incidence until 1984, with cases identified by linkage to the Danish cancer registry. In the analysis, hospitalization was used as a proxy for drug use, and analyses were not conducted for anti-epileptic drugs, either specifically or as a class. Standardized incidence rates were adjusted for age, sex, and calendar year. Among patients who were not known to have received Thorotrast (a radioactive compound used as a contrast medium for radiology), statistically significant excesses were observed in the incidence of all malignant neoplasms, and cancers of the brain and central nervous system, lung, and secondary and unspecified sites (combined). Non-statistically significant elevations (≥ 20%) were found for non-Hodgkin lymphoma, and cancers of the buccal cavity and pharynx, oesophagus, larynx, liver, biliary tract, thyroid, testes, and unspecified sites. The risk of cancer of the liver or biliary tract increased with increasing time since first admission, while no clear pattern was observed for cancer of the lung. Findings for malignant lymphoma, and cancers of the liver and biliary tract, urinary bladder, and lung were explored in subsequent nested case–control studies. A statistically significant decrease in incidence was observed for cancer of the urinary bladder. [The strengths of this study were adequate follow-up and case ascertainment. The study population consisted mainly of severe cases of epilepsy and thus it was not known whether severity of disease modified the risk of cancer. The major limitation was the lack of information on exposure to specific drugs and potential confounders at an individual level.]

Olsen *et al.* (1990) also conducted a record-linkage study among 3727 offspring of women from the Filadelfia cohort who were alive as of 1968. No increased risk of any malignant cancer was found among 2579 children born after the mother's first hospital admission and presumably exposed to anti-epileptic drugs in utero (relative risk, RR, 1.0; 95% CI, 0.6–1.7). Mothers of 2 of the 14 children with cancer had taken primidone and phenytoin during pregnancy. [Although the size of the cohort was relatively large and case ascertainment and follow-up were adequate, this study was not considered to be informative because the findings were not reported specifically for primidone, and few cancers were observed in the cohort.]

2.2 Nested case–control studies

See Table 2.1

The nested case–control studies on four types of cancer were reported in two publications: cancer of the lung and urinary bladder were reported by Olsen *et al.* (1993), and malignant lymphoma and cancer of the liver and biliary tract were reported by Olsen *et al.* (1995). The studies had similar methodologies and designs. Cancer cases identified in follow-up until 1984 were matched with two controls each from the cohort by sex, birth year, and survival time. Detailed drug information was extracted from medical records: between 23% and 27% of recorded prescriptions were for primidone, but 25% of patients had no records of prescriptions for any anticonvulsive drugs. Smoking information was surveyed among living controls, but not among cases.

Among patients who had ever used primidone, non-statistically elevated relative risks were observed for malignant lymphoma (odds ratio, OR, 1.3; Olsen *et al.*, 1995) and cancers of the lung (OR, 1.3; 95% CI, 0.7–2.3) and urinary bladder (OR, 1.6; 95% CI, 0.4–6.3) (Olsen *et al.*, 1993). The relative risk was close to unity for use of primadone and cancer of the liver and biliary tract (Olsen *et al.*, 1995). Patients exposed to Thorotrast were excluded from the reported analyses of lymphoma and cancer of the liver and biliary tract, while analyses of cancers of the lung and bladder reportedly gave similar results when repeated excluding Thorotrast-exposed patients. [The strengths of these studies were the same as those of the cohort studies. Limitations included incomplete information on exposure to primidone (with respect to duration of use; drug exposure information was collected only during the patient's stay in hospital) and on potential confounders, and small numbers of exposed cases, especially for cancers of the urinary bladder, lymphoma, and liver and biliary tract.]

Table 2.1 Nested case–control studies of cancer and exposure to primidone

Reference Study location, period	Total No. cases Total No. controls	Control source (hospital, population)	Exposure assessment	Organ site (ICD code)	Exposure categories	Exposed cases	Relative risk (95% CI)	Covariates Comments
Olsen et al. (1993) Denmark, 1932–84	104 cases 200 controls 18 cases 33 controls	Nested case–control; cohort of 8004 patients with epilepsy	Medical records from epilepsy centre; smoking information (living controls only) collected via mail survey	Lung Urinary bladder	Ever-exposed Ever-exposed	29 5	1.3 (0.7–2.3) 1.6 (0.4–6.3)	Adjusted for other anticonvulsant treatments Controls matched to cases on sex, yr of birth and survival time; analyses excluding patients given Thorotrast were also conducted; cohort smoked more than the general population
Olsen et al. (1995) Denmark, 1932–84	39 cases 73 controls 21 cases 98 controls	Nested case–control; cohort of 8004 patients with epilepsy	Medical records from epilepsy centre	Liver and biliary tract Malignant lymphoma [non-Hodgkin lymphoma and Hodgkin lymphoma]	Ever-exposed (> 10 g, 40 tablets)	NR NR	0.9 (0.4–2.3) 1.3 (0.3–5.0)	Adjusted for other anticonvulsant treatments Controls matched to cases on sex, year of birth and survival time; analyses excluding patients given Thorotrast were also conducted; cohort smoked more than the general population

NR, not reported; yr, year

Table 3.1 Studies of carcinogenicity in mice and rats given diets containing primidone

Species, strain (sex) Duration Reference	Dosing regimen Animals/group at start	Incidence of tumours	Significance	Comments
Mouse, B6C3F$_1$ (M, F) 104–105 wk NTP (2000)	Dietary concentrations of 0, 300, 600, or 1300 ppm, equivalent to daily doses of 0, 30, 65, or 150 mg/kg bw (M), or 0, 25, 50, or 100 mg/kg bw (F) 50 M and 50 F/group (age, 5–6 wk)	Hepatocellular adenoma: 22/50*, 41/50**, 39/50**, 32/50*** (M) 15/50****, 42/50**, 45/49**, 47/50** (F) Hepatocellular carcinoma: 12/50****, 31/50**, 35/50**, 38/50** (M) 3/50****, 11/50***, 19/49**, 38/50** (F) Hepatoblastoma: 0/50, 17/50**, 26/50**. 7/50***(M) 1/50, 4/50, 4/49, 4/50 (F) Hepatocellular adenoma, hepatocellular carcinoma or hepatoblastoma (combined): 31/50****, 49/50**, 49/50**, 46/50** (M) 16/50****, 42/50**, 46/49**, 50/50** (F) Thyroid follicular cell adenoma: 0/49*, 3/48, 3/50, 6/50*** (M)	*$P \leq 0.05$ (trend) **$P \leq 0.001$ ***$P \leq 0.05$ ****$P \leq 0.001$ (trend)	Purity, > 99%
Rat, F344/N (M, F) 104 wk NTP (2000)	Dietary concentrations of 0, 600, 1300, or 2500 ppm, equivalent to daily doses of 0, 25, 50, or 100 mg/kg bw 50 M and 50 F/group (age, 6 wk)	Thyroid follicular cell adenoma: 1/50, 1/50, 6/49*, 3/49 (M) Renal tubule adenoma or carcinoma (standard and extended evaluations combined): 4/50**, 2/50, 4/50, 7/50*** (M)	*$P = 0.047$ **$P = 0.025$ (trend) ***$P = 0.050$	Purity, > 99% No significant increase in the incidence of any neoplasm in females

bw, body weight; F, female; M, male; wk, week

3. Cancer in Experimental Animals

See Table 3.1

Primidone was tested for carcinogenicity by oral administration (feed) in one study in mice and one study in rats.

3.1 Mouse

In one study of carcinogenicity, groups of 50 male and 50 female B6C3F$_1$ mice (age, 5–6 weeks) were given diets containing primidone (purity, > 99%) at a concentration of 0 (control), 300, 600, or 1300 ppm for 104–105 weeks. Primidone intake was equivalent to average daily doses of approximately 0, 30, 65, or 150 mg/kg body weight (bw) in males, and 0, 25, 50 or 100 mg/kg bw in females (NTP, 2000). Survival in exposed groups was similar to that of controls, except for the group of males at the highest dose, in which survival was less than that of controls. Primidone caused significant increases in the incidence of hepatocellular adenoma, of hepatocellular carcinoma, and of hepatocellular adenoma, hepatocellular carcinoma, and hepatoblastoma (combined) in all dosed groups of males and females compared with controls. Primidone caused significant increases in the incidence of hepatoblastoma in all dosed groups of males. In males, there was also a significant positive trend in the incidence of follicular cell adenoma of the thyroid in mice receiving pyrimidone, with a significant increase in incidence in the group receiving the highest dose. There was an increased incidence in follicular cell hyperplasia of the thyroid in males and females receiving pyrimidone.

3.2 Rat

In one study of carcinogenicity, groups of 50 male and 50 female F344/N rats (age, 6 weeks) were given diet containing primidone (purity, > 99%) at a concentration of 0 (control), 600, 1300, or 2500 ppm for 104 weeks. Primidone intake was equivalent to average daily doses of approximately 0, 25, 50, or 100 mg/kg bw in males and females (NTP, 2000). Survival in exposed groups was similar to that in controls, except for males at the intermediate and highest doses, for which survival was less than that for controls. Primidone caused a significant increase in the incidence of follicular cell adenoma of the thyroid in males receiving the intermediate dose. In the extended evaluations involving additional step sections of the kidney in males, there was a small but significant increase in the incidence of renal tubule adenoma or carcinoma (single and extended evaluations combined) at the highest dose; these tumours also occurred with a small but significant positive trend. [The Working Group noted the unusually high incidence of these uncommon tumours in the controls.] The incidence of renal tubule hyperplasia was also increased in all groups of males receiving primidone. There was no significant increase in the incidence of any neoplasm in females.

4. Mechanistic and Other Relevant Data

4.1 Absorption, distribution, metabolism, and excretion

The metabolism of primidone is shown in Fig. 4.1.

Fig. 4.1 Metabolism of primidone

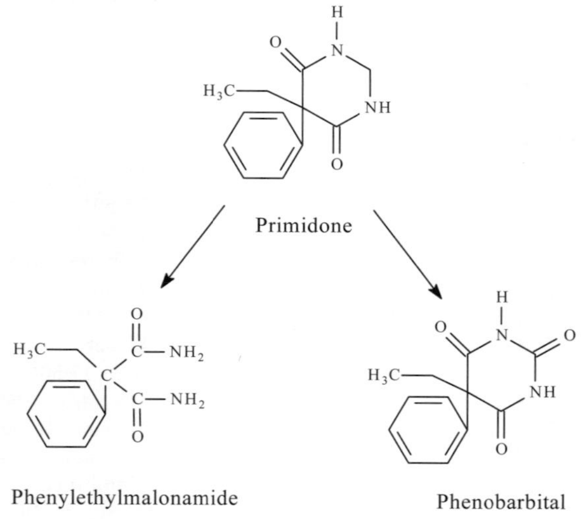

Compiled by the Working Group

4.1.1 Humans

In humans, primidone is partly eliminated unchanged via urinary excretion, and partly metabolized by hepatic cytochrome P450 (CYP) isozymes, principally to phenylethylmalonamide (PEMA) by cleavage of the pyrimidine ring, and to phenobarbital by oxidation of the methylene group (Baumel *et al.*, 1972; Martines *et al.*, 1990; Sato *et al.*, 1992; Anderson, 1998; Tanaka, 1999). The CYP isoenzymes responsible for metabolizing primidone are presently uncertain (Anderson, 1998; Tanaka, 1999).

(a) Pharmacokinetics of single doses

Baumel *et al.* (1972) reported the pharmacokinetics of primidone in two subjects given a single oral dose of 500 mg of primidone. Peak plasma concentration of primidone, measured by gas-liquid chromatography, was reached at 0.5 hours in one subject, and 4.8 hours in the other. Estimated half-lives for primidone were 5.8 and 3.3 hours, respectively. Two hours after dosing, the metabolite PEMA was detected in the plasma of both subjects, reaching peak concentrations at 7 and 8 hours before gradually declining. Estimated half-lives were 29 and

36 hours, respectively. The second metabolite, phenobarbital, was not detectable in this study.

In a study of seven volunteers given a single oral dose of 500 mg of primidone, the mean peak plasma concentration (± standard deviation) of primidone was 41.4 ± 5.2 μmol/L, reached in approximately 2 ± 1 hours. The elimination half-life was 17 ± 2.4 hours. PEMA was detected in the serum, reaching peak concentrations (4.1 ± 0.7 μmol/L) at 2–24 hours in these subjects. Phenobarbital was below the level of detection (< 2 μmol/L) of gas-liquid chromatography (Pisani *et al.*, 1984).

Subsequent studies using high-performance liquid chromatography of samples from three healthy volunteers given a single oral dose of 600 mg, showed initial slow absorption of primidone; peak concentration of unchanged primidone (mean C_{max}, 41.2 ± 5.4 μmol/mL) was achieved at 12 hours in each subject. Mean elimination half-life was 19.4 ± 2.2 hours. The metabolite PEMA was detectable at 1.3 ± 0.3 hours, and reached peak concentration (1.7 ± 0.3 μmol/L) at 36 hours. Elimination half-life was 26.5 ± 1.0 hours. The metabolite phenobarbital was detectable at 5.3 ± 1.3 hours, and reached maximal concentration (1.3 ± 0.2 μmol/L) at 52 ± 11 hours, with a long (125 ± 20 hours) elimination half-life (Sato *et al.*, 1992).

In a study of the pharmacokinetics of PEMA given as a single oral dose of 400 mg to two groups of subjects (six patients aged 10–43 years receiving long-term treatment with various anti-epileptic drugs and six "drug-free" subjects aged 22–42 years), showed no statistically significant differences between the two groups; peak serum concentrations were normally reached within 2–4 hours after dosing in both groups. In the drug-free subjects, recovery of unchanged PEMA in the urine gave an estimated oral bioavailability of at least 80%. The elimination half-life ranged from 17 to 25 hours in drug-free subjects, and from 10 to 23 hours in patients. There was no evidence for a glucuronide conjugate. The

study indicated that PEMA is readily absorbed from the gastrointestinal tract and eliminated predominantly unchanged in the urine (Cottrell *et al.*, 1982).

(b)   *Pharmacokinetics of repeated doses*

Although phenobarbital was not detected after administration of single doses of primidone, long-term administration of primidone (at "various" doses) in 46 epilepsy patients showed serum accumulation of phenobarbital, and PEMA (Baumel *et al.*, 1972). Although there was significant inter-individual variability, concentrations of the two metabolites showed correlation with those of the parent drug, and concentrations of phenobarbital were consistently higher than those of PEMA. Two of the subjects had been on a daily dose of primidone (750 mg in divided doses) for more than 3 years. After a single dose of 750 mg in this study, peak serum concentrations of primidone were achieved rapidly (by 0.5 hour), and declined slowly (half-lives, 5.3 and 7.0 hours). In both subjects, peak concentrations of metabolites, PEMA (12 and 10 μg/mL) and phenobarbital (33 and 11 μg/mL), remained relatively constant. In the cerebrospinal fluid, binding to protein by PEMA and by primidone was negligible, and approximately 60% by phenobarbital (Baumel *et al.*, 1972).

In a subsequent study in eight epileptic patients (aged 18–26 years) receiving long-term treatment with primidone (mean daily dose, 422 ± 115 mg per day), the half-life for primidone was 14.7 ± 3.5 hours (Martines *et al.*, 1990).

(c)   *Absorption, distribution, and excretion under certain conditions*

(i)   *Age-dependent effects*

The pharmacokinetics and metabolism of primidone at steady-state were studied in 18 epileptic patients who had been receiving a constant dose of primidone for at least 2 months. Data were compared in two groups: 10 elderly patients (age, 70–81 years), and 8 young patients (age, 18–26 years) (Martines *et al.*, 1990). The mean daily doses were moderately, but not significantly, higher in the elderly group, than the young (575 ± 206 mg/day and 422 ± 115 mg/day, respectively). In the elderly and young, respectively, the mean half-life of primidone was 12.1 ± 4.6 hours and 14.7 ± 3.5 hours, and the mean total clearance of primidone was 34.8 ± 9.0 mL/hour per kg and 33.2 ± 7.2 mL/hour per kg. Differences between the two groups were not statistically significant, indicating that half-life and total clearance of primidone were unaltered in elderly patients. However, some differences between the two groups were highlighted; serum concentrations of the metabolites PEMA and phenobarbital (relative to those of parent drug) were higher in the elderly than the young, significantly so in the case of PEMA ($P < 0.01$). Renal clearances of primidone, phenobarbital, and PEMA were moderately decreased (again, significantly for PEMA, $P < 0.05$) in the elderly (Martines *et al.*, 1990).

The results of this study supported previous suggestions that PEMA (unlike primidone and phenobarbital) is eliminated only by renal excretion (Cottrell *et al.*, 1982), and so its serum accumulation in the elderly probably results from moderately reduced renal elimination accompanied by an increase in the fraction of primidone metabolized (Cottrell *et al.*, 1982; Pisani *et al.*, 1984; Martines *et al.*, 1990).

The metabolism and excretion of orally administered primidone was studied in 12 children (age, 7–14 years) undergoing long-term (> 3 months) treatment for epilepsy, and were assumed to be in steady state. Four children were taking primidone only, and eight were also taking phenytoin. Plasma concentrations peaked at 4–6 hours and declined exponentially over 6–24 hours, with half-lives ranging from 4.5 to 11 hours. Mean recovery of the administered dose in the urine within 24 hours was 92% (range, 72–123%) as primidone and metabolites.

Of the total daily dose administered, 42.3% was recovered as unchanged drug, 45.2% as PEMA, and 4.9% as phenobarbital. The rate of metabolism to phenobarbital showed wide variation (25-fold) among children, which, although not influencing the overall elimination rate constant for primidine, is an important determinant of the individual patient's steady-state concentration of phenobarbital. Concomitant use of phenytoin had no detectable effect on half-life or serum concentrations of phenobarbital. Of the total primidone daily dose, approximately equal amounts of parent drug (~40%) and PEMA (~45%) were excreted, with phenobarbital as approximately 5% (Kauffman *et al.*, 1977).

(ii) Pregnancy

The placental transfer of primidone and metabolites was investigated in 14 women treated for epilepsy with primidone (and additionally phenytoin, ethosuximide or valproate in 5 women) throughout pregnancy. Primidone, PEMA, phenobarbital, and polar metabolites (*p*-hydroxyphenobarbital and *p*-hydroxyphenobarbital glucuronide) were found in similar concentrations in maternal and cord blood at birth (Nau *et al.*, 1980).

In the same study, the pharmacokinetics of primidone were studied in seven of the newborns during the first weeks of life (Nau *et al.*, 1980). Mean elimination half-lives were longer than those found in children by Kauffman *et al.* (1977): 23 ± 10 hours for primidine; 113 ± 40 hours for phenobarbital; and 35 ± 6 hours for PEMA. The shortest half-lives for primidone (8–11 hours) were detected in two neonates whose mothers had been treated with phenytoin in addition to primidone. Serum concentrations and elimination rates varied among neonates, and during the period of study. For example, serum concentrations of phenobarbital and PEMA increased in some neonates during the first few days, due to neonatal metabolism of primidine, and rate of elimination increased after a few days in some babies (Nau *et al.*, 1980).

Analyses of maternal milk of four of the mothers detected primidone and PEMA at approximately 75%, phenobarbital at approximately 50%, and total *p*-hydroxyphenobarbital (conjugated and non-conjugated) at approximately equal to concentrations measured in serum. Because of breastfeeding, all compounds were also detected in neonatal blood (Nau *et al.*, 1980).

(iii) Liver disease

The disposition of a single oral dose of 500 mg of primidone was studied in seven patients with acute viral hepatitis and in seven healthy subjects (controls). The elimination half-life and the apparent clearance of unchanged primidone in the patients did not differ significantly from that in the controls (mean elimination half-life, 18.0 ± 3.1 hours in patients, and 17.0 ± 2.4 hours in controls; mean apparent clearance of unchanged primidone, 42 ± 14 mL/hour per kg in patients, and 35 ± 8 mL/hour per kg in controls). The metabolite PEMA was detectable in serum of all healthy subjects within 2–24 hours, but undetectable (< 2 µmol/L) in sera of all except one patient. In all subjects, serum concentrations of phenobarbital remained below the limit of detection of gas-liquid chromatography. These findings indicated that accumulation of primidone is unlikely to occur in epilepsy patients who develop acute viral hepatitis (Pisani *et al.*, 1984).

(d) Pharmacokinetic and drug interactions

The CYP isozymes 1A2, 2C9, 2C19, and 3A4, and UDP-glucoronosyl transferase and epoxide hydrolases are induced by primidone and its metabolite phenobarbital [phenobarbital also induces CYP2A6] (Riva *et al.*, 1996; Anderson, 1998; Patsalos & Perucca, 2003). Thus pharmacokinetic interactions are likely to occur between primidone and other substrates for these enzymes, ultimately causing either an increase or decrease in pharmacologically active species. Primidone is frequently used in combination with such substrates (e.g. anticonvulsants such as carbamazepine, ethosuximide, valproic acid, and phenytoin). A study by Sato *et al.* (1992) showed that, in patients taking both primidone and phenytoin, metabolites of primidone in serum were detected earlier, elimination was faster, and total body clearance was increased, when compared with patients taking primidone only. In a study of seven neonates, whose mothers were treated for epilepsy throughout pregnancy, the shortest half-lives for primidone were reported in two neonates whose mothers had been treated with both phenytoin and primidone (Nau *et al.*, 1980). Conversely, Kauffman *et al.* (1977) reported that there were no effects on half-life or serum concentrations of phenobarbital in children being treated for epilepsy with phenytoin in addition to primidone.

4.1.2 Experimental systems

PEMA and phenobarbital have been identified as the major metabolites of primidone in mice (McElhatton *et al.*, 1977), rats (Baumel *et al.*, 1973; Moriyama *et al.*, 1994), rabbits (Fujimoto *et al.*, 1968; Hunt & Miller, 1978), and dogs (Frey & Löscher, 1985).

In a study by the NTP (2000), groups of B6C3F$_1$ mice were given a single dose of primidone (at 30, 80, or 200 mg/kg bw) by gavage and blood samples were collected at various time-points (ranging from 0.25 hour to 48 hours) after administration. Plasma concentrations of primidone in mice were dependent on dose and time. Absorption was rapid, and for all dose groups, plasma concentrations were detectable within 15 minutes after dosing, and remained above the limit of detection for at least 30 hours (after a dose of 30 or 80 mg/kg bw) and for at least 48 hours (after a dose of 200 mg/kg bw). Slightly higher plasma concentrations of primidone were detected in males than females.

Plasma concentrations of phenobarbital were dose-, time- and sex-dependent; phenobarbital was detected within 15 minutes after dosing. Earlier and slightly higher peak concentrations were observed in males than in females, indicating that, in mice, primidone is more rapidly metabolized to phenobarbital in males than in females (NTP, 2000).

Studies in pregnant mice given repeated intragastric doses of primidone at 100 mg/kg bw [a known teratogenic dose] over several days demonstrated no accumulation of the parent compound, or of the metabolites PEMA or phenobarbital, and all were cleared rapidly from the plasma within 24 hours. The relatively long period of dosing with primidone resulted in its more rapid rate of metabolism, resulting in higher concentrations of metabolites, than after a single dose (McElhatton *et al.*, 1977).

Studies of single doses of primidone (given by gavage) in the mouse, showed a dissimilar trend in results. The plasma half-life of phenobarbital was reported to be twice that of primidone and PEMA, and plasma : brain ratios indicated poor penetration of primidone into the brain (Leal *et al.*, 1979).

In contrast, in rats given primidone by gavage, concentrations of the parent drug peaked in the plasma after 1 hour, and in the brain after 2 hours (Baumel *et al.*, 1973). This result was supported by a subsequent study in rats given primidone by intraperitoneal injection (at a dose of 50, 100 or 200 mg/kg bw), which suggested that primidone and metabolites were able to penetrate the blood–brain barrier. Primidone was first detected in the serum (mean T_{max} range, 1.5–2.5 hours) and in the cerebrospinal fluid (mean T_{max} range, 2.0–3.5 hours), followed by its metabolites, PEMA and phenobarbital (Nagaki *et al.*, 1999).

Moriyama *et al.* (1994) reported the pharmacokinetic parameters of primidone and its major metabolites in the rat. After oral administration of primidone (at a dose of 50 mg/kg bw),

the plasma concentration of primidone rapidly increased achieving maximal levels by 1 hour, but by 12 hours had decreased to very low levels, and at 24 hours was undetectable. In contrast, concentrations of PEMA and phenobarbital gradually increased, reaching maximum levels after 4–8 hours, and these metabolites were still detected after 24 hours. T_{max} values for primidone, PEMA, and phenobarbital were 1.36, 5.70, and 6.55 hours, respectively, and C_{max} values were 18.15 µg/mL, 8.11 µg/mL, and 9.64 µg/mL, respectively. Thus concentrations of PEMA and phenobarbital were approximately 50% that of primidone. Half-lives were reported as 1.64, 4.29, and 4.96 hours for primidone, PEMA and phenobarbital, respectively.

In the study by Nagaki *et al.* (1999), the concentrations of primidone, PEMA, and phenobarbital rose in a linear and dose-dependent manner in serum and cerebrospinal fluid (mean free fraction in serum [free non-protein-bound/total concentration ratio], 0.86, 0.97, and 0.88, respectively). The respective mean values for the cerebrospinal fluid : serum ratio were 0.73, 1.06, and 0.65, suggesting rapid equilibration between blood and cerebrospinal-fluid compartments. Mean half-life values for primidone, PEMA and phenobarbital in the cerebrospinal fluid were similar to those reported in serum (Nagaki *et al.*, 1999).

In a study by the NTP (2000), groups of male and female F344/N rats were given a single dose of primidone (30, 80, or 130 mg/kg bw) by gavage, and blood samples were collected from all dose groups at various times (from 15 minutes to 30 hours) after administration (NTP, 2000). Plasma concentrations of primidone were dependent on dose and time; absorption was rapid at all doses, and primidone was detectable in the plasma within 15 minutes after dosing. Although the time-course and dose–response profiles were similar in male and female rats, plasma concentrations of primidone (at most doses and time points) were consistently higher (approximately double) and half-lives greater (two- to fivefold) in females than in males. Plasma concentrations of the metabolite phenobarbital were also dependent on dose, time, and sex; although phenobarbital was detectable in the plasma of male rats within 15 minutes after dosing, phenobarbital was undetectable in the plasma of female rats at 15 and 30 minutes, and plasma concentrations of phenobarbital, for a given dose, were consistently higher in males than in females. [Thus, the metabolism of primidone in rats appeared to be dependent on sex, with males metabolizing primidone more rapidly than females.] Phenobarbital was still detectable in the plasma of male and female rats at 30 hours after dosing (NTP, 2000).

4.2 Genetic and related effects

4.2.1 Humans

No data were available to the Working Group.

4.2.2 Experimental systems

See Table 4.1

(a) Mutagenicity

Primidone (concentration range, 33–10 000 µg/plate) was mutagenic at concentrations of 3333 µg/plate and higher in *Salmonella typhimurium* strain TA1535 in the absence of metabolic activation; no mutagenic activity was detected in TA1535 in the presence of metabolic activation, or in strains TA100, TA1537, or TA98, with or without metabolic activation (Mortelmans *et al.*, 1986).

No increases in the frequencies of sex-linked recessive lethal mutations were detected in germ cells of male *Drosophila melanogaster* treated as larvae by feeding on primidone solutions of 6–12 mM (Zolotareva *et al.*, 1979).

(b) Chromosomal damage

No increases in sister-chromatid exchange or chromosomal aberration were noted in cultured Chinese hamster ovary cells treated with primidone at concentrations ranging from 125 to 1250 µg/mL, with or without metabolic activation (NTP, 2000). Additional in-vitro studies showing no induction of sister-chromatid exchange in Chinese hamster ovary cells, or chromosomal aberration in human lymphocytes or Chinese hamster ovary cells, have been reported (Stenchever & Allen, 1973; Bishun *et al.*, 1975; Riedel & Obe, 1984).

In vivo, no induction of dominant lethal mutation was observed in germ cells of male mice treated with a single intraperitoneal injection of primidone at doses of up to 90 mg/kg bw (Epstein *et al.*, 1972) or 400 mg/kg bw (Zolotareva *et al.*, 1979). No induction of chromosomal aberrations was reported in bone-marrow cells of male mice treated with primidone at doses of up to 400 mg/kg bw by a single intraperitoneal injection (Zolotareva *et al.*, 1979). There was one report of an increased frequency of micronucleated polychromatic erythrocytes in the bone marrow of mice given 13.11 mg of primidone [dose, approximately 500 mg/kg bw] twice with an interval of 24 hours (Rao *et al.*, 1986). [The Working Group noted that the mice were sampled 6 hours after the second dose, which was too brief an interval to measure the effects of the second treatment, and possibly too long to evaluate accurately the induction of micronuclei after the initial treatment. These protocol deficiencies hindered the interpretation of the data.] Contrasting results were seen in B6C3F$_1$ male mice, in which no significant increases in the frequency of micronucleated polychromatic erythrocytes were detected in bone marrow after administration of primidone (dose range, 87.5–350 mg/kg bw) by intraperitoneal injection, three times at 24-hour intervals, in each of two replicate trials (NTP, 2000).

Table 4.1 Genetic and related effects of primidone

Test system	Results[a]		Concentration/dose (LED or HID)	Reference
	Without exogenous metabolic system	With exogenous metabolic system		
In vitro				
Salmonella typhimurium TA100, TA1537, TA98, reverse mutation	–	–[b]	10 000 µg/plate	Mortelmans *et al.* (1986)
Salmonella typhimurium TA1535, reverse mutation	+	–[b]	3333 µg/plate	Mortelmans *et al.* (1986)
Drosophila melanogaster, sex-linked recessive lethal mutation in germ cells	–	NT	12 mM in food	Zolotareva *et al.* (1979)
Sister-chromatid exchange, Chinese hamster ovary cells	–	–	1250 µg/mL	NTP (2000)
Sister-chromatid exchange, Chinese hamster ovary cells	–	–	100 µg/mL	Riedel & Obe (1984)
Chromosomal aberration, Chinese hamster ovary cells	–	–	1250 µg/mL	NTP (2000)
Chromosomal aberration, Chinese hamster ovary cells	–	–	100 µg/mL	Riedel & Obe (1984)
Chromosomal aberration, human lymphocytes	–	NT	100 µg/mL	Stenchever & Allen (1973)
Chromosomal aberration, human lymphocytes	–	NT	70 µg/mL	Bishun *et al.* (1975)
In vivo				
Dominant lethal mutation, male ICR/Ha Swiss mouse, germ cells	–		90 mg/kg bw, ip × 1	Epstein *et al.* (1972)
Dominant lethal mutation, male mouse, germ cells	–		400 mg/kg bw, ip × 1	Zolotareva *et al.* (1979)
Chromosomal aberration, male mouse, bone-marrow cells	–		400 mg/kg bw, ip × 1	Zolotareva *et al.* (1979)
Micronucleus formation, Swiss mouse, bone-marrow cells	+		13.11 mg, po × 2[c]	Rao *et al.* (1986)
Micronucleus formation, male B6C3F$_1$ mouse, bone-marrow cells	–		350 mg/kg bw, ip × 3	NTP (2000)

[a] +, positive; –, negative

[b] S9 (9000 × *g* supernatant) from Sprague-Dawley rats and Syrian hamsters treated with Aroclor 1254

[c] Dose was approximately 500 mg/kg bw; four mice per treatment group. Mice were killed 6 hours after the second treatment; 3000 polychromatic erythrocytes were scored per mouse

bw, body weight; LED, lowest effective dose; HID, highest ineffective dose; ip, intraperitoneal; NR, not reported; NT, not tested; po, oral

4.2.3 Genetic and related effects of the metabolite phenobarbital

In contrast to the limited information on primidone, there was a significant body of literature describing the results of tests for genotoxicity with phenobarbital, a major metabolite of primidone. The extensive literature on the genetic and related effects of phenobarbital was reviewed by a previous Working Group (IARC, 2001), and is summarized briefly below.

Phenobarbital did not induce sister-chromatid exchange in patients with epilepsy receiving only this drug (IARC, 2001).

In studies in which rodents were exposed to phenobarbital in vivo, no covalent binding to mouse liver DNA was observed, but the frequency of alkali-labile damage in mouse liver cells was increased. Gene mutation was not induced in a transgenic mouse strain, and sister-chromatid exchange, micronucleus formation, and chromosomal aberrations were not induced in mouse bone-marrow cells. Phenobarbital did not increase the frequency of sperm-head abnormalities in mice, but spermatogonial germ-cell chromosomal aberrations were reported in male mice in one laboratory. Further increases in the frequency of chromosomal aberration were found in liver foci cells of mice treated with phenobarbital after prior treatment with a genotoxic agent (IARC, 2001).

Chromosomal aberrations, but not gene mutations, were induced in cultured human lymphocytes treated with phenobarbital (IARC, 2001).

The numerous types of test for the genetic effects of phenobarbital in vitro included assays for DNA damage, DNA repair induction, gene mutation, and chromosomal aberration in mammalian cells, tests for gene mutation and mitotic recombination in insects and fungi, and tests for gene mutation in bacteria. Although the majority of the test results were negative, the numerous positive results could not be ignored, although they did not present a consistent pattern of genotoxicity. The inconsistency of the results, the absence of any direct evidence for an interaction with DNA, and the generally negative data in vivo led to the conclusion that phenobarbital is not genotoxic (IARC, 2001).

Phenobarbital transformed hamster embryo cells. It inhibited gap-junctional intercellular communication in hepatocytes of rats treated in vivo, and in primary cultures of hepatocytes from rats and mice, but not (in a single study) in primary cultures of hepatocytes from humans or rhesus monkey (IARC, 2001).

4.3 Other mechanistic data relevant to carcinogenesis

4.3.1 Humans

Toxicity associated with primidone in humans has been documented with reference to side-effects after use of primidone as a drug. The side-effects included nausea, vomiting, dizziness, ataxia, and somnolence, and caused early discontinuation of treatment. Smith *et al.* (1987) reported that both carbamazepine and phenytoin were associated with statistically significantly lower incidences of intolerable side-effects than were primidone or phenobarbital. Patients receiving primidone experienced the highest incidence of toxicity.

Administration of anti-epileptic drugs, such as primidone, and also carbamazepine, gabapentin, oxcarbazepine, and phenytoin affected serum concentrations of folate, homocysteine, and vitamin B_{12}. In a study involving 2730 patients treated with various anti-epileptic drugs, 170 untreated patients, and 200 healthy controls, Linnebank *et al.* (2011) reported that primidone monotherapy (10 patients) was associated with a higher frequency of folate concentrations that were below the reference range when compared with untreated patients and controls. This association was dose-dependent. Primidone monotherapy was also associated with plasma concentrations of homocysteine that were above the reference range when compared with controls (Linnebank *et al.*, 2011).

A review by Benedetti *et al.* (2005) of several studies in humans suggested that therapeutic levels of primidone or phenobarbital are not associated with an increase in thyroid-stimulating hormone levels.

4.3.2 Experimental systems

Carl *et al.* (1987a, b) studied the effects of treatment with primidone on one-carbon metabolism by measuring levels of methylene-tetrahydrofolate reductase and related parameters in the brain and liver of rats given primidone (100 mg/kg bw every 12 hours) by gastric gavage for up to 8 weeks. Primidone caused a decrease of pteroylpentaglutamates in the liver to less than half the control value within 1 week. Overall, the data suggested that primidone affects concentrations of folate in the tissue and plasma by interfering with folate-dependent metabolic processes, possibly through the interaction of primidone with the synthesis of folylpolyglutamates (Carl *et al.*, 1987a).

4.4 Susceptibility

No studies primarily addressing the susceptibility of humans to carcinogenesis induced by primidone were available to the Working Group. In a review, Singh *et al.* (2005) speculated that there might be a partly biological basis (e.g. genetic predisposition) for the association between epilepsy and cancer, possibly involving the tumour suppressor gene leucine-rich glioma inactivated 1 (*LGI1*). El-Masri & Portier (1998) have suggested that there is wide inter-individual variation in the metabolic profile of primidone, which may indicate the presence of people who produce greater amounts of primidone metabolites than the general population, and who are thus more sensitive to effects induced by primidone metabolites.

4.5 Mechanistic considerations

In humans, and in mice and rats, primidone is extensively, but not totally, metabolized to phenobarbital. Given the evidence for the carcinogenicity of primidone (see Section 3) and phenobarbital (IARC, 2001), the carcinogenic activity attributable to primidone in mice can be reasonably hypothesized to be the result of the metabolism of primidone to phenobarbital considering that both cause malignant hepatocellular tumours in this species.

The carcinogenicity of phenobarbital was evaluated by the Working Group in 2000 (IARC, 2001). Epidemiological data primarily comprised three large cohort studies of patients with epilepsy. On the basis of these and all other available studies, the Working Group concluded that there was *inadequate evidence* in humans for the carcinogenicity of phenobarbital (IARC, 2001). Singh *et al.* (2005) reviewed studies involving risk of cancer in people with epilepsy, with specific reference to the role of anti-epilepsy drugs, noting studies concerning cancer of the liver, lung, and brain. Despite considerable long-term pharmaco-epidemiological data being available for phenobarbital, evidence for carcinogenicity in humans was not consistent and phenobarbital was considered to be "possibly" carcinogenic to humans by the authors.

The Working Group in 2000 concluded that phenobarbital was *possibly carcinogenic* to humans (Group 2B) based solely on *sufficient evidence* in experimental animals (IARC, 2001).

Studies aiming to elucidate mechanisms of carcinogenesis attributable to phenobarbital in mice have been reported. Typically, these investigations exploited comparison between strains of mice that were variously sensitive and resistant to phenobarbital-induced hepatocarcinogenesis. Thus Watson & Goodman (2002) reported that there was a clear indication of more extensive changes in methylation in GC-rich regions of DNA, primarily hypermethylation, in the tumour-sensitive mice in response to treatment with phenobarbital.

Phillips *et al.* (2009) reported the effects of treatment with phenobarbital on DNA methylation and gene expression that occurred only in liver tumour-prone B6C3F$_1$ mice but not in tumour-resistant C57BL/6 mice, after 2 or 4 weeks of treatment. Differences in epigenetic control (e.g. DNA methylation) between species could, in part, underlie the enhanced propensity of rodents, as compared with humans, to develop cancer.

5. Summary of Data Reported

5.1 Exposure data

Primidone is a synthetic drug that was used commonly as an oral anticonvulsant, beginning in the 1950s. It is now only in modest use, predominantly for the treatment of essential tremor, with stable use over the past decade. Exposure is likely to be predominantly through use as a medication. Environmental contamination in groundwater has been reported.

5.2 Human carcinogenicity data

The available epidemiological studies evaluating exposure specifically to primidone were limited to two case–control studies reporting on several types of cancer nested in a cohort of epileptic patients in Denmark. Small excesses of malignant lymphoma and cancers of the lung and urinary bladder were observed among patients who were ever treated with primidone; however, the findings were based on small numbers of exposed cases. Other limitations included incomplete information on exposure to primidone (with respect to duration and post-discharge drug use) and on potential confounders. The available studies were not informative on whether exposure to primidone is a cancer hazard.

5.3 Animal carcinogenicity data

Primidone was tested for carcinogenicity in one oral administration study in mice, and one oral administration study in rats. In male and female mice, feed containing primidone caused significant increases in the incidences of hepatocellular adenoma, of hepatocellular carcinoma, and of hepatocellular adenoma, hepatocellular carcinoma and hepatoblastoma (combined). Primidone also caused a significant increase in the incidence of hepatoblastoma and of thyroid follicular cell adenoma in males. In male rats, feed containing primidone caused a significant increase in the incidence of thyroid follicular cell adenoma. Primidone also caused a small but significant increase in the incidence of renal tubule adenoma or carcinoma (combined) in males. There was no significant increase in the incidence of any neoplasm in female rats.

5.4 Mechanistic and other relevant data

In humans, primidone is partly eliminated unchanged via urinary excretion, or metabolized, by hepatic cytochrome P450 isozymes principally to phenylethylmalonamide and to phenobarbital, a non-genotoxic agent. The data on genetic toxicity for primidone in traditional assays are limited in scope and amount, but suggest that any mutagenic action of the chemical is highly specific: clear demonstration of the mutagenic activity of primidone was limited to a single report of mutation induction in *Salmonella typhimurium* strain TA1535 in the absence of metabolic activation only, and at high concentrations. The majority of well-conducted studies of chromosomal damage available for review suggested that primidone does not induce chromosomal changes in vitro or in vivo.

The reported carcinogenicity of primidone in mice is likely to be mediated through a non-genotoxic mechanism resulting from the metabolism of primidone to phenobarbital.

6. Evaluation

6.1 Cancer in humans

There is *inadequate evidence* in humans for the carcinogenicity of primidone.

6.2 Cancer in experimental animals

There is *sufficient evidence* in experimental animals for carcinogenicity of primidone.

6.3 Overall evaluation

Primidone is *possibly carcinogenic to humans (Group 2B)*.

References

Adelöw C, Ahlbom A, Feychting M, Johnsson F, Schwartzbaum J, Tomson T (2006). Epilepsy as a risk factor for cancer. *J Neurol Neurosurg Psychiatry*, 77(6):784–6. doi:10.1136/jnnp.2005.083931 PMID:16705202

Anderson GD (1998). A mechanistic approach to antiepileptic drug interactions. *Ann Pharmacother*, 32(5):554–63. doi:10.1345/aph.17332 PMID:9606477

Baumel IP, Gallagher BB, DiMicco J, Goico H (1973). Metabolism and anticonvulsant properties of primidone in the rat. *J Pharmacol Exp Ther*, 186(2):305–14. PMID:4719783

Baumel IP, Gallagher BB, Mattson RH (1972). Phenylethylmalonamide (PEMA). An important metabolite of primidone. *Arch Neurol*, 27(1):34–41. doi:10.1001/archneur.1972.00490130036005 PMID:4626105

Benedetti MS, Whomsley R, Baltes E, Tonner F (2005). Alteration of thyroid hormone homeostasis by antiepileptic drugs in humans: involvement of glucuronosyltransferase induction. *Eur J Clin Pharmacol*, 61(12):863–72. doi:10.1007/s00228-005-0056-0 PMID:16307266

Bishun NP, Smith NS, Williams DC (1975). Chromosomes and anticonvulsant drugs. *Mutat Res*, 28(1):141–3. doi:10.1016/0027-5107(75)90327-9 PMID:1143294

British Pharmacopoeia (2013). Primidone. London, United Kingdom: Medicines and Healthcare products Regulatory Agency (MHRA).

Carl GF, Eto I, Krumdieck CL (1987a). Chronic treatment of rats with primidone causes depletion of pteroylpentaglutamates in liver. *J Nutr*, 117(5):970–5. PMID:3585552

Carl GF, Gill MW, Schatz RA (1987b). Effect of chronic primidone treatment on folate-dependent one-carbon metabolism in the rat. *Biochem Pharmacol*, 36(13):2139–44. doi:10.1016/0006-2952(87)90142-0 PMID:3606631

Cottrell PR, Streete JM, Berry DJ, Schäfer H, Pisani F, Perucca E et al. (1982). Pharmacokinetics of phenylethylmalonamide (PEMA) in normal subjects and in patients treated with antiepileptic drugs. *Epilepsia*, 23(3):307–13. doi:10.1111/j.1528-1157.1982.tb06196.x PMID:7084140

Daley RD (1973). Primidone. In: Florey K, editor. Analytical Profiles of Drug Substances. Academic Press; pp. 409–437.

DrugBank (2013). Primidone. DrugBank: Open Data Drug & Drug Target Database. Version 3.0. Available from: http://www.drugbank.ca/

El-Masri HA, Portier CJ (1998). Physiologically based pharmacokinetics model of primidone and its metabolites phenobarbital and phenylethylmalonamide in humans, rats, and mice. *Drug Metab Dispos*, 26(6):585–94. PMID:9616196

eMC (2013). Primidone. Datapharm Communications Ltd., electronic Medicines Compendium (eMC). Available from: http://www.medicines.org.uk/emc, accessed 4 September 2014.

Epstein SS, Arnold E, Andrea J, Bass W, Bishop Y (1972). Detection of chemical mutagens by the dominant lethal assay in the mouse. *Toxicol Appl Pharmacol*, 23(2):288–325. doi:10.1016/0041-008X(72)90192-5 PMID:5074577

European Pharmacopoeia (2008). Primidone. European Pharmacopoeia Work Programme; pp. 2752–53. Available from: http://www.edqm.eu/en/european-pharmacopoeia-publications-1401.html, accessed 4 September 2014.

FDA (2013). Primidone. Silver Spring (MD): United States Food and Drug Administration. Available from: http://www.accessdata.fda.gov/scripts/cder/drugsatfda/index.cfm?fuseaction=Search.DrugDetails, accessed 4 September 2014.

Ferranti V, Chabenat C, Ménager S, Lafont O (1998). Simultaneous determination of primidone and its three major metabolites in rat urine by high-performance liquid chromatography using solid-phase extraction. *J Chromatogr B Biomed Sci Appl*, 718(1):199–204. doi:10.1016/S0378-4347(98)00356-9 PMID:9832377

Frey HH, Löscher W (1985). Pharmacokinetics of anti-epileptic drugs in the dog: a review. *J Vet Pharmacol Ther*, 8(3):219–33. doi:10.1111/j.1365-2885.1985.tb00951.x PMID:3932673

Fujimoto JM, Mason WH, Murphy M (1968). Urinary excretion of primidone and its metabolites in rabbits. *J Pharmacol Exp Ther*, 159(2):379–88. PMID:5638658

Hass U, Dünnbier U, Massmann G (2012). Occurrence of psychoactive compounds and their metabolites in groundwater downgradient of a decommissioned sewage farm in Berlin (Germany). *Environ Sci Pollut Res Int*, 19(6):2096–106. doi:10.1007/s11356-011-0707-x PMID:22227832

Hunt RJ, Miller KW (1978). Disposition of primidone, phenylethylmalonamide, and phenobarbital in the rabbit. *Drug Metab Dispos*, 6(1):75–81. PMID:23277

IARC (2001). Some thyrotropic agents. *IARC Monogr Eval Carcinog Risks Hum*, 79:i–iv, 1–725. http://monographs.iarc.fr/ENG/Monographs/vol79/index.php PMID:11766267

IMS Health (2012a). National Disease and Therapeutic Index (NDTI). Plymouth Meeting, Pennsylvania: IMS Health.

IMS Health (2012b). National Prescription Audit Plus (NPA). Plymouth Meeting, Pennsylvania: IMS Health.

IMS Health (2012c). Multinational Integrated Data Analysis (MIDAS). Plymouth Meeting, Pennsylvania: IMS Health

Japanese Pharmacopoeia (2007). Primidone. In: Hosokawa R editor. *The Japanese Pharmacopoeia*. 15th ed. Tokyo, Japan: Ministry of Health, Labour and Welfare; pp. 1026–7.

Kauffman RE, Habersang R, Lansky L (1977). Kinetics of primidone metabolism and excretion in children. *Clin Pharmacol Ther*, 22(2):200–5. PMID:884921

Kuhn J, Knabbe C (2013). Fully validated method for rapid and simultaneous measurement of six antiepileptic drugs in serum and plasma using ultra-performance liquid chromatography-electrospray ionization tandem mass spectrometry. *Talanta*, 110:71–80. doi:10.1016/j.talanta.2013.02.010 PMID:23618178

Lamminpää A, Pukkala E, Teppo L, Neuvonen PJ (2002). Cancer incidence among patients using antiepileptic drugs: a long-term follow-up of 28,000 patients. *Eur J Clin Pharmacol*, 58(2):137–41. doi:10.1007/s00228-002-0429-6 PMID:12012147

Lanças FM, Sozza MA, Queiroz ME (2003). Simultaneous plasma lamotrigine analysis with carbamazepine, carbamazepine 10,11 epoxide, primidone, phenytoin, phenobarbital, and PEMA by micellar electrokinetic capillary chromatography (MECC). *J Anal Toxicol*, 27(5):304–8. doi:10.1093/jat/27.5.304 PMID:12908944

Leal KW, Rapport RL, Wilensky AJ, Friel PN (1979). Single-dose pharmacokinetics and anticonvulsant efficacy of primidone in mice. *Ann Neurol*, 5(5):470–4. doi:10.1002/ana.410050512 PMID:464548

Linnebank M, Moskau S, Semmler A, Widman G, Stoffel-Wagner B, Weller M *et al.* (2011). Antiepileptic drugs interact with folate and vitamin B12 serum levels. *Ann Neurol*, 69(2):352–9. doi:10.1002/ana.22229 PMID:21246600

Martines C, Gatti G, Sasso E, Calzetti S, Perucca E (1990). The disposition of primidone in elderly patients. *Br J Clin Pharmacol*, 30(4):607–11. doi:10.1111/j.1365-2125.1990.tb03820.x PMID:2291873

McElhatton PR, Sullivan FM, Toseland PA (1977). Plasma level studies of primidone and its metabolites in the mouse at various stages of pregnancy. *Xenobiotica*, 7(10):617–22. doi:10.3109/00498257709038683 PMID:910462

MHRA (2013). UK Public Assessment Report. Mysoline 50mg tablets (primidone) PL 20132/0006. London, United Kingdom: Medicines and Heathcare Products Regulatory Agency. Available from: www.mhra.gov.uk/home/groups/par/documents/websiteresources/con088170.pdf, accessed 24 April 2015

MicroMedex (2013). Primidone. MicroMedex 2.0. Ann Arbor (MI): Truven Health Analytics Inc.

Morasch B (2013). Occurrence and dynamics of micropollutants in a karst aquifer. *Environ Pollut*, 173:133–7. doi:10.1016/j.envpol.2012.10.014 PMID:23202643

Moriyama M, Furuno K, Oishi R, Gomita Y (1994). Simultaneous determination of primidone and its active metabolites in rat plasma by high-performance liquid chromatography using a solid-phase extraction technique. *J Pharm Sci*, 83(12):1751–3. doi:10.1002/jps.2600831220 PMID:7891306

Mortelmans K, Haworth S, Lawlor T, Speck W, Tainer B, Zeiger E (1986). Salmonella mutagenicity tests: II. Results from the testing of 270 chemicals. *Environ Mutagen*, 8(S7):Suppl 7: 1–119. doi:10.1002/em.2860080802 PMID:3516675

Nagaki S, Ratnaraj N, Patsalos PN (1999). Blood and cerebrospinal fluid pharmacokinetics of primidone and its primary pharmacologically active metabolites, phenobarbital and phenylethylmalonamide in the rat. *Eur J Drug Metab Pharmacokinet*, 24(3):255–64. doi:10.1007/BF03190029 PMID:10716065

Nau H, Rating D, Häuser I, Jäger E, Koch S, Helge H (1980). Placental transfer and pharmacokinetics of primidone and its metabolites phenobarbital, PEMA and hydroxyphenobarbital in neonates and infants of epileptic mothers. *Eur J Clin Pharmacol*, 18(1):31–42. doi:10.1007/BF00561476 PMID:7398746

NTP (2000). NTP Toxicology and Carcinogenesis Studies of Primidone (CAS No. 125–33–7) in F344/N Rats and B6C3F1 Mice (Feed Studies). *Natl Toxicol Program Tech Rep Ser*, 476:1–290. PMID:12571687

O'Neil MJ (2006). The Merck Index. 14th Ed. Whitehouse Station (NJ): Merck & Co., Inc.

OEHHA (2013). Chemicals known to the state to cause cancer or reproductive toxicity. CA: Office of Environmental Health Hazard Assessment, State of California Environmental Protection Agency. Available from: http://oehha.ca.gov/prop65/prop65_list/files/P65single052413.pdf, accessed 30 June 2014.

Olsen JH, Boice JD Jr, Fraumeni JF Jr (1990). Cancer in children of epileptic mothers and the possible relation to maternal anticonvulsant therapy. *Br J Cancer*, 62(6):996–9. doi:10.1038/bjc.1990.424 PMID:2257233

Olsen JH, Boice JD Jr, Jensen JP, Fraumeni JF Jr (1989). Cancer among epileptic patients exposed to anticonvulsant drugs. *J Natl Cancer Inst*, 81(10):803–8. doi:10.1093/jnci/81.10.803 PMID:2716074

Olsen JH, Schulgen G, Boice JD Jr, Whysner J, Travis LB, Williams GM *et al.* (1995). Antiepileptic treatment and risk for hepatobiliary cancer and malignant lymphoma. *Cancer Res*, 55(2):294–7. PMID:7812960

Olsen JH, Wallin H, Boice JD Jr, Rask K, Schulgen G, Fraumeni JF Jr (1993). Phenobarbital, drug metabolism, and human cancer. *Cancer Epidemiol Biomarkers Prev*, 2(5):449–52. PMID:8220089

Özden S, Özden T, Gümül F, Tosun A (1989). Quantitative proton magnetic resonance analysis of primidone in solid dosage forms. *Spectrosc Lett*, 22(4):471–6. doi:10.1080/00387018908053896

Patsalos PN, Perucca E (2003). Clinically important drug interactions in epilepsy: general features and interactions between antiepileptic drugs. *Lancet Neurol*, 2(6):347–56. doi:10.1016/S1474-4422(03)00409-5 PMID:12849151

Phillips JM, Burgoon LD, Goodman JI (2009). The constitutive active/androstane receptor facilitates unique phenobarbital-induced expression changes of genes involved in key pathways in precancerous liver and liver tumors. *Toxicol Sci*, 110(2):319–33. doi:10.1093/toxsci/kfp108 PMID:19482888

Pisani F, Perucca E, Primerano G, D'Agostino AA, Petrelli RM, Fazio A *et al.* (1984). Single-dose kinetics of primidone in acute viral hepatitis. *Eur J Clin Pharmacol*, 27(4):465–9. doi:10.1007/BF00549596 PMID:6519155

Rao KP, Shaheen S, Usha Rani MV, Rao MS (1986). Effect of primidone in somatic and germ cells of mice. *Toxicol Lett*, 34(2-3):149–52. doi:10.1016/0378-4274(86)90204-3 PMID:3798475

Rezaei B, Jafari MT, Khademi R (2009). Selective separation and determination of primidone in pharmaceutical and human serum samples using molecular imprinted polymer-electrospray ionization ion mobility spectrometry (MIP-ESI-IMS). *Talanta*, 79(3):669–75. doi:10.1016/j.talanta.2009.04.046 PMID:19576428

Riedel L, Obe G (1984). Mutagenicity of antiepileptic drugs. II. Phenytoin, primidone and phenobarbital. *Mutat Res*, 138(1):71–4. doi:10.1016/0165-1218(84)90087-9 PMID:6541755

Riva R, Albani F, Contin M, Baruzzi A (1996). Pharmacokinetic interactions between antiepileptic drugs. Clinical considerations. *Clin Pharmacokinet*, 31(6):470–93. doi:10.2165/00003088-199631060-00005 PMID:8968658

Sato J, Sekizawa Y, Owada E, Ito K, Sakuta N, Yoshihara M *et al.* (1986). Sensitive analytical method for serum primidone and its active metabolites for single-dose pharmacokinetic analysis in human subjects. *Chem Pharm Bull (Tokyo)*, 34(7):3049–52. doi:10.1248/cpb.34.3049 PMID:3769107

Sato J, Sekizawa Y, Yoshida A, Owada E, Sakuta N, Yoshihara M *et al.* (1992). Single-dose kinetics of primidone in human subjects: effect of phenytoin on formation and elimination of active metabolites of primidone, phenobarbital and phenylethylmalonamide. *J Pharmacobiodyn*, 15(9):467–72. doi:10.1248/bpb1978.15.467 PMID:1287181

SciFinder (2013). SciFinder databases: a division of the American Chemical Society. Available from: https://www.cas.org/products/scifinder, accessed 30 June 2014.

Singh G, Driever PH, Sander JW (2005). Cancer risk in people with epilepsy: the role of antiepileptic drugs. *Brain*, 128(Pt 1):7–17. doi:10.1093/brain/awh363 PMID:15574465

Smith DB, Mattson RH, Cramer JA, Collins JF, Novelly RA, Craft B (1987). Results of a nationwide Veterans Administration Cooperative Study comparing the efficacy and toxicity of carbamazepine, phenobarbital, phenytoin, and primidone. *Epilepsia*, 28(s3):Suppl 3: S50–8. doi:10.1111/j.1528-1157.1987.tb05778.x PMID:3319543

Stenchever MA, Allen M (1973). The effect of selected antiepileptic drugs on the chromosomes of human lymphocytes in vitro. *Am J Obstet Gynecol*, 116(6):867–70. PMID:4736739

Tanaka E (1999). Clinically significant pharmacokinetic drug interactions between antiepileptic drugs. *J Clin Pharm Ther*, 24(2):87–92. doi:10.1046/j.1365-2710.1999.00201.x PMID:10380060

Thermoscientific (2004). Immonoassay products. Thermo Scientific. Available from: http://www.thermoscientific.com/en/search-results.html?keyword=primidone&matchDim=Y, accessed 30 June 2014.

Tocris (2013). Primidone safety data sheet. Tocris bioscience. Available from: http://www.tocris.com/literature/0830_sds.pdf?1432306358, accessed 4 September 2014.

US Pharmacopeia (2007). Primidone. Report No. USP30-NF25. Rockville (MD): The United States Pharmacopeial Convention; pp. 3016.

US Pharmacopeia (2009). Material Safety Data Sheet - Primidone. Rockville (MD): The United States Pharmacopeial Convention.

US Pharmacopeia (2013). Official Monographs – Primidone. Rockville (MD): The United States Pharmacopeial Convention.

Watson RE, Goodman JI (2002). Effects of phenobarbital on DNA methylation in GC-rich regions of hepatic DNA from mice that exhibit different levels of susceptibility to liver tumorigenesis. *Toxicol Sci*, 68(1):51–8. doi:10.1093/toxsci/68.1.51 PMID:12075110

WHO (2007). Cumulative List No. 14 of INN in Latin, English, French, Spanish, Arabic, Chinese and Russian (in alphabetical order of the Latin name), with supplementary information. Geneva, Switzerland: World Health Organization. Available from: http://www.vpb.gov.lt/files/539.pdf, accessed 30 June 2014.

Zesiewicz TA, Elble RJ, Louis ED, Gronseth GS, Ondo WG, Dewey RB Jr *et al.* (2011). Evidence-based guideline update: treatment of essential tremor: report of the Quality Standards subcommittee of the American Academy of Neurology. *Neurology*, 77(19):1752–5. doi:10.1212/WNL.0b013e318236f0fd PMID:22013182

Zolotareva GN, Akaeva EA, Goncharova RI (1979). Antimutagenic activity of the antispasmodic reparation hexamidine. Effect of hexamidine on level of spontaneous mutation in a number of subjects *Dokl. Acad. Nauk SSSR*, 246:469–471.[Russian]

SULFASALAZINE

1. Exposure Data

1.1 Identification of the agent

1.1.1 Nomenclature

Chem. Abstr. Serv. Reg. No.: 599-79-1 (O'Neil, 2001; SciFinder, 2013)

Chem. Abstr. Serv. Name: Benzoic acid, 2-hydroxy-5-[2-[4-[(2-pyridinylamino)sulfonyl]-phenyl]diazenyl] (O'Neil, 2001; SciFinder, 2013)

IUPAC systematic name: 2-Hydroxy-5-[2-[4-[pyridine-2-ylsulfamoyl)phenyl]diazenyl]benzoic acid (Lide, 2005; European Pharmacopoeia, 2008)

United States nonproprietary name (USAN): Sulfasalazine

Synonyms: Benzoic acid, 2-hydroxy-5-[[4-[(2-pyridinylamino)sulfonyl]phenyl]azo]-; 5-[[*p*-(2-Pyridylsulamoyl)phenyl]azo] salicylic acid (US Pharmacopeia, 2007, 2013)

See WHO (2007) for names in other languages.

1.1.2 Structural and molecular formulae and relative molecular mass

$C_{18} H_{14} N_4 O_5 S$
Relative molecular mass: 398.39
From O'Neil (2001).

1.1.3 Chemical and physical properties of the pure substance

Description: Brownish-yellow, odourless crystals (O'Neil, 2001; European Pharmacopoeia, 2008).

Melting-point: Decomposes at 240–245 °C (O'Neil, 2001)

Density: 1.48 ± 0.1 g/cm³ at 20 °C (SciFinder, 2013)

Spectroscopy data: Ultraviolet, mass, and nuclear magnetic resonance spectra have been reported (McDonnell & Klaus, 1976; European Pharmacopoeia, 2008)

Solubility: Practically insoluble in water, ether, benzene, chloroform; very slightly soluble in ethanol; soluble in alkali hydroxides (McDonnell & Klaus, 1976; O'Neil, 2001)

Octanol/water partition coefficient: Log P = 3.88 (Rosenbaum, 2011)

Stability data: The compound did not degrade when dissolved in dimethylformamide and was subjected to thermal stress at 80 °C for 196 hours (McDonnell & Klaus, 1976; Jacoby, 2000)

1.1.4 Technical products and impurities

(a) Trade names

Azulfidine EN-tabs; Azulfidine; Azaline; Sulfazine; Sulfazine EC; Apo-Sulfasalazine; PMS-Sulfasalazine; Salazopyrin En-Tabs; Salazopyrin; Azulfidina; Azulfin; Bomecon; Colo-Pleon; Disalazin; Falazine; Gastropyrin; Lazafin; Pyralin EN; Rosulfant; Salazine; Salazodin; Salazopirina; Salazopyrin Entabs; Salazopyrin-EN; Salazopyrina; Salazopyrine; Salivon; Salopyr; Salopyrine; Saridine-E; Sulcolon; Sulfasalazin; Sulfitis; Ulcol; Zopyrin (Porter & Kaplan, 2013).

(b) Impurities

Impurities as given in European Pharmacopoeia (2008):

- 4,4′-[(4-hydroxy-1,3-phenylene)bis(diazenediyl)]bis[N-(pyridin-2-yl)benzene sulfonamide
- 2-hydroxy-3,5-bis[2-[4-(pyridin-2-ylsulfamoyl)phenyl]diazenyl]benzoic acid
- 2-hydroxy-5-[2-[4-(2-iminopyridin-1(2*H*)-yl)phenyl]diazenyl]benzoic acid
- 4-[2-(2-hydroxyphenyl)diazenyl]-*N*-(pyridin-2-yl)benzenesulfonamide
- 2-hydroxy-4′-(pyridin-2-ylsulfamoyl)-5-[2-[4-(pyridin-2-ylsulfamoyl) phenyl]diazenyl] biphenyl-3-carboxylic acid

- 2-hydroxy-3-[2-[4-(pyridin-2-ylsulfamoyl)phenyl]diazenyl]benzoic acid
- 5-[2-[4′,5-bis(pyridin-2-ylsulfamoyl)biphenyl-2-yl]diazenyl]-2-hydroxy benzoic acid
- salicylic acid
- 2-hydroxy-5-[2-(4-sulfophenyl)diazenyl] benzoic acid
- 4-amino-*N*-(pyridin-2-yl)benzenesulfonamide (sulfapyridine).

1.1.5 Analysis

Selected compendial and non-compendial methods of analysis are presented in Table 1.1. Sulfasalazine in human plasma can be determined by high-performance liquid chromatography using ultraviolet detection (Fukino *et al.*, 2007). It can also be analysed through liquid chromatography-tandem mass spectrometry in human plasma using electron spray ionization techniques in multiple reaction monitoring mode, with a limit of quantification of 10 ng/mL (Gu *et al.*, 2011).

In urban water, sulfasalazine can be quantified by liquid chromatography-mass spectrometry using electron spray ionization. The limit of quantification is 65 ng/L (Tuckwell *et al.*, 2011).

1.2 Production

1.2.1 Production process

Sulfasalazine does not occur in nature. Sulfasalazine is produced by reacting sulfanilamide with salicyclic acid through a series of steps, with water as a solvent (Novacek *et al.*, 1991).

1.2.2 Use

(a) Indications

Sulfasalazine is an aminosalicylate whose chief bioactive metabolite is 5-aminosalicyclic acid (5-ASA). Sulfasalazine, mesalazine (5-ASA),

Table 1.1 Analytical methods for sulfasalazine

Sample matrix	Sample preparation	Assay method	Detection limit	Reference
Compendial methods				
Assay	–	UV-visible spectroscopy Wavelength: 359 nm		European Pharmacopoeia (2008), US Pharmacopeia (2013)
Related substances	–	LC-UV Column: C_{18} Mobile phase A: sodium dihydrogen phosphate and sodium acetate in water Mobile phase B: mobile phase A : methanol (10 : 40) Flow rate: 1 mL/min Wavelength: 320 nm		European Pharmacopoeia (2008)
Non-compendial methods Biological samples:				
Human serum, breast milk	–	LC	2.5 or 1.3 µmol/L (LOD)	Esbjörner *et al.* (1987)
Human plasma	Centrifugation	LC-UV Column: C_{18} Mobile phase: 35% acetonitrile in 25 mM phosphate buffer pH 3.0 Flow rate: 0.12 mL/min Wavelength: 365 nm		Fukino *et al.* (2007)
Human plasma	Protein precipitation using methanol treatment, solid phase extraction (1 mL of methanol containing 5% ammonia)	ELISA Buffer solutions: phosphate buffer, carbonate/bicarbonate buffer, acetate buffer	0.51 ng/mL (sensitivity) 0.02 ng/mL (LOD)	Pastor-Navarro *et al.* (2007)
Human plasma	Proteins precipitation followed by centrifugation; supernatant was mixed with 100 µL of water in polypropylene tubes and transferred to the auto-sampler	LC–ESI-MS/MS Column: phenyl Mobile phases: 0.2% formic acid, 2 mM ammonium acetate in water, 2 mM ammonium acetate in methanol MRM mode 399 *m/z*, 381 *m/z*	10 ng/mL (LOQ)	Gu *et al.* (2011)

Table 1.1 (continued)

Sample matrix	Sample preparation	Assay method	Detection limit	Reference
Mouse plasma	–	LC-UV Column: C_{18} Mobile phase: methanol and 25 mM phosphate buffer (64 : 36) pH 2.5 Flow rate: 1 mL/min	0.32 nmol/mL (LOD)	Zheng et al. (1993)
Rat plasma	–	LC-UV Column: C_{18} Mobile phase: 25 mM phosphate buffer : methanol (40 : 60) pH 3.0 Flow rate: 0.3 mL/min Wavelength: 360 nm	40 ng/mL (LOQ)	Lee et al. (2012)
Food samples:				
Pork meat	Pressurized liquid extraction with hot water, clean-up using oasis HLB cartridge (poly(divinylbenzene-co-N-pyrrolidone)	CE-ESI-MS[2] Sheath liquid: methanol, water and formic acid (49.5 : 49.5 : 1) Electrolyte: 50 mM ammonium acetate pH 4.16 MRM mode $[M+H]^+$ 398 317 *m/z*, 156 *m/z*, 108 *m/z*	6.25 µg/kg (LOD) 21.3 µg/kg (LOQ)	Font et al. (2007)
Honey	Added 10% trichloroacetic acid, heated at 65 °C, followed by liquid–liquid extraction (acetonitrile, dichloromethane), organic phase was evaporated, reconstituted using methanol : water (20 : 80)	LC-APPI-MS/MS Column: C_{18} Mobile phase: 0.5% formic acid (v/v) and 1 mM nonylfluoropentanoic acid (solvent A) and a mixture of methanol/acetonitrile (50/50, v/v), containing 0.5% formic acid (solvent B) Flow rate: 300 µL/min (SRM) positive ionization	0.4–4.5 µg/kg (LOD) 1.2–15.0 µg/kg (LOQ)	Mohamed et al. (2007)
Venalink blister packs (monitored dosage system)	Dissolve drug in dimethylformamide, dilute with methanol. Internal standard was 1 mL of 0.1% (w/v) 4-*N,N*-dimethylaminobenzaldehyde	LC-UV Column: C_{18} Mobile phase: methanol, water, and acetic acid (70 : 29 : 1) Flow rate: 1.5 mL/min Wavelength: 365 nm	0.1 ng/mL (LOD) 1 ng/mL (LOQ)	Elmasry et al. (2011)

Table 1.1 (continued)

Sample matrix	Sample preparation	Assay method	Detection limit	Reference
Environmental samples:				
Water	Aqueous sample was filtered, followed by SPE, and derivatized using acetonitrile and methanol	LC-ESI-MS^2 Column: C$_{18}$ Mobile phase A: 20 mM aqueous ammonium acetate, 0.1% formic acid Mobile phase B: 20 mM ammonium acetate in acetonitrile : methanol (2 : 1)	9–55.3 ng/mL (LOD)	Fatta *et al.* (2007)
Water	Vacuum extraction, then evaporation under gentle nitrogen stream. Reconstitution with methanol	LC-ESI-MS^n Mobile phase: water and acetonitrile with 0.1% formic acid Flow rate: 0.2 mL/min Single parent ion (positive mode) [M+H]$^+$ 399	Effluent water, 150 ng/L River water, 65 ng/L (LOQ)	Tuckwell *et al.* (2011)

APPI, atmospheric pressure photospray ionization; CE-ESI-MS^2, capillary electrophoresis-electrospray ionization-quadrupole ion trap-tandem mass spectrometry; ELISA, enzyme-linked immunosorbent assay; ESI, electrospray ionization; LC, liquid chromatography; LOD, limit of detection; LOQ, limit of quantification; MRM, multiple reaction monitoring; MS, mass spectrometry; MS^n, multistage mass spectrometry; SPE, solid-phase extraction; SPME, solid-phase microextraction; SRM, selected reaction monitoring; UV, ultraviolet

Table 1.2 Most commonly reported clinical indications for sulfasalazine in the USA, 2011–2012

Diagnosis	ICD code	Drug uses (in thousands)	Percentage of total
Rheumatoid arthritis	714.001	367	46.2
Psoriatic arthropathy	696.001	90	11.3
Colitis, ulcerative, NOS	556.004	83	10.5
Colitis, presumed infectious	009.101	69	8.7
Spondylitis, ankylopietic	720.001	28	3.5
Crohn disease	555.901	27	3.4
Surgery after intestinal disease	67.050	25	3.1
Arthritis, spine, NOS	721.901	14	1.7
Rheumatoid arthritis plus inflammatory polyarthritis, unspecified	714.901	11	1.4
All other diagnoses	–	81	10.2
Total with reported diagnoses	–	795	100

NOS, not otherwise specified
From IMS Health (2012a)

but also olsalazine and balsalazide are all 5-ASA drugs. As an anti-inflammatory and immuno-modulatory agent, sulfasalazine is used in the treatment of autoimmune and inflammatory conditions, namely inflammatory bowel disease (IBD), most prominently ulcerative colitis and Crohn disease, as well as psoriatic and rheumatoid arthritis, including juvenile rheumatoid arthritis (IMS Health, 2012a; eMC, 2013; Table 1.2). The use of sulfasalazine for the treatment of urticaria has also been reported (McGirt *et al.*, 2006). Sulfasalazine is recommended as a third-line medication in all the above conditions only when first- or second-line therapies have been ineffective.

(b) Dosage

Sulfasalazine is available as an oral dose at 250 or 500 mg, and as an oral suspension of 5 mL. There is a wide range of dosing regimens, varying from 500 mg once per day to 1000 mg four times per day, with 1000 mg twice per day being most common (35% of uses). The mean daily dosage for patients taking sulfasalazine is 2150 mg per day (IMS Health, 2012a; eMC, 2013).

(c) Trends in use

Total worldwide sales of sulfasalazine were US$ 222 million in 2012 (IMS Health, 2012b). The largest sales occurred in Japan (US$ 63 million), followed by the USA (US$ 32 million), the United Kingdom (US$ 16 million), Germany (US$ 12 million), Australia (US$ 9 million), and Canada (US$ 8 million). In the United Kingdom, 49 tonnes of sulfasalazine were prescribed in 2007 (Tuckwell *et al.*, 2011).

Use of sulfasalazine has been relatively stable in the USA since 2005, at about 360 000 drug uses per year. In the USA, approximately 100 000 patients received sulfasalazine in 2012 (IMS Health, 2012a) and 1.1 million prescriptions for sulfasalazine were dispensed each year between 2008 and 2012 (IMS Health, 2012c).

1.3 Occurrence and exposure

Sulfasalazine has been found as a persistent residue in influent and effluent of a sewage treatment plant, at concentrations of 0.1 to 0.4 µg/L (Tuckwell *et al.*, 2011).

Human exposure is largely limited to use as a medication. Workers in plants manufacturing sulfasalazine may be exposed.

1.4 Regulations and guidelines

Sulfasalazine has been widely approved by drug regulatory agencies around the world. In the USA, it was approved by the Food and Drug Administration in 1950 (FDA, 2013).

Sulfasalazine is listed as "known to cause cancer" by the State of California's Office of Environmental Health Hazard Assessment, requiring public notice of potential environmental exposure (OEHHA, 2013).

2. Cancer in Humans

2.1 Background

Sulfasalazine, a member of the family of 5-ASA drugs (see Section 1.2.2), has been used since the 1950s to treat IBD (primarily ulcerative colitis) and, to a lesser extent, Crohn disease (Hanauer, 2004). IBD is associated with an increased risk of dysplasia and cancer of the colorectum. Risk factors for IBD-associated cancer of the colorectum include duration, severity and extent of colitis, the presence of coexistent primary sclerosing cholangitis, and a family history of cancer of the colorectum (Dyson & Rutter, 2012). Chronic inflammation has been proposed as a mechanism for colorectal cancer associated with IBD (or ulcerative colitis), and thus it has been suggested that 5-ASA drugs are chemopreventive agents, because of their anti-inflammatory, anti-oxidant, and pro-apoptotic properties (Rubin *et al.*, 2006; Lakatos & Lakatos, 2008).

The available epidemiological studies included a surveillance study, two cohort studies, three nested case–control studies and three case–control studies of cancer of the colorectum among patients with IBD or ulcerative colitis. Some studies on IBD included patients with Crohn disease in addition to patients with ulcerative colitis, but none of the studies stratified by IBD subtype. A case–control study of cancer of the colorectum and exposure to dihydrofolate reductase inhibitors (sulfasalazine, triamterene, and methotrexate) was identified (Coogan & Rosenberg, 2007), but was not considered to be informative because it did not provide a risk estimate specifically for sulfasalazine; for further information, see the *Monograph* on triamterene in the present volume).

2.2 Longitudinal, cohort, and nested case–control studies

See Table 2.1 and Table 2.2

Moody *et al.* (1996) evaluated long-term treatment with sulfasalazine and risk of cancer of the colorectum in a retrospective cohort of 175 patients with ulcerative colitis diagnosed between 1972 and 1989 in Leicestershire, England. Clinical information, including compliance with sulfasalazine treatment and history of cancer, was obtained from case records. A patient was considered to be "non-compliant" if there was clear evidence that the patient had ceased taking the medication or was instructed by the physician to stop the medication without replacement by another 5-ASA drug. The crude proportion of cases of cancer of the colorectum in the sulfasalazine non-compliant group (31%) was significantly higher than in the compliant group (3%), and a significant effect of compliance was observed in survival analyses using log-ranked and Wilcoxon methods. [This study was limited by lack of a true unexposed group (the use of sulfasalazine in the non-compliant group was not known), small numbers, and limited information on use of sulfasalazine (e.g. time period, dose, duration), or other medications, and information on risk factors for cancer of the colorectum. It was not clear whether other 5-ASA drugs were used as a replacement for sulfasalazine in members of the compliant group who developed cancer, and whether the physician recommendations for stopping treatment with sulfasalazine would affect cancer outcome.]

Table 2.1 Surveillance and cohort studies of cancer and sulfasalazine

Reference Location, period	Total No. of subjects	Exposure assessment	Organ site (ICD code)	Exposure categories	Exposed cases	Relative risk (95% CI)	Covariates Comments
Moody *et al.* (1996) Leicester, England 1981–92	175	Case records – use and compliance	Colorectum	Crude proportion of cases (compliant vs non-compliant; χ^2)		$P < 0.001$	Retrospective; cohort comprised patients with total ulcerative colitis or with limited colitis who were deceased; identified via colitis database (case ascertainment, 98%). Cancer cases or dysplasia identified via case records or registry; biopsy diagnosis confirmed on 10% sample. Survival analysis adjusted for age and sex
				[OR for compliance]		[0.07 (0.02–0.30)]	
				Sulfasalazine non-compliant group	5	5/16 (31%)	
				Sulfasalazine compliant group	5	5/152 (3%)	
				Survival analysis (cancer-free) for compliance (log ranked and Wilcoxon methods)		$P < 0.001$	
Lindberg *et al.* (2001) Sweden, Follow-up, 20 yr	143	Hospital records or questionnaires	Colorectum (cancer or dysplasia)	Sulfasalazine	42	42/124 (34%)	Surveillance study; patients with ulcerative colitis participating in 20-yr colonoscopic surveillance programme; 124 patients in the treatment group
				No sulfasalazine	8	8/18 (44%)	
				Sulfasalazine vs no sulfasalazine (*t*-test)		$P = 0.38$	
				[OR for sulfasalazine]		[0.6 (0.2–1.7)]	
				Cumulative risk of CRC/dysplasia (sulfasalazine vs no treatment)		$P = 0.40$	Cumulative risk analysis adjusted for primary sclerosing cholangitis, sex, duration of ulcerative colitis, colectomy
			Colorectum (cancer only)	Sulfasalazine vs no sulfasalazine (*t*-test)		NR	Power, < 50%
				Sulfasalazine	5	5/124 (4%)	
				No sulfasalazine	2	2/18 (11%)	
				[OR for sulfasalazine]		[0.3 (0.06–1.87)]	

Table 2.1 (continued)

Reference Location, period	Total No. of subjects	Exposure assessment	Organ site (ICD code)	Exposure categories	Exposed cases	Relative risk (95% CI)	Covariates Comments
van Staa *et al.* (2005) United Kingdom, 1987–2001	33 905 with 5-ASA drug prescriptions 18 969	GPRD	Colorectum (153, 154, 159)	Reference cohort (number not reported); no history of IBD or prescription for 5-ASA drug	116	1	Patients with 5-ASA drug prescriptions and/or IBD identified from GPRD; patients with history of CRC excluded. Analysis adjusted for age and sex
				5-ASA drug/IBD cohort (5-ASA drug [excluding sulfasalazine] or sulfasalazine and IBD); *n* = 18 969	124	1.99 (1.54–2.56)	
				Sulfasalazine rheumatoid arthritis cohort (remaining sulfasalazine without IBD); number, NR	69	1.26 (0.94–1.70)	
	Nested case–control analysis (100 cases and 600 controls)			Sulfasalazine use 12 months before the index date:			Cases selected from 5-ASA drug/IBD cohort, controls randomly selected and matched for age, sex, and calendar year of index case. Analysis adjusted for BMI, IBD duration, history of colorectal polyps, NSAID, paracetamol, aspirin, immunosuppressive, glucocorticoids, prior hospitalization for gastrointestinal condition, physician visits, colonoscopy
				Regular use	22	0.67 (0.36–1.25)	
				6–12 prescriptions	3	0.95 (0.22–4.11)	
				13–30 prescriptions	5	0.41 (0.14–1.20)	
				> 30 prescriptions	14	0.77 (0.37–1.60)	
				Daily dose, < 2 g	6	0.84 (0.29–2.42)	
				Daily dose, ≥ 2 g	15	0.69 (0.35–1.37)	

5-ASA, 5-aminosalicylic acid; BMI, body mass index; CRC, colorectal cancer; GPRD, General Practice Research Database; IBD, inflammatory bowel disease; NR, not reported; NSAID, nonsteroidal anti-inflammatory drugs; OR, odds ratio; vs, versus

Table 2.2 Case–control studies of cancer of the colorectum and sulfasalazine

Reference Location, period	Total cases Total controls	Control source (hospital, population)	Exposure assessment	Organ site (ICD code)	Exposure categories	Exposed cases	Relative risk (95% CI)	Covariates Comments
Pinczowski et al. (1994) Sweden, 1965–83	102 196	Nested case–control; ulcerative colitis cohort	Medical records	Colorectum	Sulfasalazine use, one or more treatment courses (> 3 months)	48	0.38 (0.20–0.69)	Age, number of exacerbations/yr Controls matched by sex, extent of ulcerative colitis at diagnosis, and yr of diagnosis
Jess et al. (2007) Copenhagen Denmark, 1962–97; Minnesota, USA, 1940–2004	43 102	Nested case–control: IBD cohort; ulcerative colitis or Crohn disease	Medical records	Colorectum (adenocarcinoma, adenoma, or dysplasia [combined])	Sulfasalazine use, cumulative dose: 2.9/1000 g (median) for cases vs 2.2 (median) for controls	NR	1.1 (1.0–1.3)	Age and calendar yr of diagnosis Controls from the same regional cohort matched on sex, IBD (subtype, duration, calendar yr, and age of diagnosis). USA cohort followed until 2004, and Danish followed until 1997. Of the 43 cases, 23 were CRC, 13 adenoma, and 7 dysplasia
					Sulfasalazine, regular use (> 2 g/day)	36	1.1 (0.3–3.7)	
Eaden et al. (2000) England and Wales, [date, NR]	102 102	IBD patients	Medical records	Colorectum	Sulfasalazine use:			Possible selection bias, source of population patients from physician interested in study, controls from IBD Leicestershire database. Controls matched for sex, age (within 10 yr), extent and duration of disease, but not hospital or yr of diagnosis. "Adjusted for most influential variables", other 5-ASA drugs, contact with hospital doctor, colonoscopies diagnosis, relative with CRC
					< 2 g/day	7	0.93 (0.22–3.91)	
					≥ 2 g/day	32	0.85 (0.32–2.26)	

Table 2.2 (continued)

Reference Location, period	Total cases Total controls	Control source (hospital, population)	Exposure assessment	Organ site (ICD code)	Exposure categories	Exposed cases	Relative risk (95% CI)	Covariates Comments
Rutter et al. (2004) England, 1988–2002	68 136	Hospital, colonoscopy surveillance	Medical records, interviews, and postal questionnaires	Colorectum (cancer, adenoma, and dysplasia)	Sulfasalazine use: ≤ 10 yr > 10 yr	17 37	0.97 (0.41–2.26) 1.58 (0.71–3.51)	Controls matched for sex, extent and duration of ulcerative colitis, age of onset of ulcerative colitis, yr of index colonoscopy; also had to have intact colon and on surveillance within 5 yr of case diagnosis
				Colorectum (cancer)	≤ 10 yr > 10 yr	5 8	4.89 (0.47–51.00) 6.59 (0.64–67.92)	
Terdiman et al. (2007) USA, 2001–3	18 440 368 800	Population, health-care database	Administrative claims in database of large health-care insurance companies	Colorectum (ICD-9-CM)	Sulfasalazine use 1 yr before diagnosis	64	2.33 (1.80–3.01)	Controls free of cancer and bowel surgery, matched to cases by age, sex, and calendar year (20 : 1); CRC but not IBD diagnosis internally validated. No adjustment in analyses of any use 1 yr before diagnosis. Dose–response analysis adjusted for age, sex, colonoscopy, physician visits, ulcerative colitis or Crohn disease, hospitalization, NSAID, glucocorticosteroids, and immunomodulators
	364 1172	IBD patients			Sulfasalazine use 1 yr before diagnosis, IBD patients No. of prescriptions: 0 1–2 3–4 ≥ 5 *P* for trend	44 320 12 11 21	1.19 (0.83–1.72) 1.0 (ref.) 1.65 (0.80–3.39) 1.01 (0.46–2.21) 1.10 (0.63–1.92) 0.27	

5-ASA, 5-aminosalicylic acid; CRC, colorectal cancer; IBD, inflammatory bowel disease; ICD-9CM, International Classification of Diseases Ninth Revision, Clinical Modification; NR, not reported; NSAID, nonsteroidal anti-inflammatory drugs; ref., reference; vs, versus; yr, year

The association between sulfasalazine intake and colorectal cancer or dysplasia was evaluated in a study of 143 patients with ulcerative colitis who underwent regular colonoscopies and multiple biopsies in a 20-year surveillance programme in Sweden (Lindberg *et al.*, 2001). Of the 143 patients, 124 were in the group that had received treatment with sulfasalazine (treated for at least 6 months between onset of ulcerative colitis and start of surveillance by colonoscopy). Dysplasia or cancer of the colon developed in 51 patients. No statistically significant differences in the adjusted cumulative risk analysis for developing cancer or dysplasia of the colorectum, or the percentage of cancers in the two treatment groups (44% in the non-treatment group compared with 34% in the treatment group) were reported. [The study was limited by small numbers and limited exposure information.]

A cohort of users of 5-ASA drugs was identified from the General Practice Research Database in the United Kingdom (van Staa *et al.*, 2005). The cohort was divided into three subcohorts: (i) the 5-ASA drug/IBD cohort included 18 969 patients who either had a prescription for an 5-ASA drug (not including sulfasalazine) or who had taken sulfasalazine and had a diagnosis of IBD; (ii) the remaining patients who were taking sulfasalazine but did not have IBD; and (iii) a reference cohort consisting of patients without IBD or a prescription for a 5-ASA drug, matched by calendar year to participants receiving a 5-ASA drug. [The rationale for this approach was that sulfasalazine is used to treat IBD and other diseases in the United Kingdom, while the other 5-ASA drugs are only used to treat IBD.] Relative risks (RRs) for incidence of cancer of the colorectum were 1.99 (95% CI, 1.54–2.56) for the 5-ASA drug/IBD cohort, and 1.26 (95% CI, 0.94–1.70) for the sulfasalazine/non-IBD cohort.

A nested case–control analysis was conducted among the cohort of patients receiving 5-ASA drugs, which included 100 cases and 600 controls (matched to cases on age, sex, and calendar year) who had had prescriptions in the 6 months preceding the case index date. The type of 5-ASA drug was classified according to the last prescription issued before the index date. Adjusted odds ratios (ORs) were < 1 for regular use or 6–12 prescriptions, 0.41 (0.14–1.20) for 13–30 prescriptions, and 0.77 (0.37–1.60) for > 30 prescriptions in the previous 12 months, and for daily doses of < 2 g and ≥ 2 g; however, they were not statistically significant and no clear exposure–response patterns were observed (see Table 2.1). Duration of IBD was a strong risk factor for cancer of the colorectum in the study and was controlled for in the analyses. [This study had several advantages, including the prospective design, population-base selection of subjects, analyses by different exposure categories for specific 5-ASA drugs, and good clinical information on each patient. However, information on drug use was limited to the last prescription, information on lifetime drug use was not available, and there was limited information on follow-up procedures (e.g. no information was provided on tracking individuals who moved out of the region of the United Kingdom database). There was also a potential for misclassification of disease; classification appeared to be based on the General Practice Research Database with diagnosis confirmed via physician questionnaire for a small subset of patients. The study had limited statistical power. Moreover, it was unclear whether all the variables in the statistical models were potential confounders, which may have further reduced the statistical power.]

Two case–control studies were nested in population-based cohorts of patients with IBD (see Table 2.2). A Swedish study identified 102 cases of cancer of the colorectum via linkage to the national Swedish cancer registry, among a cohort of patients with ulcerative colitis (Pinczowski *et al.*, 1994). Living controls (*n* = 196), with intact or partially intact colon, were matched to cases on sex, extent of disease, and time of diagnosis of disease. Information on pharmacological therapy (including sulfasalazine), clinical features of disease, smoking, and family history of IBD, cancer of the colorectum, and other diseases, was collected from the patient's medical records. A decreased risk of cancer of the colorectum was found among individuals who had followed one or more treatment course of sulfasalazine (at least 3 months) (adjusted RR, 0.38; 95% CI, 0.20–0.69). [The strengths of the study were the prospective design, the use of a population-based cohort, and the use of controls matched for disease severity. The major limitations were the lack of detailed exposure information and small size.]

The second nested case–control study evaluated the risk of colorectal neoplasia (adenocarcinoma, adenoma, and dysplasia combined) in two cohorts of patients with IBD in Denmark and in Minnesota, USA (Jess *et al.*, 2007). Both cohorts included patients with ulcerative colitis or Crohn disease. Cases were identified via linkage with cancer registries, and controls matched for sex, vital status, and age at diagnosis, and clinical factors related to IBD were identified from each regional cohort. Exposure and clinical information was obtained from medical records. The adjusted relative risk for colorectal neoplasia was close to unity for regular use (> 2 g/day) or cumulative dose of sulfasalazine. Primary sclerosing cholangitis was a strong risk factor for colorectal neoplasia. [The advantages and limitations of this study were similar to those of the Swedish study. An additional limitation of this study was that there was not a separate analysis for cancer of the colorectum alone; of the 43 cases of colorectal neoplasia, 23 were cancer.]

2.3 Case–control studies

See Table 2.2

Three studies selected cases and controls from patients with ulcerative colitis. Eaden *et al.* (2000) evaluated the risk of colorectal cancer among patients with ulcerative colitis and controls in England and Wales. Cases (*n* = 102)

were identified from records of consenting gastroenterologists throughout England and Wales, and 102 controls matched by sex, age (categories of 10 years), extent and duration of IBD were identified from the Leicestershire database of IBD patients. Data were extracted from medical records. Sulfasalazine therapy at both < 2 g/day and ≥ 2 g/day was inversely associated with increased risk of colorectal cancer in unadjusted analyses, while adjusted odds ratios were 0.93 (95% CI, 0.22–3.91) for the group at the lower dose and 0.85 (95% CI, 0.32–2.26) for the group at higher doses. [The limitations of the study were the potential for selection bias, inadequate matching of the controls (using categories of 10 years of age, and not matching on hospital or year of diagnosis of IBD), limited exposure information, limited documentation of covariates controlled in the analyses. Odds ratios were adjusted for the use of other 5-ASA drugs, but this may not be appropriate since these drugs could work via the same mechanisms as sulfasalazine. The study population may have overlapped with the cohort reported by Moody *et al.* (1996); both studies identified patients from the same database of patients, but the years of study recruitment were not reported in the study by Eaden *et al.* (2000).]

One study evaluated risk factors for colorectal neoplasia (cancer, adenoma, and dysplasia) among patients with chronic ulcerative colitis who were part of a colonoscopy surveillance programme (Rutter *et al.*, 2004). Sixty-eight cases with neoplasia were identified and 136 controls from the surveillance population were matched on sex and clinical characteristics of IBD. Long-term use (> 10 years) of sulfasalazine was associated with a non-statistically significant elevated odds ratio for colorectal neoplasia (cancer, adenoma, or dysplasia) of 1.58 (95% CI, 0.71–3.51; 37 exposed cases); use of sulfasalazine for > 3 months to 10 years was associated with an odds ratio of 0.97 (95% CI, 0.41–2.26; 17 exposed cases). Analysis of the cancer cases only found that both exposure categories were associated with elevated, but very imprecise odds ratios based on small numbers (see Table 2.1). [A significant association between severity of inflammation and colorectal neoplasia was noted, and this hindered interpretation of the association of colorectal cancer and treatment with sulfasalazine. Other concerns included the small numbers of exposed cancer cases, lack of adjustment for risk factors, and limitations in the generalizability of the findings due to the selection of subjects from a surveillance programme. In addition, drug use may have been related to duration of ulcerative colitis, and thus matching by duration of ulcerative colitis may bias the odds ratio towards the null.]

Terdiman *et al.* (2007) evaluated use of sulfasalazine in a population based case–control study consisting of 18 440 cases of cancer of the colorectum and 368 800 controls (matched by age, sex, and calendar year) identified from two administrative databases covering all regions in the USA, including 364 cases and 1172 controls with a diagnosis of IBD. Information on claims for sulfasalazine prescriptions and other clinical variables was obtained from the claim database. A statistically significant increased risk of cancer of the colorectum was found among all patients using sulfasalazine 1 year before diagnosis (crude OR, 2.33; 95% CI, 1.80–3.01), while among patients with IBD only the adjusted odds ratio for sulfasalazine treatment was 1.19 (95% CI, 0.83–1.72); no exposure–response relationship was observed with number of prescriptions, regardless of adjustment for multiple covariates (*P* for trend, 0.27). [The strengths of this study were the large size and population-based design, and information on many (but not all) potential confounders, and some exposure–response analyses. The major limitation was the short exposure duration (1 year before diagnosis); in addition, information was not available on several key potential confounders, such as family history of colon cancer or IBD and other factors not related to medications.]

2.4 Meta-analysis

A meta-analysis of four cohort studies assessed the association between long-term treatment with sulfasalazine and risk of colorectal cancer (Diculescu *et al.*, 2003). [The Working Group could not interpret this study due to the lack of information on analytical methods and the inclusion of studies that were not specific for treatment with sulfasalazine. Furthermore, summary measures of association were not calculated.]

3. Cancer in Experimental Animals

3.1 Mouse

See Table 3.1

Oral administration

In one study, groups of 50 male and 50 female B6C3F$_1$ mice (age, 6 weeks) were given sulfasalazine (USP grade) at a dose of 0, 675, 1350, or 2700 mg/kg bw in corn oil by gavage once per day, 5 days per week, for 104 weeks. There was a 6–18% decrease in mean body weight in male and female mice at the highest dose compared with controls. The incidence of hepatocellular adenoma in males and females, and the incidence of hepatocellular adenoma or carcinoma (combined) in males and females, were significantly greater than those in controls, and the incidences increased with a positive trend. The incidence of hepatocellular carcinoma was significantly increased in female mice (Iatropoulos *et al.*, 1997; NTP, 1997a).

In a first experiment in a group of related studies, groups of 50–60 male B6C3F$_1$ mice (age, 6 weeks) were given sulfasalazine (USP grade) at a dose of 0 or 2700 mg/kg bw by gavage in corn oil once per day, 5 days per week, for 103 weeks (~2 years); in a second experiment, an unexposed

Table 3.1 Studies of carcinogenicity in mice given sulfasalazine by gavage

Strain (sex) Duration Reference	Dosing regimen, Animals/group at start	Incidence, (%) and/or multiplicity of tumours	Significance	Comments
B6C3F$_1$ (M, F) 104 wk NTP (1997a), Iatropoulos *et al.* (1997)	Sulfasalazine (in corn oil) at a dose of 0, 675, 1350, or 2700 mg/kg bw per day, 5 days per wk, for 104 wk 50 M and 50 F/group	*Males* Hepatocellular adenoma: 13/50[1], 32/50*, 28/50**, 42/50* Hepatocellular carcinoma: 13/50, 15/50, 23/50, 8/50 Hepatocellular adenoma or carcinoma (combined): 24/50[1], 38/50***, 38/50****, 44/50* *Females* Hepatocellular adenoma: 12/50[1], 28/50*, 25/50**, 28/49* Hepatocellular carcinoma: 2/50, 10/50*****, 10/50*****, 9/49***** Hepatocellular adenoma or carcinoma (combined): 14/50[2], 32/50*, 28/50*, 29/49*	*$P < 0.001$ (Poly-3 test) **$P = 0.002$ (Poly-3 test) ***$P = 0.004$ (Poly-3 test) ****$P = 0.005$ (Poly-3 test) *****$P \leq 0.05$ (Poly-3 test) [1]$P < 0.001$ (Poly-3 trend test) [2]$P = 0.005$ (Poly-3 trend test)	Purity, USP grade
B6C3F$_1$ (M) Up to 156 wk NTP (1997b), Abdo & Kari (1996)	*Exp. 1*: sulfasalazine (in corn oil) at a dose of 0 or 2700 mg/kg bw per day, 5 days per wk, for 103 wk (~2 yr), fed ad libitum *Exp. 2*: unexposed group fed such that mean body weight matched that of the treated group fed ad libitum *Exp. 3* (dietary restriction): two groups of 110 mice (one control and one dosed) were given identical quantities of feed such that the control group would attain body weights of approximately 80% that of the ad libitum-fed controls; 60 mice per group were evaluated at 103 wk (~2 yr) and the remaining 50 mice per group at 156 wk (3 yr), or when survival reached 20% 50–60 M/group	Hepatocellular adenoma: *Exp. 1*: 13/50, 42/50* *Exp. 2*: 8/50, 42/50* *Exp. 3*: 13/52, 9/50 (~2 yr) *Exp. 3*: 10/48, 14/50 (up to 3 yr) Hepatocellular carcinoma: *Exp. 1*: 13/50, 8/50 *Exp. 2*: 6/50, 8/50 *Exp. 3*: 7/52, 1/50 (~2 yr) *Exp. 3*: 16/48, 6/50 (up to 3 yr) Hepatocellular adenoma or carcinoma (combined): *Exp. 1*: 24/50, 44/50* *Exp. 2*: 14/50, 44/50* *Exp. 3*: 18/52, 9/50 (~2 yr) *Exp. 3*: 21/48, 18/50 (up to 3 yr)	*$P < 0.001$ (increase, logistic regression test)	Purity, USP grade

bw; body weight; Exp., experiment; F, female; M, male; wk, week; USP, United States Pharmacopoeia; yr, year group was fed such that the mean body weight of the group matched that of the treated group fed ad libitum. In a third experiment (dietary restriction), two groups of 110 animals, one control group and one group given sulfasalazine at a dose of 2700 mg/kg bw in corn oil were offered identical quantities of feed such that the control group would attain body weights of approximately 80% those of the control group fed ad libitum. Sixty mice from each group were evaluated at 103 weeks and the remaining 50 mice from each group were evaluated at 156 weeks (3 years), or at the time when survival reached 20%.

The mean body weight at 1 year and survival at 103 weeks (~2 years) for the mice treated with sulfasalazine were decreased by 15% and 19%, respectively, relative to controls. The body weight and survival of the weight-matched vehicle-control group were similar to those of the treated group fed ad libitum. Under the dietary restriction protocol, the control and treated groups weighed 42 g and 34 g at 1 year and had respective survival rates of 84% and 88% after 103 weeks.

Exposure to sulfasalazine under ad-libitum feeding conditions for 103 weeks (~2 years) caused significantly increased incidences of hepatocellular adenoma, and hepatocellular adenoma or carcinoma (combined) in exposed mice compared with the controls fed ad libitum and the weight-matched controls. In contrast to the findings of the first two experiments, the incidence of hepatocellular tumours in dietary-restricted mice was significantly decreased in the exposed group after 103 weeks, and was similar to that in non-treated mice after 3 years (Abdo & Kari, 1996; NTP, 1997b).

3.2 Rat

See Table 3.2

Oral administration

In one study, groups of 50 male and 50 female F344/N rats (age, 6 weeks) were given sulfasalazine (USP grade) at a dose of 0, 84, 168, or 337.5 mg/kg bw by gavage in corn oil once per day, 5 days per week, for 105 weeks (core study; continuous exposure). An additional group of male rats (stop-exposure group) was treated with sulfasalazine in corn oil at 337.5 mg/kg bw for 26 weeks, and then with corn oil only for the remainder of the study (79 weeks). Survival of male rats at the highest dose in the core study was significantly lower than that of controls, with most deaths occurring during the last 8 weeks of the study. Survival of all other treated groups was similar to that of controls.

The incidence of transitional cell papilloma of the urinary bladder in the core study was increased with a positive trend in the groups of treated male rats; the incidence in the group at the highest dose was significantly increased. The transitional cell neoplasms of the urinary tract observed in the core study were not observed in the stop-exposure group. In exposed females, there were also low incidences of [rare] transitional cell papilloma of the kidney and of the urinary bladder. All rats with transitional cell papillomas of the urinary tract also had grossly visible concretions (calculi) in the kidney and/or urinary bladder (Iatropoulos *et al.*, 1997; NTP, 1997a).

In a first experiment in a group of related studies, groups of 50–60 male F344/N rats (age, 6 weeks) were given sulfasalazine (USP grade) at a dose of 0 or 337.5 mg/kg bw in corn oil by gavage once per day, 5 days per week, for up to 104 weeks; in a second experiment, an unexposed group was fed such that the mean body weight of the group matched that of the treated group fed ad libitum. In a third experiment (dietary restriction), two groups of 110 rats, one control group and one group given sulfasalazine at a dose of 337.5 mg/kg bw in corn oil were offered identical

Table 3.2 Studies of carcinogenicity in rats given sulfasalazine by gavage

Strain (sex) Duration Reference	Dosing regimen, Animals/group at start	For each target organ: Incidence, (%) and/or multiplicity of tumours	Significance	Comments
F344/N (M, F) 105 wk NTP (1997a), Iatropoulos *et al.* (1997)	Sulfasalazine (in corn oil) at a dose of 0, 84, 168, or 337.5 mg/kg bw, once per day, 5 days per wk, for 105 wk (core study); an additional group of male rats (stop-exposure group) was treated with sulfasalazine (in corn oil) at 337.5 mg/kg bw for 26 wk and then with corn oil only for the remainder of the study (79 wk) 50 M and 50 F/group	*Males* Transitional cell papilloma of the urinary bladder: 0/50[1], 0/49, 2/50 (4%), 6/50 (12%)*; stop exposure, 0/47 *Females* Transitional cell papilloma of the urinary bladder[a]: 0/49, 0/50, 2/50 (4%), 0/50 Transitional cell papilloma of the kidney[b]: 0/50, 0/50, 0/50, 2/50 (4%)	[1]$P < 0.001$ (Poly-3 trend test) *$P =$ 0.011 (Poly-3 test)	Purity, USP grade
F344/N (M) Up to 130 wk NTP (1997b), Abdo & Kari (1996)	Exp. 1: sulfasalazine in corn oil at a dose of 0, or 337.5 mg/kg bw, once per day, 5 days per wk for up to 104 wk, fed ad libitum Exp. 2: unexposed group fed such that mean body weight matched that of the treated group fed ad libitum. Exp. 3 – dietary restriction: two groups of 110 rats (one control and one dosed) were given identical quantities of feed such that the control group would attain body weights of approximately 80% those of the ad libitum-fed controls; 60 rats/group were evaluated at 104 wk (~2 yr) and the remaining 50 rats/group at 130 wk, or when survival reached 20% 50–60 males/group	Transitional cell papilloma of the urinary bladder: *Exp. 1*: 0/50, 6/50* *Exp. 2*: 0/50, 6/50* *Exp. 3*: 0/51, 0/50 (~2 yr) *Exp. 3*: 0/49, 1/49 (up to 130 wk)	*$P =$ 0.011 (logistic regression)	Purity, USP grade

[a] Historical incidence for 2-year studies by the NTP in rats fed corn oil by gavage (vehicle control groups): 3/903 (0.3% ± 0.8%); range, 0–2%

[b] Historical incidence for 2-year studies by the NTP in rats fed corn oil by gavage (vehicle control groups): 0/920

bw, body weight; Exp., experiment; F, female; M, male; NTP, National Toxicology Program; wk, week; USP, United States Pharmacopoeia; yr, year quantities of feed such that the control group would attain body weights of approximately 80% that of the controls fed ad libitum. Sixty rats from each group were evaluated at 104 weeks and the remaining 50 rats from each group were evaluated at 130 weeks, or at the time when survival reached 20%.

After 1 year, mean body weights for the control and treated rats in the first experiment were similar. Since there was negligible body weight loss throughout the study, no adjustments were made to the weight-matched control group, thereby yielding a redundant control group. Survival at 2 years in the first experiment was 70% and 46% for the control and treated rats, respectively.

The incidence of transitional cell papilloma of the urinary bladder was significantly greater in exposed rats than in the controls fed ad libitum in the first experiment, or weight-matched controls in the second experiment. All rats with transitional cell papilloma of the urinary bladder also had grossly visible concretions in the kidney and/or urinary bladder. In the third experiment, no significant increase in the incidence of transitional cell papilloma of the urinary bladder was observed (Abdo & Kari, 1996; NTP, 1997b).

3.3 Studies of co-carcinogenicity

A group of 12 male Wistar rats was given 1,2-dimethylhydrazine at a dose of 40 mg/kg bw as a single subcutaneous injection each week, concurrently with sulfasalazine at a dose of 60 mg/kg bw per day by gavage, for 20 weeks. One control group of 11 male Wistar rats was given 1,2-dimethylhydrazine only. Development of "colon tumours" (mainly adenocarcinomas) was assessed histologically at week 21. All rats developed tumours of the intestine. In the control group receiving 1,2-dimethylhydrazine only, there were 70 tumours of the intestine with a tumour multiplicity of 6.4 ± 0.69, while in the group given 1,2-dimethylhydrazine plus

sulfasalazine there were 141 tumours of the intestine ($P \leq 0.05$, ANOVA test) with a tumour multiplicity of 11.8 ± 2.16 ($P < 0.05$, t-test) (Davis et al., 1992).

4. Mechanistic and Other Relevant Data

4.1 Absorption, distribution, metabolism, and excretion

4.1.1 Humans

(a) Absorption, distribution, metabolism, and excretion

The metabolic scheme for sulfasalazine in humans is shown in Fig. 4.1 (Das & Dubin, 1976; NTP, 1997a).

Sulfasalazine is not absorbed to any significant extent from the stomach (Das & Dubin, 1976). Slow absorption of small amounts (~10–30%) via the small intestine has been reported before enterohepatic recycling, and with the majority of unchanged drug reaching the colon (Das & Dubin, 1976; Azad Khan et al., 1982).

The sulfasalazine molecule comprises 5-ASA and sulfapyridine moieties, linked by an azo bond, which is cleaved by bacterial azoreductases in the colon, releasing 5-ASA and sulfapyridine (Azad Khan et al., 1982). This cleavage is the rate-limiting step for clearance of sulfasalazine (Das & Dubin, 1976). Most of the 5-ASA is excreted; approximately 50% directly in the faeces, and at least 25% via the kidneys (after absorption and acetylation in the liver) (Das & Dubin, 1976; Azad Khan et al., 1982). In contrast, sulfapyridine is almost completely absorbed. In the liver, sulfapyridine undergoes hydroxylation and/or N-acetylation to 5′-hydroxysulfapyridine, N^4-acetylsulfapyridine, and N^4-acetyl-5′-hydroxysulfapyridine subsequently forming glucuronic acid conjugates, before excretion

Fig. 4.1 Metabolic pathways of sulfasalazine in humans

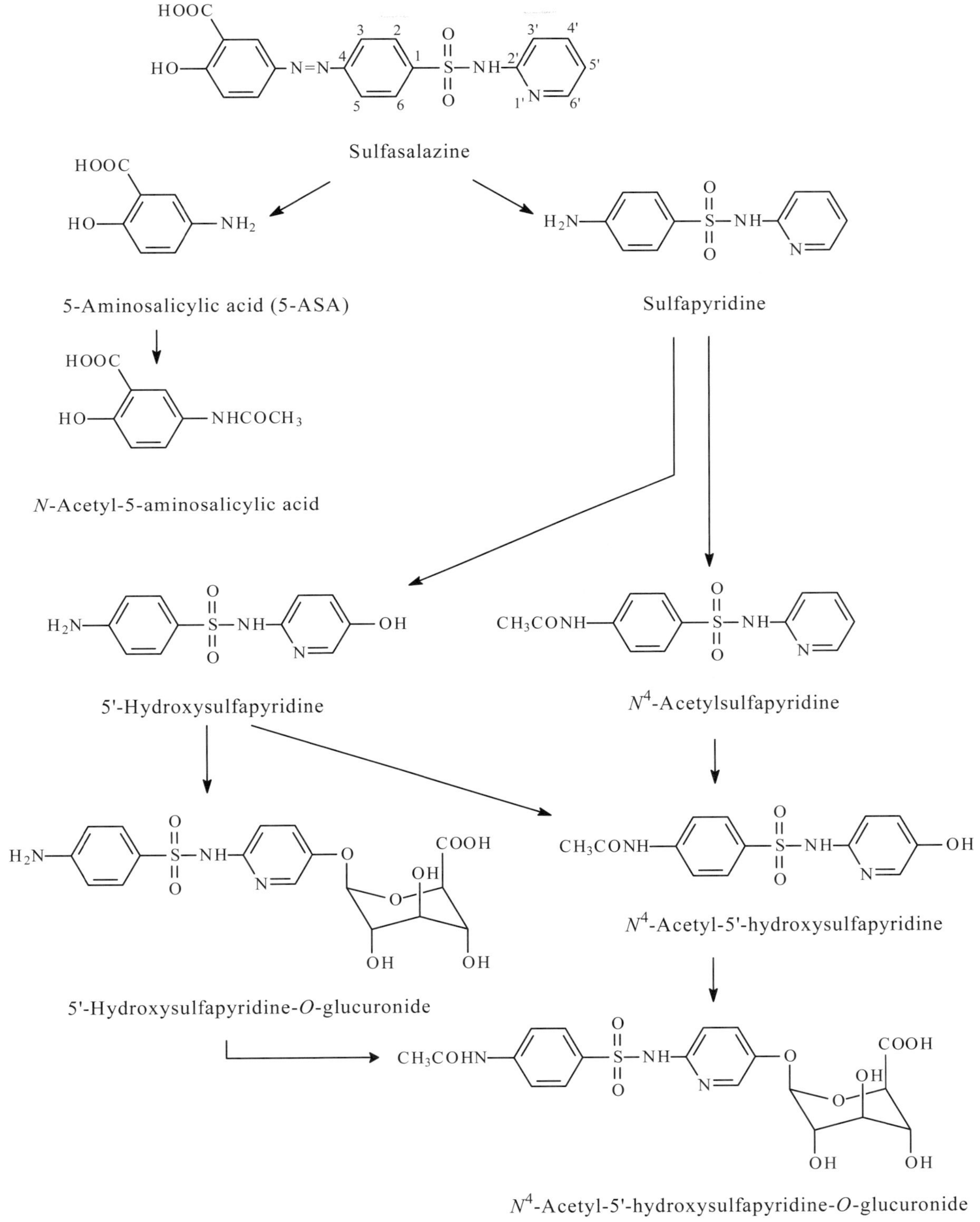

From Das & Dubin (1976), NTP (1997a). With kind permission from Springer Science and Business Media.

mainly in the urine (Das & Dubin, 1976; Azad Khan *et al.*, 1982).

In studies of serum from 10 healthy male volunteers given single oral doses of 4 g of sulfasalazine, parent drug was detectable at 1.5 hours after dosing, and at maximum concentrations at 3–5 hours in nine subjects, and after 7 hours in one subject (Schröder & Campbell, 1972). Metabolites (sulfapyridine, and acetylated and glucuronidated derivatives) were detected in the serum at 3–5 hours after dosing (Schröder & Campbell, 1972). The pharmacokinetics of rectally administered sulfasalazine have been studied in three healthy male Japanese volunteers (Tokui *et al.*, 2002). Sulfasalazine (6.5 mmol), given as a single suppository, reached maximum plasma concentration (2.5 ± 0.4 µM) in 5 hours (T_{max}), and an area under the curve (AUC) of 27.4 ± 4.8 µM.h. Parent drug was almost completely hydrolysed in the colon, and the urinary recovery was only approximately 0.2%. Maximum plasma concentration (C_{max}) of the metabolite *N*-acetyl-5-aminosalicylic acid was 0.5 ± 0.2 µM, reached in 12 hours, while that of sulfapyridine was 1.2 ± 0.4 µM, reached in 5 hours. 5-ASA was not detected in the serum. Administration of an enema containing 6.5 mmol of 5-ASA, resulted in C_{max} 5.8 ± 2.0 µM in 1 hour and an AUC of 29.4 ± 11.1 µM.h. In the urine, approximately 0.3% was recovered unchanged. The C_{max} for the acetylated metabolite, *N*-acetyl-5-aminosalicylic acid, was 13.3 ± 3.6 µM in 7 hours. More than 10% of 5-ASA was excreted in the urine as acetyl-5-aminosalicylic acid, suggesting that absorption of 5-ASA is favoured when administered rectally (Tokui *et al.*, 2002).

A study to compare the absorption and metabolism of oral preparations of sulfasalazine, mesalazine (5-ASA) and olsalazine (a dimer of 5-ASA) used regularly by patients ($n = 12, 13$, and 8, respectively) for treatment of ulcerative colitis, showed considerably greater absorption of 5-ASA and less acetylation, in patients receiving mesalazine than in those receiving olsalazine or sulfasalazine (Stretch *et al.*, 1996).

(a)   *Variation in absorption, distribution, metabolism, and excretion*

(i)   *IBD and rheumatoid arthritis*

The characteristics of absorption, metabolism, and excretion of the parent drug in four patients with IBD (ulcerative colitis or Crohn disease) were similar to those in four healthy subjects, each given a single oral dose of sulfasalazine (3 or 4 g). However, absorption and urinary excretion of the metabolite, sulfapyridine, was decreased in patients with IBD. The metabolism of sulfasalazine was markedly reduced in patients taking antibiotics and after removal of the large bowel (Azad Khan *et al.*, 1982).

Pharmacokinetic studies of sulfasalazine and its principal metabolites in 13 patients with rheumatoid arthritis and 8 patients with IBD given sulfasalazine as a single oral dose of 2 g (Astbury *et al.*, 1990), showed that patients with rheumatoid arthritis had a significantly higher (and more sustained) plasma concentration of sulfapyridine than did patients with IBD (medians of 14.0 µg/mL and 7.4 µg/mL, respectively). Two factors may have contributed to high peak plasma concentrations of sulfapyridine in patients with rheumatoid arthritis: firstly, the metabolism of sulfapyridine may be impaired, and secondly, a larger quantity of sulfasalazine may reach the lower bowel leading to higher concentrations of the subsequent cleavage compounds. The pharmacokinetics of sulfasalazine were variable among patients; maximum plasma concentrations of sulfapyridine ranged from 8 to 22 µg/mL in patients with rheumatoid arthritis, and from 5 to 18 µg/mL in patients with IBD. The elimination half-life of sulfasalazine ranged from 3 to 8 hours in patients with rheumatoid arthritis, and from 4 to 9 hours in patients with IBD (Astbury *et al.*, 1990).

(ii)   Pregnancy

Sulfasalazine and its primary metabolites are able to cross the placenta (Azad Khan & Truelove, 1979; Järnerot *et al.*, 1981). In five patients with ulcerative colitis treated with sulfasalazine (0.5 g, four times per day) throughout and after pregnancy, sulfasalazine was detected in the umbilical cord blood (mean concentration, 50% of that in maternal serum) and at very low concentrations in the amniotic fluid (Azad Khan & Truelove, 1979). Analyses of metabolites showed that total concentrations of sulfapyridine were equal in maternal and cord sera, but concentrations of free sulfapyridine were significantly lower ($P < 0.02$) in cord sera. Total concentrations of acetylated sulfapyridine were significantly higher ($P < 0.025$) in cord sera than maternal sera. Total concentrations of 5-ASA were very low in all fluids analysed (Azad Khan & Truelove, 1979). In the study by Järnerot et al. (1981) of 11 pregnant patients with IBD treated with sulfasalazine (1 g daily), concentrations of sulfasalazine were almost identical in cord and maternal serum. Seven of the women were analysed at a later date (4–24 months) after pregnancy; plasma concentrations of sulfasalazine remained the same, but concentrations of sulfapyridine had increased, probably reflecting different extents of protein binding of these compounds, and the different distribution volume in pregnancy (Järnerot *et al.*, 1981).

Small quantities of sulfasalazine and sulfapyridine have also been detected in breast milk (Azad Khan & Truelove, 1979; Järnerot & Into-Malmberg, 1979). Mean concentrations of sulfasalazine and total sulfapyridine in milk, compared with concentrations in maternal serum, were approximately 30% and 50%, respectively, as reported by Azad Khan & Truelove (1979), and negligible and 40%, respectively as reported by Järnerot & Into-Malmberg (1979). The various metabolites of sulfapyridine were present in approximately the same proportions

as in maternal serum (Azad Khan & Truelove, 1979). It was estimated that an infant would receive sulfapyridine at dose of 3–4 mg/kg bw, after a maternal dose of 2 g of sulfasalazine per day (Järnerot & Into-Malmberg, 1979). Sulfapyridine and its acetylated and glucuronidated metabolites have been shown to be excreted by babies, 1–2.5 months after maternal dosing (Järnerot & Into-Malmberg, 1979).

(c)   Genetic polymorphisms

(i)   N-Acetyltransferases

The sulfasalazine molecule may be considered as a slow-release carrier for sulfapyridine, but there is large inter-individual variation in the rate of metabolism of sulfapyridine, which can affect steady-state serum concentrations (Das & Dubin, 1976). The rate of *N*-acetylation of 5-ASA to *N*-acetyl-5-aminosalicylic acid is under genetic control (Das & Dubin, 1976). The cytosolic *N*-acetyltransferase (NAT) family comprises NAT1 and NAT2, which catalyse the transfer of acetyl groups from activated acetyl-coenzyme A to the nitrogen of primary amines, hydrazines, or hydrazides (Kuhn *et al.*, 2010). Single nucleotide polymorphisms have been detected in *NAT2*. The wildtype has been designated *NAT2*4*, but *NAT2*5*, *NAT2*6*, and *NAT2*7* alleles encode *N*-acetyltransferase enzymes with amino-acid changes that cause reduced activity (slow acetylating function). Patients with a "slow" acetylator phenotype generally show significantly higher, and more sustained plasma concentrations of sulfapyridine and its non-acetylated metabolites. The elimination half-life of sulfasalazine in patients with a slow-acetylator phenotype may be approximately 50–100% longer than in those with a fast-acetylator phenotype (Taggart *et al.*, 1992).

A 1–3 year study of 185 patients with ulcerative colitis undergoing daily treatment with sulfasalazine (2 g per day) demonstrated that serum concentrations of sulfapyridine (both free and total) were higher in patients with a slow-acetylator phenotype (Azad Khan *et al.*, 1983). Concentrations of sulfasalazine and of 5-ASA were not significantly different in fast and slow acetylators. These findings were confirmed by later studies (Taggart *et al.*, 1992).

The frequency of polymorphism in *NAT2* varies in different racial or ethnic populations (Ma *et al.*, 2009). Studies have shown that about 60% of patients with IBD, studied in Edinburgh, Scotland, are slow acetylators (Das *et al.*, 1973), and a similar proportion was found in healthy volunteers in a study in Liverpool, England (Schröder & Evans, 1972). In Germany, a study of *NAT2* genotype and acetylation, using sulfasalazine as probe drug, showed that 24 out of 44 healthy volunteers (54.5%) were slow acetylators, in accordance with the "slight prevalence of slow acetylators in central European (Caucasian) populations" which has been reported in several studies (Kuhn *et al.*, 2010).

The *NAT2* genotype has also been investigated in Asian populations. Studies in 21 Japanese subjects (8 healthy subjects and 13 patients with IBD) given a single oral dose of sulfasalazine at 40 mg/kg bw demonstrated generally good correlation between three *NAT2* genotypes (rapid, intermediate, slow acetylators) and the plasma or urinary concentrations of sulfapyridine and N^4-acetyl sulfapyridine (Tanigawara *et al.*, 2002). Similar analyses in seven healthy Japanese subjects after 8 days of continued ("multiple dosing") oral doses of 1 g of sulfasalazine once per day also demonstrated correlation with genotype (Kita *et al.*, 2001). In 18 healthy Chinese men given 1 g of sulfasalazine as a single oral dose, the *NAT2* gene was shown to be an important determinant of metabolite profiles; the frequency of slow acetylators in the Chinese population was lower than in Caucasians, but higher than in the Japanese population (Ma *et al.*, 2009).

The effects of age and acetylator status on the pharmacokinetics of sulfasalazine were compared in patients with rheumatoid arthritis (8 young and 12 elderly, with equal numbers of slow and fast acetylators in both age groups), each receiving sulfasalazine at 2 g per day for 21 days (Taggart *et al.*, 1992). In the elderly, the elimination half-life of sulfasalazine was increased [possibly partly due to slow cleavage of the azo bond (Tett, 1993)], and steady-state serum concentrations of N-acetyl-5-aminosalicylic acid were higher. The pharmacokinetics of sulfapyridine were unchanged with age, but were influenced by acetylation status, in particular, with increased steady-state serum concentrations in slow acetylators. Although age is a determinant of the steady-state concentration of salicylate moieties, the acetylator phenotype seems to play the greater role in determining serum concentrations of sulfapyridine (Taggart *et al.*, 1992).

(ii) Role of transporter proteins

An efflux ATP-binding cassette (ABC) transporter, the breast cancer resistance BCRP protein (encoded by the *ABCG2* gene), has a role in the pharmacokinetics of various drugs, including sulfasalazine. The BCRP protein is expressed at the luminal membrane of cells with key functions in drug transport, namely, placental trophoblast cells, hepatocyte bile canaliculi, kidney cells, and enterocytes.

The poor bioavailability of sulfasalazine has long been attributed to its low solubility and poor permeability (Das & Dubin, 1976). However, treatment of human T-cells with sulfasalazine was shown to cause cellular drug resistance that was mediated by induction of BCRP (*ABCG2*), suggesting that sulfasalazine may be a substrate for human BCRP (van der Heijden *et al.*, 2004; Urquhart *et al.*, 2008).

A subsequent study in vitro, using data on expression in human tissue, indicated an association between reduced cell surface expression of the 421C > A variant and reduced BCRP-mediated transport of sulfasalazine in patients carrying an A allele at position 421 of the *BCRP* [*ABCG2*] gene (Urquhart *et al.*, 2008).

Variation in the *ABCG2* gene may impair the transport of drugs that are substrates for the ABC transporter, leading to increased intestinal absorption, and/or decreased biliary excretion, and result in high plasma concentrations, as demonstrated in 37 healthy Japanese people selected according to *ABCG2* and *NAT2* genotype and given a single oral dose of 2 g of sulfasalazine (Yamasaki *et al.*, 2008). They showed that in *ABCG2-A/A* subjects, mean plasma AUC_{0-48h} and C_{max} values for sulfasalazine were significantly higher, and the AUC for sulfapyridine was lower (except in those who also had the slow-acetylator *NAT2* genotype) than in individuals without the *ABCG2* variant. The increased AUC for sulfasalazine in *ABCG2-A/A* subjects may result from increased oral availability and/or decreased hepatic clearance, since BCRP is expressed on enterocytes and hepatocytes. The ratios of $AUC_{acetylsulfapyridine}/AUC_{sulfapyridine}$ were significantly higher in subjects with the rapid-acetylator *NAT2* phenotype than in those with intermediate or slow genotypes, demonstrating that inter-individual variability in the pharmacokinetics of sulfasalazine can be attributed to genetic polymorphism in drug transport and metabolism (Yamasaki *et al.*, 2008).

4.1.2 Experimental systems

(a) Absorption, distribution, metabolism, and excretion

Experimental studies in Sprague-Dawley rats given diets containing sulfasalazine have shown that most of the sulfasalazine is reductively cleaved by intestinal bacteria to two compounds, 5-ASA (which is poorly absorbed) and sulfapyridine (which is well absorbed) (Peppercorn & Goldman, 1972). After metabolism by mammalian enzymes, 5-ASA and sulfapyridine are excreted mainly in the faeces, and in the urine, respectively (Peppercorn & Goldman, 1972).

In male and female $B6C3F_1$ mice given sulfasalazine as an intravenous dose at 5 mg/kg bw, plasma concentrations of the parent drug rapidly declined with a mean elimination half-life of 0.5 hour in males and 1.2 hour in females (Zheng *et al.*, 1993). The sex-specific differences in clearance rate were reflected in $AUC_{sulfasalazine}$ values (9.21 µM.h^{-1} and 21.39 µM.h^{-1}, in males and females, respectively).

In male and female $B6C3F_1$ mice given sulfasalazine by gavage at various doses (67.5, 675, 1350, or 2700 mg/kg bw), the bioavailability of the parent drug was approximately 17% (range, 16–18%) at the lowest dose (67.5 mg/kg bw), and was lower (range, 3–9%) at the higher doses. Both sulfapyridine and N^4-acetylsulfapyridine were identified in the plasma. Sulfapyridine was eliminated more slowly than the parent compound, and thus accumulated in all mice given multiple doses of sulfasalazine. The differential between plasma concentrations of sulfapyridine and sulfasalazine varied, however, between males and females: the AUCs for sulfapyridine, at all four doses of sulfasalazine, were higher than those of parent drug by 21–32 times in males and by 5–25 times in females, while maximum plasma concentrations were higher than those of the parent drug by 6–8 times in male mice, and up to 4 times in females. Plasma concentrations of N^4-acetylsulfapyridine were very low compared with those of sulfapyridine. [This indicated slow acetylation of sulfapyridine by $B6C3F_1$ mice, comparable to that found in humans with the slow-acetylator phenotype.] The pharmacokinetic pattern in $B6C3F_1$ mice given multiple oral doses of sulfasalazine (i.e. daily doses for three consecutive days) was similar to that in mice given a single oral dose, but accumulation of sulfapyridine was evident, producing greater $AUC_{sulfapyridine}$ values in the multiple-dose study than in the single-dose study (Zheng *et al.*, 1993).

In a study by the NTP (1997a), male F344/N rats were given sulfasalazine as an intravenous dose at 5 mg/kg bw, and pharmacokinetic parameters were compared with those in the study in male B6C3F$_1$ mice by Zheng *et al.* (1993). The rats retained sulfasalazine longer than mice; the AUC for sulfasalazine in rats was double that in mice, while values for systemic clearance and apparent volume of distribution in mice were double those in rats. The rate of elimination of sulfasalazine was similar in rats and mice; plasma elimination rate constants were 1.47 per hour and 1.28 per hour, respectively, and elimination half-lives, 0.53 hour and 0.54 hour, respectively. In F344/N rats given a low oral dose of 67.5 mg/kg bw, sulfasalazine and its metabolites were undetectable; however, after a higher dose (675 mg/kg bw), plasma concentrations of parent compound were detectable within 12 hours (NTP, 1997a).

(b) Role of transporter proteins

BCRP is a member of the ATP-dependent efflux transporters, which includes P-glycoprotein or multi-drug resistance protein 1 (*MDR1/ABCB1*) and multidrug resistance-associated protein 2 (*MRP2/ABCC2*). These transporter proteins have significant roles in the processes of drug absorption, distribution, and clearance, and are expressed at the apical membrane of cells in the liver, kidney, brain, placenta, colon, and intestine. From the latter location, on the villus tip of the apical brush-border membrane of intestinal enterocytes, they actively cause efflux of drugs from gut epithelial cells back into the intestinal lumen.

In experiments in *Bcrp$^{-/-}$* [*Abcg2$^{-/-}$*] knockout mice given sulfasalazine, the AUC for sulfasalazine was greater than in wildtype mice by 13-fold after an intravenous dose (5 mg/kg bw) and 111-fold after an oral dose (20 mg/kg bw) (Zaher *et al.*, 2006). This treatment in the *mdr1a* [*Abcb1a*] knockout mouse did not significantly change the AUC for sulfasalazine. Furthermore, studies in wildtype mice treated with an inhibitor of Bcrp (gefitinib) before an oral dose of sulfasalazine resulted in a 13-fold increase in the AUC of plasma sulfasalazine compared with nontreated

controls. This work thus demonstrated that Bcrp has a key role in controlling [i.e. maintaining a low (Dahan & Amidon, 2010)] oral bioavailability of sulfasalazine (Zaher *et al.*, 2006).

In Caco-2 cells, sulfasalazine normally exhibits a basolateral-to-apical permeability that is 19 times higher than apical-to-basolateral permeability, indicative of net mucosal secretion (Dahan & Amidon, 2009). In this study of three ATP-dependent efflux transporters (in Caco-2 cells and rat jejunum), specific inhibitors of BCRP and of MRP2 were shown to disrupt the normal direction of sulfasalazine permeability. The presence of both MRP2 and BCRP inhibitors produced an efflux ratio of 1, indicating no efflux of sulfasalazine. Inhibitors of P-glycoprotein had no effect on the movement of sulfasalazine. The results thus suggested that efflux transport of sulfasalazine is mediated by BCRP and MRP2 (Dahan & Amidon, 2009). A more recent study of sulfasalazine absorption has shown that curcumin is a potent inhibitor of human BCRP. Curcumin not only increased the plasma AUC$_{0-8h}$ eightfold in wildtype mice (but not in *Bcrp$^{-/-}$* mice), but also increased the plasma AUC$_{0-24h}$ by twofold at microdoses of sulfasalazine and by 3.2-fold at therapeutic doses in humans (Kusuhara *et al.*, 2012).

Further studies of the absorption characteristics of sulfasalazine in the isolated mouse intestine, have indicated that both influx and efflux transporters are involved in the intestinal absorption of sulfasalazine (Tomaru *et al.*, 2013). OATP2B1 is a multispecific organic anion influx transporter. Like BCRP, it is localized at the brush-border membrane of intestinal epithelial cells, and mediates uptake of many endogenous and xenobiotic substrates from the lumen. Like BCRP, sulfasalazine is a substrate for OATP2B1 (Kusuhara *et al.*, 2012; Tomaru *et al.*, 2013). The study by Kusuhara *et al.* (2012) was inspired by the finding that pharmacokinetic data (plasma AUC for parent drug) from human subjects given sulfasalazine, at either a microdose (100 µg suspension) or a therapeutic dose (2 g as tablets), demonstrated nonlinearity between doses in the AUC of plasma sulfasalazine (Kusuhara *et al.*, 2012). Investigations of sulfasalazine transport were performed in three systems in vitro, namely: (i) ATP-dependent uptake of sulfasalazine by membrane vesicles expressing human BCRP; (ii) oral bioavailability of sulfasalazine in vivo, in wildtype and *Bcrp*−/− mice; and (iii) uptake of sulfasalazine in HEK293 cells transfected with the influx transporter *OATP2B1* (*SLCO2B1*). The results indicated that sulfasalazine is a substrate for OATP2B1, and that saturation of the influx transporter OATP2B1 at the therapeutic dose is a possible mechanism underlying nonlinearity in the dose–exposure relationship for sulfasalazine (Kusuhara *et al.*, 2012).

The nonsteroidal anti-inflammatory drug indomethacin (an inhibitor of the MRP family that includes MRP2) has been shown to change, in a concentration-dependent manner, the direction of membrane permeability to sulfasalazine in Caco-2 cells; high concentrations of indomethacin substantially reduced efflux of sulfasalazine. Efflux was not however abolished, due to the contribution of BCRP to the control of absorption. Additionally, an indomethacin-induced increase in sulfasalazine permeability through the gut wall was also shown in the rat jejunal perfusion model. The concomitant intake of indomethacin and sulfasalazine may lead to increased absorption of sulfasalazine in the small intestine, reducing its concentration in the colon, and potentially altering its therapeutic effect (Dahan & Amidon, 2010).

4.2 Genetic and related effects

Several studies, particularly those conducted in vivo, have demonstrated genotoxicity associated with sulfasalazine and some of its metabolites. The mutagenicity of sulfasalazine and its two major metabolites, sulfapyridine and 5-ASA, was reviewed by Iatropoulos *et al.* (1997).

4.2.1 Humans

See Table 4.1

Mitelman *et al.* (1982) reported that there was no clear evidence of chromosomal damage in lymphocytes of patients receiving sulfasalazine for 1 month or 4 months at 3 g per day, although an effect could not be ruled out.

Increased frequencies of micronucleus formation and sister chromatid exchange in patients with IBD receiving sulfasalazine have been reported, but confounding factors were apparent in the study (Erskine *et al.*, 1984).

4.2.2 Experimental systems

See Table 4.1

(a) Mutagenicity

Sulfasalazine was not mutagenic in assays for gene mutation in bacteria, including a variety of strains of *Salmonella typhimurium*, *Escherichia coli*, and *Klebsiella pneumoniae*, in a variety of protocols, with or without metabolic activation (Voogd *et al.*, 1980; Zeiger *et al.*, 1988; Iatropoulos *et al.*, 1997). In addition, treatment with sulfasalazine did not result in an increase in mutations conferring 6-thioguanine resistance in mouse lymphoma L5178Y cells, with or without metabolic activation (Iatropoulos *et al.*, 1997).

(b) Chromosomal damage

Mackay *et al.* (1989) reported positive results in a test for induction of sister chromatid exchange in cultured human lymphocytes treated with sulfasalazine at a concentration of 20–160 µg/mL in the absence of metabolic activation. In contrast, Bishop *et al.* (1990) observed no increase in the frequency of sister chromatid exchange in Chinese hamster ovary cells treated with sulfasalazine at up to 1000 µg/mL, with or without metabolic activation. An increase in the formation of micronuclei in cultured human

Table 4.1 Genetic and related effects of sulfasalazine

Test system	Results[a]		Dose[b] (LED or HID)	Reference
	Without exogenous metabolic system	With exogenous metabolic system		
In vitro				
Salmonella typhimurium TA100, TA1535, TA97, TA98, reverse mutation	–	– [c]	6666 µg/plate	Zeiger *et al.* (1988)
Salmonella typhimurium TA100, TA1535, TA97, TA98, reverse mutation	–	–	6250 µg/plate	Iatropoulos *et al.* (1997)[d]
Escherichia coli,WP2 *uvrA*-p, reverse mutation	–	–	6250 µg/plate	Iatropoulos *et al.* (1997)[d]
Klebsiella pneumoniae, fluctuation test, base substitution mutation	–	NT	0.5 g/L	Voogd *et al.* (1980)
Mouse lymphoma L5178Y cells, 6-thioguanine resistance	–	–	700 µg/mL (–S9) 500 µg/mL (+S9)	Iatropoulos *et al.* (1997)[d]
Sister chromatid exchange, Chinese hamster ovary cells	–	–	160 µg/mL (–S9) 1000 µg/mL (+S9)	Bishop *et al.* (1990)
Sister chromatid exchange, human lymphocytes	+	NT	20 µg/mL	Mackay *et al.* (1989)
Micronucleus formation, human lymphocytes	+	NT	40 µg/mL	Mackay *et al.* (1989)
Chromosomal aberration, Chinese hamster ovary cells	–	–	1000 µg/mL	Bishop *et al.* (1990)
Chromosomal aberration, human lymphocytes	–	–	100 µg/mL	Iatropoulos *et al.* (1997)[d]
In vivo				
Micronucleus formation, male B6C3F$_1$ mouse, bone-marrow cells	+		1000 mg/kg bw, po × 2	Bishop *et al.* (1990)
Micronucleus formation, male and female B6C3F$_1$ mouse, peripheral blood erythrocytes	+		675 mg/kg bw, po × 13 wk	Bishop *et al.* (1990)
Micronucleus formation (kinetochore-positive), male B6C3F$_1$ mouse, bone-marrow cells	+		1389 mg/kg bw, po × 3	Witt *et al.* (1992a)
Micronucleus formation (total micronuclei), male B6C3F$_1$ mouse, bone-marrow cells	+		1389 mg/kg bw, po × 3	Witt *et al.* (1992a)
Micronucleus formation (kinetochore-negative), male B6C3F$_1$ mouse, bone-marrow cells	+		5634 mg/kg bw, po × 3	Witt *et al.* (1992a)
Micronucleus formation, male B6C3F$_1$ mouse, bone-marrow cells	+		1000 mg/kg bw, po × 3	NTP (1997a)
Micronucleus formation, female B6C3F$_1$ mouse, bone-marrow cells	+		1000 mg/kg bw, po × 3	NTP (1997a)
Micronucleus formation, male B6C3F$_1$ mouse, bone-marrow cells	–		4000 mg/kg bw, po × 1	NTP (1997a)

Table 4.1 (continued)

Test system	Results[a]		Dose[b] (LED or HID)	Reference
	Without exogenous metabolic system	With exogenous metabolic system		
Micronucleus formation, male F344 rat, bone-marrow cells	?		3000 mg/kg bw, po × 3[e]	NTP (1997a)
Chromosomal aberration, male B6C3F$_1$ mouse, bone marrow cells	–		1000 mg/kg bw, po × 1	Bishop *et al.* (1990)
Chromosomal aberration, male B6C3F$_1$ mouse, bone-marrow cells	–		4000 mg/kg bw, po × 3	NTP (1997a)
Chromosomal aberration, male and female Sprague-Dawley rat, bone-marrow cells	–		500 mg/kg bw, po × 1[f]	Iatropoulos *et al.* (1997)[d]
Chromosomal aberration, human lymphocytes	–		3 g/day for 4 months	Mitelman *et al.* (1980)

[a] +, positive; –, negative; ?, inconclusive
[b] In-vitro test, μg/mL; in-vivo test, mg/kg bw per day
[c] S9 from liver of Aroclor 1254-treated Sprague-Dawley rats and Syrian hamsters
[d] Studies conducted by Pharmacia, not published; results summarized in Iatropoulos *et al.* (1997)
[e] Two trials were conducted; the first trial gave positive results at the highest dose of 2700 mg/kg bw (po × 3), and the second gave negative results (HID, 3000 mg/kg bw, po × 3). The overall result was equivocal on the basis of nonreproducibility of the positive response
[f] Chromosomal aberration was measured at 6, 24, and 48 hours after treatment
HID, highest ineffective dose; LED, lowest effective dose; NT, not tested; po, oral

lymphocytes after treatment with sulfasalazine (effective concentration range, 40–160 µg/mL) in the absence of metabolic activation was reported by Mackay *et al.* (1989). No significant increases in the frequency of chromosomal aberration were observed in cultured Chinese hamster ovary cells (Bishop *et al.*, 1990), or cultured human lymphocytes (Iatropoulos *et al.*, 1997), treated with sulfasalazine (concentration, up to 1000 or 100 µg/mL, respectively). Thus the results of tests for chromosomal damage in vitro after treatment with sulfasalazine were generally negative, although sporadic positive results were reported.

In vivo, consistent with results reported in assays in vitro, no increases in the frequency of chromosomal aberration were observed in male mice or male and female rats treated with sulfasalazine by gavage at doses of up to 4000 mg/kg bw per day (Bishop *et al.*, 1990; Iatropoulos *et al.*, 1997; NTP, 1997a).

The results of assays for micronucleus formation in male and female mice treated with sulfasalazine were uniformly positive when multiple treatments (at least two) were employed (Bishop *et al.*, 1990; Witt *et al.*, 1992a, NTP, 1997a). Further investigation of the nature of the induced micronuclei revealed that the majority were kinetochore-positive, suggesting that the micronuclei contained whole chromosomes rather than fragments, and were primarily due to aneuploidy events rather than chromosome breakage (Witt *et al.*, 1992a). This observation was consistent with the negative results in assays for chromosomal aberration with sulfasalazine in vitro and in vivo (Mitelman *et al.*, 1980; Bishop *et al.*, 1990; Iatropoulos *et al.*, 1997; NTP, 1997a). The negative results of one test in male mice given a single dose of sulfasalazine at 4000 mg/kg bw underscored the need for multiple treatments to induce an observable increase in micronucleus formation (NTP, 1997a).

In addition to the necessity for multiple treatments, sulfasalazine may also demonstrate selective activity in mice; the results of a study on micronucleus formation in bone marrow of male rats given three doses of sulfasalazine (highest dose, 3000 mg/kg bw) were judged to be equivocal (NTP, 1997a); in this assay, an initial trial gave a positive response at the highest dose of 2700 mg/kg bw, but a second trial, with a highest dose of 3000 mg/kg bw, gave negative results. This apparent preferential activity in mice was consistent with the observation that mice have a greater systemic exposure than rats to sulfapyridine, the active moiety, after administration of similar doses (Zheng *et al.*, 1993).

In one study, no evidence for genotoxicity was obtained for sulfasalazine when tested for the induction of micronuclei in mouse bone marrow, with or without pretreatment with folate. Likewise, no evidence for formation of DNA adducts was detected by ^{32}P-postlabelling in rat and mouse liver and urinary bladder (Iatropoulos *et al.*, 1997). [The nuclease P1 enrichment procedure was used in the ^{32}P-postlabelling method. Assuming that *N*-hydroxylation of sulfapyridine occurred in vivo, adducts derived from this metabolite would probably be lost.]

4.2.3 Genotoxicity of sulfasalazine metabolites

See Table 4.2

Sulfasalazine has two major metabolites, sulfapyridine (a carrier molecule that allows transport of sulfasalazine to the intestine, where it is activated) and 5-ASA, the therapeutically active moiety.

(a) 5-ASA

5-ASA has not shown activity in any assay for genotoxicity in vitro or in vivo. It does not induce mutations in any of a variety of *Salmonella typhimurium* strains, with or without metabolic activation or in *Klebsiella pneumoniae* in the absence of metabolic activation (Voogd *et al.*, 1980). No induction of sister chromatid exchange, micronucleus formation, or chromosomal aberration

Table 4.2 Genetic and related effects of metabolites of sulfasalazine

Test system	Results[a]		Dose[b] (LED or HID)	Reference
	Without exogenous metabolic system	With exogenous metabolic system		
5-Aminosalicylic acid				
Salmonella typhimurium TA100, TA1537, TA98, reverse mutation	–	–	10 g/L (TA1537, TA98) 5 g/L (TA100)	Voogd *et al.* (1980)
Klebsiella pneumoniae, fluctuation test, base-substitution mutation	–	NT	0.5 g/L	Voogd *et al.* (1980)
Sister chromatid exchange, Chinese hamster ovary cells, in vitro	–	–	280 µg/mL	Witt *et al.* (1992b)
Sister chromatid exchange, human lymphocytes, in vitro	–	NT	16 µg/mL	Mackay *et al.* (1989)
Micronucleus formation, human lymphocytes, in vitro	–	NT	16 µg/mL	Mackay *et al.* (1989)
Chromosomal aberration, Chinese hamster ovary cells, in vitro	–	–	280 µg/mL	Witt *et al.* (1992b)
Micronucleus formation, male B6C3F$_1$ mouse, bone-marrow cells, in vivo	–		250 mg/kg bw, ip × 3	Witt *et al.* (1992b)
Sulfapyridine				
Sister chromatid exchange, Chinese hamster ovary cells, in vitro	+	–	1667 µg/mL	Witt *et al.* (1992b)
Chromosomal aberration, Chinese hamster ovary cells, in vitro	–	–	5000 µg/mL	Witt *et al.* (1992b)
Sister chromatid exchange, human lymphocytes, in vitro	+	NT	200 µg/mL	Mackay *et al.* (1989)
Micronucleus formation, human lymphocytes, in vitro	–	NT	400 µg/mL	Mackay *et al.* (1989)
Micronucleus formation, male B6C3F$_1$ mouse, bone-marrow cells, in vivo	+		1000 mg/kg bw, ip × 3	Witt *et al.* (1992b)
Micronucleus formation (kinetochore-positive), male B6C3F$_1$ mouse, bone-marrow cells, in vivo	+		714 mg/kg bw, po × 3	Witt *et al.* (1992a)
Micronucleus formation (total micronuclei), male B6C3F$_1$ mouse, bone-marrow cells, in vivo	+		714 mg/kg bw, po × 3	Witt *et al.* (1992a)
Micronucleus formation (kinetochore negative), male B6C3F$_1$ mouse, bone-marrow cells, in vivo	+		1429 mg/kg bw, po × 3	Witt *et al.* (1992a)
N[4]-*Acetylsulfapyridine*				
Sister chromatid exchange, human lymphocytes, in vitro	+	NT	80 µg/mL	Mackay *et al.* (1989)
Micronucleus formation, human lymphocytes, in vitro	+	NT	20 µg/mL	Mackay *et al.* (1989)
N[4]-*Acetyl-5′-hydroxysulfapyridine*				
Sister chromatid exchange, human lymphocytes, in vitro	+	NT	80 µg/mL	Mackay *et al.* (1989)
Micronucleus formation, human lymphocytes, in vitro	–	NT	80 µg/mL	Mackay *et al.* (1989)

Table 4.2 (continued)

Test system	Results[a]		Dose[b] (LED or HID)	Reference
	Without exogenous metabolic system	With exogenous metabolic system		
5'-Hydroxysulfapyridine				
Sister chromatid exchange, human lymphocytes, in vitro	–	NT	80 µg/mL	Mackay *et al.* (1989)
Micronucleus formation, human lymphocytes, in vitro	–	NT	80 µg/mL	Mackay *et al.* (1989)
N-Acetyl-5-aminosalicylic acid				
Sister chromatid exchange, human lymphocytes, in vitro	–	NT	8 µg/mL	Mackay *et al.* (1989)
Micronucleus formation, human lymphocytes, in vitro	–	NT	8 µg/mL	Mackay *et al.* (1989)

[a] +, positive; –, negative

[b] In-vitro test, µg/mL; in-vivo test, mg/kg bw per day

HID, highest ineffective dose; ip, intraperitoneal; LED, lowest effective dose; po, oral has been reported in human lymphocytes or Chinese hamster ovary cells in vitro (Mackay *et al.*, 1989; Witt *et al.*, 1992b). In vivo, no increase in the frequency of micronucleated polychromatic erythrocytes was observed in the bone marrow of male mice treated with 5-ASA (dose range, 125–250 mg/kg bw per day for 3 days) by intraperitoneal injection (Witt *et al.*, 1992b).

(b) Sulfapyridine

Sulfapyridine has been reported to induce sister chromatid exchange in Chinese hamster ovary cells and cultured human lymphocytes in the absence of metabolic activation (Mackay *et al.*, 1989; Witt *et al.*, 1992b); no increase in the frequency of sister chromatid exchange was noted in the presence of metabolic activation in Chinese hamster ovary cells (Witt *et al.*, 1992b). Sulfapyridine did not induce chromosomal aberration in Chinese hamster ovary cells, with or without metabolic activation (Witt *et al.*, 1992b). Mackay *et al.* (1989) reported that sulfapyridine did not induce micronucleus formation in cultured human lymphocytes in the absence of metabolic activation, at concentrations that reached 400 µg/mL. Sulfapyridine induced a strong, dose-related increase in the frequency of micronucleated polychromatic erythrocytes when administered either as multiple intraperitoneal injections (Witt *et al.*, 1992b) or by gavage (Witt *et al.*, 1992a). As with sulfasalazine, the majority of micronucleated erythrocytes induced by sulfapyridine in mice were shown to contain kinetochores (Witt *et al.*, 1992a), implying that sulfapyridine-induced micronucleus formation resulted from failure of mitotic chromosomal segregation, rather than chromosome breakage.

(c) Metabolites of 5-ASA and sulfapyridine

Mackay *et al.* (1989) also tested four acetylated and/or hydroxylated metabolites of sulfapyridine and 5-ASA for their ability to induce sister chromatid exchange and micronucleus formation in cultured human lymphocytes. N^4-acetylsulfapyridine was capable of inducing both sister chromatid exchange and micronucleus formation, while N^4-acetyl-5′-hydroxysulfapyridine only induced sister chromatid exchange. 5′-Hydroxysulfapyridine and N^4-acetyl-5-aminosalicylic acid did not induce either sister chromatid exchange or micronucleus formation at the concentrations tested.

4.3 Other mechanistic data relevant to carcinogenicity

4.3.1 Adverse effects

In humans, sulfasalazine is associated with a wide range of adverse side-effects that include agranulocytosis (Kaufman *et al.*, 1996), hepatotoxicity (de Abajo *et al.*, 2004; Jobanputra *et al.*, 2008), nephrotoxicity (Gisbert *et al.*, 2007), neurotoxicity (Liedorp *et al.*, 2008), and pulmonary toxicity (Parry *et al.*, 2002). Sulfasalazine is also associated with reversible infertility in men and in male experimental animals (O'Moráin *et al.*, 1984). Reactions to sulfasalazine may result from an idiosyncratic delayed-type hypersensitivity reaction that may affect internal organs in variable ways (Jobanputra *et al.*, 2008).

Case reports of serious hepatotoxicity associated with sulfasalazine are frequent and occur predominantly within the first month of starting therapy; the pattern of liver injury can be hepatocellular or cholestatic, and may lead to liver failure. Serious hepatotoxicity, which could be a part of the DRESS (drug rash, eosinophilia and systemic symptoms) syndrome is described in approximately 0.1% of users, but the estimated incidence is higher (0.4%) in patients with inflammatory arthritis (de Abajo *et al.*, 2004; Jobanputra *et al.*, 2008).

Renal toxicity associated with sulfasalazine treatment may be irreversible. Although the sulfapyridine moiety is thought to be responsible for most of the adverse effects of sulfasalazine, several case reports in patients with IBD indicate that renal toxicity in humans may occur from treatment with both sulfasalazine and 5-ASA (Gisbert *et al.*, 2007). Clinically, 5-ASA-associated nephrotoxicity is typically expressed as interstitial nephritis, glomerulonephritis, nephritic syndrome, and acute renal failure (Barbour & Williams, 1990; Birketvedt *et al.*, 2000; Augusto *et al.*, 2009). The incidence of clinically restrictive renal impairment has been estimated at < 1 per 500 patients (World *et al.*, 1996). The mechanism is unclear, although both a delayed cell-mediated response, and a dose-dependent effect have been considered (Corrigan & Stevens, 2000). 5-ASA-related nephrotoxicity appeared to be dose-related in female rats given a single intravenous injection of the sodium salt of 5-ASA at doses of up to 5.7 mmol/kg bw (Calder *et al.*, 1972); however, dose-dependency may require the administration of doses much higher than those given to humans. Of note, 5-ASA combines the structural features of a salicylate and a phenacetin, both of which have well documented nephrotoxic potential (Corrigan & Stevens, 2000).

It has been hypothesized that oxidative stress may be a factor in sulfasalazine-induced renal and hepatic injury. Treatment-related alterations in the levels of biomarkers of oxidative stress were detected in kidney and liver tissues of male Sprague-Dawley rats given sulfasalazine as daily oral doses at 0, 300, or 600 mg/kg bw for 14 days. At the highest dose, there were significant decreases in the activities of renal and hepatic superoxide dismutase, and significant increases in catalase activity, thiobarbituric acid-reactive substances, and in the oxidized/reduced glutathione ratio (Linares *et al.*, 2009).

Sulfasalazine can cause haemolytic anaemia (Das *et al.*, 1973; Mechanick, 1985) and methaemoglobinaemia (Miller *et al.*, 1971; Kater, 1974; Azad Khan *et al.*, 1983). In a group of 50 patients receiving sulfasalazine at 2.5 g per day as maintenance therapy for ulcerative colitis, approximately 40% had elevated levels of methaemoglobin (Pounder *et al.*, 1975). Although sulfonamide-induced haemolysis can be severe in patients with glucose-6-phosphate dehydrogenase deficiency, this study showed that sulfasalazine-induced erythrocyte damage also occurred in patients with normal levels of this enzyme (Pounder *et al.*, 1975).

The role of metabolites in sulfasalazine-mediated toxicity was investigated in vitro, using human erythrocytes and mononuclear leukocytes as target cells in the presence of human liver microsomes; methaemoglobin formation and cytotoxicity were selected as toxicity end-points. In addition to sulfasalazine, the study included the metabolites 5-ASA, sulfapyridine, and 5′-hydroxysulfapyridine (Pirmohamed *et al.*, 1991). Bioactivation by human liver microsomes that are dependent on reduced nicotinamide adenine dinucleotide phosphate (NADPH) to a species that caused methaemoglobinaemia and cytotoxicity was only observed with sulfapyridine. Chromatographic analysis demonstrated that sulfapyridine was converted to a short-lived intermediate ($t_{1/2}$, 8.1 minutes at pH 7.4) with elution characteristics identical to those of synthetic sulfapyridine hydroxylamine. This hydroxylamine (10–500 μM) caused a concentration-dependent increase in both methaemoglobinaemia (2.9–24.4%) and cytotoxicity in the absence of a microsomal system; neither sulfasalazine nor any of the other test metabolites had such effects. When the microsomal incubations were conducted in the presence of micromolar concentrations of reducing agents (e.g. ascorbic acid, glutathione, or *N*-acetylcysteine), sulfapyridine-induced cytotoxity was decreased in mononuclear leukocytes, but there was no effect upon the levels of methaemoglobinaemia. This suggested that sulfapyridine hydroxylamine could readily penetrate erythrocytes, where it may undergo redox cycling to nitrososulfapyridine, the species ultimately responsible for the production of methaemoglobin. These observations further suggested that

N-hydroxylation of sulfapyridine may account for some of the adverse effects associated with sulfasalazine (Pirmohamed *et al.*, 1991). [Of note, *N*-hydroxylation is thought to play a key role in the bioactivation of aromatic amine carcinogens, such as 4-aminobiphenyl (IARC, 2012).]

4.3.2 Effects upon folate pathways

Sulfasalazine has been shown to inhibit the activity of dihydrofolate reductase, methylenetetrahydrofolate reductase, and serine transhydroxymethylase, and also the cellular uptake of folate (Selhub *et al.*, 1978; Jansen *et al.*, 2004; Urquhart *et al.*, 2010).

4.3.3 Urolithiasis

An increased incidence of transitional cell papilloma of the urinary bladder in male rats treated with sulfasalazine has been correlated ($P < 0.01$) with increased incidences of concretions (calculi) in the urinary bladder (NTP, 1997a; see also Section 3). In a subsequent study, there was decreased incidence of urinary hyperplasia in male rats subjected to caloric restriction and treated with sulfasalazine, and little evidence of urinary bladder concretion, compared with rats fed ad libitum (NTP, 1997b; see also Section 3). [These data suggested that chronic inflammation associated with urolithiasis may be a factor in sulfasalazine-induced carcinogenesis of the bladder in male rats.]

4.4 Susceptibility

The adverse effects of sulfasalazine have been linked to sulfapyridine (Das *et al.*, 1973). This metabolite, which is well absorbed from the colon, is inactivated by *NAT2*-mediated *N*-acetylation. *NAT2* polymorphisms have been associated with different susceptibilities to the adverse effects of sulfasalazine. People with the slow-acetylator genotype have higher serum concentrations of free sulfapyridine and lower concentrations of acetylated sulfapyridine than fast acetylators (see also Section 4.1.1), and appear more likely to experience toxic symptoms when treated with equivalent doses of sulfasalazine (Das & Dubin, 1976; Azad Khan *et al.*, 1983; Ricart *et al.*, 2002; Tanaka *et al.*, 2002; Kumagai *et al.*, 2004; Chen *et al.*, 2007; Soejima *et al.*, 2008).

4.5 Mechanistic considerations

Sulfasalazine was reported to act as a co-carcinogen at a dose of 60 mg/kg bw per day in the 1,2-dimethylhydrazine model of colon carcinogenesis in rats. In the same study, 5-ASA, the active pharmacophore unit of sulfasalazine, acted as a co-carcinogen at a dose of 30 mg/kg bw per day, but not at 60 mg/kg bw per day, which suggested that 5-ASA exerts a protective effect on the colon mucosa, provided a sufficient amount of the compound reaches the colon (Davis *et al.*, 1992). On the basis of early proposals that localized tissue folate deficiency may account for carcinogenesis (Lashner *et al.*, 1989), it was hypothesized that sulfasalazine may be co-carcinogenic due to its anti-folate characteristics. Sulfasalazine inhibited dihydrofolate reductase, methylenetetrahydrofolate reductase, and serine transhydroxymethylase, and also the cellular uptake of folate (Selhub *et al.*, 1978; Jansen *et al.*, 2004; Urquhart *et al.*, 2010). Reduced levels of *S*-adenosylmethionine or 5,10-methylenetetrahydrofolate, required for thymidine synthesis, might account for the effect; however, colonic cells may not be completely dependent on blood stream nutrients (Meenan, 1993). In the rat, colonic bacterial folate is incorporated in the hepatic folate pool (Rong *et al.*, 1991), and this could counteract sulfasalazine-induced folate depletion (Meenan, 1993). In patients with ulcerative colitis, folate concentrations measured in colonic epithelial cells obtained from endoscopic colon biopsies were not decreased in sulfasalazine-treated patients compared with controls; this contrasted with serum concentrations of folate, which were reduced in patients receiving sulfasalazine (Meenan *et al.*, 1996). These data suggested that the potentially protective effects of folate supplementation against colorectal carcinogenesis in patients with ulcerative colitis were not due to correction of localized folate deficiency.

Two-year studies in male and female F344/N rats given sulfasalazine by gavage indicated some evidence for carcinogenic activity on the basis of increased incidences of transitional cell papilloma of the urinary bladder, and clear evidence for carcinogenic activity in male and female B6C3F$_1$ mice on the basis of increased incidences of hepatocellular adenoma and hepatocellular carcinoma (NTP, 1997a; see also Section 3). The data on mutagenicity of sulfasalazine and its metabolite, sulfapyridine, suggested that the parent drug and the metabolite are predominantly aneugens (Bishop *et al.*, 1990; Witt *et al.*, 1992a, b). Increased frequencies of micronucleus formation and sister chromatid exchange in patients with IBD receiving sulfasalazine have been reported, but confounding factors were apparent in the study (Erskine *et al.*, 1984).

Folate deficiency was considered as a possible explanation for the induction of micronucleus formation by sulfasalazine in vivo. However, patients reported to have an elevated frequency of sister chromatid exchange and micronucleus formation had serum folate concentrations that were at the low end of the normal range, and the observation of reticulocytosis in a 90-day study in mice suggested an erythropoietic effect not characteristic of folate deficiency (Bishop *et al.*, 1990).

The increased incidence of transitional cell papilloma of the urinary bladder in male rats treated orally with sulfasalazine was correlated with increased incidence of concretions (calculi) in the urinary bladder (NTP, 1997a). Chronic inflammation associated with urolithiasis may be a factor in sulfasalazine-induced carcinogenesis of the bladder in male rats.

5. Summary of Data Reported

5.1 Exposure data

Sulfasalazine is a synthetic aminosalicylate used as an oral anti-inflammatory drug. The most common use of sulfasalazine is for the treatment of autoimmune arthritis. Prescriptions have been stable over the past decade, with global sales of US$ 222 million in 2012. Environmental contamination with sulfasalazine in groundwater has been noted, but exposure is likely to be predominantly through use as a medication.

5.2 Human carcinogenicity data

The available studies of exposure to sulfasalazine included a surveillance study, two cohort studies, three nested case–control studies, and three case–control studies on cancer of the colorectum among patients with inflammatory bowel disease or ulcerative colitis. These studies were hampered in their ability to evaluate the association between exposure to sulfasalazine and risk of cancer of the colorectum by the small numbers of exposed cases, imprecise risk estimates, and little information on exposure or the dose or duration of sulfasalazine use. There were also concerns about selection bias in some studies based on clinical populations.

The best designed studies were a nested case–control study from a large cohort from the General Practice Research Database in the United Kingdom, and a large population-based case–control study among patients with inflammatory bowel disease in the USA that evaluated exposure–response relationships. Conflicting findings were reported across studies, with four studies reporting relative risks of less than unity, two studies reporting estimates close to unity, and two studies reporting a relative risk of greater than unity. Most of these relative risks were not statistically significant. In the studies that evaluated dose–response relationships, no clear patterns were observed.

5.3 Animal carcinogenicity data

In one study in male and female mice given sulfasalazine by gavage, there was a significant increase in the incidence of hepatocellular adenoma, and of hepatocellular adenoma or carcinoma (combined) in both sexes; there was also an increase in the incidence of hepatocellular carcinoma in females.

In a study of dietary restriction in male mice given diets containing sulfasalazine ad libitum, there were significant increases in the incidence of hepatocellular adenoma, and hepatocellular adenoma or carcinoma (combined) in exposed mice compared with the controls fed ad libitum and the weight-matched controls. In contrast, the incidence of hepatocellular tumours in dietary-restricted mice was significantly decreased after 2 years in the group exposed to sulfasalazine, and was similar to that in non-treated mice after 3 years.

In one study in male and female rats given sulfasalazine by gavage, there was a significant increase in the incidence of transitional cell papilloma of the urinary bladder in males; there was also a non-significant increase in the incidences of rare transitional cell papilloma of the kidney and of rare transitional cell papilloma of the urinary bladder in female rats.

In a study of dietary restriction in male rats, the incidence of transitional cell papilloma of the urinary bladder was significantly greater in rats receiving sulfasalazine than in controls fed ad libitum. No significant increase in the incidence of transitional cell papilloma of the urinary bladder was observed in rats subjected to dietary restriction and given sulfasalazine.

In a co-carcinogenicity study in male rats, sulfasalazine increased the total number and multiplicity of 1,2-dimethylhydrazine-induced intestinal tumours.

5.4 Mechanistic and other relevant data

The sulfasalazine molecule contains a 5-aminosalicylic acid moiety linked by an azo bond to a sulfapyridine moiety. Cleavage of the azo bond by bacterial azoreductases in the colon releases two pharmacologically active compounds: 5-aminosalicylic acid and sulfapyridine. Sulfapyridine is absorbed, and N-acetylated by the highly polymorphic N-acetyl transferase 2 (NAT2), resulting in considerable inter-individual variation in the pharmacokinetics of sulfasalazine.

Sulfasalazine is not mutagenic in standard bacterial assays for gene mutation, with or without exogenous metabolic activation. Tests for chromosomal damage in vitro after treatment with sulfasalazine were generally negative, although sporadic positive results have been reported. Likewise, no increases in the frequency of chromosomal aberration were observed in male mice or rats treated with sulfasalazine. Positive results were consistently obtained in assays for micronucleus formation in male and female mice in vivo when multiple treatments with sulfasalazine were given; the results suggested that these results were primarily due to aneuploidy events rather than chromosome breakage.

Sulfasalazine inhibits the activity of dihydrofolate reductase, methylenetetrahydrofolate reductase, and serine transhydroxymethylase, and also the cellular uptake of folate. However, folate deficiency does not appear to account for the effects of sulfasalazine in humans and mice.

The sulfasalazine metabolite sulfapyridine has been shown to undergo N-hydroxylation when incubated with human liver microsomes in the presence of NADPH. N-Hydroxylation is known to account for the bioactivation of carcinogenic aromatic amines to DNA-binding species, and such a pathway would be consistent with the target organs associated with sulfasalazine-induced carcinogenicity in rats. However, no evidence of DNA-adduct formation was detected in rat and mouse liver or urinary bladder.

Male rats treated orally with sulfasalazine had an increased incidence of transitional cell papilloma of the urinary bladder, and this was correlated with increased incidences of calculi in the urinary bladder. Chronic inflammation associated with urolithiasis may be a factor in sulfasalazine-induced carcinogenesis of the bladder in male rats.

6. Evaluation

6.1 Cancer in humans

There is *inadequate evidence* for the carcinogenicity of sulfasalazine in humans.

6.2 Cancer in experimental animals

There is *sufficient evidence* for the carcinogenicity of sulfasalazine in experimental animals.

6.3 Overall evaluation

Sulfasalazine is *possibly carcinogenic* to humans (*Group 2B*).

References

Abdo KM, Kari FW (1996). The sensitivity of the NTP bioassay for carcinogen hazard evaluation can be modulated by dietary restriction. *Exp Toxicol Pathol*, 48(2–3):129–37. doi:10.1016/S0940-2993(96)80033-9 PMID:8672866

Astbury C, Taggart AJ, Juby L, Zebouni L, Bird HA (1990). Comparison of the single dose pharmacokinetics of sulphasalazine in rheumatoid arthritis and inflammatory bowel disease. *Ann Rheum Dis*, 49(8):587–90. doi:10.1136/ard.49.8.587 PMID:1975737

Augusto JF, Sayegh J, Simon A, Croue A, Chennebault JM, Cousin M *et al.* (2009). A case of sulphasalazine-induced DRESS syndrome with delayed acute interstitial nephritis. *Nephrol Dial Transplant*, 24(9):2940–2. doi:10.1093/ndt/gfp277 PMID:19509026

Azad Khan AK, Nurazzaman M, Truelove SC (1983). The effect of the acetylator phenotype on the metabolism of sulphasalazine in man. *J Med Genet*, 20(1):30–6. doi:10.1136/jmg.20.1.30 PMID:6133000

Azad Khan AK, Truelove SC (1979). Placental and mammary transfer of sulfasalazine. *BMJ*, 2(6204):1553 doi:10.1136/bmj.2.6204.1553

Azad Khan AK, Truelove SC, Aronson JK (1982). The disposition and metabolism of sulphasalazine (salicylazosulphapyridine) in man. *Br J Clin Pharmacol*, 13(4):523–8. PMID:6121576

Barbour VM, Williams PF (1990). Nephrotic syndrome associated with sulphasalazine. *BMJ*, 301(6755):818 doi:10.1136/bmj.301.6755.818-b PMID:1977483

Birketvedt GS, Berg KJ, Fausa O, Florholmen J (2000). Glomerular and tubular renal functions after long-term medication of sulphasalazine, olsalazine, and mesalazine in patients with ulcerative colitis. *Inflamm Bowel Dis*, 6(4):275–9. PMID:11149559

Bishop JB, Witt KL, Gulati DK, MacGregor JT (1990). Evaluation of the mutagenicity of the anti-inflammatory drug salicylazosulfapyridine (SASP). *Mutagenesis*, 5(6):549–54. doi:10.1093/mutage/5.6.549 PMID:1979833

Calder IC, Funder CC, Green CR, Ham KN, Tange JD (1972). Nephrotoxic lesions from 5-aminosalicylic Acid. *BMJ*, 1(5793):152–4. doi:10.1136/bmj.1.5793.152 PMID:20791817

Chen M, Xia B, Chen B, Guo Q, Li J, Ye M *et al.* (2007). N-acetyltransferase 2 slow acetylator genotype associated with adverse effects of sulphasalazine in the treatment of inflammatory bowel disease. *Can J Gastroenterol*, 21(3):155–8. PMID:17377643

Coogan PF, Rosenberg L (2007). The use of folic acid antagonists and the risk of colorectal cancer. *Pharmacoepidemiol Drug Saf*, 16(10):1111–9. doi:10.1002/pds.1442 PMID:17600846

Corrigan G, Stevens PE (2000). Review article: interstitial nephritis associated with the use of mesalazine in inflammatory bowel disease. *Aliment Pharmacol Ther*, 14(1):1–6. doi:10.1046/j.1365-2036.2000.00683.x PMID:10632639

Dahan A, Amidon GL (2009). Small intestinal efflux mediated by MRP2 and BCRP shifts sulfasalazine intestinal permeability from high to low, enabling its colonic targeting. *Am J Physiol Gastrointest Liver Physiol*, 297(2):G371–7. doi:10.1152/ajpgi.00102.2009 PMID:19541926

Dahan A, Amidon GL (2010). MRP2 mediated drug-drug interaction: indomethacin increases sulfasalazine absorption in the small intestine, potentially decreasing its colonic targeting. *Int J Pharm*, 386(1–2):216–20. doi:10.1016/j.ijpharm.2009.11.021 PMID:19944137

Das KM, Dubin R (1976). Clinical pharmacokinetics of sulphasalazine. *Clin Pharmacokinet*, 1(6):406–25. doi:10.2165/00003088-197601060-00002 PMID:15752

Das KM, Eastwood MA, McManus JPA, Sircus W (1973). Adverse reactions during salicylazosulfapyridine therapy and the relation with drug metabolism and acetylator phenotype. *N Engl J Med*, 289(10):491–5. doi:10.1056/NEJM197309062891001 PMID:4146729

Davis AE, Patterson F, Crouch R (1992). The effect of therapeutic drugs used in inflammatory bowel disease on the incidence and growth of colonic cancer in the dimethylhydrazine rat model. *Br J Cancer*, 66(5):777–80. doi:10.1038/bjc.1992.359 PMID:1358165

de Abajo FJ, Montero D, Madurga M, García Rodríguez LA (2004). Acute and clinically relevant drug-induced liver injury: a population based case-control study. *Br J Clin Pharmacol*, 58(1):71–80. doi:10.1111/j.1365-2125.2004.02133.x PMID:15206996

Diculescu M, Ciocîrlan M, Ciocîrlan M, Piţigoi D, Becheanu G, Croitoru A *et al.* (2003). Folic acid and sulfasalazine for colorectal carcinoma chemoprevention in patients with ulcerative colitis: the old and new evidence. *Rom J Gastroenterol*, 12(4):283–6. PMID:14726972

Dyson JK, Rutter MD (2012). Colorectal cancer in inflammatory bowel disease: what is the real magnitude of the risk? *World J Gastroenterol*, 18(29):3839–48. doi:10.3748/wjg.v18.i29.3839 PMID:22876036

Eaden J, Abrams K, Ekbom A, Jackson E, Mayberry J (2000). Colorectal cancer prevention in ulcerative colitis: a case-control study. *Aliment Pharmacol Ther*, 14(2):145–53. doi:10.1046/j.1365-2036.2000.00698.x PMID:10651654

Elmasry MS, Blagbrough IS, Rowan MG, Saleh HM, Kheir AA, Rogers PJ (2011). Quantitative HPLC analysis of mebeverine, mesalazine, sulphasalazine and dispersible aspirin stored in a Venalink monitored dosage system with co-prescribed medicines. *J Pharm Biomed Anal*, 54(4):646–52. doi:10.1016/j.jpba.2010.10.002 PMID:21106317

eMC; electronic Medicines Compendium (2013). Sulfasalazine. Available from: http://www.medicines.org.uk, accessed 30 June 2014.

Erskine IA, Mackay JM, Fox DP (1984). Monitoring patients on long-term drug therapy for genotoxic effects. *Basic Life Sci*, 29:Pt B: 895–905. PMID:6152153

Esbjörner E, Järnerot G, Wranne L (1987). Sulphasalazine and sulphapyridine serum levels in children to mothers treated with sulphasalazine during pregnancy and lactation. *Acta Paediatr Scand*, 76(1):137–42. doi:10.1111/j.1651-2227.1987.tb10430.x PMID:2882643

European Pharmacopoeia (2008). Sulfasalazine *European Pharmacopoeia Council of Europe*, 2:2514–2516. Available from: http://www.edqm.eu/en/edqm-home-page-628.html, accessed 1 July 2014.

Fatta D, Achilleos A, Nikolaou A, Meriç S (2007). Analytical methods for tracing pharmaceutical residues in water and wastewater. *Trends Analyt Chem*, 26(6):515–33. doi:10.1016/j.trac.2007.02.001

FDA (2013). Sulfasalazine. Silver Spring (MD): US Food and Drug Administration, Drugs@FDA. Available from: http://www.accessdata.fda.gov/scripts/cder/drugsatfda/index.cfm, accessed 30 June 2014.

Font G, Juan-García A, Picó Y (2007). Pressurized liquid extraction combined with capillary electrophoresis-mass spectrometry as an improved methodology for the determination of sulfonamide residues in meat. *J Chromatogr A*, 1159(1–2):233–41. doi:10.1016/j.chroma.2007.03.062 PMID:17433345

Fukino K, Hashimoto M *et al.* (2007). Analysis between clinical efficacy of salazosulfapyridine and plasma concentrations of sulfapyridine in patients with rheumatoid arthritis. *Jpn. J. Ther. Drug Monit*, 24:113–121.

Gisbert JP, González-Lama Y, Maté J (2007). 5-Aminosalicylates and renal function in inflammatory bowel disease: a systematic review. *Inflamm Bowel Dis*, 13(5):629–38. doi:10.1002/ibd.20099 PMID:17243140

Gu G-Z, Xia H-M, Pang ZQ, Liu ZY, Jiang XG, Chen J (2011). Determination of sulphasalazine and its main metabolite sulphapyridine and 5-aminosalicylic acid in human plasma by liquid chromatography/tandem mass spectrometry and its application to a pharmacokinetic study. *J Chromatogr B Analyt Technol Biomed Life Sci*, 879(5–6):449–56. doi:10.1016/j.jchromb.2010.12.034 PMID:21251889

Hanauer SB (2004). Review article: aminosalicylates in inflammatory bowel disease. *Aliment Pharmacol Ther*, 20(s4):Suppl 4: 60–5. doi:10.1111/j.1365-2036.2004.02048.x PMID:15352896

IARC (2012). Pharmaceuticals. Volume 100 A. A review of human carcinogens. *IARC Monogr Eval Carcinog Risks Hum*, 100:Pt A: 1–401. PMID:23189749

Iatropoulos MJ, Williams GM, Abdo KM, Kari FW, Hart RW (1997). Mechanistic studies on genotoxicity and carcinogenicity of salicylazosulfapyridine an anti-inflammatory medicine. *Exp Toxicol Pathol*, 49(1–2):15–28. doi:10.1016/S0940-2993(97)80052-8 PMID:9085070

IMS Health (2012a). National Disease and Therapeutic Index (NDTI). Plymouth Meeting, Pennsylvania: IMS Health

IMS Health (2012b) Multinational Integrated Data Analysis (MIDAS). Plymouth Meeting, Pennsylvania: IMS Health

IMS Health (2012c) National Prescription Audit Plus (NPA). Plymouth Meeting, Pennsylvania: IMS Health

Jacoby HI (2000). Gastrointestinal Agents. Kirk-Othmer Encyclopedia of Chemical Technology. John Wiley & Sons, Inc. Available from: http://onlinelibrary.wiley.com/doi/10.1002/0471238961.0701192010010315.a01.pub2/abstract;jsessionid=B9EC963BD4DA13B-08CE09E6F28B43EA7.f03t04, accessed 30 June 2014.

Jansen G, van der Heijden J, Oerlemans R, Lems WF, Ifergan I, Scheper RJ et al. (2004). Sulfasalazine is a potent inhibitor of the reduced folate carrier: implications for combination therapies with methotrexate in rheumatoid arthritis. *Arthritis Rheum*, 50(7):2130–9. doi:10.1002/art.20375 PMID:15248210

Järnerot G, Into-Malmberg MB (1979). Sulphasalazine treatment during breast feeding. *Scand J Gastroenterol*, 14(7):869–71. doi:10.3109/00365527909181418 PMID:44005

Järnerot G, Into-Malmberg MB, Esbjörner E (1981). Placental transfer of sulphasalazine and sulphapyridine and some of its metabolites. *Scand J Gastroenterol*, 16(5):693–7. doi:10.3109/00365528109182032 PMID:6119765

Jess T, Loftus EV Jr, Velayos FS, Winther KV, Tremaine WJ, Zinsmeister AR et al. (2007). Risk factors for colorectal neoplasia in inflammatory bowel disease: a nested case-control study from Copenhagen county, Denmark and Olmsted county, Minnesota. *Am J Gastroenterol*, 102(4):829–36. doi:10.1111/j.1572-0241.2007.01070.x PMID:17222314

Jobanputra P, Amarasena R, Maggs F, Homer D, Bowman S, Rankin E et al. (2008). Hepatotoxicity associated with sulfasalazine in inflammatory arthritis: A case series from a local surveillance of serious adverse events. *BMC Musculoskelet Disord*, 9(1):48 doi:10.1186/1471-2474-9-48 PMID:18405372

Kater F (1974). Hemolysis, formation of Heinz bodies and of methemoglobin under therapy with Azulfidine. *Med Klin*, 69(11):466–8. [German] PMID:4151648

Kaufman DW, Kelly JP, Jurgelon JM, Anderson T, Issaragrisil S, Wiholm BE et al. (1996). Drugs in the aetiology of agranulocytosis and aplastic anaemia. *Eur J Haematol Suppl*, 60:suppl: 23–30. PMID:8987237

Kita T, Sakaeda T, Adachi S, Sakai T, Aoyama N, Hatanaka H et al. (2001). N-Acetyltransferase 2 genotype correlates with sulfasalazine pharmacokinetics after multiple dosing in healthy Japanese subjects. *Biol Pharm Bull*, 24(10):1176–80. doi:10.1248/bpb.24.1176 PMID:11642327

Kuhn UD, Anschütz M, Schmücker K, Schug BS, Hippius M, Blume HH (2010). Phenotyping with sulfasalazine - time dependence and relation to NAT2 pharmacogenetics. *Int J Clin Pharmacol Ther*, 48(1):1–10. doi:10.5414/CPP48001 PMID:20040334

Kumagai S, Komada F, Kita T, Morinobu A, Ozaki S, Ishida H et al. (2004). N-acetyltransferase 2 genotype-related efficacy of sulfasalazine in patients with rheumatoid arthritis. *Pharm Res*, 21(2):324–9. doi:10.1023/B:PHAM.0000016246.84974.ec PMID:15032315

Kusuhara H, Furuie H, Inano A, Sunagawa A, Yamada S, Wu C et al. (2012). Pharmacokinetic interaction study of sulphasalazine in healthy subjects and the impact of curcumin as an in vivo inhibitor of BCRP. *Br J Pharmacol*, 166(6):1793–803. doi:10.1111/j.1476-5381.2012.01887.x PMID:22300367

Lakatos PL, Lakatos L (2008). Risk for colorectal cancer in ulcerative colitis: changes, causes and management strategies. *World J Gastroenterol*, 14(25):3937–47. doi:10.3748/wjg.14.3937 PMID:18609676

Lashner BA, Heidenreich PA, Su GL, Kane SV, Hanauer SB (1989). Effect of folate supplementation on the incidence of dysplasia and cancer in chronic ulcerative colitis. A case-control study. *Gastroenterology*, 97(2):255–9. PMID:2568304

Lee HJ, Zhang H, Orlovich DA, Fawcett JP (2012). The influence of probiotic treatment on sulfasalazine metabolism in rat. *Xenobiotica*, 42(8):791–7. doi:10.3109/00498254.2012.660508 PMID:22348441

Lide DR, editor (2005). CRC Handbook of Chemistry and Physics. 86th ed. Boca Raton (FL), USA: CRC Press.

Liedorp M, Voskuyl AE, Van Oosten BW (2008). Axonal neuropathy with prolonged sulphasalazine use. *Clin Exp Rheumatol*, 26(4):671–2. PMID:18799104

Linares V, Alonso V, Albina ML, Bellés M, Sirvent JJ, Domingo JL et al. (2009). Lipid peroxidation and antioxidant status in kidney and liver of rats treated with sulfasalazine. *Toxicology*, 256(3):152–6. doi:10.1016/j.tox.2008.11.010 PMID:19071188

Lindberg BU, Broomé U, Persson B (2001). Proximal colorectal dysplasia or cancer in ulcerative colitis. The impact of primary sclerosing cholangitis and sulfasalazine: results from a 20-year surveillance study. *Dis Colon Rectum*, 44(1):77–85. doi:10.1007/BF02234825 PMID:11805567

Ma JJ, Liu CG, Li JH, Cao XM, Sun SL, Yao X (2009). Effects of NAT2 polymorphism on SASP pharmacokinetics in Chinese population. *Clin Chim Acta*, 407(1–2):30–5. doi:10.1016/j.cca.2009.06.025 PMID:19560446

Mackay JM, Fox DP, Brunt PW, Hawksworth GM, Brown JE (1989). In vitro induction of chromosome damage by sulphasalazine in human lymphocytes. *Mutat Res*, 222(1):27–36. doi:10.1016/0165-1218(89)90032-3 PMID:2563144

McDonnell JP, Klaus F (1976). Sulfasalazine. *Analytical Profiles of Drug Substances*, 5:515–32. doi:10.1016/S0099-5428(08)60329-9

McGirt LY, Vasagar K, Gober LM, Saini SS, Beck LA (2006). Successful treatment of recalcitrant chronic idiopathic urticaria with sulfasalazine. *Arch Dermatol*, 142(10):1337–42. doi:10.1001/archderm.142.10.1337 PMID:17043190

Mechanick JI (1985). Coombs' positive hemolytic anemia following sulfasalazine therapy in ulcerative colitis: case reports, review, and discussion of pathogenesis. *Mt Sinai J Med*, 52(8):667–70. PMID:2867466

Meenan J (1993). Co-carcinogenic effect of sulphasalazine. *Br J Cancer*, 68(5):1043–4. doi:10.1038/bjc.1993.477 PMID:8105863

Meenan J, O'Hallinan E, Scott J, Weir DG (1996). Influence of sulfasalazine and olsalamine on colonic epithelial cell folate content in patients with ulcerative colitis. *Inflamm Bowel Dis*, 2:163–7. PMID:23282560

Miller B, Engelhart A, Goebel KM, Schmidt J, Martini GA (1971). [Methemoglobin synthesis during azulfidine therapy]. *Verh Dtsch Ges Inn Med*, 77:1326–30. PMID:4405361

Mitelman F, Strömbeck B, Ursing B (1980). No cytogenic effect of metronidazole. *Lancet*, 1(8180):1249–50. doi:10.1016/S0140-6736(80)91706-7 PMID:6104060

Mitelman F, Strömbeck B, Ursing B, Nordle O, Hartley-Asp B (1982). Metronidazole exhibits no clastogenic activity in a double-blind cross-over study on Crohn's patients. *Hereditas*, 96(2):279–86. doi:10.1111/j.1601-5223.1982.tb00859.x PMID:6125490

Mohamed R, Hammel Y-A, LeBreton MH, Tabet JC, Jullien L, Guy PA (2007). Evaluation of atmospheric pressure ionization interfaces for quantitative measurement of sulfonamides in honey using isotope dilution liquid chromatography coupled with tandem mass spectrometry techniques. *J Chromatogr A*, 1160(1–2):194–205. doi:10.1016/j.chroma.2007.05.071 PMID:17560585

Moody GA, Jayanthi V, Probert CS, MacKay H, Mayberry JF (1996). Long-term therapy with sulphasalazine protects against colorectal cancer in ulcerative colitis: a retrospective study of colorectal cancer risk and compliance with treatment in Leicestershire. *Eur J Gastroenterol Hepatol*, 8(12):1179–83. doi:10.1097/00042737-199612000-00009 PMID:8980937

NTP (1997a). NTP Toxicology and Carcinogenesis Studies of Salicylazosulfapyridine (CAS No. 599–79–1) in F344/N Rats and B6C3F1 Mice (savage studies). *Natl Toxicol Program Tech Rep Ser*, 457:1–327. PMID:12587019

NTP (1997b). Effect of dietary restriction on toxicology and carcinogenesis studies in F344/N rats and B6C3F1 mice. *Natl Toxicol Program Tech Rep Ser*, 460:1–414. PMID:12587016

Novacek A *et al.* (1991). Method of producing 2-hydroxy-5-[[4-[(2-pyridinylamino)sulfonyl]phenyl]azo]benzoic acid [sulfasalazine Available from: http://www.jazdlifesciences.com/pharmatech/company/United-States-Biological/Sulfasalazine-2-Hydroxy-5-4-2-pyridinylaminosulfonylphenylazobenzoic-AcidSulfasalazine-Azulfidine-Colo-Pleon-Salaz.htm?supplierId=30001720&productId=540654

O'Moráin C, Smethurst P, Doré CJ, Levi AJ (1984). Reversible male infertility due to sulphasalazine: studies in man and rat. *Gut*, 25(10):1078–84. doi:10.1136/gut.25.10.1078 PMID:6148293

O'Neil MJ (2001). The Merck Index. 13th ed. Whitehouse Station (NJ): Merck & Co., Inc.

OEHHA; Office of Environmental Health Hazard Assessment (2013). Chemicals known to the state to cause cancer or reproductive toxicity. Available from: http://oehha.ca.gov/prop65/prop65_list/files/P65single052413.pdf, accessed 30 June 2014.

Parry SD, Barbatzas C, Peel ET, Barton JR (2002). Sulphasalazine and lung toxicity. *Eur Respir J*, 19(4):756–64. doi:10.1183/09031936.02.00267402 PMID:11999006

Pastor-Navarro N, Gallego-Iglesias E, Maquieira A, Puchades R (2007). Immunochemical method for sulfasalazine determination in human plasma. *Anal Chim Acta*, 583(2):377–83. doi:10.1016/j.aca.2006.10.028 PMID:17386570

Peppercorn MA, Goldman P (1972). The role of intestinal bacteria in the metabolism of salicylazosulfapyridine. *J Pharmacol Exp Ther*, 181(3):555–62. PMID:4402374

Pinczowski D, Ekbom A, Baron J, Yuen J, Adami HO (1994). Risk factors for colorectal cancer in patients with ulcerative colitis: a case-control study. *Gastroenterology*, 107(1):117–20. PMID:7912678

Pirmohamed M, Coleman MD, Hussain F, Breckenridge AM, Park BK (1991). Direct and metabolism-dependent toxicity of sulphasalazine and its principal metabolites towards human erythrocytes and leucocytes. *Br J Clin Pharmacol*, 32(3):303–10. doi:10.1111/j.1365-2125.1991.tb03903.x PMID:1685664

Porter RS, Kaplan JL (2013). The Merck manuals: Health care professionals. Whitehouse Station (NJ): Merck & Co., Inc. Available from: http://www.merckmanuals.com/professional/index.html, accessed 30 June 2014.

Pounder RE, Craven ER, Henthorn JS, Bannatyne JM (1975). Red cell abnormalities associated with sulphasalazine maintenance therapy for ulcerative colitis. *Gut*, 16(3):181–5. doi:10.1136/gut.16.3.181 PMID:235486

Ricart E, Taylor WR, Loftus EV, O'Kane D, Weinshilboum RM, Tremaine WJ *et al.* (2002). N-acetyltransferase 1 and 2 genotypes do not predict response or toxicity to treatment with mesalamine and sulfasalazine in patients with ulcerative colitis. *Am J Gastroenterol*, 97(7):1763–8. doi:10.1111/j.1572-0241.2002.05838.x PMID:12135032

Rong N, Selhub J, Goldin BR, Rosenberg IH (1991). Bacterially synthesized folate in rat large intestine is incorporated into host tissue folyl polyglutamates. *J Nutr*, 121(12):1955–9. PMID:1941259

Rosenbaum SE (2011). Basic pharmacokinetics and pharmacodynamics: An integrated textbook and computer simulations. Available from: http://www.theannals.com/content/46/2/305.full, accessed 5 September 2014.

Rubin DT, LoSavio A, Yadron N, Huo D, Hanauer SB (2006). Aminosalicylate therapy in the prevention of dysplasia and colorectal cancer in ulcerative colitis. *Clin Gastroenterol Hepatol*, 4(11):1346–50. doi:10.1016/j.cgh.2006.08.014 PMID:17059900

Rutter M, Saunders B, Wilkinson K, Rumbles S, Schofield G, Kamm M *et al.* (2004). Severity of inflammation is a risk factor for colorectal neoplasia in ulcerative colitis. *Gastroenterology*, 126(2):451–9. doi:10.1053/j.gastro.2003.11.010 PMID:14762782

Schröder H, Campbell DE (1972). Absorption, metabolism, and excretion of salicylazosulfapyridine in man. *Clin Pharmacol Ther*, 13(4):539–51. PMID:4402886

Schröder H, Evans DA (1972). Acetylator phenotype and adverse effects of sulphasalazine in healthy subjects. *Gut*, 13(4):278–84. doi:10.1136/gut.13.4.278 PMID:4402420

SciFinder (2013). SciFinder databases: A division of the American Chemical Society. Available from: https://www.cas.org/products/scifinder, accessed 30 June 2014.

Selhub J, Dhar GJ, Rosenberg IH (1978). Inhibition of folate enzymes by sulfasalazine. *J Clin Invest*, 61(1):221–4. doi:10.1172/JCI108921 PMID:22555

Soejima M, Kawaguchi Y, Hara M, Kamatani N (2008). Prospective study of the association between NAT2 gene haplotypes and severe adverse events with sulfasalazine therapy in patients with rheumatoid arthritis. *J Rheumatol*, 35(4):724 PMID:18398952

Stretch GL, Campbell BJ, Dwarakanath AD, Yaqoob M, Stevenson A, Morris AI et al. (1996). 5-amino salicylic acid absorption and metabolism in ulcerative colitis patients receiving maintenance sulphasalazine, olsalazine or mesalazine. *Aliment Pharmacol Ther*, 10(6):941–7. doi:10.1046/j.1365-2036.1996.85257000.x PMID:8971292

Taggart AJ, McDermott BJ, Roberts SD (1992). The effect of age and acetylator phenotype on the pharmacokinetics of sulfasalazine in patients with rheumatoid arthritis. *Clin Pharmacokinet*, 23(4):311–20. doi:10.2165/00003088-199223040-00006 PMID:1356683

Tanaka E, Taniguchi A, Urano W, Nakajima H, Matsuda Y, Kitamura Y et al. (2002). Adverse effects of sulfasalazine in patients with rheumatoid arthritis are associated with diplotype configuration at the N-acetyltransferase 2 gene. *J Rheumatol*, 29(12):2492–9. PMID:12465141

Tanigawara Y, Kita T, Aoyama N, Gobara M, Komada F, Sakai T et al. (2002). N-Acetyltransferase 2 genotype-related sulfapyridine acetylation and its adverse events. *Biol Pharm Bull*, 25(8):1058–62. doi:10.1248/bpb.25.1058 PMID:12186410

Terdiman JP, Steinbuch M, Blumentals WA, Ullman TA, Rubin DT (2007). 5-Aminosalicylic acid therapy and the risk of colorectal cancer among patients with inflammatory bowel disease. *Inflamm Bowel Dis*, 13(4):367–71. doi:10.1002/ibd.20074 PMID:17206695

Tett SE (1993). Clinical pharmacokinetics of slow-acting antirheumatic drugs. *Clin Pharmacokinet*, 25(5):392–407. doi:10.2165/00003088-199325050-00005 PMID:7904547

Tokui K, Asai Y, Arakawa T, Matsumoto T, Nabeshima T (2002). Comparative absorption of 5-aminosalicylic acid (5-ASA) after administration of a 5-ASA enema and salazosulfapyridine (SASP) after an SASP suppository

in Japanese volunteers. *Biol Pharm Bull*, 25(2):264–7. doi:10.1248/bpb.25.264 PMID:11853180

Tomaru A, Morimoto N, Morishita M, Takayama K, Fujita T, Maeda K et al. (2013). Studies on the intestinal absorption characteristics of sulfasalazine, a breast cancer resistance protein (BCRP) substrate. *Drug Metab Pharmacokinet*, 28(1):71–4. doi:10.2133/dmpk.DMPK-12-NT-024 PMID:22785334

Tuckwell R, Revitt DM, Garelick H, Jones H, Ellis B (2011). Sources and pathways for pharmaceuticals in the urban water environment. In: 12th International Conference on Urban Drainage, 11–16 September 2011, Porto Alegre, Brazil.

Urquhart BL, Gregor JC, Chande N, Knauer MJ, Tirona RG, Kim RB (2010). The human proton-coupled folate transporter (hPCFT): modulation of intestinal expression and function by drugs. *Am J Physiol Gastrointest Liver Physiol*, 298(2):G248–54. doi:10.1152/ajpgi.00224.2009 PMID:19762432

Urquhart BL, Ware JA, Tirona RG, Ho RH, Leake BF, Schwarz UI et al. (2008). Breast cancer resistance protein (ABCG2) and drug disposition: intestinal expression, polymorphisms and sulfasalazine as an in vivo probe. *Pharmacogenet Genomics*, 18(5):439–48. doi:10.1097/FPC.0b013e3282f974dc PMID:18408567

US Pharmacopeia (2007). Sulfasalazine. Report No. USP30–NF25. Rockville (MD), USA: The United States Pharmacopoeial Convention.

US Pharmacopeia (2013). Sulfasalazine. Report No. USP36. Rockville (MD), USA: The United States Pharmacopoeial Convention.

van der Heijden J, de Jong MC, Dijkmans BA, Lems WF, Oerlemans R, Kathmann I et al. (2004). Development of sulfasalazine resistance in human T cells induces expression of the multidrug resistance transporter ABCG2 (BCRP) and augmented production of TNFalpha. *Ann Rheum Dis*, 63(2):138–43. doi:10.1136/ard.2002.005249 PMID:14722201

van Staa TP, Card T, Logan RF, Leufkens HG (2005). 5-Aminosalicylate use and colorectal cancer risk in inflammatory bowel disease: a large epidemiological study. *Gut*, 54(11):1573–8. doi:10.1136/gut.2005.070896 PMID:15994215

Voogd CE, Van der Stel JJ, Jacobs JJ (1980). On the mutagenic action of some enzyme immunoassay substrates. *J Immunol Methods*, 36(1):55–61. doi:10.1016/0022-1759(80)90093-9 PMID:7009752

WHO (2007). Cumulative List No. 14 of INN in Latin, English, French, Spanish, Arabic, Chinese and Russian (in alphabetical order of the Latin name), with supplementary information. Geneva, Switzerland: World Health Organization. Available from: http://www.vpb.gov.lt/files/539.pdf, accessed 30 June 2014.

Witt KL, Bishop JB, McFee AF, Kumaroo V (1992b). Induction of chromosomal damage in mammalian cells in vitro and in vivo by sulfapyridine or 5-aminosalicylic acid. *Mutat Res*, 283(1):59–64. doi:10.1016/0165-7992(92)90122-X PMID:1380664

Witt KL, Gudi R, Bishop JB (1992a). Induction of kinetochore positive and negative micronuclei in mouse bone marrow cells by salicylazosulfapyridine and sulfapyridine. *Mutat Res*, 283(1):53–7. doi:10.1016/0165-7992(92)90121-W PMID:1380663

World MJ, Stevens PE, Ashton MA, Rainford DJ (1996). Mesalazine-associated interstitial nephritis. *Nephrol Dial Transplant*, 11(4):614–21. doi:10.1093/oxfordjournals.ndt.a027349 PMID:8671848

Yamasaki Y, Ieiri I, Kusuhara H, Sasaki T, Kimura M, Tabuchi H *et al.* (2008). Pharmacogenetic characterization of sulfasalazine disposition based on NAT2 and ABCG2 (BCRP) gene polymorphisms in humans. *Clin Pharmacol Ther*, 84(1):95–103. doi:10.1038/sj.clpt.6100459 PMID:18167504

Zaher H, Khan AA, Palandra J, Brayman TG, Yu L, Ware JA (2006). Breast cancer resistance protein (Bcrp/abcg2) is a major determinant of sulfasalazine absorption and elimination in the mouse. *Mol Pharm*, 3(1):55–61. doi:10.1021/mp050113v PMID:16686369

Zeiger E, Anderson B, Haworth S, Lawlor T, Mortelmans K (1988). Salmonella mutagenicity tests: IV. Results from the testing of 300 chemicals. *Environ Mol Mutagen*, 11(S12):Suppl 12: 1–157. doi:10.1002/em.2850110602 PMID:3277844

Zheng W, Winter SM, Mayersohn M, Bishop JB, Sipes IG (1993). Toxicokinetics of sulfasalazine (salicylazosulfapyridine) and its metabolites in B6C3F1 mice. *Drug Metab Dispos*, 21(6):1091–7. PMID:7905389

PENTOSAN POLYSULFATE SODIUM

1. Exposure Data

In this *Monograph*, pentosan polysulfate sodium will also be referred to as pentosan.

1.1 Chemical and physical data

1.1.1 Nomenclature

Chem. Abstr. Serv. Reg. No.: 37319-17-8; 140207-93-8

Chem. Abstr. Serv. Name: Xylan hydrogen sulfate, sodium salt (SciFinder, 2010)

IUPAC systematic name: [(2R,3R,4S,5R)-2-hydroxy-5-[(2S,3R,4S,5R)-5-hydroxy-3,4-di-sulfooxyoxan-2-yl]oxy-3-sulfooxyoxan-4-yl] hydrogen sulfate, sodium (PubChem, 2013)

Synonyms: Pentosan polysulfate sodium; Pentosan; Xylan hydrogen sulfate sodium salt; Xylan polysulfate sodium; Sodium pentosan polysulfate; Sodium pentosane polysulfate; Xylan sulfate sodium; Xylofuranan sulfate sodium; (1→4)-β-D-Xylan 2,3-bis(hydrogen sulfate) sodium; Sodium xylan polysulfate (O'Neil, 2006; SciFinder,2010)

Proprietary names: Elmiron, Cartrophen, Fibrase, Fibrenzym, Hemoclar, SP-54, Thrombocid

1.1.2 Structural and molecular formulae and relative molecular mass

$(C_5H_6Na_2O_{10}S_2)_n$ where n = 6–12 (US Pharmacopeial Convention, 2013)
Relative molecular mass: $[336]_n$

1.1.3 Chemical and physical properties of the pure substance

Description: White, odourless powder, slightly hygroscopic (O'Neil, 2006)

Density: 1.344 at 20 °C, 10% aqueous solution (O'Neil, 2006)

Spectroscopy data: Index of refraction is −57°at 20 °C (O'Neil, 2006)

Solubility: Soluble in water to 50% at pH 6.0 (O'Neil, 2006; RxList, 2013)

1.1.4 Technical products and impurities

Pentosan polysulfate sodium is a plant-derived, semi-synthetic mucopolysaccharide with radiochemical purity of 95.6%, with no single major impurity (Simon *et al.*, 2005; RxList, 2013).

1.2 Analysis

Several non-compendial analytical methods for the determination of pentosan polysulfate sodium in pharmaceutical formulations were available. These included normal-phase high-performance liquid chromatography with refractive index detection, capillary electrophoresis with ultraviolet detection, surface plasmon resonance, and gel-permeation chromatography with refractive index detection. The analytical methods are summarized in Table 1.1. No compendial analytical methods were available to the Working Group.

1.3 Production

1.3.1 Production process

As a semi-synthetic compound, the polysaccharide backbone of pentosan polysulfate sodium, xylan, is present in beech tree bark. Extracted xylan from beech bark or other plant sources is treated with sulfating agents (e.g. chlorosulfonic acid or sulfuryl chloride). After sulfation, pentosan polysulfate is treated with sodium hydroxide to form a sodium salt of the compound (Deshpande *et al.*, 2010).

1.3.2 Use

(a)   Indications

Orally administered pentosan polysulfate sodium is used primarily in the treatment of interstitial cystitis. It is one of only two products approved for treatment of this bladder condition and is often used after inadequate response

to the other, which is irrigation of the bladder with dimethyl sulfoxide (Hanno *et al.*, 2011). With its large, heparin-like molecular structure, pentosan has anticoagulant and fibrinolytic properties (MicroMedex, 2013), although this use was not observed in recent data from the USA. Pentosan was approved by the Food and Drug Administration for the indication of "relief of bladder pain or discomfort associated with interstitial cystitis" (FDA, 2013). In the European Union, other formulations apart from the oral form include ointment, rectal suppository, and injectable solution. Pentosan is also used in veterinary medicine as an anti-inflammatory drug to treat arthritis (MicroMedex, 2013).

(b)   Dosage

Pentosan polysulfate sodium can be administered orally, intramuscularly, rectally, or as a solution instilled into the bladder. For the treatment of interstitial cystitis, recommended dosing is an oral dose of 100 mg, three times per day, for at least 3 months (IMS Health, 2012b). Use for deep venous thrombosis prophylaxis involves intramuscular injection of 50 mg every 12 hours (MicroMedex, 2013).

(c)   Trends in use

Pentosan polysulfate sodium is not widely used in the USA, with 138 000 drug uses reported in office-based physician visits in 2012 (IMS Health, 2012b). Use had declined by 33% since 2005 (Fig. 1.1). Based on NDTI data, approximately 50 000 patients in the USA were exposed to pentosan in 2012 (IMS Health, 2012b). About 450 000 prescriptions for pentosan were dispensed in the USA in 2012, down slightly from about 490 000 in 2008 (IMS Health, 2012c).

Despite an only modest volume of use, total worldwide sales of pentosan were nonetheless US$ 276 million in 2012, with 82% occurring in the USA. The only other countries with appreciable use were Spain (US$ 16 million) and Canada (US$ 11 million) (IMS Health, 2012a).

Table 1.1 Some non-compendial analytical methods for pentosan polysulfate sodium

Sample matrix	Sample preparation	Assay method	Detection limit	Reference
Human plasma	–	Immunoassay – indirect ELISA	2.6 ng/mL (LLOQ)	Abnova (2013)
Human serum	Blood collection in tubes containing oxalate, separation of plasma by centrifugation	Amplified ELISIA using mAb 5-B-10 that recognizes 2,3-, 2,6-, and 4,6-disulfate ester ring substitution in pyranose-containing polysaccharides	50 ng/mL (LOD)	Kongtawelert & Ghosh (1990)
Human urine	Urine sample, centrifugation, incubation with equal volume CPC citrate buffer, centrifugation, dissolve precipitate in lithium chloride, addition of ethanol to mixture, centrifugation, dry precipitate with nitrogen, addition of 0.5 M HCl, hydrolysis, dry sample in vacuum oven, derivatization with TMS reagent	GC-FID Glass column Detector: FID Carrier gas: nitrogen, 30 mL/min	10 µg/mL (LOD	Lee *et al.* (1986)
Rabbit serum	Collection of blood from rabbit ear, separation of serum by centrifugation	Antiviral bioassay method based on inhibitory activity of PPS on HIV-2 virus in MT-4 cells (human T-lymphoblastoid cell line). Infection of MT-4 cells with HIV-1 or HIV-2 in culture medium, transfer to microtitre tray wells containing serum samples, 5-day incubation at 37 °C, number of viable cells by MTT	0.5 µg/mL (LOD)	Witvrouw *et al.* (1990)
Nanoparticles	Drop-wise addition of a solution of standard PPS to solution of chitosan, magnetic stirring, separation by centrifugation	CZE Buffer: Tris base in water (50–200 mM) pH 3.0–6.5 Pressure: 10–35 mbar Running voltage: −10 or 10 to −30 or 30 kV based on separation mode (normal or reversed) Injection time: 5–10 s	0.1 mg/mL (LOQ)	Abdel-Haq & Bossù (2012)
Formulation	–	HPLC Column: silica diol Mobile phase: sodium chloride (200 mM) Flow rate: 1 mL/min Detector: refractive index		Muller *et al.* (1984)
Formulation	Dilution of 10 mg of PPS with 10 mL of purified water	CZE using indirect detection Fused silica capillary Detector: UV detector (217 nm) Applied voltage: −20 kV (capillary inlet at cathode) Current: 14.4 µA Running buffer: BTC buffer, 8.75 mmol/L		Degenhardt *et al.* (1998)

Table 1.1 (continued)

Sample matrix	Sample preparation	Assay method	Detection limit	Reference
Formulation	Dilution of 10 mg PPS with 10 mL purified water	Reverse polarity CZE using a central composite design CE-UV diode-array detector Polyimide coated fused silica capillary Detector: 320 nm (reference wavelength: 217 nm) Running buffer: BTC buffer, 8.75 mmol/L	0.25 mg/mL (LOQ)	Prochazka *et al.* (2003)
Formulation	–	SPR technology, biosensor analysis with immobilized enzymes HNE, HAase or lysozyme Immobilization of enzymes: amine coupling Binding assays in HEPES-containing buffer Flow rate: 50 µL/min Regeneration: 100 mM acetic acid containing 2.0 M sodium chloride	0.3 µg/mL (LOQ)	Shen *et al.* (2003)
Formulation	Dilution in deionized water	HPLC methods (1) Column: diol GPC Mobile phase: 25 mM potassium phosphate, monobasic; 25 mM potassium phosphate, dibasic; 50 mM potassium chloride Flow rate: 0.7 mL/min Detector: refractive index (2) Column: diol GPC Mobile phase: acetonitrile in water (5 : 95); 25 mM potassium phosphate, monobasic; 25 mM potassium phosphate, dibasic; 50 mM potassium chloride Flow rate: 0.7 mL/min Detector: refractive index (3) Column: diol GPC Mobile phase: 0.9% sodium chloride in water Flow rate: 0.5 mL/min Detector: refractive index		NTP (2004)

BTC, benzene-1,2,4-tricarboxylic acid; CE, capillary electrophoresis; CPC, cetyl pyridinium chloride; CZE, capillary zone electrophoresis; ELISA, enzyme-linked immunosorbent assay; ELISIA, enzyme-linked immunosorbent inhibition assay; FID, flame ionization detector; GC, gas chromatography; GPC, gel permeation chromatography; HAase, hyaluronidase; HEPES, 4-(2-hydroxyethyl)-1-piperazineethanesulfonic acid; HIV, human immunodeficiency virus; HNE, human neutrophil elastase; HPLC, high-performance liquid chromatography; LOD, limit of detection; LLOQ, lower limit of quantitation; LOQ, limit of quantitation; MAb, monoclonal antibody; min, minute; MTT, 3′-(4,5-dimethylthiazol-2-yl)-2,5 diphenyltetrazolium bromide; PBS, phosphate buffered saline; PPS, pentosan polysulfate sodium; SPR, surface plasmon resonance; TMB, 3,3′,5,5′-tetramethylbenzidine; TMS, trimethylsilyl; UV, ultraviolet

Fig. 1.1 Reported use of pentosan by office-based physicians in the USA

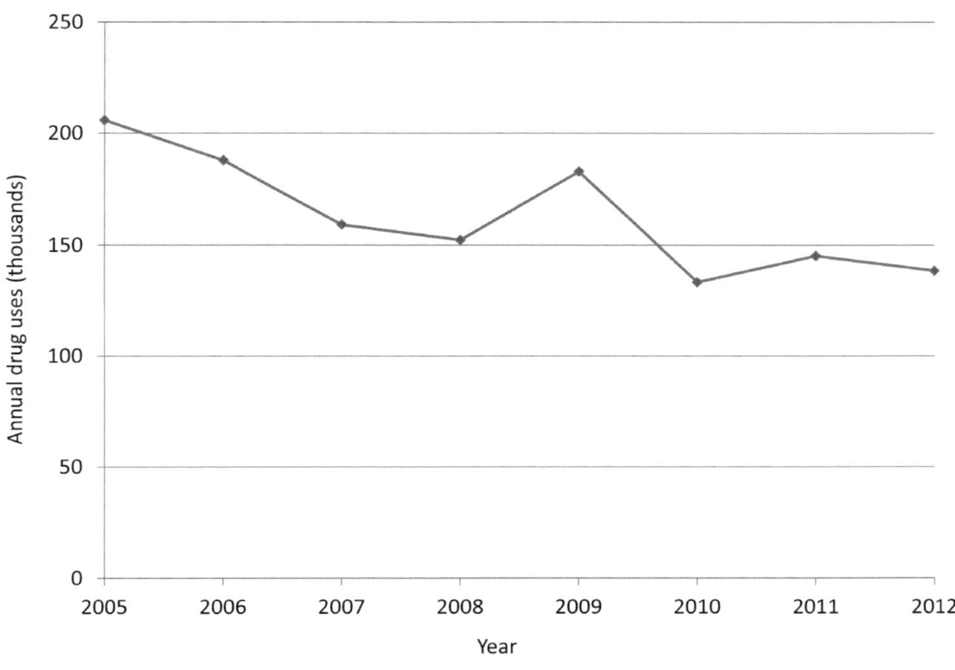

Prepared by the Working Group based on data obtained from IMS Health (2012b)

1.4 Occurrence and exposure

Pentosan polysulfate sodium does not occur in nature. Human exposure is largely limited to use as a medication. While occupational exposure in manufacturing is likely to occur, no specific studies on occupational or environmental exposure to pentosan were identified by the Working Group.

1.5 Regulations and guidelines

Pentosan has been approved by drug regulatory agencies primarily in the European Union and USA. In the USA, it was approved by the Food and Drug Administration in 1996 (FDA, 2013). The Working Group did not identify extraordinary regulatory restrictions on the use of pentosan as a medication, or regulations on environmental exposure.

2. Cancer in Humans

No data were available to the Working Group.

3. Cancer in Experimental Animals

3.1 Mouse

See Table 3.1

In one study of oral administration, groups of 50 male and 50 female B6C3F$_1$ mice (age, 6 weeks) were given pentosan polysulfate sodium (pharmaceutical grade) at doses of 0 (control), 56, 168, or 504 mg/kg body weight (bw) in deionized water by gavage once per day on 5 days per week for 104 to 105 weeks. A significant decrease in body weight was seen in females at the highest dose, but not in males or any other groups of females. Survival of all dosed groups was similar to that of controls. Liver haemangiosarcomas

Table 3.1 Studies of carcinogenicity in mice given pentosan polysulfate sodium by gavage

Strain (sex) Duration Reference	Dosing regimen, Animals/group at start	Incidence,(%) and/or multiplicity of tumours	Significance	Comments
Abdo *et al.* (2003), NTP (2004) B6C3F$_1$ (M, F) 104–105 wk	Administered at doses of 0, 56, 168, or 504 mg/kg bw in deionized water, 5 days per week, for 104–105 wk 50 M and 50 F/group	*Males* Liver haemangiosarcoma: 2/50*, 0/50, 4/50, 9/50** Hepatocellular adenoma: 19/50, 15/50, 15/50, 20/50 Hepatocellular carcinoma: 11/50, 13/50, 15/50, 13/50 Hepatocellular adenoma or carcinoma (combined): 23/50***, 23/50, 26/50, 31/50** *Female* Liver haemangiosarcoma[a]: 1/50, 1/49, 1/50, 4/49 Hepatocellular adenoma: 7/50****, 5/49, 4/50, 15/49** Hepatocellular carcinoma: 3/50, 3/50, 5/50, 3/50 Hepatocellular adenoma or carcinoma (combined): 10/50#, 8/49, 9/50, 18/49 Malignant lymphoma: 7/50##, 8/50, 6/50, 16/50**	*P < 0.001 (Poly-3 trend test) **P ≤ 0.05 (Poly-3 test) ***P = 0.031 (Poly-3 trend test) ****P = 0.003 (Poly-3 trend test) #P = 0.010 (Poly-3 trend test) ##P = 0.006 (Poly-3 trend test)	Purity, pharmaceutical grade

[a] Incidence in historical controls receiving NTP-2000 diet in 2-year studies: 24/959 (2.6% ± 1.4%); range, 0–4%

bw, body weight; F, female; M, male; wk, week

occurred with a positive trend in males, with the incidence at the highest dose significantly increased compared with controls. The incidence of liver haemangiosarcoma in females at the highest dose (4 out of 49; 8%) exceeded the incidence of this tumour in historical controls (24 out of 959, 2.6%; range, 0–4%). There was a significant increase in the incidence of malignant lymphoma in females at the highest dose.

The incidences of hepatocellular adenoma or carcinoma (combined) increased with positive trends in males and in females. The incidences of hepatocellular adenoma in females at the highest dose, and of hepatocellular adenoma or carcinoma (combined) in males at the highest dose were also significantly increased. The incidences of hepatocellular adenoma in treated males, and of hepatocellular carcinoma in treated males or treated females, were not significantly increased (Abdo *et al.*, 2003; NTP, 2004).

3.2 Rat

See Table 3.2

In one study of oral administration, groups of 50 male F344/N rats (age, 6 weeks) received pentosan polysulfate sodium (pharmaceutical grade) at oral doses of 0 (control), 14, 42, or 126 mg/kg bw, and groups of 50 female F344/N rats (age, 6 weeks) received pentosan polysulfate sodium at oral doses of 0 (control), 28, 84, or 252 mg/kg bw by gavage in deionized water, once per day, 5 days per week, for 104–105 weeks. There was no effect on body weight or survival in any of the groups of treated rats during the study. There were no significant increases in the incidence of any neoplasm in treated rats (Abdo *et al.*, 2003; NTP, 2004).

Table 3.2 Studies of carcinogenicity in rats given pentosan polysulfate sodium by gavage

Strain (sex) Duration Reference	Dosing regimen, Animals/group at start	Incidence, (%) and/or multiplicity of tumours	Significance	Comments
Abdo *et al.* (2003), NTP (2004) F344/N (M, F) 104–105 wk	Male rats were given doses of 0, 14, 42, or 126 mg/kg bw, and female rats were given doses of 0, 28, 84 or 252 mg/kg bw by gavage in deionized water, 5 days per week, for 104–105 wk 50 M and 50 F/group	See comments		Purity, pharmaceutical grade There were no significant increases in the incidence of any neoplasm

bw, body weight; F, female; M, male; wk, week

4. Mechanistic and Other Relevant Data

4.1 Absorption, distribution, metabolism, and excretion

4.1.1 Humans

Fellstrom *et al.* (1987) measured pentosan polysulfate sodium in plasma and in urine by radioassay after intravenous and oral administration in a group of eight healthy volunteers. After intravenous administration of 40 mg of pentosan, plasma clearance was 49.9 ± 6.6 mL/minute, of which renal clearance constituted 4.2 ± 1.2 mL/minute. Only 8% of the intravenous dose was recovered in the urine, suggesting that there was extensive metabolism. After daily oral dosing with 400 mg of pentosan, steady-state trough plasma concentrations were low (20–50 ng/mL), and bioavailability was 0.5–1%.

The oral bioavailability of pentosan was investigated in 18 healthy young male volunteers who received pentosan as an intravenous dose of 50 mg, or an oral dose of 1500 mg, or a placebo (Faaij *et al.*, 1999). Intravenously administered pentosan significantly increased activated partial thromboplastin time and the activity of anti-factor Xa, hepatic triglyceride lipase, and lipoprotein lipase compared with placebo in a magnitude comparable to other heparin-like compounds administered intravenously. Orally administered pentosan did not influence any of the parameters compared with placebo.

MacGregor *et al.* (1984) studied the catabolism of pentosan polysulfate sodium. Five healthy male volunteers were given [^{125}I]-labelled pentosan in conjunction with unlabelled pentosan at a dose of 0.1, 1, 7, or 50 mg intravenously. The half-lives for doses of 0.1–7 mg ranged from 13 to 18 minutes. At a dose of 50 mg, the half-life was 45 minutes. Tissue distribution studies showed that most of the radiolabelled material was localized in the liver and spleen. Pentosan was desulfated in the liver and spleen and depolymerized in the kidney, and it is likely that desulfation and depolymerization of pentosan is saturable.

Simon *et al.* (2005) studied two groups of eight healthy fasted female volunteers who sequentially received a single oral dose of 200 µCi of [^{3}H]-labelled pentosan supplemented with 300 mg of unlabelled pentosan, or 300 µCi of [^{3}H]-labelled pentosan supplemented with 450 mg of unlabelled pentosan. Most (84%) of the administered oral dose was excreted in the faeces as intact pentosan, and a smaller percentage (6%) was excreted in the urine as pentosan of low relative molecular mass and desulfated pentosan.

Excretion of pentosan was studied in 34 female patients with interstitial cystitis who were receiving long-term treatment with pentosan (Erickson *et al.*, 2006). The median concentration of pentosan in the urine of these patients was 1.2 µg/mL (range, 0.5–27.7 µg/mL). All the pentosan recovered from the urine of these patients was of low relative molecular mass.

4.1.2 Experimental systems

In a pharmacokinetic study of pentosan in New Zealand rabbits, [125I]-labelled pentosan as marker was injected simultaneously with increasing doses of unlabelled pentosan (Cadroy et al., 1987). The data indicated that prolongation of the half-life of pentosan with increasing doses resulted from progressive reduction in the clearance of the drug, with a constant volume of distribution.

Some studies of distribution were oriented towards the pharmacological application of pentosan in the treatment of interstitial cystitis. Kyker et al. (2005) used fluorescently labelled chondroitin sulfate to track the distribution of glycosaminoglycans administered intravesically to C57BL/6NHsd mouse bladder that had been damaged on the surface. Bladder damaged by trypsin or hydrochloric acid bound the labelled chondroitin sulfate extensively on the surface, with little penetration into the bladder muscle.

In rabbits given 1–1.2 mg of pentosan by intravenous administration, median recovery in the urine was 47.2% (range, 19.7–73.2%) for unfractionated pentosan, 74.6% (range, 31.4–96.3%) for pentosan of low relative molecular mass, and 3.3% (range, 2.5–5.0%) for pentosan of high relative molecular mass. In rabbits given 1.0–1.2 mg pentosan by oral administration, median recovery in the urine was 7.45% (range, 2.1–46.0%) for pentosan of low relative molecular mass, and 0.1% (range, 0.0–0.3%) for pentosan of high relative molecular mass (Erickson et al., 2006).

Sprague-Dawley rats were given [3H]-labelled pentosan orally or intravenously at a dose of 5 mg/kg bw, and killed 1 or 4 hours later, respectively. Autoradiography indicated extensive distribution of radiolabel in the whole animal after intravenous administration, with notable labelling of connective tissues, and low activity in bone and cartilage. There was a high concentration of radiolabel in the urine, and preferential localization of radiolabel to the lining of the urinary tract. After oral administration, the tissue distribution of radiolabel was similar, but activity was lower (Odlind et al., 1987).

4.2 Genetic and related effects

4.2.1 Humans

No data were available to the Working Group.

4.2.2 Experimental systems

(a) Mutagenicity

Pentosan polysulfate sodium was not mutagenic in Salmonella typhimurium strains TA97, TA98, TA100, or TA1535, with or without metabolic activation, at a concentration range of 100 to 10 000 µg/plate (NTP, 2004).

(b) Chromosomal damage

No consistent increase in the frequency of micronucleated polychromatic erythrocytes was seen in bone-marrow cells of male F344/N rats or male B6C3F$_1$ mice given pentosan at doses of 156.25–2500 mg/kg bw by gavage, three times at 24-hour intervals. An initial trial had yielded a weakly positive result (P for trend = 0.019) in male rats, but a second trial gave clearly negative results (NTP, 2004). A subsequent study in male and female B6C3F$_1$ mice given pentosan as a daily dose at 63, 125, 250, 500, or 1000 mg/kg bw by gavage for 3 months also gave negative results. There were no significant differences in the percentages of polychromatic erythrocytes in the circulating blood of mice receiving pentosan (NTP, 2004).

4.3 Other mechanistic data relevant to carcinogenicity

4.3.1 Effects on cellular physiology

Pentosan polysulfate sodium can antagonize the binding of fibroblast growth factor-2 (FGF-2) to its cell surface receptors, and has been shown to modulate the angiogenic activity of FGF-2 in tumours in humans and mice. Jerebtsova *et al.* (2007) studied the role of FGF-2 and pentosan in the pathogenesis of intestinal bleeding in mice. The results indicated that high steady-state levels of circulating FGF-2, plus anticoagulant activity, are needed to induce lethal intestinal bleeding in mice.

Treatment with pentosan prevents the progression of nephropathy in streptozotocin-induced diabetes in ageing C57B6 mice by decreasing albuminuria, renal macrophage infiltration, and expression of tumour necrosis factor-α (Wu *et al.*, 2011).

Zugmaier *et al.* (1992) concluded that pentosan is an in-vitro inhibitor of a variety of heparin-binding growth factors released from tumour cells. Of seven tumour cell lines tested, six (breast cancer: MDA-MB-231, MDA-MB-435, MDA-MB-468; lung cancer: A-549; prostate cancer: DU-145; and epidermoid carcinoma: A-431) were resistant to pentosan in soft-agar cloning assays, and did not appear to depend on autocrine stimulation by the heparin-binding growth factors. In contrast to this resistance in vitro, subcutaneous growth of tumours from all cell lines in athymic nude mice was inhibited in a dose-dependent fashion by daily intraperitoneal injections of pentosan.

Pentosan inhibits virus adsorption to cells in vitro as demonstrated by monitoring the association of radiolabelled HIV-1 virions with MT-4 cells (Baba *et al.*, 1988).

4.3.2 Effects on cell proliferation

Elliot *et al.* (2003) observed that pentosan has marked effects on the growth and extracellular matrix of smooth-muscle cells cultured from human prostate. Pentosan decreased cell proliferation and extracellular-matrix production. This suggested that the drug may have therapeutic potential in relation to benign prostatic hyperplasia.

The results of treatment of three prostate-cancer cell lines (LnCaP, PC3, and DU145) with pentosan have been reported (Zaslau *et al.*, 2006). In LnCaP cells, there was a mean inhibition of growth of 12% ± 7% at 24 hours ($P = 0.025$), and 20% ± 15% at 72 hours ($P < 0.001$). Similar inhibition was observed in the other two cell lines.

Rha *et al.* (1997) reported that growth of gastric-cancer cell lines expressing midkine, a novel heparin-binding growth/differentiation factor, was inhibited by pentosan, which was described as a heparin-binding blocking agent.

Zaslau *et al.* (2004) reported that pentosan significantly inhibited the growth of ZR75-1 breast-cancer cells; however, a significant increase in cell proliferation (25% ± 2%; $P < 0.001$) was observed in estrogen-independent MCF-7 breast-cancer cells.

The effects of pentosan on tumour growth, hyperprolactinaemia and angiogenesis in diethylstilbestrol-induced anterior pituitary adenoma in F344 rats was described by Mucha *et al.* (2002). Long-term treatment with pentosan did not cause any changes in pituitary weight, serum prolactin concentration, or density of microvessels. However, there was an increase in the number of apoptotic bodies within the anterior pituitary.

The mechanism of cell motility inhibition by pentosan appears to be independent of cytoskeletal structural alterations, including changes in microfilament and microtubule networks (Pienta *et al.*, 1992). In vitro, pentosan altered cellular contacts with the extravascular matrix and inhibited cell motility. In vivo, pentosan prolonged survival of male rats injected with highly metastatic cells.

4.4 Susceptibility

No data were available to the Working Group.

4.5 Mechanistic considerations

Most of the experimental studies on pentosan polysulfate sodium were not directed towards elucidating a possible mechanism of carcinogenesis. No mechanism of carcinogenesis was indicated by the collective findings.

5. Summary of Data Reported

5.1 Exposure data

Pentosan polysulfate sodium is a drug of high relative molecular mass that is obtained by chemically treating the bark of the beech tree. It is used in oral form to treat bladder conditions (interstitial cystitis) and in injectable form for the prevention of blood clots. A large proportion of the global use of pentosan occurs in the USA (global sales in 2012, US$ 276 million, with 82% occurring in the USA), where prescriptions have been declining over the past years.

5.2 Human carcinogenicity data

No data were available to the Working Group.

5.3 Animal carcinogenicity data

Pentosan polysulfate sodium was tested for carcinogenicity in one study in male and female mice treated by gavage, and in one study in male and female rats treated by gavage.

In mice, pentosan caused a significant increase in the incidence of liver haemangiosarcoma in males at the highest dose, and an increase in the incidence of liver haemangiosarcoma that occurred with a positive trend in males. The incidence of liver haemangiosarcoma in females at the highest dose exceeded the incidence in historical controls. It caused a significant increase in the incidence of malignant lymphoma in females at the highest dose. Exposure to pentosan increased the trend in the incidences of hepatocellular adenoma or carcinoma (combined) in males and females and also caused a significant increase in the incidence of hepatocellular adenoma in females and hepatocellular adenoma or carcinoma (combined) in males at the highest dose.

In treated rats, there were no significant increases in the incidence of any neoplasm.

5.4 Mechanistic and other relevant data

In humans, pentosan polysulfate sodium is desulfated in the liver and spleen and depolymerized in the kidney. Intravenous administration of radiolabelled pentosan to rats indicated extensive distribution of radiolabel, particularly in connective tissues, a high concentration of radiolabel in the urine, and a preferential localization of radiolabel to the lining of the urinary tract.

Pentosan was not mutagenic when tested in *Salmonella typhimurium*, with or without metabolic activation. Likewise, no evidence of chromosomal damage associated with exposure to pentosan was obtained in studies in rodents.

In vitro, pentosan is an inhibitor of a variety of heparin-binding growth factors released from tumour cells.

The data did not support any genotoxic mechanism of carcinogenesis by pentosan.

6. Evaluation

6.1 Cancer in humans

There is *inadequate evidence* in humans for the carcinogenicity of pentosan polysulfate sodium.

6.2 Cancer in experimental animals

There is *sufficient evidence* in experimental animals for the carcinogenicity of pentosan polysulfate sodium.

6.3 Overall evaluation

Pentosan polysulfate sodium is *possibly carcinogenic* to humans *(Group 2B)*.

References

Abdel-Haq H, Bossù E (2012). Capillary electrophoresis as a tool for the characterization of pentosan nanoparticles. *J Chromatogr A*, 1257:125–30. doi:10.1016/j.chroma.2012.07.096 PMID:22921360

Abdo KM, Johnson JD, Nyska A (2003). Toxicity and carcinogenicity of Elmiron in F344/N rats and B6C3F1 mice following 2 years of gavage administration. *Arch Toxicol*, 77:702–711. doi:10.1007/s00204-003-0472-9 PMID:14508637

Abnova (2013). PPS (Human) ELISA Kit. Available from: http://www.abnova.com/protocol_pdf/KA2273.pdf

Baba M, Nakajima M, Schols D *et al.* (1988). Pentosan polysulfate, a sulfated oligosaccharide, is a potent and selective anti-HIV agent in vitro. *Antiviral Res*, 9:335–343. doi:10.1016/0166-3542(88)90035-6 PMID:2465736

Cadroy Y, Dol F, Caranobe C *et al.* (1987). Pharmacokinetics of 125I-pentosan polysulfate in the rabbit. *Thromb Res*, 48:373–378. doi:10.1016/0049-3848(87)90449-X PMID:2448892

Degenhardt M, Benend H, Wätzig H (1998). Quality control of pentosane polysulfate by capillary zone electrophoresis using indirect detection. *J Chromatogr A*, 817(1–2):297–306. doi:10.1016/S0021-9673(98)00421-X PMID:9764502

Deshpande PB, Luthra P, Pandey AK, Paghdar DJ, Govardhana PSGV (2010). Process for the preparation of pentosan polysulfate or salts thereof. United States Patent No. 20100105889. Available from http://www.freepatentsonline.com/y2010/0105889.html

Elliot SJ, Zorn BH, McLeod DG *et al.* (2003). Pentosan polysulfate decreases prostate smooth muscle proliferation and extracellular matrix turnover. *Prostate Cancer Prostatic Dis*, 6:138–142. doi:10.1038/sj.pcan.4500632 PMID:12806372

Erickson DR, Sheykhnazari M, Bhavanandan VP (2006). Molecular size affects urine excretion of pentosan polysulfate. *J Urol*, 175:1143–1147. doi:10.1016/S0022-5347(05)00319-8 PMID:16469641

Faaij RA, Srivastava N, van Griensven JM *et al.* (1999). The oral bioavailability of pentosan polysulphate sodium in healthy volunteers. *Eur J Clin Pharmacol*, 54:929–935. doi:10.1007/s002280050577 PMID:10192753

FDA (2013). Pentosan Polysulfate Sodium. US Food and Drug Administration. Available from: http://www.accessdata.fda.gov/scripts/cder/drugsatfda/index.cfm

Fellstrom B, Bjorklund U, Danielson BG et al. (1987) Pertosan polysulfate (ELMIRON®): pharmacokinetics and effects on the urinary inhibition of crystal growth. Pathogenese und Klinik der Harnsteine (ed. by W. Vahlensieck & G. Gassner), pp. 340–396. Steinkopff-Verlag, Darmstadt.

Hanno PM, Burks DA, Clemens JQ, Dmochowski RR, Erickson D, Fitzgerald MP *et al.*; Interstitial Cystitis Guidelines Panel of the American Urological Association Education and Research, Inc (2011). AUA guideline for the diagnosis and treatment of interstitial cystitis/bladder pain syndrome. *J Urol*, 185(6):2162–70. doi:10.1016/j.juro.2011.03.064 PMID:21497847

IMS Health (2012a). Multinational Integrated Data Analysis (MIDAS). Plymouth Meeting, Pennsylvania: IMS Health. Available from: http://www.imshealth.com/portal/site/imshealth

IMS Health (2012b). National Disease and Therapeutic Index (NDTI). Plymouth Meeting (Pennsylvania): IMS Health, 2005–2012. Available from http://www.imshealth.com/portal/site/imshealth

IMS Health (2012c). National Prescription Audit Plus (NPA). Plymouth Meeting, Pennsylvania: IMS Health. 2008–2012.

Jerebtsova M, Wong E, Przygodzki R *et al.* (2007). A novel role of fibroblast growth factor-2 and pentosan polysulfate in the pathogenesis of intestinal bleeding in mice. *Am J Physiol Heart Circ Physiol*, 292:H743–H750. doi:10.1152/ajpheart.00969.2006 PMID:17071728

Kongtawelert P, Ghosh P (1990). A monoclonal antibody that recognizes 2,3-, 2,6-, and 4,6-disulphate ester ring substitution in pyranose-containing polysaccharides. Its production, characterization and application for the quantitation of pentosan polysulphate, dextran sulphate, glycosaminoglycan polysulphate and chondroitin sulphate E. *J Immunol Methods*, 126(1):39–49. doi:10.1016/0022-1759(90)90009-K PMID:1689359

Kyker KD, Coffman J, Hurst RE (2005). Exogenous glycosaminoglycans coat damaged bladder surfaces in experimentally damaged mouse bladder. *BMC Urol*, 5:4 doi:10.1186/1471-2490-5-4 PMID:15788101

Lee CE, Edwards HE, Navaratnam S, Phillips GO (1986). Quantitative analysis of a polysulfated xylan (SP54) in urine using gas-liquid chromatography. *Anal Biochem*, 152(1):52–8. doi:10.1016/0003-2697(86)90118-1 PMID:2420230

MacGregor IR, Dawes J, Paton L *et al.* (1984). Metabolism of sodium pentosan polysulphate in man–catabolism of iodinated derivatives. *Thromb Haemost*, 51:321–325. PMID:6208629

MicroMedex (2013) DRUGDEX® Evaluations. MicroMedex 2.0 database. Ann Arbor, Michigan: Truven Health Analytics Inc. Available from: http://micromedex. com/pharmaceutical.

Mucha S, Melen-Mucha G, Stepien T *et al.* (2002). Effects of pentosan polysulfate sodium on the estrogen-induced pituitary prolactinoma in Fischer 344 rats. *Oncol Rep*, 9:1385–1389. PMID:12375053

Muller D, Ndoume-Nze M, Jozefonvicz J (1984). High-pressure size-exclusion chromatography of anticoagulant materials. *J Chromatogr*, 297:351–8. doi:10.1016/S0021-9673(01)89055-5 PMID:6490767

NTP (2004). NTP technical report on the toxicology and carcinogenesis studies of Elmiron (CAS No. 37319–17–8) in F344/N rats and B6C3F1 mice (gavage studies). *Natl Toxicol Program Tech Rep Ser*, 512:7–289. PMID:15213766

O'Neil MJ (2006). The Merck Index - An encyclopedia of chemicals, drugs, and biologicals. 14th Ed. Whitehouse Station, NJ: Merck & Co., Inc.

Odlind B, Dencker L, Tengblad A (1987). Preferential localization of 3H-pentosanpolysulphate to the urinary tract in rats. *Pharmacol Toxicol*, 61:162–166. doi:10.1111/j.1600-0773.1987.tb01796.x PMID:2446305

Pienta KJ, Murphy BC, Isaacs WB *et al.* (1992). Effect of pentosan, a novel cancer chemotherapeutic agent, on prostate cancer cell growth and motility. *Prostate*, 20:233–241. doi:10.1002/pros.2990200308 PMID:1374181

Prochazka S, Mulholland M, Lloyd-Jones A (2003). Optimisation for the separation of the oligosaccharide, sodium pentosan polysulfate by reverse polarity capillary zone electrophoresis using a central composite design. *J Pharm Biomed Anal*, 31(1):133–41. doi:10.1016/S0731-7085(02)00569-1 PMID:12560057

PubChem (2013). Pentosan Sulfuric Polyester. Available from: http://pubchem.ncbi.nlm.nih.gov/summary/summary.cgi?cid=37720&loc=ecrcs, accessed 26 June 2014.

Rha SY, Noh SH, Kwak HJ *et al.* (1997). Comparison of biological phenotypes according to midkine expression in gastric cancer cells and their autocrine activities could be modulated by pentosan polysulfate. *Cancer Lett*, 118:37–46. doi:10.1016/S0304-3835(97)00215-2 PMID:9310258

RxList (2013). RxList - The internet drug index. Available from: http://www.rxlist.com/elmiron-drug-htm

SciFinder (2010). SciFinder Databases: Registry, Chemcats. American Chemical Society.

Shen B, Shimmon S, Smith MM, Ghosh P (2003). Biosensor analysis of the molecular interactions of pentosan polysulfate and of sulfated glycosaminoglycans with immobilized elastase, hyaluronidase and lysozyme using surface plasmon resonance (SPR) technology. *J Pharm Biomed Anal*, 31(1):83–93. doi:10.1016/S0731-7085(02)00606-4 PMID:12560052

Simon M, McClanahan RH, Shah JF *et al.* (2005). Metabolism of [3H]pentosan polysulfate sodium (PPS) in healthy human volunteers. *Xenobiotica*, 35:775–784. doi:10.1080/00498250500230586 PMID:16278190

US Pharmacopeial Convention (2013). Pentosan Polysulfate Sodium © 2013. The United States Pharmacopeial Convention. No. CAS-140207–93–8; CAS-116001–96–8 [replaced]. Available from: www.uspusan.com.

Witvrouw M, Baba M, Balzarini J, Pauwels R, De Clercq E (1990). Establishment of a bioassay to determine serum levels of dextran sulfate and pentosan polysulfate, two potent inhibitors of human immunodeficiency virus. *J Acquir Immune Defic Syndr*, 3(4):343–7. PMID:1690285

Wu J, Guan TJ, Zheng S *et al.* (2011). Inhibition of inflammation by pentosan polysulfate impedes the development and progression of severe diabetic nephropathy in aging C57B6 mice. *Lab Invest*, 91:1459–1471. doi:10.1038/labinvest.2011.93 PMID:21808238

Zaslau S, Riggs DR, Jackson BJ *et al.* (2004). In vitro effects of pentosan polysulfate against malignant breast cells. *Am J Surg*, 188:589–592. doi:10.1016/j.amjsurg.2004.07.007 PMID:15546576

Zaslau S, Sparks S, Riggs D *et al.* (2006). Pentosan polysulfate (Elmiron): in vitro effects on prostate cancer cells regarding cell growth and vascular endothelial growth factor production. *Am J Surg*, 192:640–643. doi:10.1016/j.amjsurg.2006.08.008 PMID:17071199

Zugmaier G, Lippman ME, Wellstein A (1992). Inhibition by pentosan polysulfate (PPS) of heparin-binding growth factors released from tumor cells and blockage by PPS of tumor growth in animals. *J Natl Cancer Inst*, 84:1716–1724. doi:10.1093/jnci/84.22.1716 PMID:1279186

TRIAMTERENE

1. Exposure Data

1.1 Chemical and physical data

1.1.1 Nomenclature

Chem. Abstr. Serv. Reg. No.: 396-01-0

Chem. Abstr. Serv. Name: 2,4,7-Pteridine-triamine, 6-phenyl

IUPAC systematic name: 6-Phenyl-pteridine-2,4,7-triamine

Synonyms: 6-Phenyl-2,4,7-triaminopteridine; 2,4,7-triamino-6-phenyl-pteridin

1.1.2 Structural and molecular formulae and relative molecular mass

$C_{12}H_{11}N_7$

Relative molecular mass: 253.26 (O'Neil, 2006).

1.1.3 Chemical and physical properties of the pure substance

Description: Odourless yellow powder or crystalline solid, almost tasteless at first and with a slightly bitter aftertaste, acidified solutions give a blue fluorescence (ChemicalBook, 2013)

Melting point: 316 °C

Density: 1.502 g/cm^3 (ChemSpider, 2013)

Solubility: Very slightly soluble in water and in ethanol (96%).

Stability data: Stable in formulation: acid, neutral and alkali. Slowly oxidized upon exposure to air (Bakshi & Singh, 2002; Chemical Book, 2013).

Dissociation constants: pK_a (strongest acidic) = 15.88; pK_a (strongest basic) = 3.11 (DrugBank, 2013)

1.1.4 Technical products and impurities

(a) Trade names

These are some trade names for medications with triamterene as the sole active agent: Ademine; Diren; Ditak; Diucelpin; Diurene; Diuterene; Dyazide; Dyren; Dyrenium; Dytac; Jatropur; Riyazine; Teriam; Triteren; Urinis; Urocaudal (O'Neil, 2006; DrugBank, 2013).

(b) Impurities

The following impurities are listed in the British Pharmacopoeia (2009):

- 5-Nitrosopyrimidine-2,4,6-triamine (nitrosotriaminopyrimidine)
- 2,7-Diamino-6-phenylpteridin-4-ol
- 2,4-Diamino-6-phenylpteridin-7-ol
- Phenylacetonitrile (benzyl cyanide).

1.2 Analysis

Triamterene can be identified by infrared absorption or potentiometric titration assays that use its property of producing an intense blueish fluorescence in a 1/1000 solution of formic acid. The selective estimation of triamterene in the presence of its degradation products or other compounds in biological fluids is mainly carried out by high-performance liquid chromatography (HPLC). Compendial and non-compendial analytical methods are summarized in Table 1.1.

1.3 Production and use

1.3.1 Production process

Triamterene is a synthetic compound that was first synthesized by Spickett & Timmis (1954) by the reaction of 4-amino-5-nitrosopyrimidine with phenylacetonitrile (NTP, 1993).

1.3.2 Use

(a) Indications

Triamterene has been used since 1961 as a potassium-sparing diuretic. It is still chiefly used as an antihypertension agent for the control of elevated blood pressure, as well as for the treatment of interstitial fluid accumulation (oedema), particularly when this co-exists with hypertension. Potassium-sparing diuretics, unlike other classes of diuretics, produce diuresis without loss of appreciable amounts of potassium in the urine. The most commonly reported clinical indications for triamterene in the USA in 2011–2012 are listed in Table 1.2.

Triamterene is recommended as a first-line antihypertensive in the USA (Chobanian *et al.*, 2003), and its use is recommended in combination with another class of antihypertension drug in Europe (Mansia *et al.*, 2007, Mancia *et al.*, 2009). Off-label use for Ménière disease has been reported in the medical literature (van Deelen & Huizing, 1986), and still occurs in the USA (Table 1.2; IMS Health, 2012a).

In the USA, triamterene is approved by the Food and Drug Administration (FDA, 2013) for the management of oedema and as an adjunctive diuretic where its potassium-sparing effect is desired. In 2011–12, 99.5% of its uses were as a combination product with hydrochlorothiazide. The combination of triamterene and hydrochlorothiazide is approved for the treatment of hypertension or oedema in patients who develop hypokalaemia when receiving hydrochlorothiazide alone, or for whom hypokalaemia cannot be risked. Triamterene may also be used alone or as an adjunct to other antihypertension drugs.

The European Union (eMC, 2013) lists three available formulations: triamterene alone, triamterene combined with another diuretic (hydrochlorothiazide, bemetizide, epitizide, trichlormethiazide, xipamide, or furosemide), and triamterene combined with two other antihypertension agents (propranolol/hydrochlorothiazide, reserpine/hydrochlorothiazide, or verapamil/hydrochlorothiazide). These drugs are indicated in the European Union for oedema and hypertension.

Given its use in chronic conditions, triamterene therapy would be expected to be life-long in the absence of adverse effects for the patient.

Triamterene is a weak antagonist of folic acid, and a photosensitizing drug (NTP, 1993; Vargas *et al.*, 1998).

Table 1.1 Some analytical methods for triamterene

Sample matrix	Sample preparation	Assay method	Detection limit	Reference
Compendial methods				
Identity	–	Infrared spectroscopy	–	British
Assay	–	Potentiometric titration	–	Pharmacopoeia (2009)
Non-compendial methods				
Human serum	Extraction with methyl *tert*-butyl ether, centrifugation, evaporation, reconstitution in mobile phase	HPLC-ECD Column: C_{18} Mobile phase: phosphate buffer : acetonitrile (90 : 10) Flow rate: 0.8 mL/min	5 ng/mL (LOQ)	Richter *et al.* (1996)
Human plasma	Mixing, centrifugation, gentle agitation, evaporated to dryness under N_2, extract was reconstituted with 500 μL of mobile phase	HPLC-UV Column: C_{18} Flow rate: 1 mL/min Detector: fluorescence detector Mobile phase: acetonitrile : distilled water : acetic acid Wavelength: 365 nm	20 ng/mL (LOD)	Yakatan & Cruz (1981)
Human blood, plasma, and urine	Deproteination by adding acetonitrile, mixing, centrifugation	HPLC-UV Column: C_{18} Mobile phase: acetonitrile in 0.02% phosphoric acid solvent system Flow rate: 2 mL/min Excitation wavelength: 365 nm Emission wavelength: 440 nm	20 ng/mL (plasma) 0.5 μg/mL (urine) (LOQ)	Sörgel *et al.* (1984)
Human plasma and urine	Protein precipitation (plasma), centrifugation, collection of supernatant	HPLC Column: C_{18} Fluorescence detector Mobile phase: phosphoric acid and trimethylamine buffer : acetonitrile : methanol (70 : 14 : 8) Flow rate: 0.8 mL/min	1 ng/mL (LOQ)	Swart & Botha (1987)
Human urine	Centrifugation, collection of supernatant	Matrix isopotential fluorometry	2.4 ng/mL (LOD)	Pulgarín *et al.* (2001)
Human urine	Liquid–liquid extraction with ethyl acetate, centrifugation, evaporation, reconstitution in mobile phase	LC-ESI-MS/MS Column: C_{18} Mobile phase: 1% acetic acid and acetonitrile Flow rate: 0.3 mL/min	20 ng/mL	Deventer *et al.* (2002)
Human urine	Filtration through a folded filter	CE-LIF Silica-fused capillary Phosphate buffer Wavelength: 353 nm	50 ng/mL (LOQ)	Horstkötter *et al.* (2002)

Table 1.1 (continued)

Sample matrix	Sample preparation	Assay method	Detection limit	Reference
Human urine	Extraction, preconcentration and derivatization with acetone : methyl iodide (1 : 10)	GC-MS Column: C_{18} Selected ion monitoring	130 µg/L (LOD)	Amendola *et al.* (2003)
Human urine and formulation	Solid-phase extraction	Spectrofluorimetric method Column: C_{18} Mobile phase: phosphoric acid and triethylamine buffer : acetonitrile : methanol (70 : 17 : 3)	0.8 ng/mL (LOD) 2.3 ng/mL (LOQ)	Ibañez *et al.* (2005)
Bovine milk	Extraction with acetonitrile, centrifugation, decantation of supernatant, evaporation to dryness, reconstitution with water	UPLC-ESI-MS/MS Column: C_{18} Flow rate: 0.45 mL/min Multiple reaction monitoring	0.2 µg/kg (LOD) 0.5 µg/kg (LOQ)	Shao *et al.* (2008)
Rat plasma	Tandem solid-phase extraction method by connecting two different cartridges (C_{18} and MCX)	HPLC-UV Mobile phase: acetonitrile : 0.2% acetic acid (20 : 80) Flow rate: 0.8 mL/min Detection wavelength: 265 nm	1.4 ng/mL (LOD) 4.8 ng/mL (LOQ)	Li *et al.* (2011)

CE-LIF, capillary electrophoresis-laser-induced fluorescence; GC-MS, gas chromatography-mass spectrometry; HPLC, high-performance liquid chromatography; HPLC-ECD, high performance liquid chromatography-electrochemical detection; LC-ESI-MS/MS, liquid chromatography-electrospray ionization-tandem mass spectrometry; LOD, limit of detection; LOQ, limit of quantitation; min, minute; NR, not reported; UPLC-ESI-MS/MS, ultra performance liquid chromatography-electrospray ionization- tandem mass spectrometry; UV, ultraviolet

Table 1.2 Most commonly reported clinical indications for triamterene in the USA, 2011–2012

Diagnosis[a]	ICD-9 code	Drug uses (thousands)	Percentage of total
Essential hypertension, NOS	401.90	4824	84.6
Oedema, NOS	782.30	141	2.5
Hypertensive heart disease, other	402.90	136	2.4
Hypertension, benign	401.10	60	1.0
Ménière disease	386.00	56	1.0
Chronic ischaemic disease, unspecified, with hypertension	414.50	44	0.8
Hypertensive renal disease	403.90	43	0.8
Metabolic/insulin resistance syndrome	277.70	29	0.5
Swelling of foot	729.80	24	0.4
Arteriosclerotic heart disease with hypertension	414.20	22	0.4
All other diagnoses	–	323	5.7
Total with reported diagnoses	–	5703	100.0

[a] No diagnosis was stated for 0.5% of drug uses

From IMS Health (2012a)

ICD-9, International Classification of Diseases Ninth Revision; NOS, not otherwise specified

(b) Dosage

In the USA, triamterene alone is available in doses of 50 mg and 100 mg. In combination with hydrochlorothiazide, triamterene doses of 37.5 mg, 50 mg and 75 mg are used. In 2011–12, IMS Health National Disease and Therapeutics Index (NDTI) data showed that the most commonly used form was triamterene 37.5 mg/hydrochlorothiazide 25 mg. Once-per-day dosing predominates (94%). The mean daily dosage among patients taking triamterene is 37 mg per day (IMS Health, 2012a).

In the European Union, triamterene is available as a single agent (50 mg), in combination with hydrochlorothiazide (50 mg with 25 mg hydrochlorothiazide), and in combination with furosemide (50 mg triamterene with 40 mg furosemide) (eMC, 2013).

(c) Trends in use

Triamterene is a less commonly used antihypertension agent in the USA, accounting for 3% of the medications prescribed for high blood pressure. Other members of the potassium-sparing diuretic class, spironolactone and amiloride, are chemically distinct from triamterene in several important respects (Wang *et al.*, 2007; Gu *et al.*, 2012).

In the USA, triamterene is used moderately, with 2.8 million drug uses in 2012 according to IMS Health NDTI data (IMS Health, 2012a). Its use has declined by 47% since 2005 (Fig. 1.1). Approximately 1.2 million patients in the USA received triamterene in 2012 (IMS Health, 2012a). According to the IMS Health National Prescription Audit Plus, there was a total of 5.2 million prescriptions containing triamterene dispensed in the USA in 2012, a decrease of 32% from 7.6 million prescriptions in 2008 (IMS Health, 2012b). In 2012, nearly all triamterene (99.6%) was dispensed in the form of combination products containing hydrochlorothiazide (IMS Health, 2012b).

Total worldwide sales of triamterene were US$ 141 million in 2012 according to IMS Health MIDAS data, with 80% occurring in the USA. The only other nation with sales of greater than US$ 5 million was Germany (US$ 11 million) (IMS Health, 2012c).

Fig. 1.1 Use of triamterene reported by office-based physicians, USA

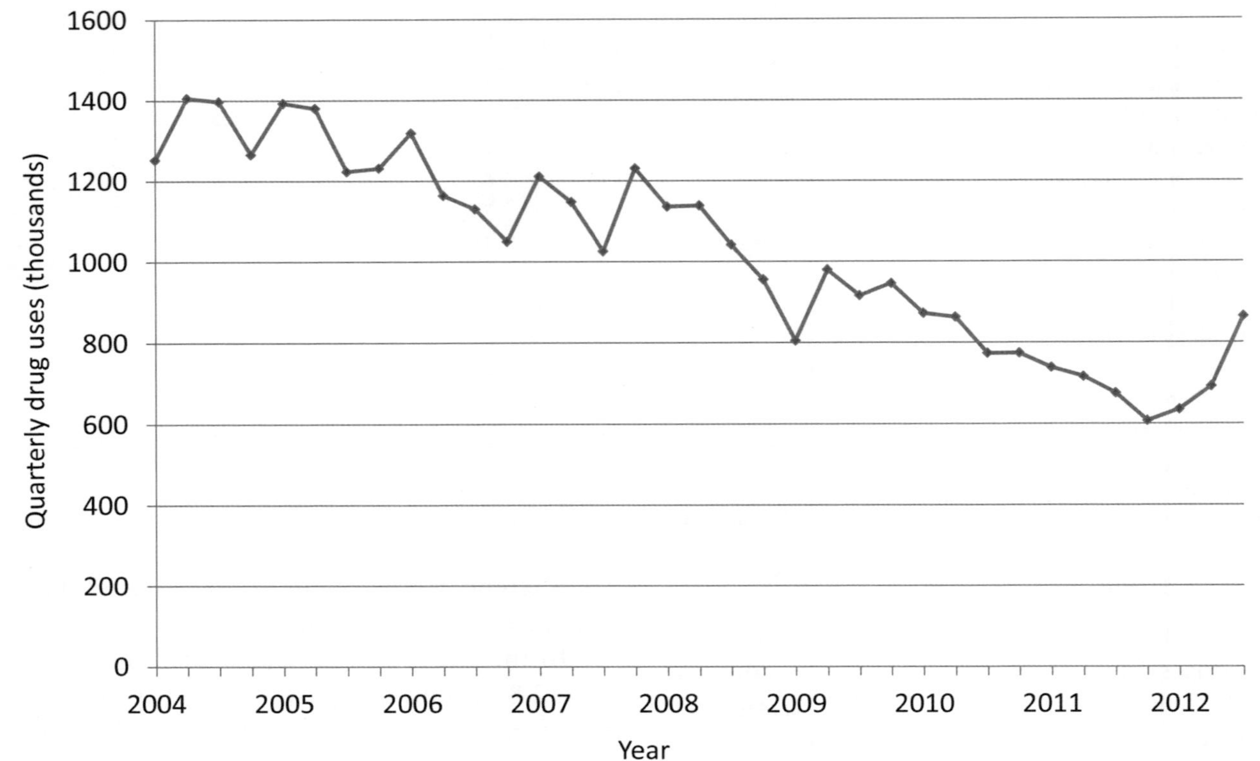

Prepared by the Working Group based on data obtained from IMS Health (2012a)

1.4   Occurrence and exposure

Triamterene does not occur in nature.

Human exposure is predominantly from use as a medication. Occupational exposure in manufacturing is also likely to occur.

1.5   Regulations and guidelines

Triamterene has been widely approved by drug regulatory agencies around the world. In the USA, it was approved by the Food and Drug Administration in 1964 (FDA, 2013). [The Working Group did not identify extraordinary regulatory restrictions on the use of triamterene as a medication, or regulations on environmental exposure.]

2.   Cancer in Humans

2.1   Background

Five case–control studies, including two nested case–control studies, assessed the association between triamterene and cancer. Cancer of the breast was investigated in three studies, and cancers of the lip and colon were each assessed in one study; however, only one study on cancer of the breast reported risk estimates specifically for triamterene. The studies are reported below, organized by relevance, and in Table 2.1.

Table 2.1 Case–control studies of cancer and triamterene

Reference Study location and period	Total No. cases Total No. controls	Control source (hospital, population)	Exposure assessment	Organ site (ICD code)	Exposure categories	Exposed cases	Relative risk (95% CI)	Covariates Comments
Williams *et al.* (1978) USA Period, NR	481 1268	Population	Mailed questionnaires to patients confirmed via physician questionnaire	Breast	Triamterene (ever-use) > 1 yr Recent use ≥ 5 yr	4 NR 0	0.4 *P* > 0.05 0.4 *P* > 0.05 NR	Age, race, centre. Other risk factors did not have confounding effects Response rate: patient questionnaire, 88%; physician questionnaire, 73%. Triamterene usually used in combination with thiazide. Only four exposed cases treated with triamterene for > 1 yr
Friedman *et al.* (2012) San Francisco, USA, 1994–2008	712 22 904	Nested case–controls; cohort of health-care subscribers	Pharmacy database (prescriptions dispensed)	Lip (squamous cell carcinoma, 97%)	HCTZ/triamterene, prescriptions before cancer diagnosis, ≥ 3 < 1 yr supply 1 to < 5 yr supply ≥ 5 yr supply	71 NR NR NR	1.98 (1.52–2.58) 0.91 (0.60–1.39) 1.87 (1.37–2.57) 2.82 (1.74–4.55)	Smoking White, non-Hispanic without HIV or organ transplant; cases identified by linking to cancer registry; controls randomly selected and matched on age, sex, and year of cohort entry; analysis, 2-yr lag
Mack *et al.* (1975) Los Angeles, USA, 1971–5	99 396	Nested case–controls (retirement community, enrolled from 1968 to 1973)	Medical records; not blinded	Breast	Hypertensive drugs (triamterene alone, 19%) – ever-use. Never used rauwolfia class of drugs Ever-used rauwolfia class of drugs	NR	0.9 [CI cannot be calculated] 2.9 [CI cannot be calculated]	Women, age 53–89 yr; controls matched by age, community entry; cases identified from community records or surrounding hospital and surveillance programmes

Table 2.1 (continued)

Reference Study location and period	Total No. cases Total No. controls	Control source (hospital, population)	Exposure assessment	Organ site (ICD code)	Exposure categories	Exposed cases	Relative risk (95% CI)	Covariates Comments
Coogan et al. (2009) Boston, New York, Philadelphia, Baltimore, USA, 1976–2007	5989 5504	Hospital medical records	Nurse administered questionnaire/ self-reported	Breast	Regular use (4×/wk for at least 3 mo) potassium-sparing diuretics that did not contain thiazide Duration (yr):	21	1.22 (0.61–2.46)	Race, education, menopausal status, parity, BMI, female-hormone use, oral contraceptives, and alcohol Women, aged 22–79 yr; controls matched to cases on age, interview year, study centre
					< 5	10	1.50 (0.57–3.96)	
					≥ 5	11	1.05 (0.38–2.88)	
					P for trend		0.64	
Coogan & Rosenberg (2007) Massachusetts, USA, 2001–4	1229 1165	Population	Telephone interview	Colorectum	Dihydrofolate reductase inhibitors (triamterene, methotrexate, and sulfasalazine)			Age, sex, NSAID use, number of doctor visits, alcohol consumption, education, vitamin use, colonoscopy, dietary factors Age, 50–74 yr. Factors considered but had little effect on odds ratio: race, exercise, BMI, family history, cholecystectomy, smoking status, hormonal replacement therapy. Most common folate antagonist: triamterene (30%)
					Regular use	34	1.6 (0.9–2.8)	
					< 5 yr	16	1.3 (0.6–3.0)	
					≥ 5 yr	18	1.9 (0.8–4.2)	
					P for trend		0.6	

BMI, body mass index; CI, confidence interval; HCTZ, hydrochlorothiazide; mo, month; NR, not reported; NSAID, nonsteroidal anti-inflammatory drug; wk, week; yr, year

2.2 Triamterene and cancer of the breast

Odds ratios (OR) specific for triamterene use were reported in a case–control study of 481 women with cancer of the breast, 421 women with benign breast lesions, and 1268 controls identified from a mammography screening project in the USA (Williams *et al.*, 1978). A small proportion of subjects were treated with triamterene, and only four women used it for more than 1 year. Most women also took other drugs. Triamterene use, both ever and recent, was associated with a decreased risk of cancer of the breast. Odds ratios adjusted for age, race, and centre were 0.4 (95% CI, not reported; $P > 0.05$) for both exposure periods. Triamterene use (ever or for 5 years) was associated with a non-significantly increased risk of benign breast lesions; however, triamterene was generally given in combination with thiazide, which was an independent risk factor for benign breast lesions in this study. [The strengths of this study were the verification of exposure information and detailed information on multiple-drug use and potential confounders. However, the study had a limited ability to evaluate the risks specific for triamterene use because only a small number of subjects were treated with triamterene and most were exposed to multiple drugs.]

2.3 Combined use of triamterene and hydrochlorothiazide, and cancer of the lip

Friedman *et al.* (2012) performed case–control analyses of the association between cancer of the lip and use of common antihypertension drugs in a cohort of medical-insurance subscribers in San Francisco, USA. Triamterene combined with hydrochlorothiazide (see *Monograph* on hydrochlorothiazide in this volume) was among the most common prescriptions for diuretics, but triamterene was not assessed separately. Cases of cancer of the lip (squamous cell carcinoma, 97%) were identified via the programme's cancer registry, and drug use was determined from pharmacy database. Analyses were based on 712 cases and 22 904 matched controls and were lagged by 2 years. The smoking-adjusted odds ratio for cancer of the lip and at least three prescriptions for hydrochlorothiazide-triamterene was 1.98 (95% CI, 1.52–2.58); and the risk increased with increasing duration of use. For prescriptions of 1 to < 5 years, the adjusted odds ratio was 1.87 (95% CI, 1.37–2.57), and for prescriptions of ≥ 5 years the adjusted odds ratio was 2.82 (95% CI, 1.74–4.55). Odds ratios for hydrochlorothiazide were higher than those for the hydrochlorothiazide-triamterene combination. [This study was relatively informative for evaluating the effects of treatment with hydrochlorothiazide-triamterene combined and risk of cancer of the lip because of its large size, nested design, use of a pharmacy database for drug usage, and consideration of potential confounders by study-selection criteria and multivariable analysis. While the study did not adjust for exposure to sunlight, it seems unlikely that exposure to sunlight was sufficiently greater in cases than controls to account for the increase in risk by up to threefold. Nevertheless, the study was not informative for evaluating specific effects of triamterene and risk of cancer.]

2.4 The drug class including triamterene, and cancer of the breast or colorectum

Mack *et al.* (1975) evaluated the association of cancer of the breast with antihypertension drugs in a nested case–control study among residents of a retirement community in Los Angeles, USA. The study included 99 cases of cancer of the breast and 396 controls matched for age and entry date, and information about medication was abstracted from medical records of the community health centre. The rauwolfia class of drugs, including reserpine, were the primary focus of the study, but some analyses were conducted for other antihypertension drugs (methyldopa alone or combined with other drugs, 35%; triamterene alone, 19%; chlorthalidone alone, 15%; hydralazine alone, 15%; spironolactone alone, 7%; guanethidine alone, 3%; and combined drugs not including methyldopa, 6%). The odds ratio for ever-use of other antihypertension drugs was 0.9 (95% CI, not reported) among women who never used the rauwolfia class of drugs, and 2.9 (95% CI, not reported) among ever-users of the rauwolfia class of drugs. [The major limitations of the study were the lack of information specific for triamterene, and the potential for confounding by other antihypertension drugs. Other limitations were the inadequate exposure information, low prevalence of exposure (14% in controls), short follow-up (in part due to the advanced age of the subjects), and the potential lack of generalizability to the general population because of the restricted subject population.]

Another study of cancer of the breast evaluated risks associated with several different classes of diuretics, including thiazides, potassium-sparing diuretics that do not contain thiazide (including triamterene), and loop diuretics, using medical records of several hospitals for 1976–2007 (Coogan *et al.*, 2009). The study included 5989 cases of invasive cancer of the breast, and 5504 matched hospital controls with diagnoses unrelated to use of diuretics. The adjusted odd ratio for cancer of the breast and regular use (defined as four times per week for at least 3 months) of potassium-sparing diuretics was 1.22 (95% CI, 0.61–2.46). The odds ratio was elevated for use for < 5 years (adjusted OR, 1.50; 95% CI, 0.57–3.96), but not for use for ≥ 5 years. [The major limitations of the study were the lack of information specific for triamterene, and the low percentage of the population using potassium-sparing diuretics (21 out of 5504 controls).

The potential for recall bias was reduced by the use of hospital controls.]

A case–control study of colorectal cancer grouped triamterene with antagonists of folic acid rather than other antihypertension drugs (Coogan & Rosenberg, 2007). The study included 1229 cases of adenocarcinoma of the colon and rectum identified from cancer registries and participating hospitals in Massachusetts, USA, and 1165 population-based controls matched for age, sex, and geographical location; cases and controls were free from Crohn disease or ulcerative colitis. Triamterene was the most commonly used folic-acid antagonist (30% of all antagonists). Elevated odds ratios were observed for regular use of dihydrofolate-reductase inhibitors, which included methotrexate and sulfasalazine in addition to triamterene (adjusted OR, 1.6; 95% CI, 0.9–2.8) and risks were somewhat higher among those who had used these drugs for 5 years or more (adjusted OR, 1.9; 95% CI, 0.8–4.2). [The study was not specific for triamterene use, and although the population was large, only a small percentage had taken dihydrofolate-reductase inhibitors including triamterene. There was also potential for misclassification of exposure due to self-reporting.]

3. Cancer in Experimental Animals

See Table 3.1

3.1 Mouse

In one study of carcinogenicity with oral administration, referred to hereafter as the first study, groups of 50–60 male and 50–60 female B6C3F$_1$ mice (age, 6 weeks) were given feed containing triamterene (purity, > 99%) at a concentration of 0 (control), 100, 200, or 400 ppm for 2 years. These concentrations were equivalent to average daily doses of approximately 0, 10, 25,

Table 3.1 Studies of carcinogenicity with triamterene in mice and rats

Species, strain (sex) Duration Reference	Dosing regimen Animals/group at start	Incidence of tumours	Significance	Comments
Mouse, B6C3F$_1$ (M, F) 104 wk NTP (1993)	*First study:* 0 (control), 100, 200 or 400 ppm in feed: 0, 10, 25, 45 mg/kg bw (M); 0, 15, 30, 60 mg/kg bw (F) *Second study:* 0 (control) or 400 ppm in feed: 0, 40 mg/kg bw (M); 0, 60 mg/kg bw (F) 50–60 M and 50–60 F/group (age, 6 wk), for both studies	*First study* Hepatocellular adenoma: 17/50 (34%), 22/50 (44%), 19/50 (38%), 20/60 (33%) (M); 10/50 (20%)*, 22/50 (44%)**, 23/50 (46%)***, 36/60 (60%)* (F) Hepatocellular carcinoma: 5/50 (10%)**, 7/50 (14%), 3/50 (6%), 13/60 (22%)** (M)[a]; 4/50 (8%), 4/50 (8%), 3/50 (6%), 8/60 (13%) (F) Hepatocellular adenoma or carcinoma (combined): 20/50 (40%), 26/50 (52%), 19/50 (38%), 29/60 (48%)** (M)[b]; 13/50 (26%)*, 26/50 (52%)**, 25/50 (50%)**, 37/60 (62%)* (F)[c] *Second study* Hepatocellular adenoma: 21/50 (42%), 36/50 (72%)* (M); 7/50 (14%), 28/51 (55%)* (F) Hepatocellular carcinoma: 9/50 (18%), 11/50 (22%) (M); 5/50 (10%), 11/51 (22%) (F)[d] Hepatocellular adenoma or carcinoma (combined): 25/50 (50%), 38/50 (76%)** (M)[b]; 10/50 (20%), 31/50 (61%)* (F)[c]	*P* < 0.001 **P* < 0.05 ***P* < 0.01 *P* < 0.001 **P* < 0.005	Purity, > 99% Second study performed because of a dosing error in mice at the highest dose in the first study [The Working Group considered that the results for the group at the highest dose could not be evaluated because of overdosing]
Rat, F344/N (M, F) 104 wk NTP (1993)	0 (control), 150, 300, 600 ppm in feed: 0, 5, 10, 25 mg/kg bw (M); 0, 5, 15, 30 mg/kg bw (F) 50 M and 50 F/group (age, 6 wk)	Hepatocellular adenoma: 0/50 (0%), 6/50 (12%)*, 4/50 (8%), 3/49 (6%) (M)[e]	*P* < 0.05	Purity, > 99% No significant increase in tumour incidence in females

[a] Historical rates of hepatocellular carcinoma in feed studies in control male mice (mean ± SD): 122/865 (14.1% ± 7.2%); range, 3–27%

[b] Historical rates of hepatocellular adenoma or carcinoma (combined) in feed studies in control male mice (mean ± SD): 249/865 (28.8% ± 10.9%); range, 17–58%

[c] Historical rates of hepatocellular adenoma and carcinoma (combined) in feed studies in control female mice (mean ± SD): 98/863 (11.4% ± 7.6%); range, 3–34%

[d] Historical rates of hepatocellular carcinoma in feed studies in control female mice (mean ± SD): 28/863 (3.2% ± 2.9%); range, 0–10%

[e] Historical rates of hepatocellular adenoma in feed studies in control male rats (mean ± SD): 19/799 (2.4% ± 2.9%); range, 0–8%

bw, body weight; F, female; M, male; SD, standard deviation; wk, week or 45 mg/kg body weight (bw) for males, and 0, 15, 30, or 60 mg/kg bw for females (NTP, 1993). Survival of exposed groups was similar to that of controls except for the group of male mice at 400 ppm. Because of a dosing error, male and female mice at the highest dietary concentration (400 ppm) actually received approximately four times the targeted concentration (approximately 1600 ppm) of triamterene for 7 days at week 40. During week 40, 12 male and 4 female mice died. The surviving mice in the group receiving the highest dose were kept in this study, but because of uncertainty regarding the effect of this 1 week of increased exposure on the outcome of the study, a second study was conducted with groups of 50–60 male and 50–60 female B6C3F$_1$ mice (age, 6 weeks) given feed containing triamterene at 0 (control) or 400 ppm (equivalent to average daily doses of approximately 40 mg/kg bw for males, and 60 mg/kg bw for females) for 2 years.

In the first study, triamterene caused significant increases in the incidences of hepatocellular adenoma in females at the lowest and intermediate doses. [The Working Group considered that the results for the group receiving the highest dose could not be evaluated because of the overdosing.] In the second study, survival of exposed groups was similar to that of controls. There were significant increases in the incidence of hepatocellular adenoma in males and females, and of hepatocellular adenoma or carcinoma (combined) in females. The incidence of liver foci was increased in some groups of treated mice in both the first and second studies. Treatment with triamterene also caused treatment-related thyroid follicular cell hyperplasia.

3.2 Rat

In one study of carcinogenicity with oral administration, groups of 50 male and 50 female F344/N rats (age, 6 weeks) were given feed containing triamterene (purity, > 99%) at a concentration of 0 (control), 150, 300, or 600 ppm.

These concentrations were equivalent to average daily doses of approximately 0, 5, 10, or 25 mg/kg bw for males, and 0, 5, 15, or 30 mg/kg bw for females (NTP, 1993). Survival of exposed groups was similar to that of controls. Triamterene caused a significant increase in the incidence of hepatocellular adenoma in male rats at the lowest dose (6 out of 50; 12%), which exceeded the range for historical controls (0–8%; 19 out of 799, 2.4%). Hepatocellular adenoma was present in all three dosed groups of males and not in males in the control group. There was no significant increase in the incidence of tumours in female rats. [Hepatocellular adenoma is a tumour that is known to progress to malignancy.]

4. Mechanistic and Other Relevant Data

4.1 Absorption, distribution, metabolism, and excretion

4.1.1 Humans

General pharmacokinetic parameters of triamterene and its major metabolite, 4′-hydroxytriamterene sulfate (see Fig. 4.1), were investigated in a randomized crossover trial with six healthy volunteers who were given triamterene by intravenous infusion (10 mg over 10 minutes), or orally (50 mg tablet) (Gilfrich *et al.*, 1983). After intravenous infusion, terminal half-lives for triamterene and 4′-hydroxytriamterene sulfate were 255 ± 42 and 188 ± 70 minutes, respectively. Total triamterene plasma clearance was 4.4 ± 1.41 L/minute, which is indicative of rapid metabolism of this compound. After oral administration, triamterene was rapidly absorbed from the gastrointestinal tract. The parent drug and 4′-hydroxytriamterene sulfate were detectable in plasma after 15 minutes, and maximum concentrations of 26.4 ± 17.7 and 779 ± 310 ng/mL, respectively, were reached after 1.5 hours. The

Fig. 4.1 Chemical structures of triamterene and its metabolites, 4′-hydroxytriamterene and 4′-hydroxytriamterene sulfate

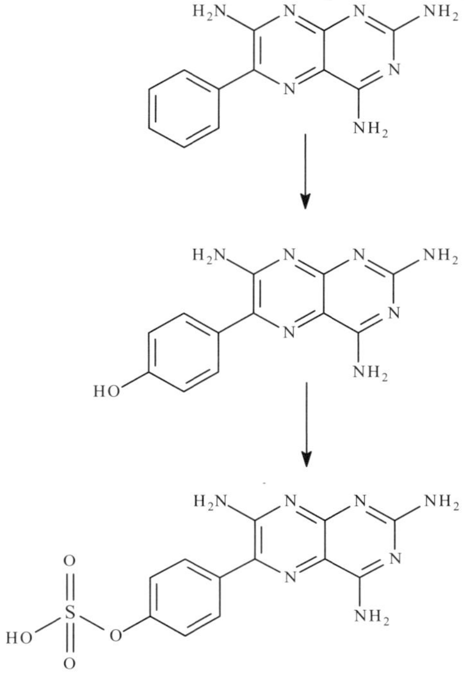

Compiled by the Working Group

half-lives of unchanged triamterene and the metabolite were not significantly different from those observed after intravenous administration.

The bioavailability of triamterene after intravenous or oral administration was calculated from plasma and urine concentrations, and found to be 52 ± 22%, demonstrating considerable inter-subject variability. By inclusion of data for total excretion of triamterene and 4′-hydroxytriamterene sulfate, the absorption was calculated to be 83.2 ± 25.9% (Gilfrich *et al.*, 1983). The high absorption of triamterene is indicative of its ability, as a weak lipid-soluble base (pK$_a$ = 6.2) to cross lipid membranes by non-ionic diffusion (Kau, 1978). Triamterene is more highly concentrated in erythrocytes than in plasma (Gilfrich *et al.*, 1983).

The pharmacokinetic interaction of triamterene and hydrochlorothiazide was investigated in a crossover study of 10 healthy volunteers given oral triamterene (doses, 0, 12.5, 25, 50, or 100 mg), and of 12 healthy volunteers given triamterene (doses, 0, 25, or 50 mg) with hydrochlorothiazide (doses, 12.5, or 25 mg). Coadministration did not affect the renal excretion of either parent drug, but significantly reduced renal excretion of 4′-hydroxytriamterene sulfate (Möhrke *et al.*, 1997).

4′-Hydroxytriamterene sulfate shows more protein binding (91% protein-bound) than triamterene (55%) (Knauf *et al.*, 1983), possibly because of ionic bonding between sulfate and protein, in addition to hydrophobic bonding (Gilfrich *et al.*, 1983). 4′-Hydroxytriamterene sulfate is almost completely eliminated by tubular secretion, while triamterene, although partly eliminated via this route, can also undergo glomerular filtration, due to the fact that a substantial proportion (45%) is not bound to protein (Knauf *et al.*, 1983).

Triamterene undergoes significant first-pass metabolism with rapid hydroxylation of the phenyl ring at the 4′-position, yielding the phase-I metabolite 4′-hydroxytriamterene (see Fig. 4.1). This intermediate metabolite is transient and is detected at most in trace amounts (< 1 ng/mL) in urine or plasma (Gilfrich *et al.*, 1983). Hydroxylation seems to be mediated virtually exclusively by cytochrome P450 1A2, and inhibition or induction of this isoenzyme will change the time-course of both triamterene and its pharmacologically active phase-II metabolite (Fuhr *et al.*, 2005).

4′-Hydroxytriamterene is rapidly conjugated via cytosolic sulfotransferases to yield the principal phase-II metabolite 4′-hydroxytriamterene sulfate (Gilfrich *et al.*, 1983; NTP, 1993; Horstkötter *et al.*, 2002). In addition, phase-II metabolism produces very small quantities of other metabolites, such as *N*-glucuronides (Lehmann, 1965).

The parent drug and its metabolite 4′-hydroxytriamterene sulfate are excreted in the urine and faeces (Kau & Sastry, 1977; NTP, 1993). Renal clearance of triamterene administered by intravenous infusion (10 mg over 10 minutes) was 0.22 ± 0.1 L/minute, and that of 4′-hydroxytriamterene sulfate was 0.17 ± 0.061 L/minute. Total urinary recovery of triamterene and of the sulfate was 4.5% and approximately 50%, respectively (Gilfrich *et al.*, 1983). Renal clearance of orally administered (50 mg) triamterene and of the sulfate was 0.18 ± 0.05 L/minute and 0.15 ± 0.03 L/minute, respectively (Gilfrich *et al.*, 1983). 4′-Hydroxytriamterene sulfate and *N*-glucuronides were also excreted into the bile (Mutschler *et al.*, 1983; NTP, 1993).

4.1.2 Experimental systems

Intestinal absorption of triamterene in the colon and the whole small intestine of the rat was shown to occur via a carrier-mediated mechanism (Montalar *et al.*, 2003) likely to comprise two carriers, and also via an efflux process (Kau & Sastry, 1977).

The tissue distribution in male Sprague-Dawley rats given [¹⁴C]triamterene intravenously showed extensive accumulation of radiolabel (Kau & Sastry, 1977). High concentrations of the parent drug were found in most tissues (except the brain, fat, and testes), and blood concentrations were low. No metabolites were detected. The highest concentrations of triamterene were reached within the first 20 minutes in highly perfused tissues such as kidneys, liver, heart, lungs, and skeletal muscle. The kidneys contained the highest concentrations of triamterene at all timed intervals and doses, but the largest dose deposition was in skeletal muscle (part of the "peripheral compartment"). Elimination was slow (estimated plasma half-life, 2.8 hours), possibly due to triamterene binding to tissue in the "central compartment" (e.g., kidneys, liver). [This study demonstrated the ability of triamterene to bind to tissue, which influences its rate of distribution and elimination.]

Studies of tissue distribution of triamterene in guinea-pigs and baboons reported triamterene concentrations in muscle and heart that were much higher than in plasma, low concentrations in the brain, active transport of triamterene in the kidney, and transfer of triamterene from mother to fetus (Pruitt *et al.*, 1975).

A quantitative study of the renal handling of [³H]triamterene in an isolated, perfused rat-kidney model showed that triamterene undergoes glomerular filtration, active tubular secretion and passive re-absorption by a pH-dependent mechanism (Kau, 1978).

When [¹⁴C]triamterene (2 mg/kg bw) was administered subcutaneously to Sprague-Dawley rats, 45% of the total radiolabel was excreted in the urine, and 50% in the faeces, over 72 hours (Kau *et al.*, 1975). In the urine and faeces, 72–79% of the administered dose was excreted as unchanged triamterene, 10–15% as free 4′-hydroxytriamterene, 1–5% as its sulfate, and 2% as a minor unidentified metabolite. [The low level of sulfate conjugation may have been a consequence of the route of administration.] The liver was identified as the major site of triamterene metabolism; triamterene was not metabolized in the kidney. No metabolites were detected in the plasma.

4.2 Genetic and related effects

4.2.1 Humans

No data were available to the Working Group.

4.2.2 Experimental systems

See Table 4.1

(a) Mutagenicity

Triamterene (up to 10 000 µg/plate) was not mutagenic in *Salmonella typhimurium* strains TA98, TA1535, TA1537 or TA100, with or without metabolic activation (S9 from rat or hamster liver) (NTP, 1993). Triamterene did not induce dominant lethal mutations in germ cells of male CD-1 mice when given at doses of up to 100 mg/kg bw per day by gavage for 5 days (Manson *et al.*, 1986).

(b) Chromosomal damage

No increase in the frequency of chromosomal aberration was induced by triamterene at concentrations of up to 600 µg/mL in Chinese hamster ovary cells in vitro in the presence or absence of metabolic activation. Triamterene did induce sister chromatid exchange in Chinese hamster ovary cells in vitro in the presence or absence of metabolic activation (NTP, 1993).

4.3 Other mechanistic data relevant to carcinogenicity

4.3.1 Effects on cell physiology

Triamterene is a potassium-sparing diuretic that blocks the epithelial sodium channel on the luminal side of the collecting tubule in the kidney. Its major physiological action is to inhibit transport of sodium ions and reduce blood volume. The action of triamterene is different from that of thiazide-based drugs, but similar to that of amiloride (Busch *et al.*, 1996). [There is no known link between sodium-channel inhibition and carcinogenesis.]

4.3.2 Effects on cell function

In cultures of the BJAB-B95–8 human lymphoma cell line, there was a dose-dependent inhibition of cell growth, with cell death following extended incubation with triamterene at 80 µM. The activity of dihydrofolate reductase was blocked by triamterene, and its metabolites 4′-hydroxytriamterene and 4′-hydroxytriamterene sulfate are less effective inhibitors of this enzyme (Schalhorn *et al.*, 1981).

Photosensitivity, a known clinical side-effect of triamterene, was demonstrated in vitro in cultures of human peripheral blood lymphocytes and neutrophils co-exposed to triamterene and ultraviolet A (UV-A) irradiation. At a concentration of 60 µg/mL, triamterene decreased cell viability to 40–50%, indicating photosensitization of twofold. Other experiments also showed that triamterene produced singlet oxygen species when irradiated with UV-A light in the presence of molecular oxygen. (Vargas *et al.*, 1998).

Table 4.1 Genetic and related effects of triamterene

Test system	Results[a]		Concentration or dose (LED or HID)	Reference
	Without exogenous metabolic system	With exogenous metabolic system		
In vitro				
Salmonella typhimurium TA100, TA98, TA1535, TA1537, reverse mutation	–	–	10 000 µg/plate	NTP (1993)
Chromosomal aberrations, Chinese hamster ovary cells	–	–	600 µg/mL	NTP (1993)
Sister chromatid exchange, Chinese hamster ovary cells	+	+	10 µg/mL, – S9 160 µg/mL, + S9	NTP (1993)
In vivo				
Dominant lethal mutations, germ cells of male CD-1 mice	–	NT	100 mg/kg bw per day for 5 days	Manson *et al.* (1986)

[a] +, positive; –, negative

bw, body weight; HID, highest ineffective dose; LED, lowest effective dose; S9, 9000 × *g* supernatant

4.4 Susceptibility

4.4.1 Liver disease

Patients with liver cirrhosis have reduced ability to hydroxylate triamterene, as evidenced by high plasma concentrations of triamterene and low concentrations of 4′-hydroxytriamterene sulfate. After administration of 200 mg of triamterene, peak plasma concentrations in eight patients without liver disease were 559 ± 48 ng/mL and 2956 ± 320 ng/mL for triamterene and 4′-hydroxytriamterene sulfate, respectively. In the seven patients with alcoholic cirrhosis, peak plasma concentrations of triamterene were increased to 1434 ± 184 ng/mL, while the concentrations of the sulfate were reduced to 469 ± 84 ng/mL. Renal clearance was also reduced in patients with cirrhosis: the clearance of triamterene and the sulfate were 2.8 ± 0.7 and 38.0 ± 6.6 mL/minute, respectively, compared with 14.4 ± 1.5 and 116.7 ± 11.6 mL/minute, respectively, in patients without liver disease (Villeneuve *et al.*, 1984).

4.4.2 Renal impairment

Although renal elimination is only a minor route of excretion for triamterene, it is the main route of elimination of 4′-hydroxytriamterene sulfate. Thus, in individuals with renal impairment, accumulation of the sulfate is substantial and progressive, but negligible for triamterene. The kinetics of triamterene were observed in 32 patients with widely varying degrees of creatinine clearance (10–135 mL/minute), an indicator of renal function. In patients with reduced renal function, significant accumulation in plasma and reduced renal clearance of the sulfate were reported. Plasma concentrations of the parent drug were not increased (Knauf *et al.*, 1983).

4.4.3 Age

Early reports concluded that the mean peak concentration of triamterene after an oral dose of 50 mg is higher in older than in younger patients (84 and 41 ng/mL, respectively), that the time to reach peak concentrations of 4′-hydroxytriamterene sulfate is prolonged [suggesting that hydroxylation decreases with age], and that the systemic clearance of the parent drug and its metabolite declines significantly with age (NTP, 1993).

In contrast, a more recent study in which an oral dose of triamterene (50 mg) was given to 11 healthy elderly individuals (mean age, 68 ± 5 years), and to 10 healthy young individuals (mean age, 25 ± 2 years) did not report a significant reduction in hydroxylation of triamterene (Fliser *et al.*, 1999). Renal clearance was similar in elderly and young individuals. This study excluded those with conditions that may adversely affect renal or hepatic function (e.g. hypertension, malnutrition, and cardiac failure) and all subjects were on a standardized diet to control intake of protein and electrolytes, particularly sodium. It was assumed by Fliser *et al.* (1999) that the subjects in previous studies may have had various conditions that affected renal and/or hepatic function.

4.5 Mechanistic consideration

Triamterene was not mutagenic in *S. typhimurium*, with or without exogenous metabolic activation, did not induce chromosomal aberrations in Chinese hamster ovary cells, with or without exogenous metabolic activation (NTP, 1993), and did not induce the dominant lethal mutation in the germ cells of male CD-1 mice in vivo (Manson *et al.*, 1986). However, positive results were obtained for induction of sister chromatid exchange in Chinese hamster ovary cells, both with and without metabolic activation (NTP, 1993). Both inhibition of dihydrofolate reductase and photosensitization are possible mechanisms for the induction of DNA damage by triamterene (Schalhorn *et al.*, 1981; Vargas *et al.*, 1998).

5. Summary of Data Reported

5.1 Exposure data

Triamterene is a synthetic potassium-sparing diuretic; unlike other diuretics, it causes limited excretion of potassium in the urine. Triamterene is most often prescribed for hypertension as a combination tablet that includes hydrochlorothiazide. In 2012, while global sales were greatest in the USA (US$ 141 million), the volume of annual prescriptions was modest and had declined over time.

5.2 Human carcinogenicity data

Five case–control studies were available to assess the association between triamterene and cancer.

In two of these studies, all subjects in the treatment group were exposed to triamterene. One of the studies reported a risk estimate that was specific for triamterene and cancer of the breast; however, most of the women took other drugs and few subjects had used triamterene for more than 1 year. The other study reported a relative risk for cancer of the lip and treatment with combined triamterene and hydrochlorothiazide, and thus any effect attributable to triamterene could not be separated from the effects attributable to hydrochlorothiazide.

The three remaining case–control studies reported findings on cancers of the breast or colorectum for triamterene in combination with other drugs (hydrochlorothiazide, other antihypertension drugs, potassium-sparing diuretics, and other inhibitors of dihydrofolate reductase).

The available studies were not informative for evaluation of the association between risk of cancer and exposure specifically to triamterene.

5.3 Animal carcinogenicity data

Triamterene was tested for carcinogenicity by oral administration in two studies in mice and one study in rats.

In a first feeding study in male and female mice, triamterene caused a significant increase in the incidence of hepatocellular adenoma in females. In a second feeding study, triamterene caused significant increases in the incidences of hepatocellular adenoma in males and females, and of hepatocellular adenoma or carcinoma (combined) in females.

In a feeding study in male and female rats, triamterene caused an increase in the incidence of hepatocellular adenoma (a tumour that is known to progress to malignancy) in males. Hepatocellular adenoma was reported in all dose groups, but not in rats in the control group. There was no significant increase in the incidence of tumours in female rats.

5.4 Mechanistic and other relevant data

In humans, triamterene is primarily metabolized to 4′-hydroxytriamterene sulfate via sulfotransferase-mediated conjugation of the phase-I metabolite, 4′-hydroxytriamterene. 4′-Hydroxytriamterene sulfate binds strongly to proteins, to a greater extent than the parent drug. Intravenous administration of radiolabelled triamterene in rats resulted in extensive accumulation of radiolabel, with the highest concentrations in highly perfused tissues, particularly the kidneys.

Triamterene was not mutagenic when tested in *Salmonella typhimurium*, in the presence or absence of exogenous metabolic activation. Triamterene also gave negative results in assays for the induction of chromosomal aberration in Chinese hamster ovary cells, in the presence or absence of exogenous metabolic activation, and did not induce dominant lethal mutation in the germ cells of male CD-1 mice in vivo. Triamterene induced sister chromatid exchange in Chinese hamster ovary cells, in the presence or absence of exogenous metabolic activation. Therefore, triamterene may produce genetic toxicity directly at the chromosomal level without metabolic activation.

Triamterene is an inhibitor of dihydrofolate reductase in vitro; its metabolites 4′-hydroxytriamterene and 4′-hydroxytriamterene sulfate are less effective inhibitors of the enzyme. When irradiated with ultraviolet A light, triamterene produced singlet oxygen species in the presence of molecular oxygen. In-vitro coexposure of human peripheral blood lymphocytes and neutrophils to triamterene and ultraviolet A resulted in decreased cell viability.

Inhibition of dihydrofolate reductase and photosensitization are possible mechanisms for the induction of DNA damage by triamterene.

6. Evaluation

6.1 Cancer in humans

There is *inadequate evidence* in humans for the carcinogenicity of triamterene.

6.2 Cancer in experimental animals

There is *sufficient evidence* in experimental animals for carcinogenicity of triamterene.

6.3 Overall evaluation

Triamterene is *possibly carcinogenic to humans (Group 2B)*.

References

Amendola L, Colamonici C, Mazzarino M, Botrè F (2003). Rapid determination of diuretics in human urine by gas chromatography-mass spectrometry following microwave assisted derivatization. *Anal Chim Acta*, 475(1-2):125–36. doi:10.1016/S0003-2670(02)01223-0

Bakshi M, Singh S (2002). Development of validated stability-indicating assay methods–critical review. *J Pharm Biomed Anal*, 28(6):1011–40. doi:10.1016/S0731-7085(02)00047-X PMID:12049968

British Pharmacopoeia (2009). Triamterene. London, UK, Medicines and healthcare products regulatory agency.

Busch AE, Suessbrich H, Kunzelmann K, Hipper A, Greger R, Waldegger S et al. (1996). Blockade of epithelial Na+ channels by triamterenes - underlying mechanisms and molecular basis. *Pflugers Arch*, 432(5):760–6. doi:10.1007/s004240050196 PMID:8772124

ChemicalBook (2013). ChemicalBook: Chemical Search Engine. Available from: http://www.chemicalbook.com.

ChemSpider (2013). ChemSpider: The free chemical database. Royal Society of Chemistry. Available from: http://www.chemspider.com.

Chobanian AV, Bakris GL, Black HR, Cushman WC, Green LA, Izzo JL Jr et al. ; Joint National Committee on Prevention, Detection, Evaluation, and Treatment of High Blood Pressure. National Heart, Lung, and Blood Institute; ; National High Blood Pressure Education Program Coordinating Committee (2003). Seventh report of the Joint National Committee on Prevention, Detection, Evaluation, and Treatment of High Blood Pressure. *Hypertension*, 42(6):1206–52. doi:10.1161/01.HYP.0000107251.49515.c2 PMID:14656957

Coogan PF, Rosenberg L (2007). The use of folic acid antagonists and the risk of colorectal cancer. *Pharmacoepidemiol Drug Saf*, 16(10):1111–9. doi:10.1002/pds.1442 PMID:17600846

Coogan PF, Strom BL, Rosenberg L (2009). Diuretic use and the risk of breast cancer. *J Hum Hypertens*, 23(3):216–8. doi:10.1038/jhh.2008.131 PMID:18971940

Deventer K, Delbeke FT, Roels K, Van Eenoo P (2002). Screening for 18 diuretics and probenecid in doping analysis by liquid chromatography-tandem mass spectrometry. *Biomed Chromatogr*, 16(8):529–35. doi:10.1002/bmc.201 PMID:12474217

DrugBank (2013). DrugBank: Open Data Drug & Drug Target Database. Version 4.2. Available from: http://www.drugbank.ca/

eMC (2013). electronic Medicines Compendium (eMC). Available from: http://www.medicines.org.uk, accessed 8 September 2014.

FDA (2013). Triamterene. US Food and Drug Administration. Available from: http://www.accessdata.fda.gov/scripts/cder/drugsatfda/index.cfm, accessed 8 September 2014.

Fliser D, Bischoff I, Hanses A, Block S, Joest M, Ritz E et al. (1999). Renal handling of drugs in the healthy elderly. Creatinine clearance underestimates renal function and pharmacokinetics remain virtually unchanged. *Eur J Clin Pharmacol*, 55(3):205–11. doi:10.1007/s002280050619 PMID:10379636

Friedman GD, Asgari MM, Warton EM, Chan J, Habel LA (2012). Antihypertensive drugs and lip cancer in non-Hispanic whites. *Arch Intern Med*, 172(16):1246–51. doi:10.1001/archinternmed.2012.2754 PMID:22869299

Fuhr U, Kober S, Zaigler M, Mutschler E, Spahn-Langguth H (2005). Rate-limiting biotransformation of triamterene is mediated by CYP1A2. *Int J Clin Pharmacol Ther*, 43(7):327–34. doi:10.5414/CPP43327 PMID:16035375

Gilfrich HJ, Kremer G, Möhrke W, Mutschler E, Völger KD (1983). Pharmacokinetics of triamterene after i.v. administration to man: determination of bioavailability. *Eur J Clin Pharmacol*, 25(2):237–41. doi:10.1007/BF00543797 PMID:6628507

Gu Q, Burt VL, Dillon CF, Yoon S (2012). Trends in antihypertensive medication use and blood pressure control among United States adults with hypertension: the National Health and Nutrition Examination Survey, 2001 to 2010. *Circulation*, 126(17):2105–14. doi:10.1161/CIRCULATIONAHA.112.096156 PMID:23091084

Horstkötter C, Kober S, Spahn-Langguth H, Mutschler E, Blaschke G (2002). Determination of triamterene and its main metabolite hydroxytriamterene sulfate in human urine by capillary electrophoresis using ultraviolet absorbance and laser-induced fluorescence detection. *J Chromatogr B Analyt Technol Biomed Life Sci*, 769(1):107–17. doi:10.1016/S1570-0232(02)00002-8 PMID:11936683

Ibañez GA, Escandar GM, Espinosa Mansilla A, Muñoz de la Peña A (2005). Determination of triamterene in pharmaceutical formulations and of triamterene and its main metabolite hydroxytriamterene sulfate in urine using solid-phase and aqueous solution luminescence. *Anal Chim Acta*, 538(1-2):77–84. doi:10.1016/j.aca.2005.02.001

IMS Health (2012a). National Disease and Therapeutic Index (NDTI). Plymouth Meeting (Pennsylvania): IMS Health, 2005–2012. Available from: http://www.imshealth.com/portal/site/imshealth, accessed 8 September 2014.

IMS Health (2012b). National Prescription Audit Plus (NPA). Plymouth Meeting, Pennsylvania: IMS Health. 2008–2012.

IMS Health (2012c). Multinational Integrated Data Analysis (MIDAS). Plymouth Meeting, Pennsylvania: IMS Health. Available from: http://www.imshealth.com/portal/site/imshealth, accessed 8 September 2014.

Kau ST (1978). Handling of triamterene by the isolated perfused rat kidney. *J Pharmacol Exp Ther*, 206(3):701–9. PMID:702330

Kau ST, Sastry BV (1977). Distribution and pharmacokinetics of triamterene in rats. *J Pharm Sci*, 66(1):53–6. doi:10.1002/jps.2600660112 PMID:833742

Kau ST, Sastry BV, Alvin JD, Bush MT (1975). Metabolism of triamterene in the rat. *Drug Metab Dispos*, 3(5):345–51. PMID:241615

Knauf H, Möhrke W, Mutschler E (1983). Delayed elimination of triamterene and its active metabolite in chronic renal failure. *Eur J Clin Pharmacol*, 24(4):453–6. doi:10.1007/BF00609885 PMID:6861860

Lehmann K (1965). [Separation, isolation and identification of metabolic products of triamterene] *Arzneimittelforschung*, 15(7):812–6. PMID:5898685

Li H, He J, Liu Q, Huo Z, Liang S, Liang Y (2011). Simultaneous analysis of hydrochlorothiazide, triamterene and reserpine in rat plasma by high performance liquid chromatography and tandem solid-phase extraction. *J Sep Sci*, 34(5):542–7. doi:10.1002/jssc.201000754 PMID:21344645

Mack TM, Henderson BE, Gerkins VR, Arthur M, Baptista J, Pike MC (1975). Reserpine and breast cancer in a retirement community. *N Engl J Med*, 292(26):1366–71. doi:10.1056/NEJM197506262922603 PMID:1138164

Mancia G, Laurent S, Agabiti-Rosei E, Ambrosioni E, Burnier M, Caulfield MJ et al. ; European Society of Hypertension(2009). Reappraisal of European guidelines on hypertension management: a European Society of Hypertension Task Force document. *J Hypertens*, 27(11):2121–58. doi:10.1097/HJH.0b013e328333146d PMID:19838131

Mansia G, De Backer G, Dominiczak A, Cifkova R, Fagard R, Germano G et al. European Society of Cardiology(2007). 2007 ESH-ESC Guidelines for the management of arterial hypertension: the task force for the management of arterial hypertension of the European Society of Hypertension (ESH) and of the European Society of Cardiology (ESC). *Blood Press*, 16(3):135–232. doi:10.1080/08037050701461084 PMID:17846925

Manson JM, Guerriero FJ, Brown T, San Sebastian J (1986). Lack of in vivo mutagenicity and testicular toxicity of triamterene in mice. *Fundam Appl Toxicol*, 7(4):533–46. doi:10.1016/0272-0590(86)90104-1 PMID:3803749

Möhrke W, Knauf H, Mutschler E (1997). Pharmacokinetics and pharmacodynamics of triamterene and hydrochlorothiazide and their combination in healthy volunteers. *Int J Clin Pharmacol Ther*, 35(10):447–52. PMID:9352394

Montalar M, Nalda-Molina R, Rodríguez-Ibáñez M, García-Valcárcel I, Garrigues TM, Merino V et al. (2003). Kinetic modeling of triamterene intestinal absorption and its inhibition by folic acid and methotrexate. *J Drug Target*, 11(4):215–23. doi:10.1080/10611860310001615947 PMID:14578108

Mutschler E, Gilfrich HJ, Knauf H, Möhrke W, Völger KD (1983). Pharmacokinetics of triamterene. *Clin Exp Hypertens A*, 5(2):249–69. doi:10.3109/10641968309048825 PMID:6831748

NTP 1993). NTP Toxicology and carcinogenesis studies of triamterene (CAS No. 396–01–0) in F344/N rats and B6C3F1 mice (feed studies). *Natl Toxicol Program Tech Rep Ser*, 420:1–367. PMID:12616291

O'Neil MJ (2006). The Merck Index - An Encyclopedia of Chemicals, Drugs, and Biologicals. 14th ed. Whitehouse Station (NJ): Merck & Co., Inc.

Pruitt AW, McNay JL, Dayton PG (1975). Transfer characteristics of triamterene and its analogs. Central nervous system, placenta, and kidney. *Drug Metab Dispos*, 3(1):30–41. PMID:234832

Pulgarín JA, Molina AA, López PF (2001). Simultaneous direct determination of amiloride and triamterene in urine using isopotential fluorometry. *Anal Biochem*, 292(1):59–68. doi:10.1006/abio.2001.5064 PMID:11319818

Richter K, Oertel R, Kirch W (1996). New sensitive method for the determination of hydrochlorothiazide in human serum by high-performance liquid chromatography with electrochemical detection. *J Chromatogr A*, 729(1-2):293–6. doi:10.1016/0021-9673(95)00900-0 PMID:9004952

Schalhorn A, Siegert W, Sauer HJ (1981). Antifolate effect of triamterene on human leucocytes and on a human lymphoma cell line. *Eur J Clin Pharmacol*, 20(3):219–24. doi:10.1007/BF00544601 PMID:7286039

Shao B, Zhang J, Yang Y, Meng J, Wu Y, Duan H (2008). Simultaneous analysis of thirteen diuretics residues in bovine milk by ultra-performance liquid chromatography/tandem mass spectrometry. *Rapid Commun Mass Spectrom*, 22(21):3427–33. doi:10.1002/rcm.3740 PMID:18837072

Sörgel F, Lin ET, Hasegawa J, Benet LZ (1984). Liquid chromatographic analysis of triamterene and its major metabolite, hydroxytriamterene sulfate, in blood, plasma, and urine. *J Pharm Sci*, 73(6):831–3. doi:10.1002/jps.2600730633 PMID:6737274

Spickett RGW, Timmis GM (1954). The synthesis of compounds with potential anti-folic acid activity. Part I. 7-Amino- and 7-hydroxy-pteridines. *J Chem Soc*, 2887–95. doi:10.1039/jr9540002887

Swart KJ, Botha H (1987). Rapid method for the determination of the diuretic triamterene and its metabolites in plasma and urine by high-performance liquid chromatography. *J Chromatogr A*, 413:315–9. doi:10.1016/0378-4347(87)80246-3 PMID:3558684

van Deelen GW, Huizing EH (1986). Use of a diuretic (Dyazide) in the treatment of Menière's disease. A double-blind cross-over placebo-controlled study.

ORL J Otorhinolaryngol Relat Spec, 48(5):287–92. doi:10.1159/000275884 PMID:3537899

Vargas F, Fuentes A, Sequera J, Méndez H, Fraile G, Velásquez M *et al.* (1998). In Vitro Approach to investigating the phototoxicity of the diuretic drug triamterene. *Toxicol In Vitro*, 12(6):661–7. doi:10.1016/S0887-2333(98)00057-5 PMID:20654456

Villeneuve JP, Rocheleau F, Raymond G (1984). Triamterene kinetics and dynamics in cirrhosis. *Clin Pharmacol Ther*, 35(6):831–7. doi:10.1038/clpt.1984.121 PMID:6734036

Wang YR, Alexander GC, Stafford RS (2007). Outpatient hypertension treatment, treatment intensification, and control in Western Europe and the United States. *Arch Intern Med*, 167(2):141–7. doi:10.1001/archinte.167.2.141 PMID:17242314

Williams RR, Feinleib M, Connor RJ, Stegens NL (1978). Case-control study of antihypertensive and diuretic use by women with malignant and benign breast lesions detected in a mammography screening program. *J Natl Cancer Inst*, 61(2):327–35.http://www.ncbi.nlm.nih.gov/entrez/query.fcgi?cmd=Retrieve&db=PubMed&list_uids=277719&dopt=Abstract PMID:277719

Yakatan GJ, Cruz JE (1981). High-performance liquid chromatographic analysis of triamterene and p-hydroxytriamterene in plasma. *J Pharm Sci*, 70(8):949–51. doi:10.1002/jps.2600700832 PMID:7310671

HYDROCHLOROTHIAZIDE

1. Exposure Data

1.1 Identification of the agent

1.1.1 Nomenclature

Chem. Abstr. Serv. Reg. No.: 58-93-5 (SciFinder, 2013)

Chem. Abstr. Serv. Name: 2*H*-1,2,4-Benzo-thiadiazine-7-sulfonamide, 6-chloro-3,4-di-hydro-1,1-dioxide (SciFinder, 2013)

IUPAC systematic name: 6-Chloro-1,1-dioxo-3,4-dihydro-2*H*-1,2,4-benzothiadiazine-7-sulfonamide

Synonyms: Dihydrochlorothiazid; Dihydro-chlorothiazide; Dihydrochlorothiazidum; Dihydrochlorurit; Dihydrochlorurite; Dihydroxychlorothiazidum; HCTZ; HCZ; Hydrochlorothiazid; Hydrochlorthiazide (DrugBank, 2013); Hidroclorotiazida; Hydrochlorothiazidum; Chlorsulfonamido-dihydrobenzothiadiazine dioxide; Chloro-sulthiadil; 3,4-dihydrochlorothiazide (IPCS, 2013)

WHO International Nonproprietary Name (INN): Hydrochlorothiazidum (WHO, 2006)

1.1.2 Structural and molecular formulae and relative molecular mass

$C_7H_8ClN_3O_4S_2$
Relative molecular mass: 297.74 (O'Neil, 2001)

1.1.3 Chemical and physical properties of the pure substance

Description: A white or almost white, crystalline powder; odourless or almost odourless (WHO, 2006)

Density: 1.693 g/cm³ (calculated) (Lookchem, 2013)

Melting point: 273–275 °C (O'Neil, 2001)

Spectroscopy data: Infrared, Raman, ultra-violet, proton nuclear magnetic resonance (¹H-NMR) and ¹³C-NMR spectral data have been reported.

Solubility: Very slightly soluble in water (722 mg/L at 25 °C; Deppeler, 1981); soluble in ethanol at ~750 g/L and in acetone (WHO, 2006); soluble in dilute ammonia; freely soluble in sodium hydroxide solution, in *n*-butylamine and in dimethylformamide; sparingly soluble in alcohol; insoluble in ether, chloroform and in dilute mineral acids (HSDB, 2013).

Octanol/water partition coefficient (log P): −0.07 (Chemspider, 2013)

Dissociation constant: pK$_a$ = 7.9 ; pK$_{a2}$ = 9.2 (O'Neil, 2001)

1.1.4 Technical products and impurities

(a) Trade names

Acuren; Adelphan; Apo-Hydro; Aquazide; Clorana; Colidur; Colonraitai; Cotrazid; Decazon; Dehydratin; Dehydrazid; Depress; Dichlotride; Dichlozid; Di-Eudrin; Dihydrochl Ozide; Dihydrochlorothiazide; Dihydrodiazid; Disalunil; Disothiazide; Dithiazide; Dithiazide; Diunorm; Diunorm; Diurace; Diural; Diuren; Diurex; Diurezin; Diuzid; Do-Hydro; Drenol; Duberzide; Edepress; Esidrex; Esidrix; H.C.T.; HCT [manufacturer]; Hexazide; Hidroclorotiazida; Hidrochlorotiazid Alkaloid; Hidromed; Hidroronol; Hidrosaluretil; Hidrotiadol; HTZ; Hybozide; Hychlozide; Hydrex; Hydride; Hydrochlorothiazide; Hydrochlorothiazidum Polpharma; Hydroklortiazid Evolan; Hydromed; Hydrozide; Hypodehydra; Hypothiazid; Hytaz; Hyzide; Keshiau; Klorzide; Koliside; Locoid; Lonpra; Microzide; Monozid; Nefrix; Newtolide; Nisidrex; Nor-Tiazida; Oretic; Ridaq; Rofucal; Tandiur; Tiazid; Urilzid; Xenia (MicroMedex, 2013).

(b) Impurities

Some impurities are described in the European Pharmacopoeia (2005):

- Chlorothiazide (active drug rarely used as an alternative to hydrochlorothiazide)
- 4-Amino-6-chlorobenzene-1,3-disulfonamide (salamide)

- 6-Chloro-*N*-[(6-chloro-7-sulfamoyl-2,3-dihydro-4*H*-1,2,4-benzothiadiazin-4-yl 1,1-dioxide)methyl]-3,4-dihydro-2*H*-1,2,4-benzothiadiazine-7-sulfonamide 1,1-dioxide.

1.2 Analysis

An overview of selected analytical methods is presented in Table 1.1.

1.3 Production and use

1.3.1 Production process

Hydrochlorothiazide is synthesized by either the reaction of *para*-formaldehyde with 5-chloro-2,4-disulfamoylaniline in nonaqueous media, or the reaction of formaldehyde with 6-chloro-7-sulfamoyl-2*H*-1,2,4-benzothiadiazine-1,1-dioxide in aqueous alkaline solution (Deppeler, 1981).

1.3.2 Use

(a) Indications

Hydrochlorothiazide is a thiazide-type diuretic chiefly used as an antihypertension agent for the control of elevated blood pressure (Table 1.2). It is often combined with other agents in the treatment of hypertension, either through separate prescriptions for hydrochlorothiazide and the other agents, or through the use of combination products in which a single tablet contains hydrochlorothiazide plus one other antihypertensive medication (more rarely, two other agents).

In the USA, hydrochlorothiazide is indicated for "the management of hypertension either as the sole therapeutic agent or in combination with other antihypertensives" and is recommended as first-line medication (Chobanian *et al.*, 2003). The Food and Drug Administration

Table 1.1 Analytical methods for hydrochlorothiazide

Sample matrix	Sample preparation	Analytical method	Detection limit	Reference
Compendial methods				
Assay	–	Potentiometry Titrant: 0.1 M TBAH Reference electrode: calomel or silver–silver chloride Indicator electrode: glass electrode 1 mL of 0.1 M TBAH is equivalent to 0.01488 g of HCTZ	–	Indian Pharmacopoeia (2010)
Assay for HCTZ tablets	–	UV-visible spectroscopy wavelength: 273 nm	–	Indian Pharmacopoeia (2010)
Assay for HCTZ tablets	–	HPLC column: C_{18} Mobile phase: monobasic sodium phosphate and acetonitrile (9 : 1) pH 3.0 ± 0.1 Flow rate: 2 mL/min	–	US Pharmacopeia (2007)
Non-compendial methods				
Human plasma	Addition of internal standard (clortalidone) and MTBE, centrifugation, addition of solvent to organic phase, evaporation and reconstitution in acetonitrile and water (1 : 1, v/v)	HPLC–tandem mass spectrometry Column: C_{18} Mobile phase: acetonitrile and water (80 : 20, v/v) SRM transition: 296.10 *m/z*, 204.85 *m/z*	5 ng/mL (LLOQ) Linearity: 5–400 ng/mL	Sousa *et al.* (2009)
Human urine	Mix urine samples with deionized water, centrifuge	HPLC–narrow bore chromatography Column: C_{18} Mobile phase: acetic acid and acetonitrile (93 : 7) pH 3 Wavelength: 272 nm Flow rate: 0.30 mL/min	1 µg/mL (LOD) Linearity: 2–50 µg/mL	Farthing *et al.* (1998)
Human serum	Gel filtration of the sera on Sephadex G-15, extraction of the protein-free fraction of the effluent with ethyl acetate	HPLC Column: C_{18} (Spherisorb ODS) Mobile phase: 15% methanol in water	50 ng/mL (LOD)	Christophersen *et al.* (1977)
Rat plasma	To plasma add internal standard (HFTZ), extraction with MTBE	LC–ESI–MS Column: C_8 Mobile phase: distilled water and acetonitrile (85 : 15) Negative ionization mode	Linearity: 4–1000 ng/mL Accuracy: 100.8–113.1% Precision: 0.28–16.4%	Takubo *et al.* (2004)

Table 1.1 (continued)

Sample matrix	Sample preparation	Analytical method	Detection limit	Reference
Human plasma, simultaneous determination of HCTZ and captopril	Derivatization with 2,4-dibromoacetophenone (pBPB) to form captopril-pBPB adduct. Extraction of HCTZ and derivatized captopril with ether and dichloromethane	Reverse phase HPLC Column: C_{18} Mobile phase: acetonitrile, trifluoroacetic acid and water (gradient elution) Flow rate:1.2 mL/min	3.3 ng/mL (LOQ)	Huang *et al.* (2006)
Human plasma, simultaneous quantitation of HCTZ and telmisartan	Liquid–liquid extraction with diethyl ether and dichloromethane (60 : 40)	LC–MS Column: C_8 Mobile phase: acetonitrile, 10 mM ammonium acetate and formic acid (gradient elution) Flow rate: 1.2 mL/min SRM transition: 295.9 *m/z* → 268.9 *m/z* Negative ionization mode	Linearity: 1.00–600 ng/mL	Yan *et al.* (2008)
Human blood and plasma	Addition of the internal standard, benzene extraction, extraction with ethyl acetate, back-extraction into NH_4OH, adjustment to pH 3.7 and extraction with ethyl acetate, evaporation, dissolution of the residue in trimethylanilinium hydroxide in methanol	GLC Column: glass U-tube Carrier gas: argon : methane (95 : 5) Flow rate: 60 mL/min Detector: electron capture detector	0.05 µg/mL (sensitivity)	Vandenheuvel *et al.* (1975)
In tablets	Dissolve drug in 0.02 M NaOH, dilute with Britton–Robinson buffer pH 3.3	Electrochemical study Electrode: glass carbon electrode pH 3.3 Oxidation potential: + 1040 mV	5.0 ng/mL (LOD)	Abdel Razak (2004)
In urine	Centrifugation at 4000 g/mL spiked with HCTZ and diluted with Britton–Robinson buffer pH 3.3	Electrochemical study Electrode: glass carbon electrode pH 3.3 Oxidation potential: + 1040 mV	14 ng/mL	Abdel Razak (2004)
In pharmaceutical formulations	Solution of HCTZ in acetone	Diffuse reflectance spectroscopy: Whatman 42 filter paper as the solid support Solvents: acetone and methanol (HPLC grade); PDAC used for spot reaction with HCTZ	1.32×10^{-2} mol/L (LOD) Linearity: 3.36×10^{-2} to 1.01×10^{-1} mol/L	Gotardo *et al.* (2005)

GLC, gas-liquid chromatography; HCTZ, hydrochlorothiazide; HFTZ, hydrofluorothiazide; HPLC, high-performance liquid chromatography; LC-MS, liquid chromatography mass spectroscopy; LC–ESI–MS, liquid chromatography–electrospray ionization–mass spectrometry; LOD, limit of detection; LLOQ, lower limit of quantification; LOQ, limit of quantification; MTBE, methyl *tert*-butyl ether; PDAC, *para*-dimethylamino cinnamaldehyde; SRM, single reaction monitoring; TBAH, tetrabutylammoniumhydroxide; UV, ultraviolet; v/v, volume per volume

Table 1.2 Most commonly reported clinical indications for hydrochlorothiazide in the USA, 2012

Diagnosis[a]	ICD-9 code	Drug uses (in thousands)	Percentage of total
Essential hypertension, NOS	401.90	21 194	86.9
Hypertensive heart disease, other	402.90	713	2.9
Chronic ischaemic disease, unspecified, with hypertension	414.50	324	1.3
Hypertension, benign	401.10	187	0.8
Surgery after heart disease	V67.03	153	0.6
Hypertensive renal disease	403.90	136	0.6
Oedema, NOS	782.30	122	0.5
Cerebrovascular accident	436.00	86	0.4
Metabolic/insulin resistance syndrome	277.70	82	0.3
All other diagnoses	–	1 332	5.5
Total with reported diagnoses	–	24 383	100

[a] No diagnosis was stated for 0.2% of drug uses.
NOS, not otherwise specified
From IMS Health (2012a)

has approved hydrochlorothiazide alone, and thirty-four combinations containing two agents, and four combinations containing three agents, although not all of these forms were currently available (FDA, 2013). The most common drugs combined with hydrochlorothiazide are triamterene (see *Monograph* on triamterene in this volume), lisinopril, losartan, and valsartan (IMS Health, 2012a).

The European Medicines Agency indication for hydrochlorothiazide is "for treatment of hypertension". Labelling includes use for hypertension and oedema for combination drugs containing hydrochlorothiazide and another diuretic agent. Hydrochlorothiazide is a recommended drug in Europe (Mansia *et al.*, 2007, 2009). Although hydrochlorothiazide is a registered product, it is generally available only in combination products. The European Union listed nineteen combination products containing hydrochlorothiazide and one other drug, and two containing two other agents, although not all are currently in use (eMC, 2013).

(b)   Dosage

Hydrochlorothiazide alone (as sold in the USA) is available in doses of 12.5 mg, 25 mg, 50 mg, and 100 mg. In combination with other pharmaceuticals, the dose of hydrochlorothiazide is generally 12.5 mg or 25 mg (eMC, 2013; MicroMedex, 2013).

When used as a single agent tablet in the USA in 2011–12, hydrochlorothiazide was most frequently used at a dose of 25 mg (69%), followed by 12.5 mg (25%) with higher doses used infrequently (5%). In combination products, a hydrochlorothiazide dosage of 12.5 mg is most common (52%), followed by 25 mg (31%) then 37.5 mg (15%). Both alone and in combination products, once-per-day dosing predominates (> 90%) with twice-per-day and less-than-daily (e.g. every second day) dosing being less common. Overall, the mean daily dosage among patients reported to be taking hydrochlorothiazide is 22 mg per day (IMS Health, 2012a).

(c)   Trends in use

Thiazide diuretics, including hydrochlorothiazide, are among the most frequently used antihypertension agents in the USA and western Europe, accounting for roughly 30%

of medications prescribed to patients with high blood pressure (Wang *et al.*, 2007). Other data confirmed that 25–30% of USA patients with hypertension were taking thiazide diuretics in 2009–2010 (Gu *et al.*, 2012). The use of hydrochlorothiazide increased modestly in the mid-2000s (Stafford *et al.*, 2006; Gu *et al.*, 2012) after publication of the results of the Antihypertensive and Lipid-Lowering Treatment to Prevent Heart Attack Trial (ALLHAT, 2002; Cushman *et al.*, 2002), which showed reasonable equivalence between chlorthalidone (a thiazide-related diuretic), amlodipine, and lisinopril. Reported uses of hydrochlorothiazide (alone or in combination products) at visits to physicians in the USA then decreased, from 28.9 million uses in 2008 to 24.3 million in 2012. Approximately 10 million patients in the USA were reported to be exposed to hydrochlorothiazide in 2012 (IMS Health, 2012a). Prescriptions containing hydrochlorothiazide dispensed in the USA in 2012 amounted to 126.5 million, a slight decrease from 136.5 million prescriptions in 2008 (IMS Health, 2012b; of these, 48.0 million prescriptions were dispensed for hydrochlorothiazide as a single-agent product (38% of the total for hydrochlorothiazide). Overall, these two data sources suggested modest declines in use over the past decade.

Total worldwide sales of hydrochlorothiazide in 2012 were US$ 10.1 billion. Sales were highest in the USA at US$ 3.4 billion, followed by Germany (US$ 0.9 billion), Japan (US$ 0.7 billion), Italy (US$ 0.6 billion), France (US$ 0.5 billion), Brazil (US$ 0.4 billion), Spain (US$ 0.4 billion), India (US$ 0.15 billion), and China (US$ 0.1 billion). The generally lower sales outside of the USA (even when adjusted for population size) reflect the greater use of other thiazide and thiazide-type diuretics in other countries (IMS Health, 2012c).

[Based on data from Wang *et al.* (2007) and Kuehlein *et al.* (2011), the Working Group calculated that 44% of patients treated for hypertension in Germany were treated with hydrochlorothiazide. This suggested that hydrochlorothiazide represented about 25% of all drugs used for hypertension in this country. These results were very consistent with previous reports that diuretics represented 39% of all drugs mentioned for German patients with hypertension, and compendium information suggesting that hydrochlorothiazide was not generally available on its own, but rather as a combination product.]

1.4 Occurrence and exposure

Human exposure to hydrochlorothiazide is largely limited to use as a medication. While occupational exposure in manufacturing is likely to occur, no specific studies on hydrochlorothiazide as an agent in occupational or environmental exposure were identified by the Working Group.

1.5 Regulations and guidelines

Hydrochlorothiazide has been widely approved by drug regulatory agencies around the world. In the USA, it was approved by the Food and Drug Administration (FDA, 2013) in 1959. The Working Group did not identify extraordinary regulatory restrictions on use of hydrochlorothiazide as a medication, or regulations on environmental exposure.

2. Cancer in Humans

Hydrochlorothiazide is a diuretic in a class of thiazide compounds primarily used to treat hypertension, but also oedema and congestive heart failure. In addition to diuretic effects on the kidney, hydrochlorothiazide has photosensitizing properties, enhancing skin sensitivity to sunlight exposure.

Epidemiological studies have investigated associations with use of hydrochlorothiazide using pharmacy information in pre-paid health plans and data from national databases linking with physician and/or cancer registry information. Some studies evaluated thiazides as a class of drugs either through prescription records or self-reported use. The types of cancers investigated or observed in these studies included those related to exposure to sunlight (e.g. lip or cutaneous malignancies), and those of the kidney (e.g. renal cell carcinoma), with a few reports of other malignancies (e.g. cancers of the prostate, colon, breast, and endometrium). See Table 2.1 and Table 2.2.

2.1 Cancers of the lip and skin

Using data from 1994 to 2006 from the Kaiser Permanente Medical Care Program in northern California, USA, Friedman *et al.* (2009) screened for drugs potentially related to cancer occurrence by analysing cancer cases and controls matched on age (same year), sex, year of starting drug coverage, and index date (matched to the case's date of diagnosis). The analysis considered the potentially confounding effects of HIV positivity, and other medical conditions. Elevated risks were observed for cancers of the lip (odds ratio, OR, 2.29; 95% CI, 1.84–2.86) and all other types of cancer of the skin combined, including Merkel cell, malignant fibrous histiocytoma, dermatofibrosarcoma, skin appendage carcinoma and other rarer types (OR, 1.56; 95% CI, 1.20–2.01) in relation to three or more prescriptions of hydrochlorothiazide at least 2 years before diagnosis. No association was observed with cutaneous melanoma or other cancers. [Many comparisons were made. Risk estimates were only provided if they indicated an association with an odds ratio > 1.50 with three or more prescription with a 2-year lag, *P* < 0.01 for difference from odds ratio 1.00, or a higher odds ratio for three or more prescriptions compared with

one prescription. Limitations further included the heterogeneity of "other skin cancers" and inability to examine basal cell and squamous cell skin cancers. Also, information was lacking to evaluate the potential confounding or effect modification by factors related to sun exposure. For cancers of the lip and other sites, the results referred to hydrochlorothiazide in combination with other drugs. Since computerized pharmacy records only began in 1994, only a limited latency period could be observed.]

On the basis of the findings from Friedman *et al.* (2009), a similarly designed nested case–control study on cancer of the lip was carried out from 1994 to 2008; the study included 712 cases (of which 97.2% were squamous cell carcinomas of the lip) and 22 904 non-Hispanic, white controls (Friedman *et al.*, 2012). An increased odds ratio for cancer of the lip was observed for people having three or more prescriptions of any medicine containing hydrochlorothiazide (OR, 2.19; 95% CI, 1.74–2.76) or exclusively hydrochlorothiazide (OR, 2.03; 95% CI, 1.23–3.36) at least 2 years before the reference date. Odds ratios were higher with longer duration of prescriptions. [A strength of this study was the large sample size that allowed them to look at hydrochlorothiazide alone; however, there were no data on potentially modifying or confounding factors, including factors related to sun exposure. The definition of cancer of the lip presumably used the definition provided by the Surveillance, Epidemiology, and End Results Program (SEER) of the National Cancer Institute, USA.]

In a population-based nested case–control study from North Jutland, Denmark, diagnoses of melanoma, squamous cell carcinoma, and basal cell carcinoma from 1989 to 2003 were identified through the Danish cancer registry, which includes non-melanoma as well as melanoma of the skin (Jensen *et al.*, 2008). Four controls per case were selected from the Danish Civil Registration System, matched on age (exact), sex, and area of residence. Prescriptions

Table 2.1 Case–control studies of thiazides (including hydrochlorothiazide) and cancer

Reference Location; period	Total cases Total controls	Control source (hospital, population)	Exposure assessment	Organ site (ICD code)	Exposure categories	Exposed cases	Relative risk (95% CI)	Covariates Comments
Friedman *et al.* (2009) Northern California, USA; August 1994–December 2006	NR NR	KPMCP subscribers	KPMCP computerized prescription records		HCTZ use, including combinations, ≥ 3 dispensings, 2-yr lag[a]			Controls matched on sex, year of birth, and year of starting drug coverage
				Kidney (renal pelvis)	No		1.00 (ref.)	
					Yes	537	1.71 (1.54–1.91)	Nested case–control study of 10 controls to each case identified by the KPMCP cancer registry
				Lip	No		1.00 (ref.)	Uncertainty as to whether the association with kidney cancer was due to hypertension or the drug
					Yes	147	2.29 (1.84–2.86)	Lung cancer only weakly related to lip cancer, making confounding by smoking less likely to be an explanation
				Skin (other than lip)	No		1.00 (ref.)	Other types of cancer of the skin included: 35 Merkel cell carcinoma, 14 malignant fibrous histiocytoma, 8 dermatofibrosarcoma, 7 skin appendage carcinoma, 5 or fewer of 14 other rarer types
					Yes	95	1.56 (1.20–2.01)	

Table 2.1 (continued)

Reference Location; period	Total cases Total controls	Control source (hospital, population)	Exposure assessment	Organ site (ICD code)	Exposure categories	Exposed cases	Relative risk (95% CI)	Covariates Comments
Friedman *et al.* (2012) Northern California, USA; 1994–2008	712 22 904 controls	Subscribers to KPMCP	KPMCP computerized prescription records	Lip	HCTZ use, including combinations, ≥ 3 dispensings, 2-yr lag[a]			Matched on age, sex, year of cohort entry. Adjusted for cigarette smoking Non-Hispanic whites only; age, ≥ 30 yr; excludes transplant recipients and HIV-positive; 3 : 1, men : women
					HCTZ prescriptions[b]	103		
					No HCTZ prescriptions		1.00 (ref.)	
					≥ 3 HCTZ prescriptions		2.19 (1.74–2.76)	No stratum-specific numbers provided, just the overall number of cases prescribed HCTZ alone, only and with triamterene
					HCTZ prescriptions only[a]	19		
					No HCTZ prescriptions		1.0 (ref.)	
					≥ 3 HCTZ prescriptions		2.03 (1.23–3.36)	
					Years of supply:			
					HCTZ:[b]	103		
					< 1 yr		0.98 (0.66–1.45)	
					1 to < 5 yr		2.03 (1.54–2.68)	
					≥ 5 yr		4.22 (2.82–6.31)	
					HCTZ-triamterene:[b]	71		
					< 1 yr		0.91 (0.60–1.39)	
					1 to < 5 yr		1.87 (1.37–2.57)	
					≥ 5 yr		2.82 (1.74–4.55)	

Table 2.1 (continued)

Reference Location; period	Total cases Total controls	Control source (hospital, population)	Exposure assessment	Organ site (ICD code)	Exposure categories	Exposed cases	Relative risk (95% CI)	Covariates Comments
Jensen *et al.* (2008) North Jutland County, Denmark; 1989–2003	5964 BCC, 1129 SCC, 1151 MM 32 412 controls	Population	North Jutland County's prescription database	Skin (BCC, SCC, MM)	HCTZ prescriptions before diagnosis			Chronic medical conditions, previous use of oral glucocorticoids, prescriptions for other photosensitizing diuretics
					MM:			Sparse data for HCTZ only (*n* = 13 cases); no association with MM in this limited group
					None		1.00 (ref.)	
					Any	98	1.32 (1.03–1.70)	
					Prescriptions > 1 yr since diagnosis		1.30 (0.99–1.71)	
					Prescriptions > 5 yr since diagnosis		1.24 (0.86–1.78)	
					Linear per 10 000 mg		0.99 (0.95–1.03)	
					SCC:			Sparse data for HCTZ only (*n* = 5 cases); no clear association with SCC in this limited group
					None		1.00 (ref.)	
					Any	159	1.58 (1.29–1.93)	
					Prescriptions > 1 yr since diagnosis		1.67 (1.36–2.07)	
					Prescriptions > 5 yr since diagnosis		1.92 (1.46–2.54)	
					Linear per 10 000 mg		1.03 (1.01–1.06)	
					BCC:			Wider CIs for HCTZ only (*n* = 84 cases); no clear association with BCC
					None		1.00 (ref.)	
					Any	542	1.05 (0.95–1.16)	
					Prescriptions > 1 yr since diagnosis		1.05 (0.94–1.17)	
					Prescriptions > 5 yr since diagnosis		1.10 (0.95–1.26)	
					Linear per 10 000 mg		1.02 (1.00–1.03)	

Table 2.1 (continued)

Reference Location; period	Total cases Total controls	Control source (hospital, population)	Exposure assessment	Organ site (ICD code)	Exposure categories	Exposed cases	Relative risk (95% CI)	Covariates Comments
Robinson et al. (2013) New Hampshire, USA; 1993–2009	1637 SCC, 1605 BCC 1906 controls	Population	Personal interview	Skin (BCC, SCC)	Thiazides (diuretics)	239		Age, sex, number of previous episodes of painful sunburn OR for photosensitizing cardiovascular drugs (mainly thiazides), 1.3 (95% CI, 1.0–1.6)
					SCC		1.0 (ref.) 1.3 (0.7–2.4)	OR restricted to HCTZ was similar
					BCC		"No association"	
de Vries et al. (2012) Multicentre (Finland, Germany, Greece, Italy, Malta, Poland, Scotland and Spain)	1371 (602 BCC; 409 SCC; 360 CMM) 1550 controls	Hospital (same dermatology outpatient clinics and hospital departments as the cases)	Questionnaire	Skin (BCC, SCC, CMM)	Thiazide (bendroflumethiazide) CMM BCC SCC	33 94 99	1.22 (0.77–1.93) 1.27 (0.92–1.75) 1.66 (1.16–2.37)	Age, sex, phototype, and country Study period not reported. Age- and sex-matched controls
Hiatt et al. (1994) Northern California, USA; 1964–89	257 (167 men, 90 women) 257 controls (167 men, 90 women)	Subscribers to KPMCP	KPMCP prescription records and chart review	Kidney (renal cell carcinoma)	Thiazide, ever-use Men: No Yes Women: No Yes		1.0 (ref.) 1.2 (0.6–2.1) 1.0 (ref.) 4.0 (1.5–10.8)	History of smoking, BMI, hypertension, history of kidney infection at check-up ORs were highest for the category of longest time since first use, duration of use, number of mentions, and grams, but trends were not statistically significant
Stanford et al. (1986) USA (BCDDP); 1973–7	1362	Population	Home interview	Breast	Thiazide, ever-use	167	1.22 (0.9–1.6)	Age at diagnosis Exposure information for antihypertensive and oedema medications was truncated at the time of diagnosis for cases or at an equivalent time for controls

Table 2.1 (continued)

Reference Location; period	Total cases Total controls	Control source (hospital, population)	Exposure assessment	Organ site (ICD code)	Exposure categories	Exposed cases	Relative risk (95% CI)	Covariates Comments
Li et al. (2003) Washington state, USA; April 1997– May 1999	975 1007 controls	Population (CMS list)	In-person interview	Breast	Thiazides Ever-use 6 mo to 5 yr > 5 yr	246 81 159	1.4 (1.1–1.8) 1.5 (1.1–2.2) 1.3 (1.0–1.7)	Age Of 1210 eligible cases identified, 975 women (80.6%) were interviewed (14% refused, 4% died, 1% moved away, 1% refused contact with patients). Of the 1365 eligible women who were selected as controls, 1007 women (73.8%) were interviewed (22% refused, 2% died, 2% moved away, 1% not located)
Fortuny et al. (2009) New Jersey, USA; 2001–5	469 467 controls	Population	Personal interview	Endometrium	Thiazides No Yes Duration of use: < 3 yr 3–6 yr > 6 yr P (trend test)	369 100 28 23 48	1.0 (ref.) 1.8 (1.1–3.0) 1.6 (0.8–3.5) 1.2 (0.6–2.8) 2.4 (1.2–4.8) 0.39	Adjusted for age (linear spline), BMI (four categories), demographic factors (education, race), other estrogen-related variables (menarche, hormone therapy, oral contraceptives, age at menopause, parity), smoking, family history of endometrial cancer, plus all other variables included in table Three methods were used to locate controls (random-digit dialling for women aged < 65 yr, CMS lists for women aged ≥ 65 yr, area sampling for women aged ≥ 55 yr)

Table 2.1 (continued)

Reference Location; period	Total cases Total controls	Control source (hospital, population)	Exposure assessment	Organ site (ICD code)	Exposure categories	Exposed cases	Relative risk (95% CI)	Covariates Comments
Hallas *et al.* (2012) Denmark; 2000–5	149 417 597 668 controls	Population (Danish cancer registry, Danish national registry of patients, prescription database of the Danish Medicines Agency, and Danish person registry)	Prescription records (database of the Danish Medicines Agency)	Any cancer	Thiazides All malignancies	11 509	1.25 (1.22–1.28)	Prior discharge diagnosis of COPD or inflammatory bowel disease, modified Charlson index that contains 19 categories of comorbidity Four controls matched by age and sex were selected for each case by a risk-set sampling. For all drug classes, those exposed who had taken at least 1000 defined daily doses during the past 5 yr before the index date were considered

[a] Users of other drugs excluded

[b] All use of drug, regardless of other drugs dispensed

BCDDP, Breast Cancer Detection Demonstration Project; BCC, basal cell carcinoma; BMI, body mass index; CI, confidence interval; COPD, chronic obstructive pulmonary disease; CMM, cutaneous malignant melanoma; CMS, Centers for Medicare & Medicaid Services; HCTZ, hydrochlorothiazide; KPMCP, Kaiser Permanente Medical Care Program; mo, month; MM, malignant melanoma; NR, not reported; ref., reference; RR, relative risk; SCC, squamous cell carcinoma; yr, year

Table 2.2 Cohort studies of thiazides (including hydrochlorothiazide) and cancer

Reference Location; period	Total No. of subjects	Exposure assessment	Organ site (ICD code)	Exposure categories	No. of cases/ deaths	Relative risk (95% CI)	Covariates Comments
cited in Friedman et al. (2009) USA; 1969–2002	NR	KPMCP computerized prescription records	Kidney	Thiazide use Any use	 55	SMR[a] 1.36 (1.03–1.77)	Limited details on study design. Limited data on potential confounding factors
Ruiter et al. (2010) The Netherlands; 1986–2007	10 692 with no prescriptions for diuretics before April 1991	Computerized pharmacy records	Skin (BCC)	Thiazide use Never used Ever used Days of use: < 94 94–524 524–1646 > 1646	 385 137 34 35 34 34	Hazard ratio 1.0 (ref.) 1.0 (0.95–1.05) 1.02 (0.72–1.45) 0.98 (0.69–1.39) 0.86 (0.60–1.22) 1.10 (0.77–1.58)	Age, sex, smoking, tendency to sunburn, residence in a country with high ambient UV radiation, hair and eye colour, other photosensitizing drugs Cases identified from general practitioners and linkage with national cancer registry. Unclear how many BCC cases may have been missed
Flaherty et al. (2005) United States Nurses' Health Study, USA; 1980–2000; and HPFS, USA; 1998	118 191 women and 48 953 men	Self-report in 1980, then every 2 yr	Kidney (renal cell carcinoma)	Thiazide use Current use in 1980, women Current use in 1986, men	 22 22 20 20	 1.5 (1.0–2.4) 1.4 (0.9–2.3) 1.5 (0.9–2.5) 0.8 (0.5–1.5)	Limited exposure information, hypertension an independent risk factor Age-adjusted Age, BMI, hypertension Age-adjusted Age, BMI, hypertension
Friedman & Ury (1980) Northern California, USA; 1969–76	143 574 outpatients with at least one prescription filled in 1969–73	KPMCP computerized prescription records	All cancers, prostate	Thiazides Prostate cancer P for trend All cancers P for trend	 53 585	SMR 1.4 < 0.05 1.1 NS	Age-, sex-standardized SMR based on expected rates from the 3rd National Cancer Survey in the San Francisco Bay Area. Drugs not specifically HCTZ
van den Eeden & Friedman (1995) San Francisco, USA; 1969–88	143 574	KPMCP prescription records	All cancers (56 cancer sites) Gall bladder	Thiazides 	1464 16	SMR 1.07 (1984) SMR 1.02 (1988) SMR 1.8 (P < 0.05)	

Table 2.2 (continued)

Reference Location; period	Total No. of subjects	Exposure assessment	Organ site (ICD code)	Exposure categories	No. of cases/ deaths	Relative risk (95% CI)	Covariates Comments
Tenenbaum et al. (2001) Tel Aviv, Israel; 1992–6	14 166 patients with previous myocardial infarction and/ or stable angina syndrome, screened for participation in BIP study (2153 on diuretics; 375 on HCTZ alone; 199 on amiloride/ HCTZ combination)	Derived from intake examination [unclear from paper]	All cancers, colon	All cancers: No diuretics HCTZ HCTZ/ Amiloride Colon cancer: No diuretics HCTZ Amiloride/ HCTZ	622 29 16 73 5 4	Hazard ratio 1.00 (ref.) 1.41 (0.97–2.05) 1.45 (0.88–2.38) Hazard ratio 1.00 (ref.) 2.12 (0.85–5.26) 3.15 (1.15–8.65)	Significant covariates were included: age, sex, smoking, and triglycerides No information available on duration or doses of drugs administered

[a] HCTZ not distinguished from other thiazides in previous screenings in a smaller cohort, but elevated risk of kidney cancer detected for thiazides as a group.
BCC, basal cell carcinoma; BIP, Bezafibrate Infarction Prevention; HCTZ, hydrochlorothiazide; HPFS, Health Professionals Follow-up Study; KPMCP, Kaiser Permanente Medical Care Program; NR, not reported; NS, not significant; ref., reference; SMR, standardized morbidity ratio; UV, ultraviolet; yr, year

for diuretics were obtained from a database of ambulatory patient prescriptions that began in 1989 and had full coverage of the population in 1991. Taking into account history of chronic disease, prescriptions for oral glucocorticoids and other photosensitizing diuretics, elevated odds ratios were found for squamous cell carcinoma (OR, 1.58; 95% CI, 1.29–1.93) and melanoma (OR, 1.32; 95% CI, 1.03–1.70) in relation to prescriptions for hydrochlorothiazide. A weak association was observed for basal cell carcinoma (OR, 1.05; 95% CI, 0.95–1.16). For squamous cell carcinoma, the odds ratios increased linearly with increasing total dose of prescriptions; the dose trend was weak for basal cell carcinoma, and was not present for melanoma. Additionally, for squamous cell carcinoma, the association was stronger, with a longer lag period from time of prescription to diagnosis. A sensitivity analysis indicated that underascertainment of skin-cancer diagnosis could have led to an underestimate of risk. [A limitation of this study was that it relied on data from medical records and on prescriptions, and thus was not able to assess the potential confounding or modifying effects of factors related to sun exposure. Additionally, hydrochlorothiazide was frequently given with amiloride, and there were too few subjects to evaluate the effects of therapy with hydrochlorothiazide only.]

In a prospective cohort study from the Netherlands, Ruiter *et al.* (2010) used computerized outpatient pharmacy records to assess the relation between thiazide use and basal cell carcinoma. The analysis included 10 692 individuals, largely Caucasian, with no diuretic prescriptions before April 1991. Basal cell carcinomas were identified by general practitioners and linkage with the national cancer registry for 1986 to 2007. After adjustment for multiple potentially confounding factors, no excess risk of basal cell carcinoma was observed with either cumulative duration of use or average grams of thiazide prescription (Ruiter *et al.*, 2010). [It was

uncertain whether complete ascertainment of basal cell carcinoma was achieved.]

A population-based case–control study of cases of basal cell carcinoma (*n* = 1605) and squamous cell carcinoma (*n* = 1637) and controls that were frequency-matched on age and sex (*n* = 1906) from New Hampshire, USA, included self-reported use of photosensitizing drugs such as hydrochlorothiazide (Robinson *et al.*, 2013). Elevated odds ratios for squamous cell carcinoma of the skin were observed for reported use of photosensitizing cardiovascular drugs (the majority of which were thiazides) (OR, 1.3; 95% CI, 1.0–1.6), and specifically for thiazides (OR, 1.3; 95% CI, 0.7–2.4); the manuscript indicated that the odds ratio for hydrochlorothiazide was "similar" [which was not surprising since hydrochlorothiazide comprised the majority of the thiazides sold in the USA]. Multiple potentially confounding factors were considered in the analysis, including risk factors related to sun exposure, and history of cigarette smoking. No associations were observed with use of thiazides and basal cell carcinoma. [Limitations of this study were the reliance on self-reported drug use information, lack of statistical power to evaluate effect modification by sunlight-related factors, and failure to report the risk estimate for hydrochlorothiazide.]

A multicentre, hospital-based study of cancer of the skin carried out in Europe (Finland, Germany, Greece, Italy, Malta, Poland, Scotland, and Spain) examined thiazide use determined through questionnaires completed partly by the participant and partly by a dermatology department. The study included 409 cases of squamous cell carcinoma, 602 cases of basal cell carcinoma, 360 cases of cutaneous malignant melanoma, and 1550 controls. Cases were consecutive patients, recently diagnosed (within 3 months of study entry), aged 18 years or older, from one of the participating dermatology practices. Controls were patients visiting the hospital clinics for reasons other than cancer of the skin and were frequency-matched to cases on age (as far as possible in 5-year strata) and sex. Cases and controls were excluded if they were unable to complete the questionnaire, did not agree to take part, had Fitzpatrick skin types V–VI, had ever received phototherapy, or had photoallergies or lupus erythematosus. A minimum of 3 months, daily intake of self-reported thiazide (bendroflumethiazide) was associated with an odds ratio of 1.66 (95% CI, 1.16–2.37) for squamous cell carcinoma, an odds ratio of 1.27 (95% CI, 0.92–1.75) for basal cell carcinoma, and an odds ratio of 1.22 (95% CI, 0.77–1.93) for cutaneous melanoma (de Vries *et al.*, 2012).

2.2 Renal cell carcinoma

A standardized morbidity ratio (SMR) analysis was conducted of outpatients enrolled in the Kaiser Permanente Medical Care Program with at least one prescription for thiazide filled between 1969–1973 who were followed for cancer until 2002 A total of 55 observed versus 40.34 expected cancers of the kidney were observed among those with thiazide prescriptions (SMR, 1.36; 95% CI, 1.03–1.77) (Friedman *et al.*, 2009). [Limited details on the study design were provided, and there were limited data available on potentially confounding or modifying factors.]

In the nested case–control analyses of data from the Kaiser Permanente Medical Care Program from 1994–2006 conducted by Friedman *et al.* (2009), an increased risk of cancer of the renal pelvis (OR, 1.71; 95% CI, 1.54–1.91) was observed in association with three or more prescriptions of hydrochlorothiazide at least 2 years before diagnosis. [This observation was one of many comparisons. The study reported limited data on potentially confounding factors, i.e. those not available in medical records, e.g. cigarette smoking history. While hypertension was evaluated in the analysis, it was uncertain whether findings for cancer of the renal pelvis could be attributed to hydrochlorothiazide use

or to hypertension, since use of other cardiovascular drugs, e.g. Clonidine, Diltiazem, and Gemfibrozil, were also related to risk of renal cell cancer.]

Also using records from the Kaiser Permanente Medical Care Program, Hiatt *et al.* (1994) conducted a nested case–control study of 257 cases of renal cell carcinoma and one-to-one matched controls. Cases included members enrolled in the programme with documented renal cell carcinoma diagnosed between 1964 and 1989 and who had received a standardized multiphasic health check-up (offered from 1964 to 1988) before diagnosis. Controls who had also undergone the multiphasic health check-up were matched to cases on the age (± 1 year) when they had the check-up, and were required to be enrolled in the Kaiser Permanente Medical Care Program when their case was diagnosed. Data on thiazide use up to 6 months before diagnosis (and a matched date for controls), were abstracted from the medical records. An association was found between thiazide use and renal cell carcinoma among women (OR, 4.0; 95% CI, 1.5–10.8) but not men (OR, 1.2; 95% CI, 0.6–2.1) adjusted for multiple potentially confounding factors, including hypertension (Hiatt *et al.*, 1994). Odds ratios did not increase with estimated number of grams used (based on time since first use, duration, and number of mentions of use in the chart). [Data on potentially confounding or modifying factors were available through the multiphasic check-up.]

A cohort analysis of renal cell carcinoma was conducted in the United States Nurses' Health Study and Health Professionals Follow-up Study (HPFS) of 118 191 women and 48 953 men without a history of cancer (Flaherty *et al.*, 2005). Renal cell carcinomas self-reported (up to 2000 in the Nurses' Health Study, and 1998 in the HPFS) were confirmed by medical record in more than 80% of cases, and the 156 women and 110 men with histologically verified (via biopsy, nephrectomy or autopsy) renal cell carcinoma were included in the analysis. Thiazide use was based on self-report (beginning in 1980 for the Nurses' Health Study, and 1986 for the HPFS) and was updated every 2–4 years. For women, the age-adjusted relative risk estimate was 1.5 (95% CI, 1.0–2.4), and after adjustment for history of hypertension, and updated body mass index was 1.4 (95% CI, 0.9–2.3); among men, the relative risks were 1.5 (95% CI, 0.9–2.5), and 0.8 (95% CI, 0.5–1.5), respectively. The result was not altered when using updated information on thiazide use. [There was limited information on thiazide use derived from a postal questionnaire. As in other studies, it was not possible to exclude the possibility of confounding by hypertension, since hypertension is a major indication for hydrochlorothiazide use. Hypertension was reported to be an independent risk factor for renal cell carcinoma in this study.]

2.3 Other cancers

Other cancers were assessed in analyses of standardized morbidity ratio using the Kaiser Permanente Medical Care Program prescription pharmacy database and the Kaiser Permanente cancer registry with the northern California (USA) cancer registry as the referent population. Among 143 574 outpatients, with at least one prescription filled between 1969–1973 who were followed for cancer until 1976 using hospital-discharge records for the programme and the cancer registry, Friedman & Ury (1980) found an elevated age- and sex-standardized morbidity ratio for cancer of the prostate (SMR, 1.4; $P < 0.05$). In a subsequent analysis, with follow-up data until 1988, van den Eeden & Friedman (1995) reported a greater than expected incidence of tumours of the gall bladder with thiazide use (16 observed, 8.9 expected; SMR, 1.8; $P < 0.05$). [The limitations of these hypothesis-generating analyses are mentioned in Sections 2.1 and 2.2. Additionally, in the 1995 study, other hypertension drugs also were related to elevated standardized morbidity

ratio for cancer of the gall bladder, raising the possibility the association was due to the indication rather the specific drug.]

Two case–control studies of cancer of the breast evaluated self-reported use of thiazides. A case–control analysis of thiazides was conducted in the USA within the Breast Cancer Detection Demonstration Project, a multicentre breast-screening trial involving in-person interviews with women with cancer of the breast (diagnosed between 1973 and 1977) and controls (neither recommended for a biopsy nor had a biopsy during participation in the programme) (Stanford et al., 1986). Response rates were 86% for cases and 74% for controls. Self-reported use of thiazides for at least 6 months compared with women without a history of hypertension was associated with an age-adjusted odds ratio of 1.22 (95% CI, 0.9–1.6). Odds ratios by duration of use were 1.28 for < 5 years, 1.50 for 5–9 years, and 1.33 for ≥ 10 years (P for trend, 0.06). For years since first use were 1.27 for < 5 years, 1.70 for 5–9 years, and 1.06 for ≥ 10 years (P for trend, 0.12).

A more recent population-based case–control study from western Washington State, USA, included 975 cases of cancer of the breast in women aged 65–79 years diagnosed between 1997 and 1999, and identified through the cancer registry for the region (Li et al., 2003). Controls ($n = 1007$) were identified through Center for Medicare and Medicaid services, and cases were limited to those who were registered in this system. Response rates were 81% of cases and 74% of controls. In-person interviews encompassed a detailed history of cardiovascular medications used, and included duration and dose, using a life-events calendar and photographs of medicines to enhance recall. Ever-use of hydrochlorothiazide was reported by 19% of controls. The odds ratio for cancer of the breast among women who reported use of thiazides for 6 months or more compared with women who had never used any antihypertension medication was 1.4 (95% CI, 1.1–1.8), and 1.5 (95% CI, 1.1.–2.2) for 6 months to 5 years of use, and 1.3 (95% CI, 1.0–1.7) for > 5 years of use. Multiple potentially confounding factors were taken into consideration, including race, income, marital status, education, age at menarche, parity, age at first birth, type of menopause, age at menopause, duration of oral contraceptive use, ever-use of hormone replacement therapy, first-degree family history of breast carcinoma, smoking status, average daily intake of alcohol, and body mass index. However, none changed the estimate by more than 10%, and thus estimates were only adjusted for age. [This study was large and had relatively extensive information on exposure. The use of recall aids to prompt reporting of drug use was an additional strength. The lack of clear trends with duration could be due to poorer recall for use further in the past, or to lack of a true association.]

A population-based case–control study of invasive epithelial endometrial cancer evaluated thiazide use in New Jersey, USA (Fortuny *et al.*, 2009). Cases were derived from The Estrogen, Diet, Genetics, and Endometrial Cancer (EDGE) study – a population-based case–control study conducted in six counties in northern New Jersey. Cases diagnosed with endometrial cancer between 1 July 2001 and 30 June 2005 were identified by the cancer registries for the region and state. To be eligible, cases were required to be aged 21 years and over and residing in one of the six counties (Bergen, Essex, Hudson, Middlesex, Morris, and Union). Controls, without a history of hysterectomy, were identified through random-digit dialling (age, < 65 years) and Centers for Medicare and Medicaid records. Response rates were 30% for the cases and 39% for the controls. After adjustment for multiple potentially confounding factors, including age, sex, level of education, smoking, body mass index, hypertension, diabetes, and use of other drugs, the overall odds ratio for use of thiazides for at least 6 months was 1.8 (95%

CI, 1.1–3.0) [compared with those with no use or use for less than 6 months]. Odds ratios were 1.6 (95% CI, 0.8–3.5), 1.2 (95% CI, 0.6–2.8), 2.4 (95% CI, 1.2–4.8) for < 3, 3–6, and > 6 years of use, respectively (*P* for trend, 0.39). [Low response rates could have introduced selection bias.]

A cohort analysis was conducted of 14 166 individuals recruited between 1990 and 1992 to participate in the Bezafibrate Infarction Prevention study in Israel (Tenenbaum *et al.*, 2001). Participants were followed for incidence and mortality from cancer until 1996 using the Israel population registry and national cancer registry. Participants included those with a history of heart disease (myocardial infarction, stable angina syndrome) but without a permanent pacemaker implantation, cerebrovascular disease, chronic hepatic or renal disease, peripheral vascular disease, malignant disease, estrogen therapy, type 1 diabetes mellitus, or use of lipid-modifying drugs. Incidence of all cancers was increased among those who used hydrochlorothiazide (hazard ratio, HR, 1.41; 95% CI, 0.97–2.05) or a combination hydrochlorothiazide/amiloride therapy (HR, 1.45; 95% CI, 0.88–2.38). An elevated incidence of cancer of the colon was observed among those who used hydrochlorothiazide (*n* = 5 cases; HR, 2.12; 95% CI, 0.85–5.26) or a combination hydrochlorothiazide/amiloride therapy (*n* = 4 cases; HR, 3.15; 95% CI, 1.15–8.65). Age, sex, smoking status, and triglycerides were included in the models if they were statistically significant using stepwise Cox models. [No other specific cancer types were mentioned in relation to hydrochlorothiazide. The limitations of this study included the small number of cancers of the colon. There was no information about use, i.e. dose or duration. The precise method of ascertaining medication use was not explained and was assumed to be derived from the intake examination. Given that the cohort was part of a clinical trial, the results may not be generalizable.]

A population-based case–control study was conducted on cancers from 2000 to 2005 using the Danish cancer registry, and drug use was estimated from the Prescription Database of the Danish Medicines Agency (Hallas *et al.*, 2012). A thiazide user was defined as a person having taken 1000 defined daily doses of the drug, and the comparison group was never-users. The odds ratio for all cancers combined was 1.25 (95% CI, 1.22–1.28). [This was a large study with no details on the types of cancer among subjects exposed to thiazides. The association with all cancers combined could be due to confounding by indication as other antihypertension drugs also were related to overall cancer incidence.]

3. Cancer in Experimental Animals

3.1 Oral administration

See Table 3.1

3.1.1 Mouse

In a feeding study, groups of 50 male and 50 female mice (age, 7–8 weeks) were given diets containing hydrochlorothiazide [USP grade] at dietary concentrations of 0 (control), 2500, or 5000 ppm and held until death or completion of the 103–104-week exposure period (NTP, 1989; Bucher *et al.*, 1990). No changes in survival, changes in group mean body weight, or gross clinical evidence of toxicity were identified in male or females exposed to hydrochlorothiazide. A significant increase in the incidences of hepatocellular adenoma, and hepatocellular adenoma or carcinoma (combined) was seen in males at the highest dose; an increase in the incidence of hepatocellular carcinoma in mice at the highest dose (9 out of 50 versus 4 out of 48) was not statistically significant ($P = 0.161$). Statistically significant, dose-related increases in the incidence of hepatocellular adenoma, and hepatocellular

adenoma or carcinoma (combined) were seen in males. No significant increases in the incidence of any neoplasms were seen in females. [Although significant increases in the incidences of hepatocellular adenoma, and hepatocellular adenoma or carcinoma (combined) were observed in male mice exposed to hydrochlorothiazide, these findings may have been the result of an unusually low incidence of hepatocellular neoplasms in the dietary control group in this study (15%) compared with those seen in control groups (30%) from the National Toxicology Program (NTP) historical database. The Working Group noted that no data on historical controls were available from the laboratory where this agent was tested.]

3.1.2 Rat

In a feeding study, groups of 24 male and 24 female rats (age, 6–8 weeks) were given diets containing hydrochlorothiazide [USP grade] at a dietary concentration of 0 (control), or 0.1% (1000 ppm) for 104 weeks (Lijinsky & Reuber, 1987). The rats were observed until natural death or moribundity occurred, or the end of the study at 130 weeks. Although the total observation period was not specified, median times of death in male and female rats exposed to hydrochlorothiazide were 111 and 114 weeks, respectively. Median times of death in untreated controls were 107 weeks in males and 122 weeks in females. Dietary administration of hydrochlorothiazide at 1000 ppm was well tolerated. Although body weights were not reported, a high incidence of chronic progressive nephropathy was seen in male and female rats exposed to hydrochlorothiazide; this finding suggested that the dose of 1000 ppm used in the study approached the maximum tolerated dose for this agent. No statistical analyses of the incidences of preneoplastic or neoplastic lesions were reported. The incidence of adrenal pheochromocytoma was increased [$P < 0.005$] from 0 out of 24 in control

Table 3.1 Studies of carcinogenicity in mice and rats given diets containing hydrochlorothiazide

Species, strain (sex) Duration Reference	Dosing regimen, Animals/group at start	Incidence of tumours	Significance	Comments
Mouse, B6C3F$_1$ (M, F) 103–104 wk NTP (1989), Bucher *et al.* (1990)	Diets containing hydrochlorothiazide at 0 (control), 2500, or 5000 ppm 50 M and 50 F/group (age, 7–8-wk)	Hepatocellular adenoma: 3/48 (6%)*, 8/49 (16%), 14/50 (28%)** (M) Hepatocellular carcinoma: 4/48 (8%), 4/49 (8%), 9/50 (18%) (M) Hepatocellular adenoma or carcinoma (combined): 7/48 (15%)*, 10/49 (20%), 21/50 (42%)** (M)	*$P < 0.01$ (trend) **$P \leq 0.012$	Purity, USP grade No historical control data from the laboratory where this agent was tested Unusually low incidence of hepatocellular neoplasms in the male control group (15%) compared with control groups from the NTP historical database (30%) No significant increases in the incidence of any neoplasm were reported in females
Rat, F344 (M, F) 130 wk Lijinsky & Reuber (1987)	Diets containing hydrochlorothiazide at 0 (control), or 1000 ppm for 104 wk. Rats were held untreated for up to an additional 26 wk 24 M and 24 F/group (age, 6–8 wk)	Adrenal pheochromocytoma: 6/24, 9/24 (M); 0/24, 9/24* (F)	*[$P < 0.005$]	Purity, USP grade No statistical analyses were reported
Rat, F344 (M, F) 105–106 wk NTP (1989), Bucher *et al.* (1990)	Diets containing hydrochlorothiazide at 0 (control), 250, 500, or 2000 ppm 50 M and 50 F/group (age, 7–8-wk)	–	–	Purity, USP grade Decreased body weight in all exposed groups may have reduced sensitivity to neoplastic development No significant increases in the incidence of any neoplasm were reported in either sex

F, female, M, male; USP, United States Pharmacopeia; wk, week females to 9 out of 24 in exposed females; the incidences of adrenal pheochromocytoma in males were 6 out of 24 and 9 out of 24 in control and treated animals, respectively. [The Working Group noted the unusually high incidence of adrenal pheochromocytoma in males in the control group.] Exposure to hydrochlorothiazide also induced significant increases [$P < 0.001$] in the incidence of parathyroid hyperplasia in males and females.

In a feeding study, groups of 50 male and 50 female rats (age, 7–8 weeks) were given diets containing hydrochlorothiazide [USP grade] at dietary concentrations of 0 (control), 250, 500, or 2000 ppm, and maintained until death or completion of the 105–106-week exposure period (NTP, 1989; Bucher *et al.* 1990). No gross clinical evidence of agent toxicity was identified in either male or female rats exposed to hydrochlorothiazide. Survival curves were very similar in all groups of males. Although an apparent trend towards early mortality was seen in females exposed to hydrochlorothiazide, the differences in survival curves were not statistically significant. Mean body weights in all groups of rats exposed to hydrochlorothiazide were below those in the control groups; at study termination, body weight suppression in both sexes was greater than 15%. This reduction in mean body weight was apparently secondary to suppression of food intake, but was not clearly dose-related. No significant increases in the incidence of any neoplasms were reported in all groups of exposed rats. [The Working Group noted that decreased body weight in all groups exposed to hydrochlorothiazide may have reduced the sensitivity of these animals to neoplastic development.] Confirming the results of Lijinsky & Reuber (1987), significant increases in the incidence of hyperplasia of the parathyroid gland were seen in all groups of exposed rats of males and females.

3.2 Coexposure with modifying agents

In experimental groups that were components of the study described above, Lijinsky & Reuber (1987) exposed groups of 24 male and 24 female F344 rats to diets containing hydrochlorothiazide at 0 ppm (control) or 1000 ppm in combination with sodium nitrite at 2000 ppm for 104 weeks, and maintained until 130 weeks. The study was designed to determine whether exposure to hydrochlorothiazide associated with sodium nitrite could result in the formation of carcinogenic *N*-nitroso compounds in the stomach. No significant increases in neoplastic or preneoplastic lesions were reported. [No statistical analyses of the incidence of preneoplastic or neoplastic lesions were reported.]

4. Mechanistic and Other Relevant Data

4.1 Absorption, distribution, metabolism, and excretion

4.1.1 Humans

(a) Pharmacokinetics of single doses

Pharmacokinetic studies using [^{14}C]hydrochlorothiazide given orally ($n = 4$) or intravenously ($n = 2$) to healthy subjects have shown that hydrochlorothiazide is absorbed mainly (~70%) via the duodenum and upper jejunum, and only to a minor extent via the stomach (Beermann *et al.*, 1976).

High-performance liquid chromatography (HPLC) analysis of plasma and urine samples from 12 healthy volunteers given single oral doses of hydrochlorothiazide (25, 50, 100, or 200 mg as tablets or suspensions) showed that plasma profiles (i.e. mean peak plasma concentrations, times of peak concentrations, areas under plasma curves) and recovery of unchanged drug in the urine were linearly related to dose (Patel *et al.*, 1984). This was consistent with a previous report from Beermann & Groschinsky-Grind (1977), who used gas-liquid chromatography (GLC) analyses. Absorption from all doses was rapid; peak plasma concentrations were achieved at approximately 2 hours. These findings were common to both tablet and suspension formulations (Patel *et al.*, 1984).

A study in healthy volunteers to evaluate the urinary excretion of hydrochlorothiazide from 25 mg and 50 mg tablets sourced from seven different distributors and at least six manufacturers demonstrated equivalent bioavailability for all products (Meyer *et al.*, 1975). Thus, the bioavailability of hydrochlorothiazide did not appear to differ between different oral preparations (Beermann, 1984).

Absorption of hydrochlorothiazide is generally considered to follow first-order kinetics (Barbhaiya *et al.*, 1982); however, one study of plasma concentrations over the 48 hours following an oral dose of 100 mg in four healthy volunteers (Redalieu *et al.*, 1985) suggested zero-order absorption. [Zero-order kinetics implies accumulation of excess dissolved drug at the absorption site, or saturable absorption, neither of which have so far been demonstrated with hydrochlorothiazide.]

Reports on the influence of ingested food on the absorption of hydrochlorothiazide were conflicting. In a study reporting increased absorption in the presence of food (Beermann & Groschinsky-Grind, 1978b), the mean urinary recovery of an oral dose of 75 mg of hydrochlorothiazide in eight subjects, under both fasting and non-fasting conditions, was found by GLC to be 47% and 55%, respectively. In contrast, a study of eight healthy volunteers each given 50 mg of hydrochlorothiazide reported reduction in plasma absorption (modestly affected by varying accompanying fluid volumes) and reduction in urinary recovery of hydrochlorothiazide taken after (rather than before) food (Barbhaiya *et al.*, 1982). [The inconsistency between these studies was due to procedural differences, for example, differing doses used, and variation in times when food was permitted after dosing. Fasting and non-fasting subjects were permitted food 4 hours after dosing in the later study (Barbhaiya *et al.*, 1982) but not until 10 hours after dosing, in the fasted subjects only, in the earlier study (Beermann & Groschinsky-Grind, 1978b).] It was suggested that prolonged abstinence from food in the fasted group had altered gastrointestinal secretion and motility, affecting drug absorption (Barbhaiya *et al.*, 1982).

Hydrochlorothiazide, in all therapeutic doses, is approximately 40% bound to plasma protein, and accumulates in erythrocytes. The ratio of uptake between erythrocytes and plasma is approximately 3.5 : 1 (Beermann *et al.*, 1976). Equilibrium of hydrochlorothiazide between plasma and erythrocytes is reached 4 hours after an oral dose (Beermann *et al.*, 1976). HPLC analyses in seven healthy volunteers showed that 24 hours after a single oral dose of hydrochlorothiazide of 100 mg, the concentration of hydrochlorothiazide bound to erythrocytes was approximately ninefold the concentration in plasma (Yamazaki *et al.*, 1989).

The study by Beermann *et al.* (1976) of [^{14}C] hydrochlorothiazide given as oral ($n = 4$) or intravenous ($n = 2$) doses to healthy subjects demonstrated negligible recovery in the faeces and duodenal bile, and showed that the main excretory route of hydrochlorothiazide was via the kidneys. Mean renal clearance was approximately 300 mL/minute. There was no reabsorption (Beermann *et al.*, 1976). Clearance was by glomerular filtration and active secretion via the organic anion transport system at the proximal tubules (Beermann *et al.*, 1976; Barbhaiya *et al.*, 1982; Kim *et al.*, 2003).

Elimination of hydrochlorothiazide from plasma was biphasic over 24–27 hours; plasma concentrations fell rapidly over the initial 12 hours, and then more slowly (Beermann *et al.*, 1976; Barbhaiya *et al.*, 1982; Patel *et al.*, 1984). The urinary excretion rate closely resembled this time course (Barbhaiya *et al.* 1982). The plasma elimination half-life was about 6 hours initially, but up to 15 hours terminally (Barbhaiya *et al.*, 1982; Patel *et al.*, 1984). Approximately 70% and 90% of the oral and intravenous administered doses, respectively, were recovered unchanged in the urine of healthy volunteers (Beermann *et al.*, 1976), and thus reflected gastrointestinal absorption of hydrochlorothiazide.

(b) Pharmacokinetics of repeated doses

Three patients who had been receiving hydrochlorothiazide only for a minimum of 3 months to treat hypertension (without cardiac failure), were given an oral dose of 50 mg of [^{14}C] hydrochlorothiazide after an overnight fast. Peak concentrations occurred at 3–4 hours in plasma and at 4 to 5 hours in blood cells, and urinary recovery for two of the patients was of the same magnitude as that in healthy subjects, but lower in one patient (who had decreased renal function) (Beermann *et al.*, 1976).

(c) Metabolism

It is generally considered that since hydrochlorothiazide is excreted in urine almost entirely as unchanged drug, it is not metabolized in humans (Beermann *et al.*, 1976). Radiographic analysis of urine extracts ($n = 110$) collected from five healthy subjects and three patients given [^{14}C]hydrochlorothiazide orally revealed a single spot with the same chromatographic properties as hydrochlorothiazide and representing > 95% of the radiolabel. However, two samples from one subject collected on the second and third days after dosing revealed some radiolabelled material (< 0.5% of total radiolabel excreted) that did not correspond to hydrochlorothiazide (Beermann *et al.*, 1976). The nature of this material was found by Okuda *et al.* (1987) to be 2-amino-4-chloro-1,3-benzenedisulfonamide

(ACBS), a hydrolysis product of hydrochlorothiazide. Concentrations of this metabolite were higher (4.3% of hydrochlorothiazide excreted) in patients' urine 24 hours after taking hydrochlorothiazide than in the same batch of bulk tablets (0.4%), so it was unlikely to be a tablet contaminant.

Okuda *et al.*, (1987) also demonstrated that, while concentrations of hydrochlorothiazide in erythrocytes and plasma peaked at 6 hours after dosing and then slowly declined, the concentrations of ACBS were continuing to rise at 24 hours. Thus it seems ACBS is formed by hydrolysis after administration of hydrochlorothiazide, and is excreted more slowly than it is produced. Furthermore, ACBS appears to have a stronger affinity to erythrocytes than does hydrochlorothiazide; concentrations of ACBS and hydrochlorothiazide in erythrocytes were approximately equal, but ACBS concentrations in plasma were approximately 10 times lower than those of hydrochlorothiazide (Okuda *et al.*, 1987).

Metabolites of hydrochlorothiazide were also investigated in urine of six healthy volunteers after oral administration of a single tablet containing 25 mg of hydrochlorothiazide and 25 mg of spironolactone. Hydrochlorothiazide and ACBS (at a concentration at least 10 times higher than the parent drug) and the minor metabolite, chlorothiazide, were detected in the urine by liquid chromatography-mass spectrometry 120 hours after administration (Deventer *et al.*, 2009).

(d) Variation in absorption, distribution, and excretion

(i) Pregnancy

A study of 10 pregnant women given a daily dose of hydrochlorothiazide of 50 mg for at least 2 weeks (to treat oedema and/or hypertension) demonstrated that the diuretic crossed the human placenta, resulting in concentrations in the umbilical cord plasma that were similar to those in maternal plasma. In amniotic fluid, the concentration of hydrochlorothiazide was higher than that in maternal or umbilical cord plasma by up to 5 and 19 times, respectively (Beermann *et al.*, 1980).

A subsequent case report confirmed these findings, and also reported very low concentrations of hydrochlorothiazide in breast milk (relative to maternal blood). Hydrochlorothiazide was not however detectable (detection limit, 20 ng/mL) in the blood of the nursing infant (Miller *et al.*, 1982).

(ii)   Impaired renal function

A study in 23 patients with varying degrees of impaired renal function showed reduction in the extent and rate of elimination of hydrochlorothiazide; only about 10% of an oral dose was recovered, and the elimination half-life was increased from a mean value of 6.4 hours in healthy individuals to 11.5 hours (in patients with a mean creatinine clearance of 60 mL/minute) and to 21 hours (in patients with a mean creatinine clearance of 19 mL/minute). Intestinal absorption was considered not to be reduced in these patients, since the area-under-the-curve values were greater in those with low creatinine clearance than in healthy subjects. In patients with severe renal impairment, the elimination half-life was prolonged further to approximately 34 hours and recovery of hydrochlorothiazide was greatly reduced even after extending the collection period (Niemeyer *et al.*, 1983).

(iii)   Gastrointestinal surgery

Absorption of hydrochlorothiazide has been shown to be impaired in patients who have undergone intestinal-shunt surgery for obesity. GLC urine analysis (Backman *et al.*, 1979) for five patients who received an oral dose of hydrochlorothiazide of 775 mg (at times ranging from 1.5 to 6 years after surgery) showed that the recovery of unchanged drug was only 31% of the administered dose (i.e. approximately half the amount normally recovered in the urine).

(iv)   Cardiac conditions

The pharmacokinetics of hydrochlorothiazide have been shown to be altered in patients with congestive heart failure (Beermann & Groschinsky-Grind, 1979). GLC analysis of plasma and urine of seven patients given oral hydrochlorothiazide (50–75 mg) indicated substantial reduction in the extent and rate of absorption of hydrochlorothiazide (recovery of only 21–37% of the administered dose in three patients, and delayed plasma peak in another). The total urinary excretion of hydrochlorothiazide in two other patients was approximately 50% of the administered dose. Since the reduced intestinal mobility shown in cardiac failure would be expected to promote the uptake of hydrochlorothiazide, the observed decrease in absorption was suggested to be due to changes in the intestinal wall and/or in blood.

This study also highlighted a substantial reduction in renal clearance (range, 10–187 mL/minute) in these cardiac patients. These patients were older than those studied previously (age, 40–60 years), and it was considered that reduced renal function and age may have been factors in the reduction of absorption (Beermann & Groschinsky-Grind, 1979).

Absorption of hydrochlorothiazide was reported to be unchanged in patients with hypertension (Beermann *et al.*, 1976).

(v)   Racial differences

Racial differences in the pharmacokinetics of hydrochlorothiazide have been investigated in a matched group of (nine black and nine white) hypertensive patients given a single dose of 25 mg of hydrochlorothiazide. Analyses of serial samples of blood and urine collected over 36 hours demonstrated that the pharmacokinetics of hydrochlorothiazide did not differ according to race (Ripley *et al.*, 2000).

(vi) Pharmacokinetic and drug interactions

Absorption of an oral dose of 75 mg of hydrochlorothiazide given to six healthy volunteers was shown to be increased by concomitant administration of propantheline. This effect was attributed to the reduction in gastrointestinal motility caused by this anticholinergic drug (Beermann & Groschinsky-Grind, 1978a). The centrally-acting α-adrenergic agonist guanabenz and the excipient polyvinylpyrrolidone 10 000, increased the absorption of hydrochlorothiazide. Cholestyramine and colestipol reduced mean peak plasma concentrations of hydrochlorothiazide (Welling, 1986).

No significant pharmacokinetic interactions have been noted between hydrochlorothiazide and propranolol, metoprolol, sotalol, or acebutolol. A similar lack of significant interactions has been noted between hydrochlorothiazide and spironolactone and indomethacin, allopurinol and its metabolite, oxipurinol, and phenytoin (Welling, 1986).

Early studies on hydrochlorothiazide and triamterene as components of a fixed drug combination revealed differences in bioavailability from combination tablets and capsules, but subsequent work suggested that these differences may have been due to the effects of formulation rather than drug interaction (Welling, 1986).

4.1.2 Experimental systems

A study of intrahepatic distribution in rats demonstrated that, after steady-state intravenous infusion, hydrochlorothiazide distributes homogeneously but not instantaneously throughout the liver. This was proposed to be because hydrochlorothiazide does not undergo metabolism in the liver (AbdelHameed et al., 1993).

In a study in isolated perfused rat kidney, Masereeuw et al. (1997) demonstrated that renal clearance of hydrochlorothiazide exceeded clearance by glomerular filtration only at low perfusate concentrations. At higher concentrations (> 100 µg/mL), the renal excretion changed from net secretion to net reabsorption due to saturation of the secretory system and substantial passive tubular reabsorption.

4.2 Genetic and related effects

4.2.1 Humans

No data were available to the Working Group.

4.2.2 Experimental systems

See Table 4.1

(a) Mutagenicity

The Working Group did not identify any new data on the mutagenicity of hydrochlorothiazide published since the previous IARC Working Group review (IARC, 1990). In two studies, hydrochlorothiazide was not mutagenic to *Salmonella typhimurium* in the presence or absence of an exogenous metabolic system (Waskell, 1978; Andrews et al., 1984). Hydrochlorothiazide was not mutagenic in bacterial screening systems, with or without enzymatic activation, but can form chemically reactive mutagenic products after reaction with nitrite, a product of nitric oxide (Andrews et al., 1984). [The Working Group noted that only one concentration was used in both studies.] In a third study, in strain TA98, but not in TA1535, TA1537, or TA100, a small, reproducible, concentration-dependent increase in the mean number of revertants was observed in the absence but not in the presence of an exogenous metabolic system (Mortelmans et al., 1986). Hydrochlorothiazide did not induce reversion in an *arg⁻* strain of *Escherichia coli* (Hs30R) (Fujita, 1985). At concentrations greater than 500 µg/mL, hydrochlorothiazide produced cytotoxic effects and induced mutations resulting in resistance to trifluorothymidine in L5178Y mouse lymphoma cells in the absence of an exogenous metabolic system (NTP, 1989).

Table 4.1 Genetic and related effects of hydrochlorothiazide

Test system	Results[a]		Concentration or dose (LED or HID)	Reference
	Without exogenous metabolic system	With exogenous metabolic system		
In vitro				
Salmonella typhimurium TA1535, reverse mutation assay	–	–	10 000 µg/plate	Mortelmans *et al.* (1986)
Salmonella typhimurium TA1535, reverse mutation assay	–	–	1000 µg/plate	Andrews *et al.* (1984)
Salmonella typhimurium TA100, reverse mutation assay	–	–	10 000 µg/plate	Mortelmans *et al.* (1986)
Salmonella typhimurium TA100, reverse mutation assay	–	–	5000 µg/plate	Waskell (1978)
Salmonella typhimurium TA100, reverse mutation assay	–	–	1000 µg/plate	Andrews *et al.* (1984)
Salmonella typhimurium TA1537, reverse mutation assay	–	–	10 000 µg/plate	Mortelmans *et al.* (1986)
Salmonella typhimurium TA1538, reverse mutation assay	–	–	1000 µg/plate	Andrews *et al.* (1984)
Salmonella typhimurium TA98, reverse mutation assay	+	–	3333 µg/plate	Mortelmans *et al.* (1986)
Salmonella typhimurium TA98, reverse mutation assay	–	–	5000 µg/plate	Waskell (1978)
Salmonella typhimurium TA98, reverse mutation assay	–	–	1000 µg/plate	Andrews *et al.* (1984)
Escherichia coli (Hs30R) reversion assay in an *arg⁻* strain	–	NT	0.26 mM	Fujita (1985)
Nondisjunction in *Aspergillus nidulans* spot test	–	NT	NR	Bignami *et al.* (1974)
Chromosome aberration, Chinese hamster ovary cells	–	–	1250 µg/mL	Galloway *et al.* (1987)
Chromosome aberration, Chinese hamster lung cell line	(+)	–	0.5 mg/mL	Ishidate *et al.* (1981)
Sister chromatid exchange, Chinese hamster ovary cells	+	+	900 µg/mL	Galloway *et al.* (1987)
Mutations resulting in trifluorothymidine resistance, L5178Y mouse lymphoma cells	+	NT	500 µg/mL	NTP (1989)
Cytokinesis blocked micronucleus assay, cultured human lymphocytes	+	NT	40 µg/mL	Andrianopoulos *et al.* (2006)
In vivo				
Drosophila melanogaster, sex-linked recessive lethal mutation	–		10 000 ppm in diet	Valencia *et al.* (1985)
Drosophila melanogaster, sex-linked recessive lethal mutation	–		10 000 µg/kg, injection	Valencia *et al.* (1985)

[a] +, positive; (+), weakly positive; –, negative

HID, highest ineffective dose; LED, lowest effective dose; NR, not reported; NT, not tested

In the presence of ultraviolet A irradiation, hydrochlorothiazide significantly enhanced the production of DNA cyclobutane pyrimidine dimers (thymine–thymine dimers, detected by

HPLC) in isolated DNA and in the skin of mice defective in DNA repair (Kunisada *et al.*, 2013).

(b)   Chromosomal damage

Chromosomal damage caused by hydrochlorothiazide was reviewed by a previous IARC Working Group (IARC, 1990). In a spot test, hydrochlorothiazide did not induce nondisjunction and mitotic crossing-over in *Aspergillus nidulans* (Bignami *et al.*, 1974). Hydrochlorothiazide did not induce sex-linked recessive lethal mutation in *Drosophila melanogaster* fed or injected with hydrochlorothiazide solutions at 10 mg/mL (Valencia *et al.*, 1985). Significant increases in the frequency of sister chromatid exchange were observed in Chinese hamster ovary cells in the presence and absence of an exogenous metabolic system (Galloway *et al.*, 1987). Although the results of tests for chromosomal aberration were considered to be negative, very high frequencies of chromatid gaps were noted at 900 and 1000 µg/mL (Galloway *et al.*, 1987). Chromosomal aberrations were not found in Chinese hamster lung cells, but polyploidy was observed after treatment with hydrochlorothiazide for 48 hours (Ishidate *et al.*, 1981).

One new study was identified since the previous IARC (1990) evaluation. Hydrochlorothiazide was found to induce micronucleus formation and chromosome breakage in cultured human lymphocytes via chromosome delay (Andrianopoulos *et al.*, 2006).

4.3   Other mechanistic data relevant to carcinogenicity

Effects on cell physiology

Hydrochlorothiazide is a thiazide-based diuretic that acts on an electroneutral Na^+/Cl^- cotransporter in the distal convoluted tubules of kidney nephrons. The major physiological action of hydrochlorothiazide is to compete for the chloride site on this transporter, thus inhibiting Na^+ transport and reducing blood volume. Clinical evidence also indicates that hydrochlorothiazide can act as a photosensitizer in the presence of irradiation by ultraviolet A or ultraviolet B (Addo *et al.*, 1987). The incidence of phototoxic exanthem is "occasional" (> 1/1000 to < 1/100) (Rote Liste Service GmbH, 2012)

4.4   Susceptibility

No data were available to the Working Group.

4.5   Mechanistic considerations

The possible association between exposure to hydrochlorothiazide and cancer of the skin may result from drug-related photosensitization, which would cause DNA damage (production of dimers by hydrochlorothiazide in the presence of sunlight) and may also lead to a chronic inflammatory reaction in the skin.

5.   Summary of Data Reported

5.1   Exposure data

Hydrochlorothiazide is a thiazide-based diuretic that is recommended as a first-line therapy for hypertension. Most frequently, hydrochlorothiazide is used with other drugs that lower blood pressure, including in combination products. In the USA, use of hydrochlorothiazide has declined slightly over the past decade.

5.2 Human carcinogenicity data

The occurrence of cancer among patients using hydrochlorothiazide has been examined in cohort and case–control studies from the USA and Denmark, and in an observational cohort within an intervention trial of heart disease patients from Israel. Other cohort and case–control studies have examined use of thiazides (but not specifically hydrochlorothiazide) in multiple regions of Europe and in the USA.

5.2.1 Cancers of the skin and lip

Associations between use of hydrochlorothiazide and squamous cell carcinoma of the skin or lip were assessed in two case–control studies in Denmark, and California, USA. The case–control study from Denmark reported an excess risk of squamous cell carcinoma of the skin associated with hydrochlorothiazide use, and risk increased with increasing dose; cancer of the lip was not evaluated. A case–control analysis of a cohort study from California detected an excess risk of cancer of the lip and "other skin cancers" (not including squamous cell carcinoma, basal cell carcinoma, or melanoma) among users of hydrochlorothiazide. This was followed by a nested case–control study of cancer of the lip in the same population, which reported a statistically significant twofold increase in risk for three or more prescriptions, and increasing odds ratios with duration of use. This was the only study with adequate statistical power to assess use of hydrochlorothiazide alone. Two other case–control studies of cancer of the skin in Europe and the USA reported increased odds ratios for squamous cell carcinoma of the skin associated with use of thiazide or photosensitizing cardiovascular drugs (mainly thiazides); these findings supported the results of studies reporting on hydrochlorothiazide specifically.

While the available data on hydrochlorothiazide and skin cancer generally suggested associations with squamous cell carcinoma for sites potentially exposed to sunlight (i.e. skin and lip), only a few studies have evaluated the association between hydrochlorothiazide exposure and cancer of the skin and lip, and even fewer studies have examined dose or duration effects. The Working Group considered that the potential confounding effect of sunlight exposure, a major risk factor for squamous cell carcinoma, was minimal, since positive associations were observed in studies that could account for this effect. Effect modification by sun exposure is potentially important, but had not been thoroughly examined.

In contrast to the results for squamous cell carcinoma, results from case–control and cohort studies that examined basal cell carcinoma and malignant melanoma of the skin were weaker, lacked dose–response relationships, or gave results that were close to unity.

5.2.2 Other cancer sites

An increased risk of cancer of the kidney associated with use of hydrochlorothiazide (one study) or thiazide was reported in three studies in two independent study populations in the USA; an earlier study in one of those populations had also found an increased risk of renal cell carcinoma among women with unspecified thiazide use. This association was difficult to interpret owing to potential confounding by hypertension, an independent risk factor for renal disease.

Two case–control studies on cancer of the breast assessed thiazide use: the odds ratios found were 1.2, and 1.4, respectively. Increased risks of cancer of the gall bladder, colon, prostate, and endometrium associated with thiazide use were reported each in a single study.

In conclusion, there were few studies on the risk of other cancers in relation to use of hydrochlorothiazide, and results had the potential to be confounded by drug indication.

5.3 Animal carcinogenicity data

Hydrochlorothiazide was tested for carcinogenicity in one feeding study in male and female mice, in two feeding studies in male and female rats, and in one feeding study with coexposure to sodium nitrite in male and female rats. In the first study, hydrochlorothiazide caused a significant increase in the incidence of hepatocellular adenoma, and of hepatocellular adenoma or carcinoma (combined) in male mice; there were no significant increases in the incidence of any neoplasm in female mice. In the second study, there was an increased incidence of adrenal pheochromocytoma in female rats. No significant increase in the incidence of any neoplasm was observed in male rats in the second study, or in male and female rats in the third study. The study of coexposure also gave negative results.

5.4 Mechanistic and other relevant data

Hydrochlorothiazide is excreted essentially unchanged in humans.

Hydrochlorothiazide was not mutagenic in standard bacterial screening assays, but produced cytotoxic effects and induced mutation in L5178Y mouse lymphoma cells in the absence of exogenous metabolic activation. Hydrochlorothiazide increased the frequency of sister chromatid exchange, but not chromosomal aberration, in Chinese hamster ovary cells, both in the presence and absence of an exogenous metabolic system. Hydrochlorothiazide induced polyploidy, but not chromosomal aberration, in Chinese hamster lung cells. In-vitro induction of micronucleus formation and chromosome breakage via chromosome delay were observed in human lymphocytes exposed to hydrochlorothiazide.

In the presence of ultraviolet A irradiation, hydrochlorothiazide enhanced the production of DNA cyclobutane–pyrimidine dimers, both in isolated DNA and in the skin of DNA repair-deficient mice.

The possible association between exposure to hydrochlorothiazide and cancer of the skin may result from drug-related photosensitization, which would cause DNA damage (production of dimers by hydrochlorothiazide in the presence of sunlight) and may also lead to a chronic inflammatory reaction in the skin.

6. Evaluation

6.1 Cancer in humans

There is *limited evidence* in humans for the carcinogenicity of hydrochlorothiazide. Positive associations were observed for squamous cell carcinoma of the skin and lip.

6.2 Cancer in experimental animals

There is *limited evidence* in experimental animals for the carcinogenicity of hydrochlorothiazide.

6.3 Overall evaluation

Hydrochlorothiazide is *possibly carcinogenic to humans (Group 2B)*.

References

Abdel Razak O (2004). Electrochemical study of hydrochlorothiazide and its determination in urine and tablets. *J Pharm Biomed Anal*, 34(2):433–40. doi:10.1016/S0731-7085(03)00497-7 PMID:15013158

AbdelHameed MH, Chen TM, Chiou WL (1993). Intrahepatic distribution of hydrochlorothiazide and quinidine in rats: implications in pharmacokinetics. *J Pharm Sci*, 82(10):992–6. doi:10.1002/jps.2600821004 PMID:8254499

Addo HA, Ferguson J, Frain-Bell W (1987). Thiazide-induced photosensitivity: a study of 33 subjects. *Br J Dermatol*, 116(6):749–60. doi:10.1111/j.1365-2133.1987.tb04893.x PMID:3620339

ALLHAT (2002). Major outcomes in high-risk hypertensive patients randomized to angiotensin-converting enzyme inhibitor or calcium channel blocker vs diuretic: The Antihypertensive and Lipid-Lowering Treatment to Prevent Heart Attack Trial (ALLHAT). *JAMA*, 288(23):2981–97. doi:10.1001/jama.288.23.2981 PMID:12479763

Andrews AW, Lijinsky W, Snyder SW (1984). Mutagenicity of amine drugs and their products of nitrosation. *Mutat Res*, 135(2):105–8. doi:10.1016/0165-1218(84)90162-9 PMID:6363913

Andrianopoulos C, Stephanou G, Demopoulos NA (2006). Genotoxicity of hydrochlorothiazide in cultured human lymphocytes. I. Evaluation of chromosome delay and chromosome breakage. *Environ Mol Mutagen*, 47(3):169–78. doi:10.1002/em.20180 PMID:16304670

Backman L, Beerman B, Groschinsky-Grind M, Hallberg D (1979). Malabsorption of hydrochlorothiazide following intestinal shunt surgery. *Clin Pharmacokinet*, 4(1):63–8. doi:10.2165/00003088-197904010-00006 PMID:421412

Barbhaiya RH, Craig WA, Corrick-West HP, Welling PG (1982). Pharmacokinetics of hydrochlorothiazide in fasted and nonfasted subjects: a comparison of plasma level and urinary excretion methods. *J Pharm Sci*, 71(2):245–8. doi:10.1002/jps.2600710226 PMID:7062255

Beermann B (1984). Aspects on pharmacokinetics of some diuretics. *Acta Pharmacol Toxicol (Copenh)*, 54:Suppl 1: 17–29. doi:10.1111/j.1600-0773.1984.tb03626.x PMID:6369882

Beermann B, Fåhraeus L, Groschinsky-Grind M, Lindström B (1980). Placental transfer of hydrochlorothiazide. *Gynecol Obstet Invest*, 11(1):45–8. doi:10.1159/000299817 PMID:7390276

Beermann B, Groschinsky-Grind M (1977). Pharmacokinetics of hydrochlorothiazide in man. *Eur J Clin Pharmacol*, 12(4):297–303. doi:10.1007/BF00607430 PMID:590315

Beermann B, Groschinsky-Grind M (1978a). Enhancement of the gastrointestinal absorption of hydrochlorothiazide by propantheline. *Eur J Clin Pharmacol*, 13(5):385–7. doi:10.1007/BF00644613 PMID:668798

Beermann B, Groschinsky-Grind M (1978b). Gastrointestinal absorption of hydrochlorothiazide enhanced by concomitant intake of food. *Eur J Clin Pharmacol*, 13(2):125–8. doi:10.1007/BF00609756 PMID:658108

Beermann B, Groschinsky-Grind M (1979). Pharmacokinetics of hydrochlorothiazide in patients with congestive heart failure. *Br J Clin Pharmacol*, 7(6):579–83. doi:10.1111/j.1365-2125.1979.tb04646.x PMID:465280

Beermann B, Groschinsky-Grind M, Rosén A (1976). Absorption, metabolism, and excretion of hydrochlorothiazide. *Clin Pharmacol Ther*, 19(5 Pt 1):531–7. PMID:1277708

Bignami M, Morpurgo G, Pagliani R, Carere A, Conti G, Di Giuseppe G (1974). Non-disjunction and crossing-over induced by pharmaceutical drugs in Aspergillus nidulans. *Mutat Res*, 26(3):159–70. doi:10.1016/S0027-5107(74)80070-9 PMID:4604824

Bucher JR, Huff J, Haseman JK, Eustis SL, Elwell MR, Davis WE Jr *et al.* (1990). Toxicology and carcinogenicity studies of diuretics in F344 rats and B6C3F1 mice. 1. Hydrochlorothiazide. *J Appl Toxicol*, 10(5):359–67. doi:10.1002/jat.2550100509 PMID:2254588

Chemspider (2013). ChemSpider: The free chemical database. Royal Society of Chemistry. http://www.chemspider.com/chemical-structure.3513.html

Chobanian AV, Bakris GL, Black HR, Cushman WC, Green LA, Izzo JL Jr *et al.*; Joint National Committee on Prevention, Detection, Evaluation, and Treatment of High Blood Pressure. National Heart, Lung, and Blood Institute; National High Blood Pressure Education Program Coordinating Committee (2003). Seventh report of the Joint National Committee on Prevention, Detection, Evaluation, and Treatment of High Blood Pressure. *Hypertension*, 42(6):1206–52. doi:10.1161/01.HYP.0000107251.49515.c2 PMID:14656957

Christophersen AS, Rasmussen KE, Salvesen B (1977). Determination of hydrochlorothiazide in serum by high-pressure liquid chromatography. *J Chromatogr*, 132(1):91–7. doi:10.1016/S0021-9673(00)93774-9 PMID:833234

Cushman WC, Ford CE, Cutler JA, Margolis KL, Davis BR, Grimm RH *et al.*; ALLHAT Collaborative Research Group(2002). Success and predictors of blood pressure control in diverse North American settings: the antihypertensive and lipid-lowering treatment to prevent heart attack trial (ALLHAT). *J Clin Hypertens (Greenwich)*, 4(6):393–404. doi:10.1111/j.1524-6175.2002.02045.x PMID:12461301

de Vries E, Trakatelli M, Kalabalikis D, Ferrandiz L, Ruiz-de-Casas A, Moreno-Ramirez D *et al.*; EPIDERM Group (2012). Known and potential new risk factors for skin cancer in European populations: a multicentre case-control study. *Br J Dermatol*, 167:Suppl 2: 1–13. doi:10.1111/j.1365-2133.2012.11081.x PMID:22881582

Deppeler HP (1981). Hydrochlorothiazide. In: Analytical Profiles of Drug Substances, Volume 10:405–441.

Deventer K, Pozo OJ, Van Eenoo P, Delbeke FT (2009). Detection of urinary markers for thiazide diuretics after oral administration of hydrochlorothiazide and altizide-relevance to doping control analysis. *J Chromatogr A*, 1216(12):2466–73. doi:10.1016/j.chroma.2009.01.032 PMID:19187939

DrugBank (2013). Open Data Drug & Drug Target Database. Version 4.1. Available from: http://www.drugbank.ca

eMC (2013). Electronic Medicines Compendium. Available from: http://www.medicines.org.uk

European Pharmacopoeia (2005). Ed. 6.0. Strasbourg: Europe Directorate for the Quality of Medicines of the Council of Europe (EDQM).

Farthing D, Fakhry I, Ripley EB, Sica D (1998). Simple method for determination of hydrochlorothiazide in human urine by high performance liquid chromatography utilizing narrowbore chromatography. *J Pharm Biomed Anal*, 17(8):1455–9. doi:10.1016/S0731-7085(98)00021-1 PMID:9800665

FDA (2013). Drugs@FDA. Available from: http://www.accessdata.fda.gov/scripts/cder/drugsatfda/index.cfm, accessed 8 September 2014.

Flaherty KT, Fuchs CS, Colditz GA, Stampfer MJ, Speizer FE, Willett WC et al. (2005). A prospective study of body mass index, hypertension, and smoking and the risk of renal cell carcinoma (United States). *Cancer Causes Control*, 16(9):1099–106. doi:10.1007/s10552-005-0349-8 PMID:16184476

Fortuny J, Sima C, Bayuga S, Wilcox H, Pulick K, Faulkner S et al. (2009). Risk of endometrial cancer in relation to medical conditions and medication use. *Cancer Epidemiol Biomarkers Prev*, 18(5):1448–56. doi:10.1158/1055-9965.EPI-08-0936 PMID:19383893

Friedman GD, Asgari MM, Warton EM, Chan J, Habel LA (2012). Antihypertensive drugs and lip cancer in non-Hispanic whites. *Arch Intern Med*, 172(16):1246–51. doi:10.1001/archinternmed.2012.2754 PMID:22869299

Friedman GD, Udaltsova N, Chan J, Quesenberry CP Jr, Habel LA (2009). Screening pharmaceuticals for possible carcinogenic effects: initial positive results for drugs not previously screened. *Cancer Causes Control*, 20(10):1821–35. doi:10.1007/s10552-009-9375-2 PMID:19582585

Friedman GD, Ury HK (1980). Initial screening for carcinogenicity of commonly used drugs. *J Natl Cancer Inst*, 65(4):723–33. PMID:6932525

Fujita H (1985). Arginine reversion and lambda induction in E. coli with benzothiadiazine diuretics irradiated with near-ultraviolet light. *Mutat Res*, 158(3):135–9. doi:10.1016/0165-1218(85)90076-X PMID:2934628

Galloway SM, Armstrong MJ, Reuben C, Colman S, Brown B, Cannon C et al. (1987). Chromosome aberrations and sister chromatid exchanges in Chinese hamster ovary cells: evaluations of 108 chemicals. *Environ Mol Mutagen*, 10(S10):Suppl 10: 1–175. doi:10.1002/em.2850100502 PMID:3319609

Gotardo MA, Pezza L, Pezza HR (2005). Determination of hydrochlorothiazide in pharmaceutical formulations by diffuse reflectance spectroscopy. *Ecletica Quimica*, 30(2):17–24. doi:10.1590/S0100-46702005000200002

Gu Q, Burt VL, Dillon CF, Yoon S (2012). Trends in antihypertensive medication use and blood pressure control among United States adults with hypertension: the National Health And Nutrition Examination Survey, 2001 to 2010. *Circulation*, 126(17):2105–14. doi:10.1161/CIRCULATIONAHA.112.096156 PMID:23091084

Hallas J, Christensen R, Andersen M, Friis S, Bjerrum L (2012). Long term use of drugs affecting the renin-angiotensin system and the risk of cancer: a population-based case-control study. *Br J Clin Pharmacol*, 74(1):180–8. doi:10.1111/j.1365-2125.2012.04170.x PMID:22243442

Hiatt RA, Tolan K, Quesenberry CP Jr (1994). Renal cell carcinoma and thiazide use: a historical, case-control study (California, USA). *Cancer Causes Control*, 5(4):319–25. doi:10.1007/BF01804982 PMID:8080943

HSDB (2013) Hazardous Substances Data Bank. Hydrochlorothiazide. United States National Library of Medicine. Available from: http://www.toxnet.nlm.nih.gov, accessed 8 September 2014.

Huang T, He Z, Yang B, Shao L, Zheng X, Duan G (2006). Simultaneous determination of captopril and hydrochlorothiazide in human plasma by reverse-phase HPLC from linear gradient elution. *J Pharm Biomed Anal*, 41(2):644–8. doi:10.1016/j.jpba.2005.12.007 PMID:16413728

IARC (1990). Hydrochlorothiazide. *IARC Monogr Eval Carcinog Risks Hum*, 50:293–305. PMID:2292804

IMS Health (2012a). National Disease and Therapeutic Index (NDTI). Plymouth Meeting, Pennsylvania: IMS Health; 2005–12.

IMS Health (2012b). National Prescription Audit Plus (NPA). Plymouth Meeting, Pennsylvania: IMS Health; 2008–12.

IMS Health (2012c). Multinational Integrated Data Analysis (MIDAS). Plymouth Meeting, Pennsylvania: IMS Health. Available from: http://www.imshealth.com/portal/site/imshealth

Indian Pharmacopoeia (2010). The Indian Pharmacopoeia Commission. Ghaziabad, India.

IPCS (2013). Hydrochlorothiazide. Geneva: International Programme on Chemical Safety, World Health Organization. Available from: http://www.inchem.org/documents/pims/pharm/hydrochl.htm.

Ishidate M, Sofuni T, Yoshikawa K (1981). Chromosomal aberration tests *in vitro* as a primary screening tool for environmental mutagens and/or carcinogens. *GANN Monograph on Cancer Research*, 27:95–108.

Jensen AO, Thomsen HF, Engebjerg MC, Olesen AB, Sørensen HT, Karagas MR (2008). Use of photosensitising diuretics and risk of skin cancer: a population-based case-control study. *Br J Cancer*, 99(9):1522–8. doi:10.1038/sj.bjc.6604686 PMID:18813314

Kim GH, Na KY, Kim SY, Joo KW, Oh YK, Chae SW et al. (2003). Up-regulation of organic anion transporter 1 protein is induced by chronic furosemide or hydrochlorothiazide infusion in rat kidney. *Nephrol Dial Transplant*, 18(8):1505–11. doi:10.1093/ndt/gfg186 PMID:12897087

Kuehlein T, Laux G, Gutscher A, Goetz K, Szecsenyi J, Campbell S et al. (2011). Diuretics for hypertension–an inconsistency in primary care prescribing behaviour. *Curr Med Res Opin*, 27(3):497–502. doi:10.1185/03007995.2010.547932 PMID:21208153

Kunisada M, Masaki T, Ono R, Morinaga H, Nakano E, Yogianti F et al. (2013). Hydrochlorothiazide enhances UVA-induced DNA damage. *Photochem Photobiol*, 89(3):649–54. doi:10.1111/php.12048 PMID:23331297

Li CI, Malone KE, Weiss NS, Boudreau DM, Cushing-Haugen KL, Daling JR (2003). Relation between use of antihypertensive medications and risk of breast carcinoma among women ages 65–79 years. *Cancer*, 98(7):1504–13. doi:10.1002/cncr.11663 PMID:14508839

Lijinsky W, Reuber MD (1987). Pathologic effects of chronic administration of hydrochlorothiazide, with and without sodium nitrite, to F344 rats. *Toxicol Ind Health*, 3(3):413–22. doi:10.1177/074823378700300313 PMID:3686543

Lookchem (2013). Lookchem database. Hydrochlorothiazide. Available from: http://www.lookchem.com, accessed 8 September 2014.

Mansia G, De Backer G, Dominiczak A, Cifkova R, Fagard R, Germano G et al.; European Society of Hypertension; European Society of Cardiology (2007). 2007 ESH-ESC Guidelines for the management of arterial hypertension: the task force for the management of arterial hypertension of the European Society of Hypertension (ESH) and of the European Society of Cardiology (ESC). *Blood Press*, 16(3):135–232. doi:10.1080/08037050701461084 PMID:17846925

Mansia G, Laurent S, Agabiti-Rosei E, Ambrosioni E, Burnier M, Caulfield MJ et al.; European Society of Hypertension (2009). Reappraisal of European guidelines on hypertension management: a European Society of Hypertension Task Force document. *J Hypertens*, 27(11):2121–58. doi:10.1097/HJH.0b013e328333146d PMID:19838131

Masereeuw R, Moons WM, Russel FG (1997). Saturable accumulation and diuretic activity of hydrochlorothiazide in the isolated perfused rat kidney. *Pharmacology*, 54(1):33–42. doi:10.1159/000139467 PMID:9065959

Meyer MC, Melikian AP, Whyatt PL, Slywka GW (1975). Hydrochlorothiazide bioavailability: an evaluation of thirteen products. *Curr Ther Res Clin Exp*, 17(6):570–7. PMID:808380

MicroMedex (2013). 2.0. Ann Arbor, Michigan: Truven Health Analytics Inc.

Miller ME, Cohn RD, Burghart PH (1982). Hydrochlorothiazide disposition in a mother and her breast-fed infant. *J Pediatr*, 101(5):789–91. doi:10.1016/S0022-3476(82)80323-5 PMID:7131161

Mortelmans K, Haworth S, Lawlor T, Speck W, Tainer B, Zeiger E (1986). Salmonella mutagenicity tests: II. Results from the testing of 270 chemicals. *Environ Mutagen*, 8(S7):Suppl 7: 1–119. doi:10.1002/em.2860080802 PMID:3516675

Niemeyer C, Hasenfuss G, Wais U, Knauf H, Schäfer-Korting M, Mutschler E (1983). Pharmacokinetics of hydrochlorothiazide in relation to renal function. *Eur J Clin Pharmacol*, 24(5):661–5. doi:10.1007/BF00542218 PMID:6873147

NTP (1989). Toxicology and carcinogenesis studies of hydrochlorothiazide (CAS No. 58–93–5) in F344/N rats and B6C3F1 mice (feed studies). *Natl Toxicol Program Tech Rep Ser*, 357:1–194. PMID:12695784

O'Neil MJ (2001). The Merck Index - An Encyclopedia of Chemicals, Drugs, and Biologicals, 13th ed. Whitehouse Station (NJ): Merck & Co., Inc.

Okuda T, Itoh S, Yamazaki M, Nakahama H, Fukuhara Y, Orita Y (1987). Biopharmaceutical studies of thiazide diuretics. III. In vivo formation of 2-amino-4-chloro-m-benzenedisulfonamide as a metabolite of hydrochlorothiazide in a patient. *Chem Pharm Bull (Tokyo)*, 35(8):3516–8. doi:10.1248/cpb.35.3516 PMID:3427729

Patel RB, Patel UR, Rogge MC, Shah VP, Prasad VK, Selen A et al. (1984). Bioavailability of hydrochlorothiazide from tablets and suspensions. *J Pharm Sci*, 73(3):359–61. doi:10.1002/jps.2600730317 PMID:6716243

Redalieu E, Chan KK, Tipnis V, Zak SB, Gilleran TG, Wagner WE Jr et al. (1985). Kinetics of hydrochlorothiazide absorption in humans. *J Pharm Sci*, 74(7):765–7. doi:10.1002/jps.2600740714 PMID:4032251

Ripley E, King K, Sica DA (2000). Racial differences in response to acute dosing with hydrochlorothiazide. *Am J Hypertens*, 13(2):157–64. doi:10.1016/S0895-7061(99)00168-5 PMID:10701815

Robinson SN, Zens MS, Perry AE, Spencer SK, Duell EJ, Karagas MR (2013). Photosensitizing agents and the risk of non-melanoma skin cancer: a population-based case-control study. *J Invest Dermatol*, 133(8):1950–5. doi:10.1038/jid.2013.33 PMID:23344461

Rote Liste Service GmbH (2012). HCT-ratiopharm 12,5 mg Tabletten.

Ruiter R, Visser LE, Eijgelsheim M, Rodenburg EM, Hofman A, Coebergh JW et al. (2010). High-ceiling diuretics are associated with an increased risk of basal cell carcinoma in a population-based follow-up study. *Eur J Cancer*, 46(13):2467–72. doi:10.1016/j.ejca.2010.04.024 PMID:20605443

SciFinder (2013). SciFinder Databases: Registry, Chemcats. American Chemical Society. Available from: http://www.cas.org/products/scifinder

Sousa CEM, Bedor DCG, Gonçalves TM et al. (2009). Rapid determination of hydrochlorothiazide in human plasma by high performance liquid chromatography-tandem mass spectrometry. *Lat Am J Pharm*, 28:793–7.

Stafford RS, Monti V, Furberg CD, Ma J (2006). Long-term and short-term changes in antihypertensive prescribing by office-based physicians in the United States. *Hypertension*, 48(2):213–8. doi:10.1161/01.HYP.0000229653.73128.b6 PMID:16785334

Stanford JL, Martin EJ, Brinton LA, Hoover RN (1986). Rauwolfia use and breast cancer: a case-control study. *J Natl Cancer Inst*, 76(5):817–22. PMID:3457968

Takubo T, Okada H, Ishii M, Hara K, Ishii Y (2004). Sensitive and selective liquid chromatography-electrospray ionization tandem mass spectrometry analysis of hydrochlorothiazide in rat plasma. *J Chromatogr*

B Analyt Technol Biomed Life Sci, 806(2):199–203. doi:10.1016/j.jchromb.2004.03.060 PMID:15171930

Tenenbaum A, Grossman E, Fisman EZ, Adler Y, Boyko V, Jonas M et al. (2001). Long-term diuretic therapy in patients with coronary disease: increased colon cancer-related mortality over a 5-year follow-up. J Hum Hypertens, 15(6):373–9. doi:10.1038/sj.jhh.1001192 PMID:11439311

US Pharmacopeia (2007). Hydrochlorothiazide, USP28-NF23. Rockville (MD), USA: The United States Pharmacopoeial Convention.

Valencia R, Mason JM, Woodruff RC, Zimmering S (1985). Chemical mutagenesis testing in Drosophila. III. Results of 48 coded compounds tested for the National Toxicology Program. Environ Mutagen, 7(3):325–48. doi:10.1002/em.2860070309 PMID:3930234

van den Eeden SK, Friedman GD (1995). Prescription drug screening for subsequent carcinogenicity. Pharmacoepidemiol Drug Saf, 4(5):275–87. doi:10.1002/pds.2630040504

Vandenheuvel WJA, Gruber VF, Walker RW, Wolf FJ (1975). GLC analysis of hydrochlorothiazide in blood and plasma. J Pharm Sci, 64(8):1309–12. doi:10.1002/jps.2600640810 PMID:1151702

Wang YR, Alexander GC, Stafford RS (2007). Outpatient hypertension treatment, treatment intensification, and control in Western Europe and the United States. Arch Intern Med, 167(2):141–7. doi:10.1001/archinte.167.2.141 PMID:17242314

Waskell L (1978). A study of the mutagenicity of anesthetics and their metabolites. Mutat Res, 57(2):141–53. doi:10.1016/0027-5107(78)90261-0 PMID:351387

Welling PG (1986). Pharmacokinetics of the thiazide diuretics. Biopharm Drug Dispos, 7(6):501–35. doi:10.1002/bdd.2510070602 PMID:3828483

WHO(2006). The International Pharmacopoeia, . 4th ed. Geneva, Switzerland: World Health Organization.

Yamazaki M, Itoh S, Okuda T, Tanabe K, Nakahama H, Fukuhara Y et al. (1989). Binding of hydrochlorothiazide to erythrocytes. J Pharmacobiodyn, 12(7):423–8. doi:10.1248/bpb1978.12.423 PMID:2593083

Yan T, Li H, Deng L, Guo Y, Yu W, Fawcett JP et al. (2008). Liquid chromatographic-tandem mass spectrometric method for the simultaneous quantitation of telmisartan and hydrochlorothiazide in human plasma. J Pharm Biomed Anal, 48(4):1225–9. doi:10.1016/j.jpba.2008.08.021 PMID:18838240

PIOGLITAZONE AND ROSIGLITAZONE

1. Exposure Data

Thiazolidinediones are a class of synthetic compounds that exert direct effects on the mechanisms of insulin resistance, and result in improved insulin action and reduced hyper-insulinaemia. In the present *Monograph*, the Working Group evaluated pioglitazone and rosiglitazone, two thiazolidinediones that initially showed great promise as receptor-mediated oral therapy for type 2 diabetes mellitus. Rosiglitazone and pioglitazone were introduced to the market at about the same time (1999 in the USA, and 2001–2002 in Taiwan, China; Tseng, 2012d). Some patients may therefore have been exposed to both drugs, which were sometimes prescribed sequentially. The Working Group did not consider other thiazolidinediones, such as troglitazone, which was marketed for only a short period (1997–2000), before being withdrawn from the world market subsequent to reports of fatal hepatotoxicity (Julie *et al.*, 2008).

1.1 Chemical and physical data on pioglitazone

1.1.1 Nomenclature

(a) Pioglitazone

Chem. Abstr. Serv. Reg. No.: 111025-46-8 (SciFinder, 2013).

Chem. Abstr. Serv. Name: 2,4-Thiazolidine-dione, 5-[[4-[2-(5-ethyl-2-pyridinyl)ethoxy]phenyl]methyl]- (SciFinder, 2013).

IUPAC systematic Name: 5-[[4-[2-(5-Ethylpyridin-2-yl)ethoxy]phenyl]methyl]-1,3-thiazolidine-2,4-dione (Drugbank, 2013; Pubchem, 2013).

WHO International Nonproprietary Name (INN): Pioglitazonum (WHO, 2007).

(b) Pioglitazone hydrochloride

Chem. Abstr. Serv. Reg. No.: 112529-15-4 (SciFinder, 2013).

Chem. Abstr. Serv. Name: 2,4-Thiazolidine-dione,5-[[4-[2-(5-ethyl-2-pyridinyl)ethoxy]phenyl]methyl]-, hydrochloride (1:1) (SciFinder, 2013).

Proprietary Names: Actos; Glustin; Zactose (Drugbank, 2013; Pubchem, 2013).

United States Nonproprietary Name (USAN): Pioglitazone hydrochloride

1.1.2 Structural and molecular formulae and relative molecular mass

(a)   Pioglitazone

$C_{19}H_{20}N_2O_3S$ (O'Neil, 2006)
Relative molecular mass: 356.44

(b)   Pioglitazone hydrochloride

$C_{19}H_{20}N_2O_3S. HCl$
Relative molecular mass: 392.90

1.1.3 Chemical and physical properties of the pure substance

(a)   Pioglitazone

Description: Colourless needles from dimethylformamide and water (O'Neil, 2006)

Density: 1.260 g/cm³ at 20 °C (Langchem, 2013)

Melting point: 183–184 °C (O'Neil, 2006; Milne, 2000)

Spectroscopy data: Ultraviolet (UV) (Venkatesh *et al.*, 2006), proton nuclear magnetic resonance (^{1}H NMR) (Madivada *et al.*, 2009), ^{13}C NMR (Madivada *et al.*, 2009), infrared (IR) (Madivada *et al.*, 2009), and mass spectrometry (MS) (Wang & Miksa, 2007; Thevis *et al.*, 2005) have been reported

Solubility: 14.05 µg/mL (water); 25.07 µg/mL (0.15 M NaCl); 10.61 µg/mL (0.1 M phosphate buffer) (Seedher & Kanojia, 2008); 46.85 mg/L at 25 °C (EMA CHMP, 2012)

The solubility is highly dependent on pH, and is greater at lower pH. Solubility according to pH: 52.60 µg/mL (pH 1.83); 38.63 µg/mL (pH 2.57); 4.55 µg/mL (pH 3.92); 6.35 µg/mL (pH 7.39); 19.19 µg/mL (pH 8.82); 49.96 µg/mL (pH 9.52) (Seedher & Kanojia, 2009); 100 µg/mL in 1:1 dimethyl sulfoxide:phosphate-buffered saline (pH 7.2); 2.5 mg/mL in dimethylformamide and dimethyl sulfoxide (Cayman SDS, 2013)

Stability data: Exposure to heat (105 °C) results in a change of appearance; exposure to heat and UV light results in a slight drop (1.5–2%) in assay; exposure to 0.1 N sodium hydroxide results in degradation; exposure to heat (105 °C) and peroxide results in a slight increase in total impurities (EMA CHMP, 2012)

Octanol/water partition coefficient: Log P = 2.72–3.73 (Giaginis *et al.*, 2007)

Vapour pressure: 2.88 × 10⁻¹⁴ mm Hg at 25 °C, estimated (EMA CHMP, 2012)

(b)   Pioglitazone hydrochloride

Description: White crystalline powder, odourless (Physicians Desk Reference, 2012); colourless prisms from ethanol (O'Neil, 2006)

Density: 1.26 g/cm³ (ChemicalBook, 2013)

Melting point: 193–194 °C (O'Neil, 2006; Milne, 2000)

Solubility: Practically insoluble in water, insoluble in ether, slightly soluble in ethanol, very slightly soluble in acetone and acetonitrile (O'Neil, 2006); very soluble in dimethylformamide (Physicians Desk Reference, 2012)

Vapour pressure: 3.0 × 10⁻¹³ mm Hg at 25 °C (ChemicalBook, 2013)

1.1.4 Technical products and impurities

Pioglitazone hydrochloride is used to formulate the finished dosage forms described below.

(a) Trade names

Actos; Glustin; Glizone; Pioz; Zactose (Rx List, 2013).

(b) Impurities

Three impurities were detected up to concentration of 0.1% by reversed-phase high-performance liquid chromatography (HPLC) and were characterized by ^{1}H NMR, ^{13}C NMR, MS, and IR spectral data (Kumar *et al.*, 2004):

- 5-(4-Hydroxybenzyl)-1,3-thiazolidine-2,4-dione
- 5-(4-Fluorobenzyl)-1,3-thiazolidine-2,4-dione
- 2-[2-(4-Bromophenoxy)   ethyl-5-ethyl] pyridine.

Four impurities in pioglitazone were prepared and characterized by NMR spectroscopy (Richter *et al.*, 2007):

- 5-{4-[2-(5-Ethyl-6-{4-[2-(5-ethylpyridin-2-yl)-ethoxy]phenyl}pyrid-2-yl)ethoxy]benzyl}-1,3-thiazolidine-2,4-dione
- 5-{4-[2-(5-Ethyl-4-{4-[2-(5-ethylpyridin-2-yl)ethoxy]phenyl}pyrid-2-yl)ethoxy]benzyl}-1,3-thiazolidine-2,4-dione
- 5-{6,4'-bis-[2-(5-Ethyl-pyridin-2-yl)ethoxy]biphenyl-3-ylmethyl}-1,3-thiazolidine-2,4-dione
- 5-{4-[2-(5-Ethyl-pyridin-2-yl)ethoxy]benzyl}-3-[2-(5-ethyl-pyridin-2-yl)ethyl]-1,3-thiazolidine-2,4-dione.

1.2 Analysis of pioglitazone

Physical properties used for the identification of the substance, e.g. IR and melting point, are presented in Section 1.1.3. Selected non-compendial methods are presented in Table 1.1.

There are numerous methods including HPLC with UV or MS detection for the analysis of pioglitazone in different matrices, such as formulations, plasma, and serum. The limit of quantitation (LOQ) in serum using the method by Palem *et al.* (2011) is 1 ng/mL; Lin *et al.* (2003) reported a LOQ of 0.5 ng/mL in human plasma. Other reported techniques for analysing formulations include capillary electrophoresis (Radhakrishna *et al.*, 2002a) and potentiometric sensors (Mostafa & Al-Majed, 2008).

1.3 Production and use of pioglitazone

1.3.1 Production

Pioglitazone exists in two polymorphic crystal forms. Polymorph 1 is used in the manufacture of the finished drug product. The manufacture of pioglitazone consists of six steps, the last in combination with hydrochloride to yield pioglitazone hydrochloride (EMEA, 2012).

1.3.2 Use

(a) Indications

Pioglitazone acts as an "insulin sensitizer", providing a means to improve glycaemic control by reducing insulin resistance and thus decreasing hyperglycaemia in patients with type 2 diabetes mellitus (Sweetman, 2011; FDA, 2013a). Pioglitazone acts only in the presence of endogenous insulin. It is indicated particularly for overweight patients as an adjunct to diet and exercise to improve glycaemic control. It is contraindicated in patients with type 1 diabetes mellitus, and for the treatment of diabetic ketoacidosis. It

Table 1.1 Analytical methods for pioglitazone and rosiglitazone

Sample matrix	Sample preparation	Assay method	Detection limit	Reference
Non-compendial methods				
Human plasma	Pre-activation of SPE column with acetonitrile and KH_2PO_4, addition of IS and KH_2PO_4 to pioglitazone solution in plasma, extraction using SPE column, elution using acetonitrile and water, filtration, and analysis of filtrate	LC-UV Column: C_{18} Mobile phase: methanol, acetonitrile and mixed phosphate buffer (pH 2.6, 10 mM) (40 : 12 : 48, v/v/v) Flow rate: 1.2 mL/min Wavelength: 269 nm	50 ng/mL (LLOQ)	Sripalakit *et al.* (2006)
Human plasma	Addition of pioglitazone standard solutions, IS, diethylether, mixing, centrifugation, addition of NaOH to organic layer, mixing, centrifugation, and injection of aqueous layer in HPLC	LC-UV Column: C_{18} Mobile phase: acetonitrile and 140 mM KH_2PO_4 (pH 4.45) (40 : 60, v/v) Flow rate : 1.4 mL/min Wavelength: 269 nm	25 ng/mL (LLOQ)	Souri *et al.* (2008)
Human plasma	Addition of IS, 0.1 M ammonium acetate, pH adjustment, extraction with methyl *tert*-butyl ether and butyl chloride, centrifugation, evaporation, residues dissolved in mobile phase, centrifugation	LC-ESI-MS Column: C_{18} Mobile phase: acetonitrile : water (60 : 40) with 10 mM ammonium acetate and 0.02% TFA Flow rate: 0.2 mL/min SRM transition: 357 m/z →134 m/z (positive mode)	0.5 ng/mL (LLOQ)	Lin *et al.* (2003)
Human serum	Samples diluted 1 : 1 (v/v) with acetonitrile containing IS	LC-ESI-MS Column: C_{18} Mobile phase: 50% of 10 mM ammonium acetate in acetonitrile: water (10 : 90) and 50% of water : acetonitrile (10 : 90) Flow rate: 1/35 mL/min SRM transition: 357 m/z → 134 m/z (positive mode)	9 ng/mL (LLOQ)	Xue *et al.* (2003)
Pig serum	Addition of IS, NaOH solution (1 M), dichloromethane, centrifugation, separation of organic layer, evaporation, reconstitution with methanol and analysis	LC-UV Column: C_{18} Mobile phase: acetonitrile : 50 mM ammonium acetate buffer (pH 5) (67 : 33, v/v) Flow rate: 1 mL/min Wavelength: 240 nm	1 ng/mL (LLOQ)	Palem *et al.* (2011)
Dog serum	Serum samples loaded on the column, elution with acetonitrile, eluate mixed with purified water, and analysis	LC-UV Column: C_{18} Mobile phase: Acetonitrile : water (41 : 59, v/v) containing 1.2 mL/L acetic acid (pH 6.0 ± 0.05) Flow rate: 1.0 mL/min Wavelength: 229 nm	25 ng/mL (LLOQ)	Zhong & Lakings (1989)

Table 1.1   (continued)

Sample matrix	Sample preparation	Assay method	Detection limit	Reference
Rat serum	Addition of IS solution (rosiglitazone), precipitation by addition of ethylacetate, centrifugation, and analysis	LC-UV Column: C_{18} Mobile phase: Methanol : ammonium acetate (30 mM, pH 5) (60 : 40, v/v) Flow rate: 1.0 mL/min Wavelength: 269 nm	15 ng/mL (LOD) 50 ng/mL (LOQ)	Ravikanth *et al.* (2011)
Human serum and urine	Serum sample: activation of SPE column, addition of phosphate buffer, elution with methanol and 0.02 M sodium acetate, addition of acetic acid, evaporation, dissolve residue in 0.1 M KH_2PO_4, extraction in diethylether, evaporation and addition of IS Urine sample: addition of 0.1 M KH_2PO_4, extraction with mixture of diethylether and dichloromethane (4 : 1, v/v), evaporation, dissolution in IS solution, and analysis	LC-UV Column: C_{18} Mobile phase: 0.05 M phosphate buffer (pH 6.0) : methanol (9 : 1, v/v) and 0.05 M phosphate buffer (pH 6.0): methanol : acetonitrile (4 : 2 : 4, v/v) Flow rate: 1.0 mL/min Wavelength: 269 nm	Serum: 0.01–0.05 µg/mL Urine: 0.1–0.5 µg/mL	Yamashita *et al.* (1996)
Bulk and pharmaceutical formulation	Bulk sample: sample in mixture of aqueous 0.1% *ortho*-phosphoric acid and acetonitrile at 1 : 1 (v/v) Formulation: 20 weighed tablets ground to a fine powder, extraction with diluting solution, centrifugation	HPLC Column: C_{18} Mobile phase: 10 mM KH_2PO_4 : acetonitrile (pH 6.0) Flow rate: 1 mL/min Wavelength: 225 nm		Radhakrishna *et al.* (2002a)
Tablet formulation	Tablets ground to fine powder, dissolve in methanol, sonication, filtration, dilution, and analysis	HPLC Column: C_{18} Mobile phase: methanol : phosphate buffer (pH 4.3) (75 : 25, v/v) Flow rate: 1.0 mL/min Wavelength: 258 nm		Jain *et al.* (2008)
Tablet	Finely powdered tablets, addition of methanol, sonication, centrifugation, supernatant diluted with 60% methanol, injection on column	HPLC Column: C_{18} Mobile phase: ammonium formate buffer (0.05 M, pH 4.1) : acetonitrile (45 : 55, v/v) Flow rate 1.0 mL/min Wavelength: 266 nm	42 ng/mL (LOD)	Jedlicka *et al.* (2004)

Table 1.1   (continued)

Sample matrix	Sample preparation	Assay method	Detection limit	Reference
Formulation	Powder transferred to volumetric flask, volume adjustment with acetonitrile and methanol (1 : 1), sonication, filtration, addition of IS and injection onto HPLC column	HPLC Column: C_{18} Mobile phase: formic acid, (0.05 M, pH 3.0), water : acetonitrile (5 : 95, v/v) and water : methanol (10 : 90, v/v) Flow rate : 1.0 mL/min Wavelength: 260 nm		Venkatesh *et al.* (2006)
Environmental sample	Addition of acetonitrile to stabilize sample, store at 4 °C, filtration, addition of rosiglitazone as IS, and analysis	HPLC-TOF-MS Column: C_{18} Mobile phase: acetonitrile (containing formic acid 0.1%, v/v) and an aqueous 10 mM ammonium formate solution (containing formic acid 0.1%, v/v) Flow rate: 0.7 mL/min	LOQ Waste water: 1.1 ng/L River water: 1.2 ng/L Tap water: 3.1 ng/L	Martín *et al.* (2012)
Formulation	Addition of mobile phase to flask containing tablet powder, sonication, filtration, and analysis	RP-UPLC Column: C_{18} Mobile phase: acetonitrile:buffer (pH 3.2) (20 : 80, v/v) Flow rate: 0.2 mL/min Wavelength: 220 nm	0.01 µg/mL (LOD) 0.05 µg/mL (LOQ)	Xavier & Basavaiah (2012)
Formulation	Crushing of tablet, transfer of powder to beaker, dissolve in acidic water solution, sonication, pH adjustment to 3.0 using phosphate buffer	Potentiometric sensors The sensing membranes incorporate ion association complexes of pioglitazone cation and sodium tetraphenylborate or phosphomolybdic acid or phosphotungstic acid as electroactive material.		Mostafa & Al-Majed (2008)
Marketed formulation	Tablet finely powdered, extraction with methanol, further dilutions to achieve a concentration of 100 µg/mL of pioglitazone using methanol	Chiral normal-phase HPLC Column: chiral Mobile phase: hexane and *n*-propyl alcohol (80 : 20, v/v) Flow rate: 1.0 mL/min Wavelength: 233 nm	100 ng/mL (LOD) 400 ng/mL (LOQ)	Gowramma *et al.* (2012a, b)
Bulk and pharmaceutical formulation	Twenty weighed tablets ground to a fine powder, extraction with diluting solution, centrifugation	Capillary electrophoresis Separation mode: micellar electrokinetic chromatographic fused-silica capillary Background electrolyte: 80 parts of 20 mM sodium borate (pH 9.3) containing 50 mM SDS and 20 parts of acetonitrile. Wavelength: 210 nm Voltage: 25 kV	Pioglitazone unsaturated impurity: 0.29 µg/mL (LOD) 0.74 µg/mL (LOQ)	Radhakrishna *et al.* (2002a)

HPLC, high-performance liquid chromatography; HPLC-TOF-MS, high-performance liquid chromatography time of flight mass spectrometry; IS, internal standard; KH_2PO_4, monopotassium phosphate; LC-UV, liquid chromatography ultraviolet spectroscopy; LC-ESI-MS, liquid chromatography electrospray ionization mass spectrometry; LOD, limit of detection; LLOQ, lower limit of quantification; LOQ, limit of quantification; NaOH, sodium hydroxide; RP-UPLC, reverse phase-ultra high pressure liquid chromatography; SDS, sodium dodecyl sulfate; SPE, solid-phase extraction; SRM, selected reaction monitoring; TFA, trifluoroacetic acid; UV, ultraviolet

Table 1.2 Most commonly reported clinical indications for pioglitazone and rosiglitazone in the USA, 2011–2012

Diagnosis[a]	ICD-9 code[b]	Drug uses (in thousands)		Percentage of total	
		Pioglitazone	Rosiglitazone	Pioglitazone	Rosiglitazone
Diabetes mellitus NOS	250.001	3500	90	54.0	28.4
Diabetes type II, non-insulin dependent	250.003	2585	126	39.9	39.8
Diabetic nephropathy	250.302	66	7	1.0	2.1
Diabetic neuropathy	250.503	60	–	0.9	–
Diabetic kidney disease	250.301	57	13	0.9	4.1
Diabetes type I, insulin dependent	250.002	45	–	0.7	–
Metabolic/insulin resistant syndrome	277.701	35	60	0.5	18.9
Elevated glucose	790.201	27	–	0.4	–
Polycystic ovary syndrome	256.401	–	7	–	2.1
All other diagnoses	–	110	14	1.7	–
Total with reported diagnoses	–	6484	316	100.0	100.0

[a] No diagnosis was stated for 0.3% of drug uses.

[b] The ICD-9 codes given are a more detailed, proprietary version developed by IMS Health.

NOS, not otherwise specified

From IMS Health (2012b)

is also contraindicated in patients with advanced congestive heart failure (FDA, 2013a).

Apart from its approved indication for treatment of type 2 diabetes mellitus, pioglitazone is also used for other off-label indications (Table 1.2).

(b) Dosage

Pioglitazone is available as tablets of 15, 30 and 45 mg dosage titrated on adequacy of therapeutic response (Sweetman, 2011). Pioglitazone is also available in combination products, including pioglitazone and metformin (Actoplus Met), pioglitazone and glimeperide (Duetact), and pioglitazone and alogliptin (Oseni) (FDA, 2013a; ChemSpider, 2013).

(c) Trends in use

Pioglitazone was one of the most widely used drugs for the treatment of type 2 diabetes among adults in 2000–2005. However, prescription sales of thiazolidinediones in general, and of pioglitazone in particular, have declined following several studies that suggested links to congestive heart failure (Singh *et al.*, 2007a), and fractures (Loke *et al.*, 2009), and subsequent warnings about the risk of cancer of the bladder (FDA, 2013a). Prescription trends from the Netherlands also declined after regulatory warnings concerning fractures and development of cancer of the bladder (Ruiter *et al.*, 2012).

Total worldwide sales of pioglitazone were US$ 3.34 billion in 2012, with 71% occurring in the USA (US$ 2.37 billion). Other nations with significant sales of pioglitazone included Japan (US$ 322 million), India (US$ 106 million), United Kingdom (US$ 71 million) and Italy (US$ 66 million) (IMS Health, 2012a).

Pioglitazone was reported in 2.4 million drug uses in the USA in 2012, a decline from 6.7 million reported uses in 2006, according to IMS Health National Disease and Therapeutic Index data. Based on these same data, approximately 600 000 patients in the USA were taking pioglitazone in 2012 (IMS Health, 2012b). See also Fig. 1.1.

Fig. 1.1 Trends in use of pioglitazone by office-based physicians in the USA

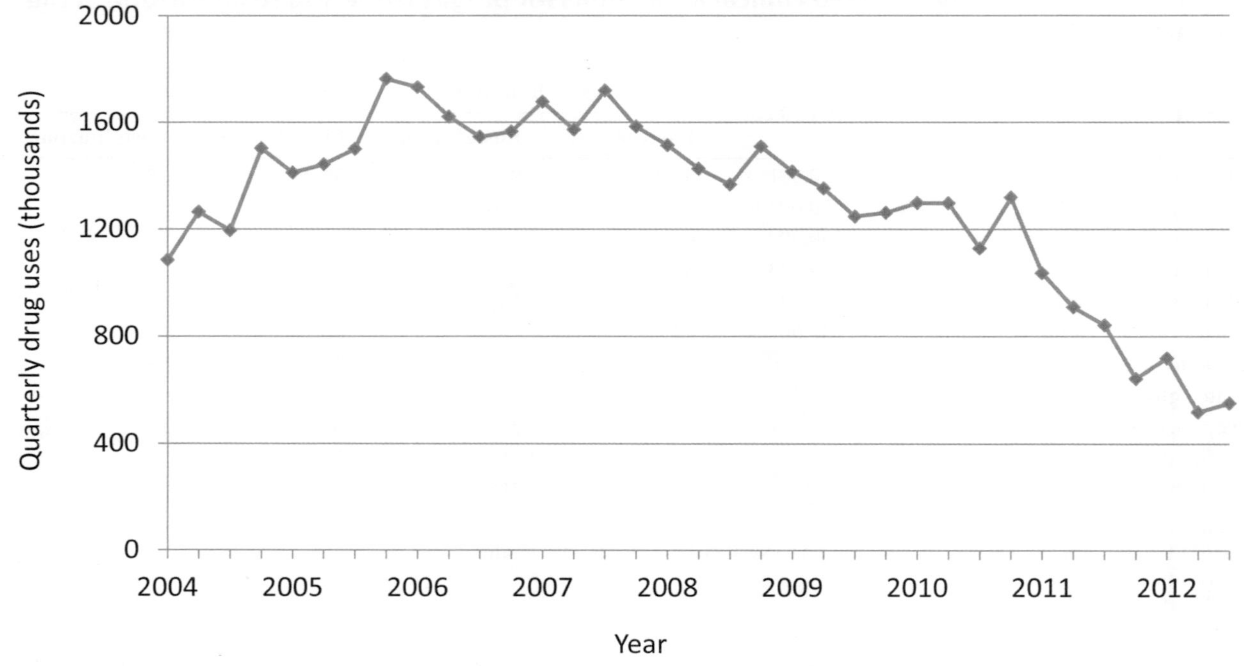

Prepared by the Working Group from data obtained from IMS Health, National Disease and Therapeutic Index (IMS Health, 2012b).

1.4 Occurrence and exposure to pioglitazone

1.4.1 Natural occurrence

Pioglitazone is not reported to occur naturally. The production and medicinal use of pioglitazone may contaminate the environment through various waste streams (Pubchem, 2013). If released into the air, pioglitazone is removed by wet or dry deposition, since it exists solely in the particulate phase in the atmosphere. Pioglitazone does not volatilize from dry soil surfaces based upon its vapour pressure. If released into the water, pioglitazone is expected to adsorb to suspended solids and sediment.

1.4.2 Occupational exposure

Occupational exposure to pioglitazone may occur through inhalation and dermal contact at workplaces where pioglitazone is produced or used (Pubchem, 2013). No information was available to the Working Group on the potential number of workers exposed.

1.5 Regulations and guidelines for pioglitazone

Pioglitazone was first approved for use in the USA on 15 July 1999 (FDA, 2013b). The Food and Drug Administration (FDA) approved a risk evaluation and mitigation strategy (REMS) for pioglitazone to ensure that the benefits of this drug outweighed the risks; however, this REMS was later rescinded.

The French Agency for the Safety of Health Products (AFFSAPS) suspended the use of medications containing pioglitazone in 2011, on the basis of a French study linking pioglitazone to cancer of the bladder (AFFSAPS, 2013). Following this study, the Federal Institute for Drugs and Medical Devices (BrFAM) in Germany also recommended the suspension of sales of pioglitazone (BrFAM, 2011).

1.6 Chemical and physical data on rosiglitazone

1.6.1 Nomenclature

(a)   Rosiglitazone

Chem. Abstr. Serv. Reg. No.: 122320-73-4 (SciFinder, 2013)

Chem. Abstr. Serv. name: 2,4-Thiazolidinedione, 5-[[4-[2-(methyl-2-pyridinylamino)ethoxy]phenyl]methyl] (SciFinder, 2013)

IUPAC Systematic Name: 5-[[4-[2-[Methyl(pyridin-2-yl)amino]ethoxy]phenyl]methyl]-1,3-thiazolidine-2,4-dione (Pubchem, 2013)

WHO INN: Rosiglitazone (WHO, 2007)

(b)   Rosiglitazone maleate

Chem. Abstr. Serv. Reg. No.: 155141-29-0 (SciFinder, 2013)

Chem. Abstr. Serv. Name: 2,4-Thiazolidinedione, 5-[[4-[2-(methyl-2-pyridinylamino)ethoxy]phenyl]methyl]-, (2Z)-2-butenedioate (1:1) (SciFinder, 2013)

IUPAC Systematic Name: (Z)-But-2-enedioic acid;5-[[4-[2-[methyl(pyridin-2-yl)amino]ethoxy]phenyl]methyl]-1,3-thiazolidine-2,4-dione (Pubchem, 2013)

Proprietary Names: Gaudil (Pubchem, 2013); Rezult (SciFinder, 2013); Avandia (GSK, 2012)

1.6.2 Structural and molecular formulae and relative molecular mass

(a)   Rosiglitazone

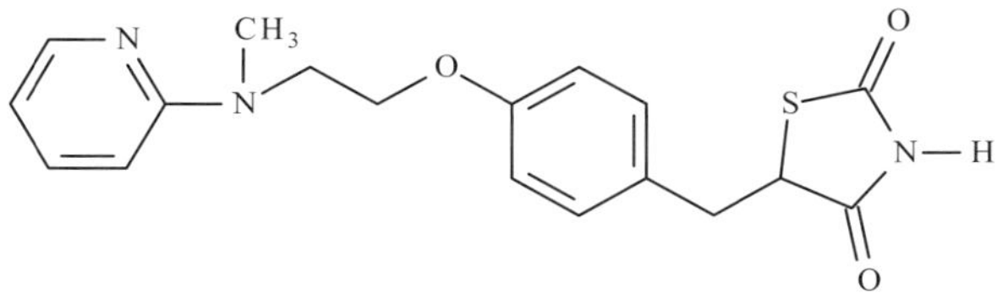

$C_{18}H_{19}N_3O_3S$
Relative molecular mass: 357.43

(b)   Rosiglitazone maleate

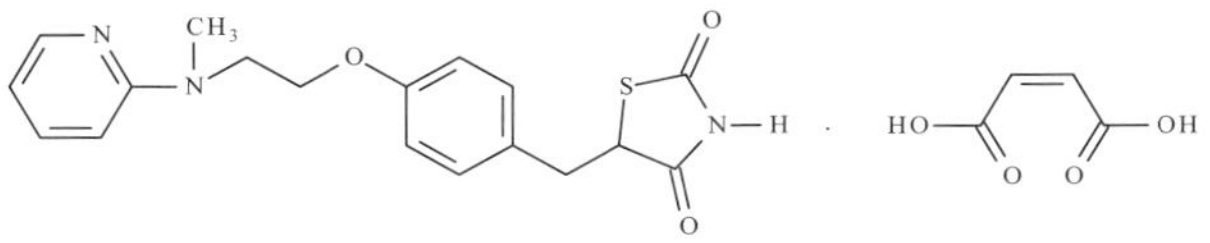

$C_{18}H_{19}N_3O_3S. C_4H_4O_4$
Relative molecular mass: 473.50
From O'Neil (2006), SciFinder (2013)

1.6.3 Chemical and physical properties of the pure substance

(a)   Rosiglitazone

Description: Solid, colourless crystals from methanol (O'Neil, 2006)

Melting point: Rosiglitazone: 151–155 °C (O'Neil, 2006)

Density: 1.315 ± 0.06 g/cm³ at 20 °C and pressure 760 Torr (SciFinder, 2013)

Spectroscopy data: UV (Venkatesh *et al.*, 2006), ¹H NMR, ¹³C NMR, IR (potassium bromide), and MS have been reported. (Pang *et al.*, 2009; Wang & Miksa, 2007)

Solubility: 30.67 µg/mL in water at 25 °C; 3.79 µg/mL in 0.1 M phosphate buffer at 25 °C (Seedher & Kanojia, 2008; Seedher & Kanojia, 2009); 35.09 µg/mL in 0.15 M NaCl at 25 °C (Seedher & Kanojia, 2008); soluble in the mg/mL range in ethanol, dimethyl sulfoxide, and dimethylformamide (Cayman SDS, 2013); 10.45 mg/L in water at 25 °C (NLM, 2013)

Octanol/water partition coefficient: Log P = 2.78–3.02 (Giaginis *et al.*, 2007)

Vapour pressure: 1.14×10^{-13} mm Hg at 25 °C (SciFinder, 2013)

(b)   Rosiglitazone maleate

Description: White to off-white solid (O'Neil, 2006; GSK, 2012)

Melting point: 122–123 °C (O'Neil, 2006)

Solubility: Readily soluble in ethanol and in buffered aqueous solution at pH 2.3; solubility decreases with increasing pH in the physiological range (O'Neil, 2006; GSK, 2012)

Stability data: Stable for 2 years when stored at 4 °C. Stock solutions are stable for up to 3 months when stored at –20 °C (Enzo PDS, 2012)

1.6.4 Technical products and impurities

Rosiglitazone maleate is used to formulate the finished dosage forms described below.

(a)   Trade names

Avandia (GSK, 2012); Roglit 4; Romerol; Rosit-2; Sensulin; Tazone-4 (BDdrugs, 2013)

(b)   Impurities

- Desmethyl impurity or 5-(4-(2-(pyridin-2-yl-amino)ethoxy)benzyl)thiazolidine-2,4-dione (Krishna *et al.*, 2008)

- Dimer impurity or 5-((2,4-dioxothiazolidin-5-yl)(4-(2-(methyl(pyridin-2-yl)amino)ethoxy)phenyl)methyl)-5-(4-(2-(methyl(pyridin-2-yl)amino)ethoxy)benzyl)thiazolidine-2,4-dione (Krishna *et al.*, 2008)

- Succinate impurity or 2-(5-(4-(2-(methyl-(pyridin-2-yl)amino)ethoxy)benzyl)-2,4-dioxothiazolidin-3-yl)succinic acid (Krishna *et al.*, 2008)

- 4-(2-(Methyl(pyridin-2-yl)amino)ethoxy)benzaldehyde (Radhakrishna *et al.*, 2002b)

1.7   Analysis of rosiglitazone

Physical properties used for the identification of the substance, e.g. IR and melting point, are presented in Section 1.6.3.

Selected non-compendial methods are presented in Table 1.1. Rosiglitazone can be analysed in different matrices such as plasma, serum, urine and formulations, by HPLC and with detection by UV or MS. Detection and quantification limits for determination of rosiglitazone in human serum by HPLC method with UV detection are 0.033 µg/mL and 0.102 µg/mL, respectively (Sultana *et al.*, 2011). Rosiglitazone can be analysed in human plasma with lower limit of quantification of 1.00 ng/mL using liquid chromatography electrospray ionization mass spectrometry (LC-ESI-MS) (O'Maille *et al.*, 2008). Other analytical methods for detection in human urine include square-wave adsorptive stripping voltammetry method (Al-Ghamdi & Hefnawy, 2012); analysis of formulation can be also achieved with capillary electrophoresis with UV detection (Yardımcı *et al.*, 2007) or by UV spectroscopy (Sireesha *et al.*, 2011).

1.8   Production and use of rosiglitazone

1.8.1 Production

Rosiglitazone is produced by dissolving 2-*N*-methyl-2-pyridylaminoethanol in dimethylformamide and adding sodium hydroxide under atmospheric nitrogen (Cantello *et al.*, 1994; Pubchem Substance, 2013). 4-Fluorobenzaldehyde is added. The resulting mixture is then dissolved in toluene and piperidine is added. The compound obtained is dissolved in dioxane and hydrogenated at room temperature and atmospheric pressure. Rosiglitazone is separated by filtration, vacuum concentration and recrystallization.

1.8.2 Use

(a) Indications

Rosiglitazone maleate is an antidiabetic agent indicated for the improvement of glycaemic control in adults with type 2 diabetes mellitus, as an adjunct to diet and exercise. Rosiglitazone maleate decreases hyperglycaemia by reducing insulin resistance in the presence of endogenous insulin (Avandia, 2010; Sweetman, 2011).

In the USA, rosiglitazone maleate is only indicated for patients already using rosiglitazone, or for those not taking rosiglitazone and who have been unable to achieve adequate glycaemic control using other diabetes medications, or who have decided not to take pioglitazone (Avandia, 2010). In the USA, the most commonly reported indication for rosiglitazone is type 2 diabetes mellitus (see Table 1.2).

Rosiglitazone is also used for off-label indications such as polycystic ovarian syndrome and insulin resistance syndrome.

Side-effects include fluid retention, congestive heart failure, and liver disease (Pubchem Substance, 2013).

(b) Dosage

Rosiglitazone is available as tablets of 2 mg, 4 mg, and 8 mg. Rosiglitazone is also available in combination with glimeperide or with metformin. Rosiglitazone is started at a dose of 4 mg and can be titrated up to a dose of 8 mg, if inadequate response is obtained in combination with metformin or sulfonylureas (Sweetman, 2011).

(c) Trends in use

Total worldwide sales of rosiglitazone in 2012 were US$ 43 million, a decline from much higher levels in the previous decade (IMS Health,

2012a). In 2012, there were limited, if any, sales in most countries of the European Union as a consequence of the decision of the European Medicines Agency to suspend marketing of this medication in September 2010 (EMA, 2010). Countries with appreciable continuing sales included China (US$ 12 million), Canada (US$ 11 million), Mexico (US$ 7 million), Australia (US$ 3 million), USA (US$ 3 million), and Argentina (US$ 3 million). The use of rosiglitazone rapidly declined in the USA after increased risk of cardiovascular disease associated with use of rosiglitazone was reported in May 2007 (Nissen & Wolski, 2007; Singh *et al.*, 2007b).

Rosiglitazone was reported as 105 000 drug uses in the USA in 2012, down from 6.7 million uses in 2005 (IMS Health, 2012b; see Fig. 1.2). Approximately 10 000 patients in the USA were taking rosiglitazone in 2012, down from about 40 000 in 2011 (IMS Health, 2012b).

Prescribing trends from the Netherlands show a decline in prescriptions for rosiglitazone after regulatory warnings (Ruiter *et al.*, 2012). Since the marketing authorization for rosiglitazone was suspended, rosiglitazone is no longer available for use in Europe (EMA, 2010). Prescriptions for rosiglitazone have also declined in several other countries across Asia, such as Taiwan, China (Lu & Li, 2013).

1.9 Occurrence and exposure to rosiglitazone

1.9.1 Natural occurrence and environmental fate

Rosiglitazone is not reported to occur naturally. The production and use of rosiglitazone may result in its release to the environment through various waste streams. If released to air, it will exist solely in the particulate phase and will be removed from the atmosphere by wet or dry deposition (Pubchem Substance, 2013).

Fig. 1.2 Trends in use of rosiglitazone by office-based physicians in the USA

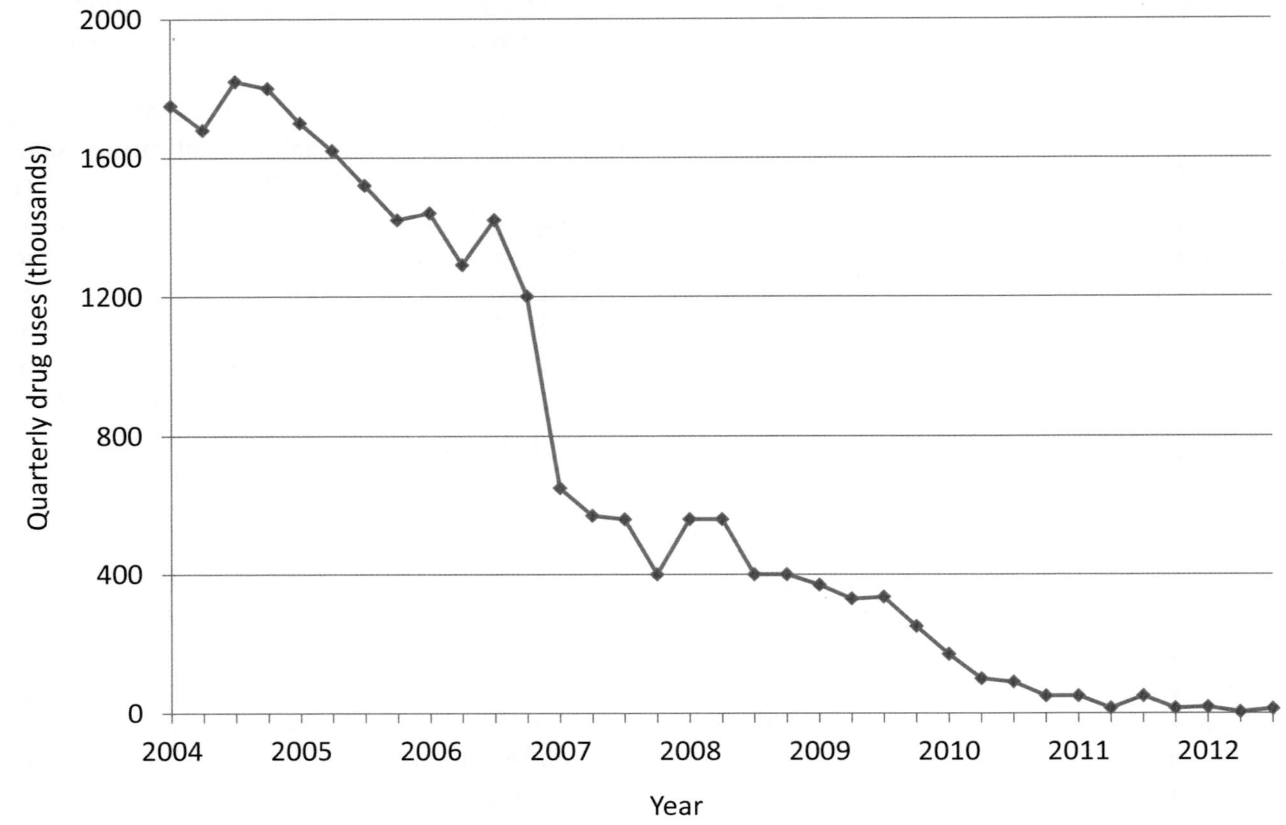

Prepared by the Working Group from data obtained from IMS Health, National Disease and Therapeutic Index (IMS Health, 2012b).

1.9.2 Occupational exposure

Occupational exposure to rosiglitazone may occur through inhalation of dust and via dermal contact at workplaces where rosiglitazone is produced or used (Pubchem Substance, 2013). No information was available to the Working Group on the potential number of workers exposed.

1.10 Regulations and guidelines for rosiglitazone

In the USA, rosiglitazone is only available under a REMS, and approved by FDA on the basis of safety and effectiveness (DHHS/FDA, 2007; Woodcock *et al.*, 2010). The marketing authorization for rosiglitazone was withdrawn in Europe (EMA, 2010), where rosiglitazone is no longer in use after being linked in several studies to an increase in the risk of myocardial infarction (Nissen & Wolski, 2007; Singh *et al.*, 2007b).

In June 2013, an FDA advisory committee meeting was held to discuss the re-adjudication of data on cardiovascular events associated with rosiglitazone from a large randomized controlled trial (FDA, 2013c). The advisory committee recommended that restrictions on rosiglitazone be lessened, since re-adjudication did not reveal a statistically significant increase in the risk of cardiovascular events.

2. Cancer in Humans

Thiazolidinediones (rosiglitazone, pioglitazone and troglitazone) have been used as orally administered glucose-lowering drugs in patients with type 2 diabetes mellitus. Rosiglitazone and pioglitazone were introduced to the market at about the same time (1999 in the USA, and 2001 and 2002 for rosiglitazone and pioglitazone, respectively, in Taiwan, China; Tseng, 2012d). Some patients may therefore have been exposed to both drugs, which were sometimes prescribed sequentially. Troglitazone was marketed for only a short period (1997–2000), before being withdrawn from the world market subsequent to reports of fatal hepatotoxicity (Julie *et al.*, 2008).

There was a concern regarding the potential for ascertainment bias in the observational studies, since differences in the intensity and frequency of ascertainment between the pioglitazone and control groups were unknown. Since pioglitazone is associated with an increased risk of oedema and congestive heart failure, patients taking pioglitazone were potentially more likely to undergo more frequent urine analysis, which could lead to detection of microscopic haematuria, more frequent cystoscopies, and eventually a diagnosis of cancer of the bladder.

Pioglitazone and rosiglitazone may have different effects on the risk of cancer and the Working Group therefore evaluated these compounds separately, whenever data were available. Studies that reported results for non-specific thiazolidinediones were considered uninformative by the Working Group and are not cited in this *Monograph*.

Several of the studies on these agents were based on analyses of large databases from France, the United Kingdom, the USA, and Taiwan, China, which are briefly described below. Associations of multiple cancers with specific thiazolidinediones were reported (see Table 2.1)

The French health insurance databases SNIIRAM (*Système national d'information inter-régimes de l'Assurance maladie*) and PMSI (*Programme de médicalisation des systèmes d'information*) cover all employees and represent approximately 75% of the French population. These databases contain all reimbursement data for the patients' health expenditure, including medication and outpatient medical and nursing care prescribed or performed by health-care professionals. International Classification of Diseases 10th Revision (ICD-10) codes are applied in the databases and hospital discharge information can be linked. To evaluate the association between the use of pioglitazone or rosiglitazone and risk of various cancers, a cohort of 1 491 060 diabetic patients (aged 40–79 years on 31 December 2006) from this national health insurance scheme was created. Patients included had filled at least one prescription for an antidiabetic drug (i.e. metformin, sulfonylurea, pioglitazone, rosiglitazone, other oral antidiabetic drugs and/or insulin) in 2006. Patients were excluded if they had cancer of the bladder diagnosed before study entry or within the first 6 months after study entry. Diagnosis of cancer of the bladder or other cancers was followed up until 31 December 2009 (Neumann *et al.*, 2012). [The Working Group noted that the period of follow-up was only 3 years. It was unclear which drugs patients may have used in the past, before enrollment into the cohort.]

In the United Kingdom, The Health Improvement Network (THIN) database (since 2003), managed by the Medicines and Healthcare Products Regulatory Agency, MHRA) is similar in structure and content to the General Practice Research Database (GPRD, 1994–2002), which provides electronic medical records of approximately 10 million patients living in the United Kingdom [the Working Group estimated a 50% overlap in the two databases]. Data available include demographic information, medical diagnoses (using Read codes, a standard classification

Table 2.1 Cohort studies of cancer and exposure to pioglitazone or rosiglitazone

Reference Location, follow-up period	Total No. of subjects	Exposure assessment	Organ site (ICD code)	Exposure categories	Exposed cases	Relative risk (95% CI)	Covariates Comments
Bladder cancer							
Lewis *et al.* (2011)[a] KPNC, USA, 1997–2008	193 099	Prescription records	Bladder (linkage with KPNC cancer registry)	*Pioglitazone*			Included diabetic patients aged ≥ 40 yr between 1997 and 2002. Numbers of cases reported as median incidence rate per 100 000 person-years.
				Never use	791	1.00 (ref.)	
				Ever use	90	1.2 (0.9–1.5)	
				Time since starting (mo):			
				< 18	NR	1.2 (0.8–1.7)	
				18–36	NR	1.4 (0.9–2.1)	
				> 36	NR	1.3 (0.9–1.8)	
				P for trend		0.07	
				Duration of therapy (mo):			
				< 12	NR	0.8 (0.6–1.3)	
				12–24	NR	1.4 (0.9–2.1)	
				> 24	NR	1.4 (1.03–2.0)	
				P for trend		0.03	
				Cumulative dose (mg):			
				1–10 500	NR	1.0 (0.7–1.5)	
				10 501–28 000	NR	1.2 (0.8–1.8)	
				> 28 000	NR	1.4 (0.96–2.1)	
				P for trend		0.08	
Neumann *et al.* (2012) France, 2006–9	1 491 060 (pioglitazone exposed: *n* = 155 535)	Prescription records	Bladder (discharge diagnosis with ICD-10 C67, combined with specific aggressive treatment)	*Pioglitazone (+) vs (–):*			Age, sex (when applicable), and exposure to glucose-lowering drugs. Patients with diabetes in two large national linked databases: health insurance system (SNIIRAM) and hospitalization (PMSI), 2006–2009. Age range: 40–79 yr; lack of consideration of potential confounders like smoking and comorbidities.
				Both sexes	2016	1.22 (1.05–1.43)	
				Men	1790	1.28 (1.09–1.51)	
				Women	226	0.78 (0.44–1.37)	
				Rosiglitazone (+) vs (–):			
				Both sexes	2016	1.08 (0.92–1.26)	
				Men	1790	1.10 (0.93–1.30)	
				Women	226	0.89 (0.53–1.49)	

Table 2.1 (continued)

Reference Location, follow-up period	Total No. of subjects	Exposure assessment	Organ site (ICD code)	Exposure categories	Exposed cases	Relative risk (95% CI)	Covariates Comments
Neumann et al. (2012) France, 2006–9 (cont.)				*Pioglitazone (–), both sexes*		1.00 (ref.)	Age, sex (when applicable), level of pioglitazone use (i.e. cumulative dose and duration of exposure, respectively) and exposure to other glucose-lowering drugs
				Cumulative dose (mg):			
				< 10 500	NR	1.12 (0.89–1.40)	
				10 500–27 999	NR	1.20 (0.93–1.53)	
				≥ 28 000	NR	1.75 (1.22–2.50)	
				Duration of exposure (d):			
				< 360	NR	1.05 (0.82–1.36)	
				360–719	NR	1.34 (1.02–1.75)	
				≥ 720	NR	1.36 (1.04–1.79)	
				Pioglitazone (–), men		1.00 (ref.)	
				Cumulative dose (mg):			
				< 10 500	NR	1.17 (0.92–1.48)	
				10 500–27 999	NR	1.24 (0.96–1.60)	
				≥ 28 000	NR	1.88 (1.30–2.71)	
				Duration of exposure (d):			
				< 360	NR	1.10 (0.84–1.43)	
				360–719	NR	1.39 (1.06–1.84)	
				≥ 720	NR	1.44 (1.09–1.91)	
				Pioglitazone (–), women		1.00 (ref.)	
				Cumulative dose (mg):			
				< 10 500	NR	0.77 (0.36–1.65)	
				10 500–27 999	NR	0.84 (0.35–2.06)	
				≥ 28 000	NR	0.57 (0.08–4.11)	
				Duration of exposure (d):			
				< 360	NR	0.76 (0.34–1.72)	
				360–719	NR	0.87 (0.32–2.35)	
				≥ 720	NR	0.71 (0.22–2.23)	

Table 2.1 (continued)

Reference Location, follow-up period	Total No. of subjects	Exposure assessment	Organ site (ICD code)	Exposure categories	Exposed cases	Relative risk (95% CI)	Covariates Comments
Wei et al. (2013)[b] General Practice Research Database, United Kingdom, 2001–10	207 714 (pioglitazone exposed, 23 548; unexposed, 184 166)	Prescription records	Bladder (database records)	Pioglitazone (yes vs no)	869	1.16 (0.83–1.62)	Type 2 diabetes patients aged ≥ 40 yr. HR, 1.22 (95% CI, 0.80–1.84) in a propensity-matched analysis done in a group of patients without missing data on baseline characteristics
Tseng (2012a)[c] Taiwan, China, 2006–9	54 928	Medical reimbursement records in the Taiwan, China, National Health Insurance database	Bladder (ICD-9 188)	*Pioglitazone*			
				Never-users	155	1.00 (ref.)	
				Ever-users	10	1.31 (0.66–2.58)	
				Time since starting (mo):			
				< 18	4	1.38 (0.49–3.83)	
				18–36	5	1.54 (0.62–3.84)	
				> 36	1	0.65 (0.09–4.77)	
				P for trend		0.6352	
				Duration of therapy (mo):			
				< 12	8	1.54 (0.73–3.26)	
				≥ 12	2	0.82 (0.20–3.35)	
				P for trend		0.6919	
				Cumulative dose (mg):			
				1–10 500	8	1.45 (0.69–3.06)	
				> 10 500	2	0.94 (0.23–3.84)	
				P for trend		0.7125	

Table 2.1 (continued)

Reference Location, follow-up period	Total No. of subjects	Exposure assessment	Organ site (ICD code)	Exposure categories	Exposed cases	Relative risk (95% CI)	Covariates Comments
Tseng (2013a)[d] Taiwan, China, 2006–9	547 584 diabetic men	Medical reimbursement records in the Taiwan, China, National Health Insurance database	Bladder (ICD-9 188)	Pioglitazone (yes vs no) Rosiglitazone (yes vs no)	1869 1869	1.02 (0.75–1.39) 1.12 (0.92–1.37)	Benign prostatic hyperplasia is a significant risk factor for bladder cancer in diabetic men. The hazard ratios for pioglitazone and rosiglitazone are estimated in diabetic men with benign prostatic hyperplasia.
Fujimoto et al. (2013) Japan, 2000–11	21 335	Hospital records	Bladder	Pioglitazone (yes vs no)	170	1.75 (0.89–3.45)	NR, probably not adjusted. Single centre, lack of adjustment for confounders.
Colorectal cancer							
Neumann et al. (2012)[e] France, 2006–9	1 485 146	Prescription records	Colorectum (ICD-10 C18 to C21)	Pioglitazone (+) vs (–) Rosiglitazone (+) vs (–)	10 618 10 618	0.97 (0.90–1.05) 0.88 (0.82–0.95)	Age, sex (when applicable), and exposure to glucose-lowering drugs
Tseng (2012b)[e] Taiwan, China, 2003–5	995 843	Reimbursement databases	Colon (ICD-9 153)	Pioglitazone (yes vs no) Rosiglitazone (yes vs no)	3 versus 2386 29 vs 2360	0.78 (0.25–2.49) 1.22 (0.81–1.84)	
Ferrara et al. (2011) KPNC, USA, 1997–2005	252 467	Prescription records	Colon	Never-use of other TZD Ever-use of other TZD Never-use of pioglitazone Ever-use of pioglitazone	1260 1260	1.00 (ref.) 1.1 (0.8–1.5) 1.00 (ref.) 0.9 (0.7–1.1)	
Lung cancer							
Ferrara et al. (2011)[f] KPNC, USA, 1997–2005	252 467	Prescription records	Lung/bronchus (linkage with KPNC cancer registry)	Never-use of other TZD Ever-use of other TZD Never-use of pioglitazone Ever-use of pioglitazone	1637 1637	1.00 (ref) 0.9 (0.6–1.3) 1.00 (ref.) 1.0 (0.8–1.3)	Ten categories of cancer sites, diabetic patients aged ≥ 40 yr
Neumann et al. (2012) France, 2006–9	1 493 472	Prescription records	Lung (ICD-10 C33 and C34)	Pioglitazone (+) vs (–) Rosiglitazone (+) vs (–)	9298 9298	0.94 (0.87–1.02) 0.91 (0.84–0.99)	Age, sex, and exposure to glucose-lowering drugs

Table 2.1 (continued)

Reference Location, follow-up period	Total No. of subjects	Exposure assessment	Organ site (ICD code)	Exposure categories	Exposed cases	Relative risk (95% CI)	Covariates Comments
Prostate cancer							
Ferrara *et al.* (2011)[f] KPNC, USA, 1997–2005	252 467	Prescription records	Prostate (linkage with KPNC cancer registry)	Never-use of other TZD Ever-use of other TZD Never-use of pioglitazone Ever-use of pioglitazone	2105 2105	1.00 (ref.) 1.0 (0.7–1.3) 1.00 (ref.) 1.0 (0.8–1.2)	Ten categories of cancer sites. Diabetic patients aged ≥ 40 yr
Tseng (2011)[g] Taiwan, China, 2003–5	494 630	Medical reimbursement records in the Taiwan, China, National Health Insurance database	Prostate (ICD-9 185)	Pioglitazone (yes vs no) Rosiglitazone (yes vs no)	889 889	0.77 (0.10–5.75) 0.88 (0.43–1.80)	
Breast cancer							
Ferrara *et al.* (2011) KPNC, USA, 1997–2005	252 467	Prescription records	Female breast (linkage with KPNC cancer registry)	Never-use of other TZD Ever-use of other TZD Never-use of pioglitazone Ever-use of pioglitazone	1561 1561	1.0 (ref.) 0.9 (0.7–1.2) 1.0 (ref.) 1.0 (0.8–1.3)	
Neumann *et al.* (2012) France, 2006–9	671 510	Prescription records	Female breast (ICD-10 C50)	Pioglitazone (+) vs (–) Rosiglitazone (+) vs (–)	6820 6820	0.91 (0.83–1.00) 0.80 (0.73–0.88)	Age, sex, and exposure to glucose-lowering drugs

Table 2.1 (continued)

Reference Location, follow-up period	Total No. of subjects	Exposure assessment	Organ site (ICD code)	Exposure categories	Exposed cases	Relative risk (95% CI)	Covariates Comments
Other cancers							
Ferrara *et al.* (2011) KPNC, USA, 1997–2005	252 467	Prescription records	Linkage with KPNC cancer registry	Never-use of other TZD		1.00 (ref.)	
			NHL	Ever-use of other TZD	569	0.7 (0.4–1.2)	
			Corpus uterus	Ever-use of other TZD	552	1.2 (0.8–1.9)	
			Pancreas	Ever-use of other TZD	431	1.0 (0.6–1.8)	
			Kidney/renal pelvis	Ever-use of other TZD	430	1.3 (0.7–2.3)	
			Rectum	Ever-use of other TZD	390	0.7 (0.4–1.5)	
			Melanoma	Ever-use of other TZD	373	1.0 (0.5–1.8)	
				Never-use of pioglitazone		1.00 (ref.)	
			NHL	Ever-use of pioglitazone	569	1.3 (1.0–1.8)	
			Corpus uterus	Ever-use of pioglitazone	552	1.1 (0.8–1.5)	
			Pancreas	Ever-use of pioglitazone	431	1.2 (0.8–1.7)	
			Kidney/renal pelvis	Ever-use of pioglitazone	430	0.7 (0.4–1.1)	
			Rectum	Ever-use of pioglitazone	390	1.2 (0.8–1.8)	
			Melanoma	Ever-use of pioglitazone	373	1.3 (0.9–2.0)	
Neumann *et al.* (2012) France, 2006–9	1 495 787	Prescription records	Kidney (ICD-10 C64)	Pioglitazone (+) vs (−)	2861	0.91 (0.79–1.06)	Age, sex, and exposure to glucose-lowering drugs
				Rosiglitazone (+) vs (−)	2861	0.98 (0.86–1.13)	
	1 495 411		Head and neck (ICD-10 C00 to C14)	Pioglitazone (+) vs (−)	2868	0.85 (0.73–0.99)	Age, sex, and exposure to glucose-lowering drugs
				Rosiglitazone (+) vs (−)	2868	0.79 (0.67–0.92)	
Tseng (2012c)[h] Taiwan, China, 1996–2005	999 730	Reimbursement databases	Thyroid (ICD-9 193)	Pioglitazone (yes vs no)	943	0.52 (0.07–3.93)	
				Rosiglitazone (yes vs no)		0.67 (0.23–1.95)	

Table 2.1 (continued)

Reference Location, follow-up period	Total No. of subjects	Exposure assessment	Organ site (ICD code)	Exposure categories	Exposed cases	Relative risk (95% CI)	Covariates Comments
Tseng (2013c)[i] Taiwan, China, 2003–5	998 540	Reimbursement databases	Oral cavity, lip, and pharynx (ICD-9 140, 141, 143, 144, 145, 146, 148, and 149)	Pioglitazone (yes vs no) Men Women Rosiglitazone (yes vs no) Men Women	766	1.70 (0.22–13.20) no incident cases of oral cancer 1.15 (0.44–3.04) 0.90 (0.20–3.98)	

[a] Age, sex, race/ethnicity, current smoking, renal function, bladder condition, congestive heart failure, income, baseline A1C, newly diagnosed with diabetes at start of follow-up, duration of diabetes, other cancer before baseline, other diabetic medications (other TZDs, metformin, sulfonylureas, other oral hypoglycaemic drugs, insulin).

[b] Age, sex, duration of diabetes, smoking status and BMI before entry into the study, and insulin treatment and number and type of different oral hypoglycaemic drug classes used during the follow-up period.

[c] Age, sex, diabetes duration, nephropathy, urinary-tract disease, hypertension, COPD, cerebrovascular disease, IHD, peripheral arterial disease, eye disease, dyslipidaemia, heart failure, rosiglitazone, sulfonylurea, meglitinide, metformin, acarbose, insulin, statin, fibrate, angiotensin-converting enzyme inhibitor/angiotensin-receptor blocker, Ca-channel blocker, region of residence, occupation, and other cancer before baseline.

[d] Age, diabetes duration, nephropathy, urinary-tract diseases, hypertension, COPD, cerebrovascular disease, IHD, peripheral arterial disease, eye disease, dyslipidaemia, heart failure, obesity, alcohol-related diagnosis, non-alcohol-related chronic liver disease, rosiglitazone/pioglitazone, sulfonylurea, meglitinide, metformin, acarbose, insulin, statin, fibrate, ACEI/ARB, Ca-channel blockers, α-blockers, 5-α reductase inhibitors, clopidogrel, ticlopidine, dipyridamole, cyclophosphamide, diuretics, other cancer before baseline and potential detection examinations.

[e] Age, sex, diabetes, hypertension, COPD, asthma, stroke, nephropathy, IHD, peripheral arterial disease, eye disease, dyslipidaemia, obesity, statin, fibrate, ACEI/ARB, Ca-channel blocker, aspirin, dipyridamole, clopidogrel/ticlopidine, NSAIDs, sulfonylurea, metformin, insulin, acarbose, rosiglitazone, region of residence, occupation, and colon-cancer detection examinations.

[f] Age, ever use of other diabetes medications, year of cohort entry, sex, race/ethnicity, income, current smoking, baseline HbA1c, diabetes duration, new diabetes diagnosis, creatinine, and congestive heart failure.

[g] Age, diabetes duration, hypertension, COPD, stroke, nephropathy, IHD, peripheral arterial disease, eye disease, obesity, dyslipidaemia, statin, fibrate, ACEI/ARB, Ca-channel blocker, sulfonylurea, metformin, insulin, acarbose, rosiglitazone, region of residence, and occupation.

[h] Age, sex, diabetes, living region, occupation, detection examination, hypertension, COPD, stroke, nephropathy, IHD, peripheral arterial disease, eye disease, obesity, dyslipidaemia, benign thyroid disease, other cancer, sulfonylurea, metformin, insulin, acarbose, pioglitazone/rosiglitazone, statin, fibrate, ACEI/ARB, Ca-channel blocker, aspirin, ticlopidine, clopidogrel, NSAIDs.

[i] Age, diabetes, obesity, hypertension, COPD, alcohol-related diagnoses, stroke, nephropathy, IHD, peripheral arterial disease, eye disease, dyslipidaemia, statin, fibrate, ACEI/ARB, Ca-channel blockers, sulfonylurea, metformin, insulin, acarbose, pioglitazone/rosiglitazone, living region, occupation, potential detection.

ACEI/ARB, angiotensin-converting enzyme inhibitors/angiotensin receptor blockers; BMI, body mass index; Ca, calcium; COPD, chronic obstructive pulmonary disease; d, day; HbA1c, glycated haemoglobin; HR, hazard ratio; IHD, ischaemic heart disease; KPNC, Kaiser Permanente Northern California; mo, month; NHL, non-Hodgkin lymphoma; NR, not reported; NSAIDs, nonsteroidal anti-inflammatory drugs; PMSI, *Programme de médicalisation des systèmes d'information*; ref., reference; SNIIRAM, *Système national d'information inter-régimes de l'Assurance maladie*; TZD, thiazolidinediones; vs, versus; yr; year system used in the United Kingdom primary-care settings), lifestyle, and measures taken during clinical practice. The database is regularly updated and practitioners contributing data receive training for consistency in data recording. Studies conducted by Wei *et al.* (2013) and Azoulay *et al.* (2012) used this database.

In the USA, the Kaiser Permanente Northern California (KPNC) pharmacy database covers 3.2 million members of this health plan (approximately 30% of the population of the area) and includes outpatient prescriptions dispensed at a KPNC pharmacy. Approximately 95% of members fill their prescriptions at KPNC pharmacies. The KPNC diabetes registry gathers longitudinal electronic medical records and clinically related data for patients with diabetes from the following sources: primary hospital-discharge diagnoses of diabetes, two or more outpatient-visit diagnoses of diabetes, any prescription of a diabetes-related medication, or any record of glycated haemoglobin (HbA1c) > 6.7%. The database includes information of cancer registries, pharmacy records, laboratory records, and inpatient and outpatient medical diagnoses. Patients who met any of the following criteria were eligible for forming a cohort for the analysis of the association between pioglitazone use and risk of cancer referred to in this Monograph: (i) as of 1 January 1997, diagnosed with diabetes, aged $\geq$ 40 years, and members of KPNC; (ii) diagnosed with diabetes, reached age 40 years between 1 January 1997 and 31 December 2002, and were KPNC members on their 40th birthday; or (iii) having diabetes and aged $\geq$ 40 years when joining KPNC between 1 January 1997 and 31 December 2002. A total of 193 099 patients (30 173 ever-users and 162 926 never-users of pioglitazone) were followed and a mid-point interim analysis was published in 2011 (Lewis *et al.*, 2011).

Several independent groups (Tseng, 2011, 2012a, 2012b, 2013a; Chang *et al.*, 2012) used the reimbursement databases of the National Health Insurance of Taiwan, China, for evaluating the association between use of thiazolidinediones and risk of various cancers. Since March 1995, a compulsory and universal system of health insurance (National Health Insurance) has been implemented in Taiwan, China. All contracted medical institutes must submit computerized and standard claim documents for reimbursement. More than 99% of the population of 23 million people were enrolled in this insurance system, and > 98% of the hospitals nationwide were under contract with the insurance. The average number of annual physician visits in Taiwan, China, is one of the highest around the world, at approximately 15 visits per year per capita in 2009. The National Health Research Institute is the only institute approved, as per local regulations, for handling these reimbursement databases for academic research. The databases contain detailed records on every visit for each patient, including outpatient visits, emergency-department visits, and hospital admission. The databases also include principal and secondary diagnostic codes, prescription orders, and claimed expenses. Certain computerized databases, including a database from the national cancer registry (with a high level of completeness), are also available for data linkage. Most studies used the International Classification of Diseases Ninth Revision, Clinical Modification (ICD-9-CM) codes for disease or cancer diagnosis, with or without data linkage with the cancer registry. [The Working Group noted that there may have been a detection bias associated with this database because of the high number of patient visits per capita.]

2.1 Cancer of the bladder

See Fig. 2.1

Fig. 2.1 Risk of cancer of the bladder associated with ever-use or never-use of pioglitazone or rosiglitazone, by study design[a]

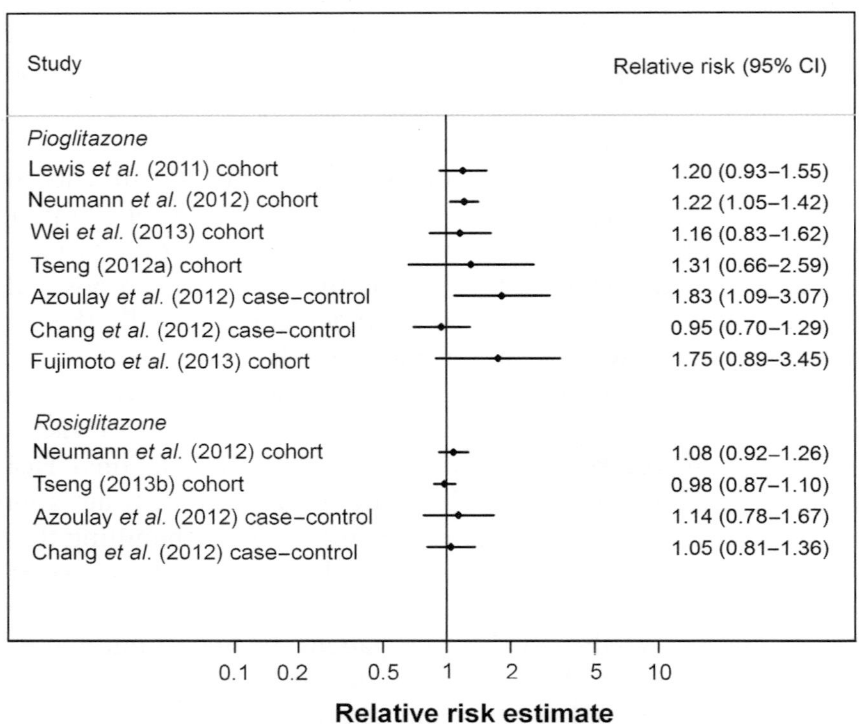

[a] Weights are from random-effects analysis
Compiled by the Working Group

2.1.1 Clinical trial

The potential risk of cancer of the bladder associated with exposure to pioglitazone in humans was first raised by the large randomized PROspective pioglitAzone Clinical Trial In macroVascular Events (PROactive), which showed an imbalance of incident cases of cancer of the bladder, with greater number in patients randomized to pioglitazone than to placebo (14 cases versus 6 cases, or 0.5% versus 0.2%; $P = 0.069$) (Dormandy et al., 2005). [Insufficient data were provided to calculate a risk estimate. The aim of the PROactive clinical trial was primarily to evaluate macrovascular events associated with use of pioglitazone. The Working Group also noted that 11 out of the 20 cases of cancer of the bladder were diagnosed within 1 year of randomization, which might have precluded a cause–effect relationship.] After excluding one case of previously diagnosed cancer of the bladder in the placebo group (found later to show benign histology), Hillaire-Buys et al. (2011) recalculated the crude relative risk of cancer of the bladder for pioglitazone versus placebo in PROactive as 2.83 (95% CI, 1.02–7.85; P value for Fisher exact test = 0.04). [In a randomized controlled trial, the confounders are balanced at baseline and any differences in ascertainment are likely to be non-differential. The Working Group noted these findings in light of the very low incidence of cancer of the bladder. After excluding the eleven cases of cancer of the bladder diagnosed within 1 year of randomization, one with benign histology in the placebo group, and six with known risk factors for cancer of the bladder, only three cases remained – two in the group receiving pioglitazone and one in the placebo group.]

2.1.2 Cohort studies

See Table 2.1

Lewis *et al.* (2011) studied the incidence of cancer of the bladder among 193 099 members of the KPNC health plan who were enrolled in the plan's diabetes registry and were aged ≥ 40 years between 1997 and 2002. The registry routinely compiled electronic medical records data from various sources, including cancer registries, pharmacy records, laboratory records, and medical diagnoses. Incident cases of cancer of the bladder were identified from 2002 to 2008 via the KPNC cancer registry and ever-use of specific diabetes medications (defined as two or more prescriptions within 6 months) was determined from the pharmacy database. In the mid-point interim analysis of a 10-year longitudinal KPNC cohort study in the USA (Lewis *et al.*, 2011), the overall hazard ratio was 1.2 (95% CI, 0.9–1.5) for cancer of the bladder for ever-users of pioglitazone versus never-users; patients who used pioglitazone for > 24 months showed a risk with adjusted hazard ratio of 1.4 (95% CI, 1.03–2.0). [Although adjustment for smoking was a strength of this study, only current smoking was considered, which may not have fully controlled for confounding.]

Neumann *et al.* (2012) analysed the risk of cancer of the bladder associated with exposure to pioglitazone and rosiglitazone in a cohort of 1 491 060 diabetic patients aged 40–79 years who had been prescribed at least one dose of glucose-lowering drugs in 2006. Subjects were followed between 2006 and 2009 using the French national health insurance information system (SNIIRAM) linked with the French hospital discharge database (PMSI). Overall, 2016 cases of cancer of the bladder were identified (men, 1790 cases; and women, 226 cases). Patients were excluded if they had an occupationally related cancer of the bladder, or if they were diagnosed before entry or within the first 6 months after study entry. Patients were followed up for a mean of 39.9 months (27.4 months due to exposure), starting 6 months after study entry. Ten percent of the patients (155 535 out of 1 491 060) took a minimum of two prescriptions for pioglitazone over 6 consecutive months. Compared with non-use, the estimated hazard rate ratio for cancer of the bladder associated with use of pioglitazone was 1.22 (95% CI, 1.05–1.43) and for rosiglitazone was 1.08 (95% CI, 0.92–1.26), after adjustment for age, sex, and exposure to glucose-lowering drugs. Dose–response analyses were available only for pioglitazone and showed increasing hazard ratios with increasing duration and cumulative dose. The hazard ratios for cumulative doses of < 10 500, 10 500–27 999 and ≥ 28 000 mg compared with never-users of pioglitazone was 1.12 (95% CI, 0.89–1.40), 1.20 (95% CI, 0.93–1.53) and 1.75 (95% CI, 1.22–2.50), respectively; and were 1.05 (95% CI, 0.82–1.36), 1.34 (95% CI, 1.02–1.75) and 1.36 (95% CI, 1.04–1.79), respectively, for duration of exposure < 360, 360–719 and ≥ 720 days compared with never-users. [Smoking was not accounted for in the analyses and therefore may have confounded the reported results. Sex-specific analyses suggested an association observed only in men, but not in women. Data on smoking were not available for adjustment. Since pioglitazone is usually used as a second- or third-line antidiabetic drug, users of pioglitazone may have had longer duration of diabetes, poorer glycaemic control, and higher rates of chronic diabetic complications and comorbidities. All these characteristics may affect the risk of cancer of the bladder (Perez, 2013; Tseng, 2012d). The length of follow-up limited evaluation of the long-term impact of treatment.]

In a matched cohort study by Wei *et al.* (2013) that used a propensity score approach (derived from baseline characteristics of age, sex, smoking, body mass index, and diabetes duration), the association between use of pioglitazone and risk of cancer of the bladder was assessed in patients with type 2 diabetes using the General Practice Research Database. Between 2001 and 2010, 207 714 patients aged ≥ 40 years were studied: 23 548 users of pioglitazone and 184 166 patients receiving other antidiabetic medications. Follow-up started at the date of first prescription for pioglitazone or other oral antidiabetic drugs during the study period and ended in December 2010. Patients with a cancer diagnosis before the entry date or less than 90 days of follow-up time were excluded. Incident cases of cancer of the bladder were obtained from general practitioner records during follow-up. Hazard ratios were computed, comparing the risk of developing cancer of the bladder in the group receiving pioglitazone and in the group receiving treatment with other oral antidiabetic drugs. A propensity score matched analysis was used in patients without missing data on baseline characteristics to minimize confounding by indication (n = 34 498). The following potential confounders were included: smoking status, age, sex, duration of diabetes from first diagnosis to the first treatment with oral antidiabetic drug during the study period, body mass index before entry into the study, and insulin treatment and number and type of different oral antidiabetic drug classes used during follow-up. During the study period, 66 new cases of cancer of the bladder (mean follow-up time, 3.5 years) occurred in the pioglitazone group, and 803 cases in the group receiving other oral antidiabetic drugs (mean follow-up time, 5.3 years) (adjusted HR, 1.16; 95% CI, 0.83–1.62). [The use of a propensity score to control for confounding by adjustment was a strength of this study. There was a potential overlap in the studied population because the authors used a similar database to that used by Azoulay *et al.* (2012).]

The National Health Insurance of Taiwan, China, was used to conduct several analyses of cancer of the bladder associated with the use of thiazolidinediones (Tseng, 2012a, 2013a, b).

Tseng (2012a) followed a random sample of 54 928 patients with type 2 diabetes in the reimbursement databases of the National Health Insurance for 4 years from 1 January 2006 to 31 December 2009. Among 165 incident cases of cancer of the bladder, 10 (0.39%) were ever-users and 155 (0.30%) were never-users of pioglitazone, and were not necessarily using other antidiabetic drugs. The hazard ratio for ever-users versus never-users of pioglitazone was 1.31 (95% CI, 0.66–2.58) after adjustment for age, sex, diabetes duration, various comorbidities, and medications. Dose–response relationships were also evaluated, but no trend was observed. [Smoking and body mass index were not available for analyses from the databases.]

In a second study drawn from the entire database of the National Health Insurance of Taiwan, China, Tseng (2013a) evaluated the risk of cancer of the bladder associated with use of pioglitazone and rosiglitazone in a subgroup of 85 152 men with type 2 diabetes and benign prostatic hyperplasia. The hazard ratios (HR) for cancer of the bladder among the diabetic patients with benign prostatic hyperplasia for ever-users of pioglitazone (HR, 1.02; 95% CI, 0.75–1.39) and rosiglitazone (HR, 1.12; 95% CI, 0.92–1.37) were close to 1.0. [The study was not primarily aimed at analysing the risk of cancer of the bladder associated with use of pioglitazone or rosiglitazone, and therefore no dose–response relationship was assessed. Smoking and body mass index could not be adjusted for because of lack of such information in the databases. There was a concern over overlapping of the study population with that of Tseng (2012a).]

In a third study drawn from the entire database of the National Health Insurance of Taiwan, China, Tseng (2013b) evaluated the association between use of rosiglitazone and risk of cancer of the bladder after excluding patients who had ever been exposed to pioglitazone. A total of 885 236 patients with type 2 diabetes and receiving oral antidiabetic agents (except pioglitazone) and/or insulin were studied for incidence of cancer of the bladder from 1 January 2006 to 31 December 2009. Among these patients, 102 926 were ever-users and 782 310 were never-users of rosiglitazone, with 356 and 2753 incident cases of cancer of the bladder, respectively. The hazard ratio for cancer of the bladder for ever-users versus never-users of rosiglitazone was 0.98 (95% CI, 0.87–1.104) after adjustment for age, sex, diabetes duration, various comorbidities, and medications. Dose–response relationships were also evaluated, but neither the P values for the hazard ratios of the categories nor the P values for trends were significant. [This study evaluated use of rosiglitazone and risk of cancer of the bladder after excluding potential residual confounding from pioglitazone. The study used databases covering the whole nation and spanning the whole period since the start of rosiglitazone use in Taiwan, China. However, data on smoking and body mass index were not available for analyses. There was a concern regarding overlapping of the study population with that of Tseng (2012a). The follow-up duration of 4 years may also have been too short.]

Fujimoto *et al.* (2013) identified nine cases of cancer of the bladder in a cohort of 663 patients who had taken pioglitazone, in a database of 21 335 patients with type 2 diabetes from a single Japanese hospital between 2000 and 2011. They reported a hazard ratio of 1.75 (95% CI, 0.89–3.45) for cancer of the bladder among pioglitazone users compared with all patients with diabetes. [The Working Group noted that incident cases were defined as any bladder cancers diagnosed after onset of drug therapy. No information was given about total follow-up time. Duration and dose of drug were only given for identified cases, as were data about smoking status. No other details were given about confounders.]

2.1.3 Nested case–control studies

See Table 2.2

To determine whether the use of pioglitazone was associated with an increased risk of incident cancer of the bladder in people with type 2 diabetes, Azoulay *et al.* (2012) conducted a nested case–control analysis within a cohort of 115 727 people with type 2 diabetes in the United Kingdom General Practice Research Database. Participants were newly treated with oral hypoglycaemic agents between 1 January 1988 and 31 December 2009. All incident cases of cancer of the bladder occurring during follow-up ($n = 470$) were identified and 376 cases were matched to up to 20 controls ($n = 6699$) on year of birth, year of cohort entry, sex, and duration of follow-up. Exposure was defined as ever-use of pioglitazone and/or rosiglitazone (defined by the presence of at least one prescription between cohort entry and the year before the index date), along with measures of duration and cumulative dosage. Analyses were adjusted for smoking status, excessive alcohol use, obesity, HbA1c, previous bladder conditions, previous cancer (other than non-melanoma skin cancer), Charlson comorbidity score, and ever-use of other antidiabetic agents (metformin, sulfonylureas, insulin, and other oral hypoglycaemic agents). Overall, ever-use of pioglitazone was associated with an increased rate of cancer of the bladder (rate ratio, 1.83; 95% CI, 1.10–3.05), with a positive exposure–response trend ($P = 0.030$). The highest risk was observed in patients exposed for > 24 months (RR, 1.99; 95% CI, 1.14–3.45) and in those with a cumulative dosage > 28 000 mg (RR, 2.54; 95% CI, 1.05–6.14). [Enrolment of new users of diabetes medications, who may have had less severe disease, and adjustment for smoking were potential strengths of this study. However, there was a potential overlap in the study population with that of Wei *et al.* (2013).]

Table 2.2 Case–control studies of cancer and exposure to pioglitazone or rosiglitazone

Reference Study location and period	Total No. cases No. of controls	Control source (hospital, population)	Exposure assessment	Organ site (ICD code)	Exposure categories	Exposed cases	Relative risk (95% CI)	Covariates Comments
Bladder cancer								
Azoulay et al. (2012)[a] United Kingdom, 1988–2009	376 6699	General Practice Research Database	Prescription records	Bladder (Read codes)	Never-use of any TZD	319	1.00 (ref.)	Up to 20 controls per case, matched on year of birth, year of cohort entry, sex, and duration of follow-up
					Exclusive ever-use of pioglitazone	19	1.83 (1.10–3.05)	
					Exclusive ever-use of rosiglitazone	36	1.14 (0.78–1.68)	
					Ever-use of both pioglitazone and rosiglitazone	2	0.78 (0.18–3.29)	
					Pioglitazone			
					Cumulative duration (mo):			
					≤ 12	1	0.56 (0.07–4.42)	
					13–24	2	3.03 (0.63–14.52)	
					> 24	16	1.99 (1.14–3.45)	
					P for trend		0.050	
					Cumulative dosage (mg):			
					≤ 10 500	7	1.58 (0.69–3.62)	
					10 501–28 000	6	1.66 (0.70–3.94)	
					> 28 000	6	2.54 (1.05–6.14)	
					P for trend		0.030	
					Rosiglitazone			
					Cumulative duration (d):			
					≤ 519	9	0.80 (0.40–1.62)	
					> 519–1022	13	1.33 (0.73–2.40)	
					> 1022	14	1.34 (0.75–2.40)	
					P for trend		0.32	
					Cumulative dosage (mg):			
					≤ 2464	8	0.71 (0.34–1.49)	
					> 2464–5152	15	1.50 (0.86–2.62)	
					> 5152	13	1.27 (0.69–2.32)	
					P for trend		0.49	

Table 2.2 (continued)

Reference Study location and period	Total No. cases No. of controls	Control source (hospital, population)	Exposure assessment	Organ site (ICD code)	Exposure categories	Exposed cases	Relative risk (95% CI)	Covariates Comments
Chang et al. (2012)[b] Taiwan, China, 2000–7	1583 6308	Population	Reimbursement databases	Bladder (linkage through national cancer registry)	*Pioglitazone*			
					Never-user	NR	1.00 (ref)	
					Ever-user	NR	0.95 (0.70–1.29)	
					Cumulative dosage (DDD):			
					< 120	NR	0.83 (0.54–1.27)	
					≥ 120	NR	1.07 (0.72–1.57)	
					Cumulative duration (yr):			
					≤ 1	NR	0.87 (0.61–1.25)	
					1–2	NR	1.20 (0.65–2.22)	
					2–3	NR	0.84 (0.30–2.36)	
					≥ 3	NR	1.56 (0.51–4.74)	
					Cumulative dose duration:			
					High	NR	1.13 (0.69–1.83)	
					Intermediate	NR	1.06 (0.65–1.71)	
					Low	NR	0.77 (0.48–1.25)	
					Rosiglitazone			
					Never-user	NR	1.00 (ref.)	
					Ever-user	NR	1.05 (0.81–1.36)	
					Cumulative dosage (DDD):			
					< 120	NR	1.05 (0.77–1.45)	
					≥ 120	NR	1.05 (0.78–1.40)	
					Cumulative duration (yr):			
					≤ 1	NR	1.07 (0.80–1.42)	
					1–2	NR	1.26 (0.86–1.86)	
					2–3	NR	0.60 (0.33–1.08)	
					≥ 3	NR	1.14 (0.65–1.99)	
					Cumulative dose duration:			
					High	NR	1.09 (0.77–1.54)	
					Intermediate	NR	0.92 (0.65–1.29)	
					Low	NR	1.14 (0.82–1.58)	

Table 2.2   (continued)

Reference Study location and period	Total No. cases No. of controls	Control source (hospital, population)	Exposure assessment	Organ site (ICD code)	Exposure categories	Exposed cases	Relative risk (95% CI)	Covariates Comments
Song et al. (2012) Republic of Korea, 2005–11	329 658	Hospital	Electronic medical records	Bladder (confirmed by cytology)	Pioglitazone (–) Pioglitazone (+)	308 21	1.00 (ref.) 2.09 (0.26–16.81)	Alcohol, smoking, coexisting cancer, haemoglobin and albumin Single centre (severance hospital), 1 : 2 age-sex-matched cases:controls; age, > 20 yr. No significant differences in diabetes duration, BMI, and renal function between cases and controls
Hassan et al. (2010) USA, 2000–8	122 86	Hospital	Interviewed with a structured and validated questionnaire	Liver (pathologically confirmed)	TZD (–) TZD (+)	116 6	1.00 (ref.) 0.3 (0.1–0.7)	Age, sex, race, education, cigarette smoking, alcohol drinking, HCV, HBV, and family history of cancer
Chang et al. (2012)c Taiwan, China, 2000–7	10 741 41 847	Population		Liver (linkage through national cancer registry)	*Pioglitazone* Never-user Ever-user Cumulative dosage (DDD): < 120 ≥ 120 Cumulative duration (yr): ≤ 1 1–2 2–3 ≥ 3	 10 267 (non-use) 474 225 249 352 79 30 13	 1.00 (ref.) 0.83 (0.72–0.95) 0.87 (0.72–1.05) 0.80 (0.67–0.95) 0.87 (0.74–1.02) 0.80 (0.59–1.07) 0.71 (0.45–1.14) 0.44 (0.23–0.86)	Age- and sex-matched controls (≥ 4 controls per case). A significantly lower risk of liver cancer was mainly observed in diabetic patients with chronic liver disease and with higher cumulative dosage or longer duration of use

Table 2.2 (continued)

Reference Study location and period	Total No. cases No. of controls	Control source (hospital, population)	Exposure assessment	Organ site (ICD code)	Exposure categories	Exposed cases	Relative risk (95% CI)	Covariates Comments
Chang et al. (2012)[c] Taiwan, China, 2000–7 (cont.)					Rosiglitazone			Age- and sex-matched controls (≥ 4 controls per case). A significantly lower risk of liver cancer was mainly observed in diabetic patients with chronic liver disease and with higher cumulative dosage or longer duration of use
					Never-user of rosiglitazone	9154 (non-use)	1.00 (ref.)	
					Ever-user of rosiglitazone	1587	0.73 (0.65–0.81)	
					Cumulative dosage (DDD):			
					< 120	725	0.86 (0.75–0.98)	
					≥ 120	862	0.64 (0.56–0.72)	
					Cumulative duration (yr):			
					≤ 1	1034	0.78 (0.69–0.88)	
					1–2	330	0.66 (0.56–0.79)	
					2–3	135	0.59 (0.46–0.74)	
					≥ 3	88	0.64 (0.49–0.85)	
Colorectal cancer								
Chang et al. (2012)[d] Taiwan, China, 2000–7	7200 28 712	Population	Reimbursement databases	Colorectum (linkage through national cancer registry)	*Pioglitazone*			Age- and sex-matched controls (≥ 4 controls per case)
					Never-user	6822 (non-use)	1.00 (ref.)	
					Ever-user	378	1.04 (0.91–1.20)	
					Cumulative dosage (DDD):			
					< 120	170	1.15 (0.95–1.39)	
					≥ 120	280	0.97 (0.82–1.16)	
					Cumulative duration (yr):			
					≤ 1	278	1.15 (0.98–1.34)	
					1–2	60	0.82 (0.61–1.11)	
					2–3	26	0.86 (0.55–1.33)	
					≥ 3	14	0.77 (0.43–1.39)	
					Rosiglitazone			
					Never-user	6127	1.00 (ref.)	
					Ever-user	1073	0.86 (0.76–0.96)	
					Cumulative dosage (DDD):			
					< 120	434	0.89 (0.77–1.03)	
					≥ 120	639	0.83 (0.73–0.95)	

Table 2.2 (continued)

Reference Study location and period	Total No. cases No. of controls	Control source (hospital, population)	Exposure assessment	Organ site (ICD code)	Exposure categories	Exposed cases	Relative risk (95% CI)	Covariates Comments
Chang et al. (2012)[d] Taiwan, China, 2000–7 (cont.)					Cumulative duration (yr):			
					≤ 1	678	0.91 (0.80–1.04)	
					1–2	220	0.78 (0.65–0.94)	
					2–3	99	0.69 (0.54–0.88)	
					≥ 3	76	0.83 (0.63–1.10)	
Lung cancer								
Chang et al. (2012)[e] Taiwan, China, 2000–7	5361 21 313	Population	Reimbursement databases	Lung (linkage through national cancer registry)	*Pioglitazone*			
					Never-user	NR	1.00 (ref.)	
					Ever-user	NR	1.14 (0.95–1.37)	
					Cumulative dosage (DDD):			
					< 120	NR	1.13 (0.89–1.44)	
					≥ 120	NR	1.20 (0.96–1.50)	
					Cumulative duration (yr)			
					≤ 1	NR	1.25 (1.01–1.53)	
					1–2	NR	1.09 (0.77–1.53)	
					2–3	NR	0.91 (0.51–1.61)	
					≥ 3	NR	0.20 (0.05–0.86)	
					Cumulative dose duration:			
					High	NR	1.00 (0.75–1.33)	
					Intermediate	NR	1.32 (1.01–1.73)	
					Low	NR	1.16 (0.88–1.51)	
					Rosiglitazone			
					Never-user	NR	1.00 (ref)	
					Ever-user	NR	1.12 (0.90–1.39)	
					Cumulative dosage (DDD):			
					< 120	NR	1.37 (1.08–1.74)	
					≥ 120	NR	1.00 (0.80–1.25)	

Table 2.2 (continued)

Reference Study location and period	Total No. cases No. of controls	Control source (hospital, population)	Exposure assessment	Organ site (ICD code)	Exposure categories	Exposed cases	Relative risk (95% CI)	Covariates Comments
Chang et al. (2012)[e] Taiwan, China, 2000–7 (cont.)					Cumulative duration (yr):			
					≤ 1	NR	1.26 (1.01–1.58)	
					1–2	NR	0.83 (0.63–1.09)	
					2–3	NR	0.96 (0.70–1.33)	
					≥ 3 years	NR	1.17 (0.82–1.67)	
					Cumulative dose duration			
					High	NR	0.95 (0.74–1.22)	
					Intermediate	NR	1.13 (0.89–1.43)	
					Low	NR	1.34 (1.05–1.72)	

[a] Alcohol, obesity, smoking, HbA1c, previous bladder conditions, previous cancer (other than non-melanoma skin cancer), Charlson comorbidity score, and ever-use of other antidiabetic agents (metformin, sulfonylureas, insulin, and other oral hypoglycaemic agents).

[b] Multivariable model with stepwise selection of covariates, including pioglitazone, rosiglitazone, short-acting human insulin, metformin (mean daily dosage in quartiles), sulfonylurea (mean daily dosage in quartiles), number of oral antidiabetic agents, nephropathy, glinides, ACE inhibitors, chronic kidney disease, Ca-channel blockers, neuropathy.

[c] Multivariate model with stepwise selection of covariates, including pioglitazone, rosiglitazone, short-acting human insulin, metformin (mean daily dosage in quartiles), sulfonylurea (mean daily dosage in quartiles), number of oral antidiabetic agents, chronic liver disease, statins, aspirin, β-blockers, chronic kidney disease, glinides (oral antidiabetic agent), nephropathy, cerebrovascular disease, Ca-channel blockers, cardiovascular disease, chronic lung disease.

[d] Multivariate model with stepwise selection of covariates, including pioglitazone, rosiglitazone, short-acting human insulin, metformin (mean daily dosage in quartiles), sulfonylurea (mean daily dosage in quartiles), number of oral antidiabetic agents, glinides, nephropathy, neuropathy, chronic liver disease, statins, retinopathy, Ca-channel blockers, ACE inhibitors, peripheral vascular disease, depression, β-blockers, aspirin, chronic kidney disease, chronic lung disease, cerebrovascular disease.

[e] Multivariable model with stepwise selection of covariates, including pioglitazone, rosiglitazone, short-acting human insulin, metformin (mean daily dosage in quartiles), sulfonylurea (mean daily dosage in quartiles), number of oral antidiabetic agents, chronic lung disease, glinides, retinopathy, Ca-channel blockers, chronic kidney disease, statins, angiotensin receptor blockers, chronic liver disease, α-glucosidase inhibitors.

ACE, angiotensin-converting enzyme; BMI, body mass index; Ca, calcium; d, day; DDD, defined daily doses; HbA1c, glycated haemoglobin; HBV, hepatitis B virus; HCV, hepatitis C virus; mo, month; NR, not reported; ref., reference; TZD, thiazolidinediones; yr, year

2.1.4 Case–control studies

See Table 2.2

Chang *et al.* (2012) conducted a nationwide case–control study to evaluate the risk of several malignancies in diabetic patients who received thiazolidinediones (pioglitazone or rosiglitazone). A total of 606 583 patients with type 2 diabetes, aged ≥ 30 years, without a history of cancer, were identified from the National Health Insurance claims database, Taiwan, China, between 1 January 2000 and 31 December 2000. As of 31 December 2007, patients with incident cancer of the liver, colorectum, lung, or urinary bladder were included as cases, and up to four age- and sex-matched controls were selected by risk-set sampling. Information was collected on prescribed drug types (according to the Anatomic Therapeutic Chemical classification system, A10BG02 for rosiglitazone and A10BG03 for pioglitazone), dosage, date of prescription, supply days, and total number of pills dispensed from the outpatient pharmacy-prescription database. Approximately 26.1% of patients had ever received rosiglitazone, and 14.1% had received pioglitazone. The mean cumulative duration was 522 days, and the mean daily dosage was 0.14 defined daily doses per day for rosiglitazone, compared with 375 days and 0.11 defined daily doses per day for pioglitazone.

With 1583 cases of cancer of the bladder and 70 559 diabetic controls, an increased risk of cancer of the bladder was associated with only ≥ 3 years of pioglitazone use (1.56; 95% CI, 0.51–4.74). The hazard ratio for the highest category of cumulative dose duration was 1.13 (95% CI, 0.69–1.83). [This study had a longer follow-up period than several others evaluating rosiglitazone and pioglitazone, but these drugs did not become available in Taiwan, China, until after follow-up began. The methods were not clearly described and it was not clear how cumulative dose was estimated. The investigators included chronic kidney disease and various drugs in the models. The important risk factor of tobacco smoking could not be adjusted for, but chronic lung disease, a proxy indicator of smoking, was included as a covariate. The study population potentially overlapped with that of Tseng (2012a, 2013a, b).]

In the Republic of Korea, Song *et al.* (2012) conducted a case–control study in diabetic patients with cancer of the bladder (*n* = 329) who presented at one hospital between November 2005 and June 2011. Cases exposed to pioglitazone were matched by sex and age to 658 control patients without cancer of the bladder who were listed on the hospital diabetes registry. The odds ratio for cancer of the bladder associated with a history of pioglitazone use was 2.09 (95% CI, 0.26–16.81) [but it was unclear whether this model was adjusted for potential confounders]. [The Working Group considered that the description of the methods and statistical analysis was inadequate, with conflicting information and some elements of the design (i.e. case–control study in a single tertiary hospital, history of pioglitazone or other medications prescribed before visiting this tertiary centre was not available, recall bias in information on confounders from the retrospective nature of the study, opposite association between pioglitazone use and cancer of the bladder in univariate and multivariate analyses) gave cause for concern.]

2.1.5 Other study designs

A study was conducted by Piccinni *et al.* (2011) using the FDA Adverse Event Reporting System, in the USA. Cases of cancer of the bladder were compared with all other reports of adverse effects within the system; a reporting odds ratio of 4.30 (95% CI, 2.82–6.52) was estimated for cancer of the bladder associated with pioglitazone compared with other antidiabetic drugs, and was elevated in each sex separately. [The Working Group noted that interpretation of these results was challenging because there was no information about the population at risk: adverse event reports for drugs may not be a representative sample of the population. Analyses using the Adverse Events Reporting System may suffer from notoriety bias, but this study was conducted before concerns about pioglitazone were well known.]

2.1.6 Meta-analyses

Several meta-analyses have evaluated the association between the use of thiazolidinediones and cancer of the bladder (Zhu *et al.*, 2012; Colmers *et al.*, 2012b; Bosetti *et al.*, 2013; Ferwana *et al.*, 2013). [The Working Group found it difficult to compare meta-analyses since each included different, but partially overlapping, studies, some of which were unpublished.]

Zhu *et al.* (2012) conducted a meta-analysis on the association between pioglitazone and cancer of the bladder from five studies, including one prospective, randomized, controlled study (Dormandy *et al.*, 2005), three cohort studies (Lewis *et al.*, 2011; Neumann *et al.*, 2012; Tseng, 2012a), and one case–control study (Chang *et al.*, 2012). There was no evidence for the presence of significant heterogeneity between the five studies ($Q = 2.68$, $P = 0.61$; $I^2 = 0.0\%$). The meta-relative risk was 1.17 (95% CI, 1.03–1.32) for all studies. In patients with cumulative treatment exposure to pioglitazone for > 24 months, the meta-relative risk was 1.38 (95% CI, 1.12–1.70), and in those with a cumulative dose of > 28 000 mg, the meta-relative risk was 1.58 (95% CI, 1.12–2.06).

A meta-analysis by Colmers *et al.* (2012b) included unpublished results for cancer of the bladder associated with specific thiazolidinediones. The meta-relative risk for pioglitazone was 1.22 (95% CI, 1.07–1.39) and for rosiglitazone was 0.87 (95% CI, 0.34–2.23).

In a meta-analysis by Bosetti *et al.* (2013), the meta-relative risk was 1.20 (95% CI, 1.07–1.34) from six studies on pioglitazone, and 1.08 (95% CI, 0.95–1.23) from three studies on rosiglitazone.

Longer duration of treatment (> 24 months) (1.42, 1.17–1.72) and higher cumulative dose (> 28 000 mg) of pioglitazone (1.64, 1.28–2.12) were associated with a significantly higher risk.

A meta-analysis by Ferwana *et al.* (2013) included six studies and reported a hazard ratio of 1.23 (95% CI, 1.09–1.39) associated with use of pioglitazone.

2.2 Cancer of the liver

There were no cohort studies evaluating the association between cancer of the liver and specific drugs of the thiazolidinedione class.

In a case–control study, Chang *et al.* (2012) (see Section 2.1.4 for description of study; see Table 2.2), reported a lower risk of cancer of the liver associated with both pioglitazone and rosiglitazone. The adjusted odds ratio (OR) for pioglitazone was 0.83 (95% CI, 0.72–0.95), and for rosiglitazone was 0.73 (95% CI, 0.65–0.81). Odds ratios decreased with increasing categories of duration of pioglitazone use (OR, 0.44; 95% CI, 0.23–0.86 for ≥ 3 years). [Although several risk factors for cancer of the liver were accounted for in the analysis, important potential confounders such as smoking, alcohol use, and hepatitis status, were not accounted for.]

2.3 Cancer of the colorectum

2.3.1 Case–control studies

See Table 2.2

In a multivariate analysis for risk of cancer of the colorectum associated with use of pioglitazone or rosiglitazone, Chang *et al.* (2012) (see Section 2.1.4 for description of study) reported odds ratios of 1.04 (95% CI, 0.91–1.20) associated with pioglitazone use, and 0.86 (95% CI, 0.76–0.96) associated with rosiglitazone use. The magnitude of the odds ratio for the highest exposure duration of ≥ 3 years was very similar for rosiglitazone (OR, 0.83; 95% CI, 0.63–1.10) and for pioglitazone (OR, 0.77; 95% CI, 0.43–1.39). Furthermore, a trend of decreasing odds ratios with increasing cumulative duration of exposure was observed for both rosiglitazone and pioglitazone. [See Section 2.1.4 for the strengths and limitations of this study.]

2.3.2 Cohort studies

See Table 2.1

Ferrara *et al.* (2011) evaluated risk of cancer of the colorectum associated with pioglitazone use in a cohort of 252 467 male and female patients aged ≥ 40 years in the KPNC diabetes registry (see Section 2, introduction, for description). Data on use of diabetes medications were obtained from the pharmacy clinical database, and the filling of two prescriptions of pioglitazone within 6 months was defined as "ever used". Information was collected from electronic medical records about all confounders, except smoking, which was supplemented by postal-survey data. The hazard ratio for cancer of the colorectum associated with ever-use versus never-use of pioglitazone was 0.9 (95% CI, 0.7–1.1), after adjusting for a large number of potential confounders including current smoking, age, and ever-use of other diabetes medications. [This study was based on the same population as Lewis *et al.* (2012). The authors were only able to examine recently initiated therapy and short-term use (median, 1.6 years) of pioglitazone, although the latency period until development of cancer of the bladder may be longer.]

Neumann *et al.* (2012) (see Section 2.1.2 for description of study) investigated risk of cancer of the colorectum in users of pioglitazone or rosiglitazone compared with non-users, and reported hazard ratios of 0.97 (95% CI, 0.90–1.05) for pioglitazone, and 0.88 (95% CI, 0.82–0.95) for rosiglitazone.

Tseng (2012b) (see Section 2.1.2 for description of study) assessed risk of cancer of the colon in thiazolidinedione users versus non-users in a multivariable analysis. Hazard ratios of 0.78 (95% CI, 0.25–2.49) for pioglitazone users, and 1.22 (95% CI, 0.81–1.84) for rosiglitazone users were reported.

2.3.3 Meta-analyses

A meta-analysis derived from three observational studies (Colmers *et al.*, 2012a) calculated a meta-risk ratio of 0.97 (95% CI, 0.90–1.04) for cancer of the colorectum associated with pioglitazone use (see Section 2.1.6 for further description).

2.4 Cancer of the lung

2.4.1 Case–control studies

See Table 2.2

In a multivariable analysis for cancer of the lung, Chang *et al.* (2012) (see Section 2.1.4 for description of study) reported an odds ratio for pioglitazone use of 1.14 (95% CI, 0.95–1.37) and 1.12 (95% CI, 0.90–1.39) associated with rosiglitazone use. A higher risk was reported with a cumulative duration of ≥ 1 year for use of either pioglitazone or rosiglitazone, with adjusted odds ratios of 1.25 (95% CI, 1.01–1.53) and 1.26 (95% CI, 1.01–1.58), respectively. [The investigators included chronic kidney disease and various drugs in the models. The important risk factor of tobacco smoking could not be adjusted for, but chronic lung disease, a proxy indicator of smoking, was included as a covariate.]

2.4.2 Cohort studies

See Table 2.1

In a multivariable analysis in the study by Ferrara *et al.* (2011) (see Section 2.3.2 for description of study), no effect was found on the incidence of cancer of the lung or bronchus in pioglitazone users when compared with never-users (adjusted HR, 1.0; 95% CI, 0.8–1.3). [Adjustment for smoking was a strength of this study, but only current smoking was considered, which may not have fully controlled for confounding.]

Similarly, in a cohort study of diabetic patients in France Neumann *et al.* (2012) (see Section 2.1.2 for description of study) reported no significant difference in the risk of cancer of the lung in users compared with non-exposed controls for pioglitazone (adjusted HR, 0.94; 95% CI, 0.87–1.02), or for rosiglitazone (adjusted HR, 0.91; 95% CI, 0.84–0.99). Hazard ratios were not adjusted for smoking.

2.4.3 Meta-analyses

A meta-analysis of "pulmonary malignancies" by Monami *et al.* (2008) showed that the meta-odds ratio for rosiglitazone versus comparators in clinical trials was 0.67 (95% CI, 0.30–1.51).

Colmers *et al.* (2012a) reported a meta-relative risk for ever-users of pioglitazone versus never-users of 0.95 (95% CI, 0.88–1.02) from two observational studies.

2.5 Cancer of the prostate

See Table 2.1

No case–control studies evaluated the association between use of pioglitazone or rosiglitazone and cancer of the prostate.

A cohort study by Ferrara *et al.* (2011) (see Section 2.3.2 for description of study) found no association when comparing ever-use of pioglitazone versus never-use (adjusted HR, 1.0; 95% CI, 0.8–1.2). Tseng (2011) (see Section 2 introduction for description of study) reported an inverse association for ever-use of pioglitazone versus never-use (adjusted HR, 0.77; 95% CI, 0.10–5.75) and for rosiglitazone (adjusted HR, 0.88; 95% CI, 0.43–1.80).

Two meta-analyses (Monami *et al.*, 2008; Colmers *et al.*, 2012a) reported meta-relative risks of around unity for cancer of the prostate associated with the use of pioglitazone or rosiglitazone.

2.6 Cancer of the breast

In the PROactive clinical trial (Dormandy *et al.*, 2005; see Section 2.1.1 for description of study), an imbalance in the number of cases of cancer of the breast was noted, with three cases in the pioglitazone group and eleven in the placebo group. [Insufficient data were provided to calculate a risk estimate. The PROactive trial was primarily aimed at evaluating macrovascular events associated with pioglitazone use.]

In a multivariable analysis in the study by Ferrara *et al.* (2011) (see Section 2.3.2 and 2.4.2 for comments and description of study; see Table 2.1), no effect was found in the incidence of cancer of the breast in pioglitazone users when compared with never-users (adjusted HR, 1.0; 95% CI, 0.8–1.3).

Similarly, a cohort study of diabetic patients in France (Neumann *et al.*, 2012; see Section 2.3.2 for comments and description of study; see Table 2.1) reported no significant difference in the risk of cancer of the breast in pioglitazone users when compared with non-exposed controls (adjusted HR, 0.91; 95% CI, 0.83–1.00). A significantly reduced risk of cancer of the breast was found in rosiglitazone users when compared with non-exposed controls (adjusted HR, 0.80; 95% CI, 0.73–0.88).

The meta-relative risk estimated by Colmers *et al.* (2012a) for cancer of the breast in ever-users of pioglitazone versus never-users from two observational studies was 0.93 (95% CI, 0.85–1.01).

2.7 Other site-specific cancers

See Table 2.1

Several of the studies described above also reported on other site-specific cancers. The study by Ferrara *et al.* (2011) reported relative risks of > 1 for some other cancers.

Neumann *et al.* (2012) reported a hazard ratio of near unity for cancer of the kidney among users of pioglitazone or rosiglitazone, and hazard ratios of approximately 0.8 for both agents for cancer of the head and neck.

By using the National Health Insurance database of Taiwan, China, Tseng evaluated the association of pioglitazone and rosiglitazone with the risk of cancer of the thyroid (Tseng, 2012c), and cancer of the oral cavity, lip, and pharynx (Tseng, 2013c), respectively. The hazard ratio for cancer of the thyroid was 0.52 (95% CI, 0.07–3.93) for pioglitazone and 0.67 (95% CI, 0.23–1.95) for rosiglitazone (Tseng, 2012c); for cancer of the oral cavity, lip, and pharynx, the hazard ratio was 1.70 (95% CI, 0.22–13.20) for pioglitazone and 1.15 (95% CI, 0.44–3.04) for rosiglitazone (Tseng, 2013c).

In a meta-analysis by Colmers *et al.* (2012a), the meta-risk ratio for cancer of the kidney was 0.89 (95% CI, 0.76–1.04) for ever-users of pioglitazone versus never-users from two observational studies.

3. Cancer in Experimental Animals

3.1 Pioglitazone

3.1.1 Oral administration

(a) Mouse

See Table 3.1

As part of its pharmacology review of the New Drug Application package (NDA 21–073) for pioglitazone submitted by the Takeda America Research and Development Center, the FDA summarized the results of a 2-year study that was performed to evaluate the potential carcinogenicity of pioglitazone in mice (FDA, 1999a). In this study, groups of 60 male and 60 female CD-1 mice [age not reported] received pioglitazone by gavage at doses of 0 (vehicle), 0 (placebo suspension), 3, 10, 30, or 100 mg/kg body weight (bw) per day for 104 weeks. [Vehicle and placebo suspension were not specified.]

There was a significant positive trend towards increased mortality with increasing dose in male mice. Increased incidences of benign pheochromocytoma of the adrenal gland were seen in exposed male mice, and increased incidences of leiomyosarcoma of the uterine cervix were seen in exposed female mice when compared with controls. [Although it was noted that the FDA identified these differences as being statistically significant, the Working Group could not confirm the statistical analyses because original study data (e.g. mortality) were not available (FDA, 1999a).]

(b) Genetically engineered mouse

Pino *et al.* (2004) reported increased incidence and multiplicity of adenoma of the large intestine in Apc^{Min}/+ mice (a genetically engineered mouse model that overexpresses the *Apc* gene, leading to rapid development of intestinal neoplasms) with dietary exposure to any of several peroxisome proliferator-activated receptor γ (PPARγ) agonists, including pioglitazone. In this study, male C57BL/6J-Apc^{Min}/+ mice (age, 6–7 weeks) were fed diets containing pioglitazone at a concentration selected to achieve a dose of 150 mg/kg bw per day for 8 weeks. All mice exposed to pioglitazone (15 out of 15, 100% [$P < 0.01$]) developed adenoma of the large intestine, compared with 60% (9 out of 15 mice) in the dietary control group. Pioglitazone increased the multiplicity of tumours of the large intestine, but not of the small intestine [data and statistics were provided in graphical form]. [The Working Group noted that, although used extensively as a model system for cancer chemoprevention, the predictive value of the Apc^{Min}/+ mouse in the identification of agents that may promote or otherwise stimulate carcinogenesis in the human colon was unknown.]

(c) Rat

See Table 3.2

Table 3.1 Studies of carcinogenicity in mice given pioglitazone orally

Strain (sex) Duration Reference	Dosing regimen, Animals/group at start	Incidence of tumours	Significance	Comments
CD-1 (M, F) 104 wk FDA (1999a)	0 (vehicle control), 0 (placebo suspension), 3, 10, 30, 100 mg/kg bw per day by gavage in an unspecified vehicle or suspension. 60 M and 60 F/group	Benign pheochromocytoma of the adrenal gland: 0/60, 0/60, 0/60, 0/60, 2/60*, 1/60* (M) Leiomyosarcoma of the uterine cervix: 0/60, 0/60, 0/60, 0/60, 1/60*, 1/60* (F)	*$P < 0.05$ (Peto test)	The Working Group was unable to confirm the statistical analyses. Increase in mortality in exposed males.
C57BL6J-Apc^{Min}/+ (M) 8 wk Pino et al. (2004)	Pioglitazone mixed in feed and given to achieve daily doses of 0 or ~150 mg/kg bw 15/group	Large intestine adenoma : 9/15, 15/15*	*[$P < 0.01$] $P \leq 0.05$ for increased multiplicity of large intestine tumour [data and statistics read from graph]	Genetically engineered mouse sensitive to intestinal carcinogenesis. No increases in the multiplicity of small intestine tumours.

bw, body weight; F, female, M, male; wk, week

Table 3.2 Studies of carcinogenicity in rats given pioglitazone orally

Strain (sex) Duration Reference	Dosing regimen, Animals/group at start	Incidence of tumours	Significance	Comments
Sprague-Dawley (M, F) 104 wk FDA (1999a)	0 (vehicle control), 0 (placebo suspension), 1, 4, 8 (M only), 16, or 63 mg/kg bw per day by gavage in an unspecified vehicle or suspension 60 M and 60 F/group	Transitional cell carcinoma of urinary bladder: 0/60, 0/60, 0/60, 2/60, 3/60, 5/60, 4/60 (M) 0/60, 0/60, 0/60, 0/60, –, 0/60, 0/60 (F)	$P < 0.025$ (trend) (M)	Increase in mortality in exposed M and F
		Transitional cell papilloma of urinary bladder: 0/60, 0/60, 0/60, 0/60, 4/60, 2/60, 2/60 (M); 0/60, 0/60, 1/60, 1/60, –, 1/60, 0/60 (F)	NS	
		Fibrosarcoma of subcutis: 0/60, 0/60, 0/60, 0/60, 0/60, 2/60, 2/60 (M)	$P < 0.025$ (trend)	
		Subcutaneous lipoma: 0/60, 0/60, 1/60, 0/60, –, 1/60, 3/60 (F)	$P < 0.025$ (trend)	
CD (M) 104 wk Sato et al. (2011)	0 (control) or 16 mg/kg bw by gavage in citric acid granules for 85 wk 90/group	Urinary bladder Papilloma: 0/78, 7/82* Carcinoma: 0/78, 1/82	*$P \leq 0.05$ (Peto test)	

bw, body weight; F, female, M, male; NS, not significant; wk, week

As part of its pharmacology review of the New Drug Application package (NDA 21–073) for pioglitazone submitted by the Takeda America Research and Development Center, the FDA summarized the results of a 2-year study that was performed to evaluate the potential carcinogenicity of pioglitazone in rats (FDA, 1999a). In this study, groups of 60 male and 60 female Sprague-Dawley rats [age not reported] received pioglitazone by gavage at doses of 0 (vehicle), 0 (placebo suspension), 1, 4, 8 (males only), 16, or 63 mg/kg bw per day for 104 weeks. [Vehicle and placebo suspension were not specified.] There was a significant positive trend towards increased mortality with increasing dose in male and female rats.

Treatment with pioglitazone caused a significant positive trend in the incidence of transitional cell carcinoma of the urinary bladder in male rats. Although female rats did not demonstrate an increased incidence of transitional cell tumours of the urinary bladder, urothelial hyperplastic lesions were identified in male and female rats exposed to pioglitazone. In addition, pioglitazone induced a small but significant positive trend in the incidence of fibrosarcoma of the subcutis in male rats, and a significant positive trend in the incidence of subcutaneous lipoma in female rats (FDA, 1999a).

Sato *et al.* (2011) reported a study in which two groups of 90 male CD rats (age, 6 weeks) received pioglitazone (in citric acid granules) by gavage at a dose of 0 (control), or 16 mg/kg bw per day for 85 weeks, followed by a 19-week observation period. There was a significant increase in the incidence of papilloma of the urinary bladder in the exposed group (7 out of 82 rats) compared with the controls (0 out of 78 rats). There was also one carcinoma of the urinary bladder in the exposed group compared with none in the controls.

3.1.2 Coexposure with modifying agents

See Table 3.3

A group of 34 male and 35 female strain H Swiss mice was exposed by whole-body inhalation to mainstream cigarette smoke for 4 months, starting 12 hours after birth, and then kept in filtered air until the experiment was terminated at age 7 months. After weaning (at age 4–5 weeks), the mice also received diets containing pioglitazone at a concentration of 120 mg/kg. A control group of 34 male and 38 female mice was exposed to mainstream cigarette smoke only. In females, 5 out of 35 ($P < 0.01$) mice exposed to pioglitazone developed adenoma of the kidney versus 0 out of 38 controls. In males, 3 out of 32 mice developed kidney adenoma versus 0 out of 34 controls (La Maestra *et al.*, 2013).

3.2 Rosiglitazone

3.2.1 Oral administration

(a) Mouse

See Table 3.4

As part of its pharmacology review of the New Drug Application package (NDA 21–071) for rosiglitazone that was submitted by SmithKline Beecham Pharmaceuticals, the FDA summarized the results of a 2-year feeding study that was performed to evaluate the potential carcinogenicity of rosiglitazone in mice (FDA, 1999b). In this study, groups of 60 male and 60 female CD-1 mice [age not reported] received diet supplemented with rosiglitazone at concentrations that were selected to provide doses of 0 (control), 0.4, 1.5, or 6.0 mg/kg bw for 105 weeks. A significant positive trend towards increased mortality with increasing dose was seen in male and female mice. The reduction in survival of male mice in the group at the highest dose necessitated early termination of this dose group at week 95, instead of week 105. The only significant increase in the incidence of any neoplasm

Table 3.3 Studies of carcinogenicity involving exposure to pioglitazone or rosiglitazone with modifying agents

Species, strain (sex) Duration Reference	Modifying agent	Dosing regimen, Animals/group at start	Incidence of tumours	Significance
Mouse, H Swiss (M, F) 7 mo La Maestra *et al.* (2013)	Mainstream cigarette smoke by whole-body inhalation for 4 mo, starting 12 hours after birth, followed by filtered air for 3 mo	After weaning (at age, 4–5 wk), mice were also fed diets containing pioglitazone at a concentration of 0 (control) or 120 mg/kg. 34, 34/group (M) 38, 35/group (F)	Kidney adenoma: 0/34, 3/32 (M) 0/38, 5/35* (F)	*$P < 0.01$
Rat, F344 (F) 7 mo Lubet *et al.* (2008)	*N*-Butyl-*N*-(4-hydroxybutyl)nitrosamine (150 mg) by gavage in thanol : water, 2×/wk for 8 wk	After 2 wk, rats were given rosiglitazone by gavage at 0 (control), 50 mg/kg bw per day 35, 35/group	Urinary bladder carcinoma: 20/35, 34/34*	*$P < 0.01$
Rat, F344 (F) 8 mo Lubet *et al.* (2008)	*N*-Butyl-*N*-(4-hydroxybutyl)nitrosamine (150 mg) by gavage in ethanol : water, 2×/wk for 8 wk	2 wk later, rats were given rosiglitazone by gavage at 0 (control), 10 mg/kg bw per day 29, 30/group	Urinary bladder carcinoma: 8/29, 28/30*	*$P < 0.01$
Rat, F344 (F) 10 mo Lubet *et al.* (2008)	*N*-Butyl-*N*-(4-hydroxybutyl)nitrosamine (150 mg) by gavage in ethanol : water, 2×/wk for 8 wk	2 wk later, rats were given rosiglitazone by gavage at 0 (control), 0.4, or 2 mg/kg bw per day 25, 29, 30/group	Urinary bladder carcinoma : 12/25, 19/29, 24/30*	*$P < 0.05$

bw, body weight; F, female, mo, month; M, male; wk, week

Table 3.4 Studies of carcinogenicity in mice given diets containing rosiglitazone

Strain (sex) Duration Reference	Dosing regimen, Animals/group at start	Incidence of tumours	Significance	Comments
CD-1 (M, F) 105 wk FDA (1999b)	Rosiglitazone mixed in feed to achieve doses of 0 (control), 0.4, 1.5, or 6.0 mg/kg bw per day 60 M and 60 F/group	Liver haemangiosarcoma: 0/60, 4/60*, 0/60, 0/60 (M)	*$P = 0.013$	There was a significant trend for increasing mortality with increasing dose in M and F. High-dose males were killed at wk 95. No increase in the incidence of any type of neoplasm in females
C57BL6J-Apc[Min]/+ (M) 8 wk Pino et al. (2004)	Rosiglitazone mixed in feed to achieve doses of 0 or ~20 mg/kg bw per day 15/group	Large intestine adenoma : 9/15, 14/14*	*$[P < 0.01]$ $P \leq 0.05$ for increased multiplicity of large intestine tumours [data and statistics read from graph]	Genetically engineered mouse sensitive to intestinal carcinogenesis. No increases in multiplicity of small intestine tumours.

bw, body weight; F, female, M, male; wk, week; NR, not reported in any dose group was an increased incidence of liver haemangiosarcoma in male mice at the lowest dose (FDA, 1999b). [Because no significant evidence of a dose–response relationship was seen, the Working Group concluded that there was no treatment-related positive trend in the incidence of liver haemangiosarcoma, or of any other tumour type in either sex.]

(b) Genetically engineered mouse

Pino *et al.* (2004) reported increased incidence and multiplicity of adenoma of the large intestine in Apc^{Min}/+ mice (a genetically engineered mouse model that overexpresses the *Apc* gene, leading to rapid development of intestinal neoplasms) with dietary exposure to rosiglitazone. In this study, male C57BL6J-Apc^{Min}/+ mice (age, 6–7 weeks) were fed rosiglitazone at a dietary concentration selected to achieve a dose of 20 mg/kg bw per day, for 8 weeks. All mice exposed to rosiglitazone (14 out of 14, 100% [$P < 0.01$]) developed adenoma of the large intestine, compared with 60% (9 out of 15 mice) in the dietary controls group. Rosiglitazone increased the multiplicity of tumours of the large intestine, but not of the small intestine [data and statistics were provided in in graphical form]. [The Working Group noted that, although used extensively as a model system for cancer chemoprevention, the predictive value of the Apc^{Min}/+ mouse in the identification of agents that may promote or otherwise stimulate carcinogenesis in the human colon was unknown.]

(c) Rat

See Table 3.5

As part of its pharmacology review of the New Drug Application package (NDA 21–071) for rosiglitazone submitted by SmithKline Beecham Pharmaceuticals, the FDA summarized the results of a 2-year study that was performed to evaluate the potential carcinogenicity of rosiglitazone in rats (FDA, 1999b). In this study, groups of 60 male and 60 female Sprague-Dawley rats

[age not reported] received rosiglitazone by gavage at doses of 0 (control), 0.05, 0.3, or 2.0 mg/kg bw per day in 1% methylcellulose for 2 years. In comparison to vehicle controls, a significant increase in mortality was seen in males at the highest dose. Significant increases in the incidence of subcutaneous lipoma were seen in males at the intermediate dose, and in females at the highest dose. [Increases in the incidence of subcutaneous lipoma and adipocyte hyperplasia (a putative preneoplastic lesion that is linked to lipoma) in males and females, were considered to be treatment-related.]

3.2.2 Coexposure with modifying agents

See Table 3.3

In two studies evaluating the activity of rosiglitazone as a chemopreventive agent for cancer of the urinary bladder, groups of female F344 rats received *N*-butyl-*N*-(4-hydroxybutyl) nitrosamine (BBN) by gavage in 0.1 mL ethanol : water (25 : 75, v/v), twice per week, for 8 weeks. Beginning 2 weeks after the last dose of BBN, parallel groups of rats were given rosiglitazone at a dose of 0.4, 2, 10, or 50 mg/kg bw per day by gavage, or the vehicle (carboxymethylcellulose : polyethylene glycol 400; 50 : 50, v/v) only, for 7–10 months, followed by necropsy and histopathological examination of the urinary bladder (Lubet *et al.*, 2008).

In the first study, the incidence of carcinoma of the urinary bladder in rats exposed to BBN plus rosiglitazone (50 mg/kg bw per day) for 7 months was 100% (34 out of 34; $P < 0.01$), compared with 57% (20 out of 35) in the group exposed to BBN only. In the follow-up study with lower doses of rosiglitazone, the incidence of carcinoma of the urinary bladder at 8 months in the group receiving BBN plus rosiglitazone (10 mg/kg bw per day) was 93% (28 out of 30; $P < 0.01$), compared with 28% (8 out of 29) in the group exposed to BBN only. In the same study, the incidence of carcinoma of the urinary bladder at 10 months in groups treated

Table 3.5 Studies of carcinogenicity in rats given rosiglitazone by gavage

Strain (sex) Duration Reference	Dosing regimen, Animals/group at start	Incidence of tumours	Significance	Comments
Sprague-Dawley (M, F) 104 wk FDA (1999b)	Rosiglitazone given at doses of 0, 0 (second control group), 0.05, 0.3, or 2.0 mg/kg bw in 1% methylcellulose 60 M and 60 F/group	Subcutaneous lipoma: 3/60, 4/60, 5/59, 13/58*, 6/60 (M) 1/60, 2/60, 3/60, 1/59, 9/60** (F)	*$P = 0.001$ **$P = 0.003$	Significantly increased mortality in high-dose males Second control group reported, but no information on how it differed from the first control group

bw, body weight; F, female, M, male; wk, week

with BBN plus rosiglitazone (2 or 0.4 mg/kg bw per day) group was 80% (24 out of 30; $P < 0.05$) and 67% (19 out of 29), versus 48% (12 out of 25) in BBN-treated vehicle controls. When administered alone (without prior exposure to BNN), rosiglitazone (10 mg/kg bw) did not induce carcinoma of the urinary bladder during the 8-month observation period. [The Working Group noted that the predictive value of the BBN model for the identification of agents that can enhance or promote cancer of the human bladder had not been established.]

4. Mechanistic and Other Relevant Data

4.1 Absorption, distribution, metabolism, and excretion of pioglitazone

4.1.1 Humans

(a) Absorption, distribution, and excretion

In fasting individuals, pioglitazone was measurable in the serum within 30 minutes after oral administration, with peak concentrations observed within 2 hours. Administration with food slightly delayed the time to peak serum concentration (to 3–4 hours), but did not alter the extent of absorption. The mean serum half-life of pioglitazone ranged from 3 to 7 hours, while the

mean serum half-life of the pharmacologically active metabolites M-III and M-IV ranged from 16 to 24 hours. Serum concentrations of total pioglitazone (pioglitazone plus active metabolites) remained elevated 24 hours after dosing (Takeda Pharmaceuticals, 2013).

The apparent oral clearance (CL/F) of pioglitazone has been calculated as 5–7 L per hour. The mean apparent volume of distribution (Vd/F) of pioglitazone after administration of a single oral dose was 0.63 ± 0.41 (mean ± standard deviation) L/kg bw. Pioglitazone binds extensively (> 99%) to protein in human serum, principally to serum albumin. Pioglitazone also binds other serum proteins, but with lower affinity. Metabolites M-III and M-IV also are extensively bound (> 98%) to serum albumin (Takeda Pharmaceuticals, 2013).

Steady-state serum concentrations of pioglitazone and total pioglitazone were achieved within 7 days. At steady state, M-III and M-IV reached serum concentrations equal to or greater than that of pioglitazone. In healthy volunteers and in patients with type 2 diabetes, pioglitazone comprised approximately 30–50% of the peak total pioglitazone serum concentrations and 20–25% of the total area under the curve (AUC) for serum concentration–time. Maximum serum concentration (C_{max}), AUC, and trough serum concentration (C_{min}) for pioglitazone and total pioglitazone increased proportionally at doses of 15 mg and 30 mg per day (Takeda Pharmaceuticals, 2013).

After oral administration, 15–30% of the administered dose of pioglitazone was recovered in the urine. Most of the oral dose was excreted into the bile either unchanged or as metabolites, and eliminated in the faeces. Renal elimination of pioglitazone was negligible (Takeda Pharmaceuticals, 2013).

There was no significant difference in the pharmacokinetic profile of pioglitazone in subjects with normal or with moderately impaired renal function. In patients with moderate and severe renal impairment, although mean serum concentrations of pioglitazone and its metabolites were increased, no dose adjustment is needed. After repeated oral doses of pioglitazone, mean AUC values were decreased in patients with severe renal impairment compared with healthy subjects with normal renal function for pioglitazone (Budde *et al.*, 2003).

In a multi-dosing study, pioglitazone was rapidly absorbed, with median time to maximal serum concentration (C_{max}) occurring within 2 hours. Serum concentrations of pioglitazone and its active metabolites remained elevated 24 hours after exposure (Christensen *et al.*, 2005).

(b) Metabolism

Pioglitazone is extensively metabolized by hydroxylation and oxidation to its active metabolites, which are keto and hydroxy derivatives. The active metabolites include M-II active (hydroxy), M-III active (keto), and M-IV active (hydroxy) (Fig. 4.1; Takeda Pharmaceuticals, 2013).

In-vitro data have demonstrated that multiple isoforms of cytochrome P450 (CYP) are involved in the metabolism of pioglitazone, including CYP2C8 and, to a lesser degree, CYP3A4 (Kirchheiner *et al.*, 2005). CYP2C9 is not significantly involved in the elimination of pioglitazone (Jaakkola *et al.*, 2006). Pioglitazone is not a strong inducer of CYP3A4, and pioglitazone was not shown to induce CYPs (Nowak *et al.*, 2002).

4.1.2 Experimental systems

In pharmacokinetic studies with male rats, peak plasma concentrations of pioglitazone were reported at 1 hour, and the plasma terminal half-life of pioglitazone was 7.5 hours. The distribution of pioglitazone was not extensive; the tissue/plasma ratio was low (< 0.5), except for the gastrointestinal tract (Krieter *et al.*, 1994).

The AUCs for pioglitazone metabolites M-III and M-IV were higher in female rats than in males, while levels of M-II were similar in both sexes (Fujita *et al.*, 2003).

4.2 Absorption, distribution, metabolism, and excretion of rosiglitazone

4.2.1 Humans

(a) Absorption, distribution, and excretion

In a study in healthy volunteers, the absorption of rosiglitazone was relatively rapid, with 99% oral bioavailability after oral absorption (Cox *et al.*, 2000).

Peak plasma concentrations were observed about 1 hour after single oral doses. Maximum plasma concentration (C_{max}) and the AUC of rosiglitazone increased in a dose-proportional manner over the therapeutic dose range (National Library of Medicine, 2010).

The mean oral volume of distribution of rosiglitazone was approximately 17.6 L, based on a population pharmacokinetic analysis. Rosiglitazone is approximately 99.8% bound to plasma proteins, primarily albumin (National Library of Medicine, 2010).

The elimination half-life of rosiglitazone was 3–4 hours and was independent of dose. The time to C_{max} and the elimination half-life for two metabolites in plasma were significantly longer than for rosiglitazone itself (4–6 hours versus 0.5–1 hours, and about 5 days versus 3–7 hours) (Cox *et al.*, 2000).

Fig. 4.1 Pioglitazone and metabolites

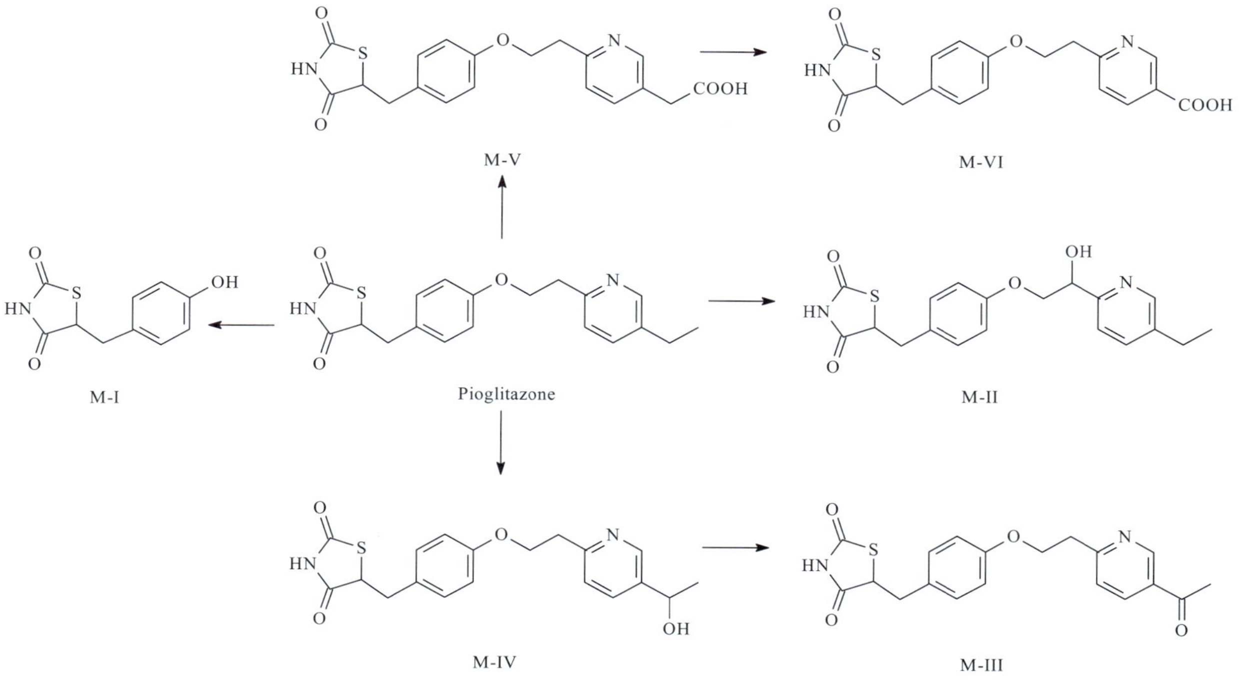

Compiled by the Working Group

After oral or intravenous administration of rosiglitazone maleate, approximately 64% and 23% of the administered dose was eliminated in the urine and in the faeces, respectively (National Library of Medicine, 2010). No unchanged drug was eliminated in the urine.

In a pharmacokinetics study of administration of rosiglitazone with food, absorption measured via T_{max} was delayed by 1.75 hours. The C_{max} was reduced by approximately 20%, but the geometric mean ratio of AUC for the fed/fasted state was 0.94. No dose adjustment is required for administration of rosiglitazone with food (Freed *et al.*, 1999).

The half-life values of rosiglitazone are similar in fasted and fed subjects (Bulliman *et al.*, 1995).

Ethnicity had no impact on the pharmacokinetics of rosiglitazone among healthy subjects (Chu *et al.*, 2007).

In patients with mild, moderate, or severe renal insufficiency there are slight increases in AUC for rosiglitazone (10–20%), which were not deemed to be clinically relevant (Chapelsky *et al.*, 2003).

In a placental transfer study, the risk of placental transfer of rosiglitazone was higher after 10 weeks of gestation (Chan *et al.*, 2005).

(b)   Metabolism

Rosiglitazone is extensively metabolized by CYP2C9 and CYP2C8, with no unchanged drug excreted in the urine (Kirchheiner *et al.*, 2005). The major routes of metabolism were *N*-demethylation and hydroxylation, leading to *N*-desmethyl-rosiglitazone and 3-hydroxy-rosiglitazone, followed by conjugation with sulfate and glucuronic acid. All the circulating metabolites were considerably less potent than the parent compound and, therefore, are not expected to contribute to the activity of rosiglitazone (National Library of Medicine, 2010; see Fig. 4.2).

Fig. 4.2 Rosiglitazone and metabolites

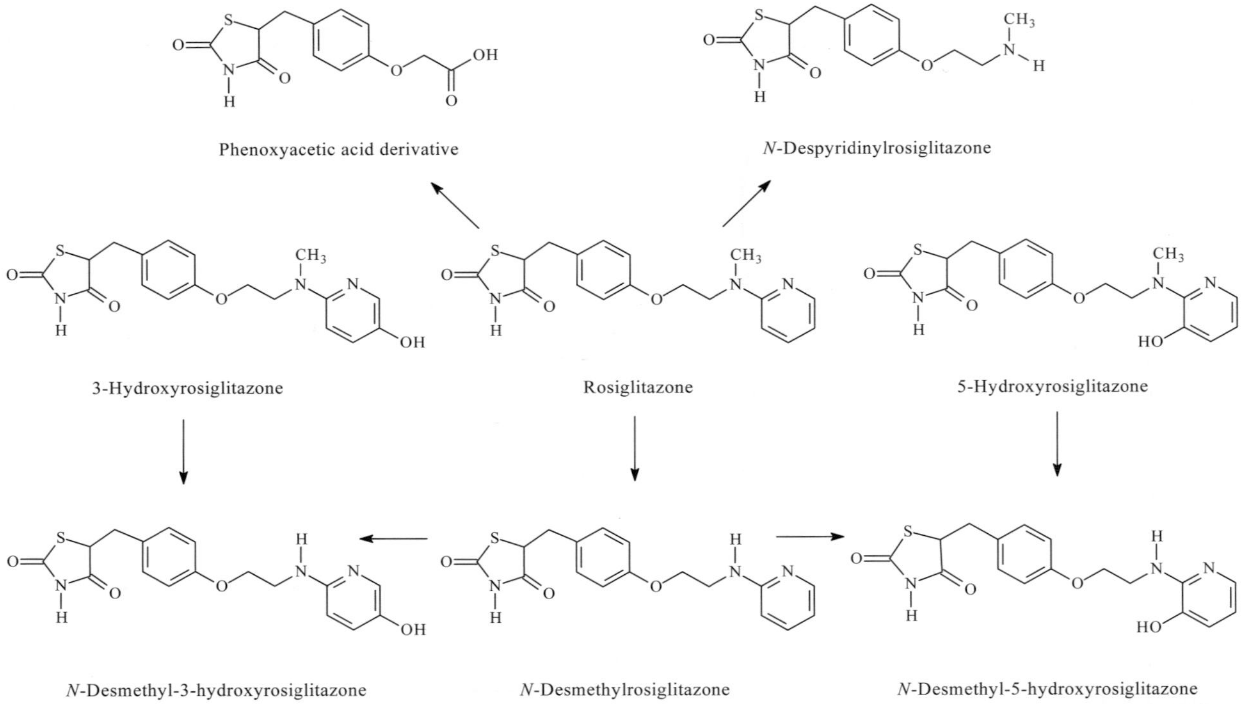

Compiled by the Working Group

4.2.2 Experimental systems

Rosigilitazone was extensively metabolized after oral administration in mice. Mean bioavailability was found to be 100%, 60%, and 95% in rats, dogs, and humans, respectively (EMEA, 2005).

The main metabolites observed in humans are also observed in rats; however, the clearance in rats was almost ten times higher than in humans, probably due to the higher levels of CYP2C in rat microsomes (EMEA, 2005; Calixto *et al.*, 2011).

4.3 Genetic and related effects

4.3.1 Humans

DNA damage

Incubating pioglitazone (100 μM) with human peripheral blood lymphocytes significantly increased the frequency of chromosomal aberrations, sister chromatid exchanges, and increased levels of 8-oxodeoxyguanosine (Table 4.1; Alzoubi *et al.*, 2012).

4.3.2 Experimental systems

(a) DNA damage

Male Sprague-Dawley rats treated with pioglitazone by gavage had a dose-dependent increase in the frequency of DNA damage in peripheral blood lymphoctyes and liver cells, as measured by comet assays. The addition of an enzyme mixture containing endonuclease III and formamidopyrimidine glycosylase significantly increased the frequency of DNA damage, suggesting that DNA damage was due to oxidation of DNA bases (Table 4.1; Bedir *et al.*, 2008).

Pioglitazone did not increase the frequency of chromosomal aberrations in Chinese hamster lung cells. Pioglitazone did not induce unscheduled DNA synthesis in primary rat hepatocytes,

Table 4.1 Genetic and related effects of pioglitazone

Test system	Results		Dose or concentration (LED or HID)	Reference
	Without exogenous metabolic system	With exogenous metabolic system		
In vitro				
Salmonella typhimurium, TA98, TA100, TA1535, TA1537, with 20-minute pre-incubation, reverse mutation	–	–	5000 µg/plate	FDA Drug Approval Package (1999a)
Salmonella typhimurium, TA98, TA100, TA1535, TA1537, TA1538, reverse mutation	–	–	2000 µg/plate	FDA Drug Approval Package (1999a)
Escherichia coli WP2 *uvrA*, with 20-minute pre-incubation, mutation	–	–	5000 µg/plate	FDA Drug Approval Package (1999a)
Gene mutation, Chinese hamster ovary cells, *Hprt* gene	–	–	200 µg/mL – S9; 500 µg/mL + S9	FDA Drug Approval Package (1999a)
Gene mutation, AS52 Chinese hamster cells, *Xprt* gene	–	–	200 µg/mL – S9; 200 µg/mL + S9	FDA Drug Approval Package (1999a)
Unscheduled DNA synthesis, male F344 rat primary hepatocytes	–	NT	100 µg/mL	FDA Drug Approval Package (1999a)
Chromosomal aberration, Chinese hamster lung cells	–	–	5 mM	FDA Drug Approval Package (1999a)
Chromosomal aberration, human peripheral blood lymphocytes	+	NT	100 µM	Alzoubi *et al.* (2012)
Sister chromatid exchange, human peripheral blood lymphocytes	+	NT	100 µM	Alzoubi *et al.* (2012)
8-Oxodeoxyguanosine, human peripheral blood lymphocytes	+	NT	100 µM	Alzoubi *et al.* (2012)
In vivo				
Micronucleus formation, CD-1 mice	–		5000 mg/kg bw per day, single intraperitoneal injection, up to 72 hours	FDA Drug Approval Package (1999a)
Comet assay, male Sprague-Dawley rat peripheral blood lymphocytes	+		10 mg/kg bw per day, by gavage, for 14 days	Bedir *et al.* (2008)
Comet assay, male Sprague-Dawley rat liver cells	+		10 mg/kg bw per day, by gavage, for 14 days	Bedir *et al.* (2008)

+, positive; –, negative; HID, highest ineffective dose; LED, lowest effective dose; NR, not reported; NT, not tested or micronucleus formation in CD-1 mice (Table 4.1; FDA Drug Approval Package, 1999a).

Male Sprague-Dawley rats treated with rosiglitazone by gavage showed a dose-dependent increase in the frequency of DNA damage in peripheral blood lymphoctyes and liver cells, as measured by comet assays (Table 4.2; Bedir *et al.*, 2006).

In-vitro assays for chromosomal aberration and unscheduled DNA synthesis, and in-vivo assays for micronucleus formation gave negative results with rosiglitazone (Table 4.2; FDA Drug Approval Package, 1999b).

Rosiglitazone gave negative results in the Growth Arrest and DNA Damage gene 45α-Green Fluorescent Protein (GADD45α-GFP) GreenScreen Human Cell genotoxicity assay in the presence or absence of metabolic activation (Table 4.2; Luzy *et al.*, 2012).

(b)   Gene mutations

Pioglitazone and its metabolites M-I, M-IV, M-V, and M-VI were not mutagenic in *Salmonella typhimurium* strains TA98, TA100, TA1535, or TA1537, or in *Escherichia coli* strain WP2 *uvrA*, in either the presence or absence of metabolic activation. Pioglitazone was not mutagenic at the *Hprt* gene of Chinese hamster ovary cells, or at the *Xprt* gene of AS52 Chinese hamster cells. Pioglitazone metabolites M-I and M-VI were mutagenic in mouse lymphoma L5178Y cells in the presence of metabolic activation; metabolites M-IV and M-V gave negative results, and the assay conducted with pioglitazone was considered inadequate (Table 4.1; Table 4.3; FDA Drug Approval Package, 1999a).

Rosiglitazone was not mutagenic in *S. typhimurium* strains TA98, TA100, TA1535, TA1537, or TA1538, or in *E. coli* strain WP2 *uvrA*, in either the presence or absence of an exogenous metabolic activation system. Rosiglitazone was mutagenic in mouse lymphoma L5178Y cells in the presence of metabolic activation (Table 4.2; FDA Drug Approval Package, 1999b).

4.4   Other mechanistic data

Pioglitazone selectively stimulates PPARγ, and to a lesser extent PPARα (Smith, 2001). Acidification of the urine, as a result of ammonium chloride administration in male rats, did not alter PPARα, PPARβ (PPARδ), or PPARγ mRNA or protein expression, PPARα- or PPARγ-regulated gene expression, total or phosphorylated epidermal growth factor receptor (Egfr) protein, *Egfr* or *Akt2* gene expression, or urothelial-cell proliferation. These results suggested that the suppression of bladder tumorigenesis by acidifying the urine of rats exposed to PPARγ agonists, such as pioglitazone, was not due to alterations in PPARα, PPARβ, or Egfr expression or PPAR signalling in the bladder epithelium of rats (Achanzar *et al.*, 2007; Sato *et al.*, 2011).

Roglitazone significantly increased the incidence of tumours of the bladder induced BBN in female F344 rats. The mechanism for the induction of these tumours was not known (Lubet *et al.*, 2008).

Strain H Swiss mice exposed to mainstream cigarette smoke since birth for 4 months, and subsequently exposed to pioglitazone, had lower levels of DNA damage in exfoliated bladder cells, as measured by comet assays, than mice exposed to mainstream cigarette smoke and fed control diet. However, the mice exposed to mainstream cigarette smoke and then pioglitazone had an increased incidence of kidney tubular epithelium hyperplasia, kidney adenoma, kidney lesions, and/or urinary tract lesions, compared with mice exposed to mainstream cigarette smoke only, or sham-treated mice. These data suggested that pioglitazone can act as a promoter of tumours of the kidney in mice. Mice exposed to mainstream cigarette smoke and pioglitazone had more acidic urine than sham-exposed mice (La Maestra *et al.*, 2013). [There was not a group that received pioglitazone only.]

In male C57BL/6J-Apc[Min]/+ mice, a heterozygous mouse strain susceptible to intestinal

Table 4.2 Genetic and related effects of rosiglitazone

Test system	Results		Dose or concentration (LED or HID)	Reference
	Without exogenous metabolic system	With exogenous metabolic system		
In vitro				
Salmonella typhimurium, TA98, TA100, TA1535, TA1537, TA1538, reverse mutation	–	–	5000 µg/plate	FDA Drug Approval Package (1999b)
Escherichia coli WP2 *uvrA*, mutation	–	–	5000 µg/plate	FDA Drug Approval Package (1999b)
Gene mutation, mouse lymphoma L5178Y cells, *Tk* locus	?	+	100 µg/mL – S9; 200 µg/mL + S9	FDA Drug Approval Package (1999b)
Chromosomal aberration, human lymphocytes	–	–	240 µg/mL	FDA Drug Approval Package (1999b)
GADD45α-GFP GreenScreen Human Cell, genotoxicity assay	–	–	NR	Luzy *et al.* (2012)
In vivo				
Micronucleus formation, CD-1 mice	–		700 mg/kg bw, single intraperitoneal injection, up to 72 hours	FDA Drug Approval Package (1999b)
Unscheduled DNA synthesis, male Sprague-Dawley rat primary hepatocytes	–		2000 µg/mL	FDA Drug Approval Package (1999b)
Comet assay, male Sprague-Dawley rat peripheral blood lymphocytes	+		1.0 mg/kg bw per day, for 14 days	Bedir *et al.* (2006)
Comet assay, male Sprague-Dawley rat liver cells	+		0.5 mg/kg bw per day, for 14 days	Bedir *et al.* (2006)

+, positive; –, negative; ?, inconclusive; GADD45, growth arrest and DNA damage gene; GFP, green fluorescent protein; HID, highest ineffective dose; LED, lowest effective dose; S9, supernatant fraction of liver homogenate × 9000 *g*

Table 4.3 Genetic and related effects of metabolites of pioglitazone

Test system	Results		Dose or concentration (LED or HID)	Reference
	Without exogenous metabolic system	With exogenous metabolic system		
M-I				
Salmonella typhimurium, TA98, TA100, TA1535, TA1537, reverse mutation	–	–	NR	FDA Drug Approval Package (1999a)
Escherichia coli WP2 *uvrA* mutations	–	–	NR	FDA Drug Approval Package (1999a)
Gene mutation, mouse lymphoma L5178Y cells, *Tk* locus	?	+	NR	FDA Drug Approval Package (1999a)
M-IV				
Salmonella typhimurium, TA98, TA100, TA1535, TA1537, reverse mutation	–	–	NR	FDA Drug Approval Package (1999a)
Escherichia coli WP2 *uvrA*, mutation	–	–	NR	FDA Drug Approval Package (1999a)
Gene mutation, mouse lymphoma L5178Y cells, *Tk* locus	–	–	NR	FDA Drug Approval Package (1999a)
M-V				
Salmonella typhimurium, TA98, TA100, TA1535, TA1537, reverse mutation	–	–	2000 µg/plate	FDA Drug Approval Package (1999a)
Escherichia coli WP2 *uvrA*, mutation	–	–	2000 µg/plate	FDA Drug Approval Package (1999a)
Gene mutation, mouse lymphoma L5178Y cells, *Tk* locus	–	–	NR	FDA Drug Approval Package (1999a)
M-VI				
Salmonella typhimurium, TA98, TA100, TA1535, TA1537, reverse mutation	–	–	2000 µg/plate	FDA Drug Approval Package (1999a)
Escherichia coli WP2 *uvrA*, mutation	–	–	2000 µg/plate	FDA Drug Approval Package (1999a)
Gene mutation, mouse lymphoma L5178Y cells, *Tk* locus	?	+	NR	FDA Drug Approval Package (1999a)

+, positive; –, negative;?, inconclusive; LED, lowest effective dose; HID, highest ineffective dose; NR, not reported; NT, not tested neoplasms, PPARγ agonists (troglitazone, 150 mg/kg bw per day; rosiglitazone, 20 mg/kg bw per day; or NID525, 150 mg/kg bw per day) significantly increased the multiplicity of neoplasms (primarily adenomas) in the large intestine. The mechanism was not explored (Pino *et al.*, 2004).

The administration of rosiglitazone (20 mg/kg bw per day for 8 weeks) to male C57BL/6J-Apc^Min/+ mice significantly increased the multiplicity of tumours of the large intestine, and increased expression of PPARγ in the large intestine, and increased expression of β-catenin. A similar increase in tumour multiplicity, and β-catenin expression, was observed with troglitazone, another PPARγ agonist (150 mg/kg bw per day) (Lefebvre *et al.*, 1998).

Male Sprague-Dawley rats were treated with rosiglitazone at 8 mg/kg bw per day by gavage for up to 16 days. Treatment with rosiglitazone had modest effects on levels of the transcription factor Egr-1 in the bladder urothelium. Likewise, there was minimal effect with fenofibrate, a PPARα agonist. In contrast, ragaglitazar, a dual-action agonist of PPARα and γ, and a rat bladder carcinogen, caused a substantial increase in the level of Egr-1. These data suggested that the co-activation of both PPARα and γ is required for the increased expression of Egr-1 (Egerod *et al.*, 2005).

The relationship between nuclear EGR-1 protein levels and stage of human bladder tumour was investigated using tissue microarrays. The extent of nuclear EGR-1 immunostaining was associated with a higher risk of progression to stage T2–T4 cancer of the bladder (Egerod *et al.*, 2009a).

Male Sprague-Dawley rats given rosiglitazone plus fenofibrate expressed Egr-1 protein on both the dorsal and ventral regions of the urinary bladder (Egerod *et al.*, 2009b).

In male Sprague-Dawley rats, rosiglitazone (given by gavage at 8 or 20 mg/kg bw per day for 7 days) had minimal effects on the levels of the transcription factor Egr-1 in the bladder urothelium, heart, or liver. In contrast, fenofibrate, a PPARα agonist, increased the levels of Egr-1 in the liver and heart (Egerod *et al.*, 2010).

4.5 Susceptibility

No data were available to the Working Group.

4.6 Mechanistic considerations

Pioglitazone, a PPARγ agonist, has been implicated in cancer of the urinary bladder in rats, and rosiglitazone, which is also a PPARγ agonist, promotes cancer of the urinary bladder in rats, and possibly tumours of the kidney in mice. Four mechanisms of carcinogenicity have been considered in rats treated with PPARγ agonists: (i) genotoxicity of metabolites formed from the agonists; (ii) cytotoxicity of the agonists or their metabolites in the urothelium, causing cancer due to a proliferation-driven chronic "wound-healing response"; (iii) formation of urinary solids (urolithiasis), due to urinary changes induced by the agonists or their metabolites, which results in chronic irritation of the urothelium; and (iv) a receptor-mediated effect of the agonists, with carcinogenesis caused by activation of PPARγ transcription factors in the urothelium. These mechanisms may not be mutually exclusive.

4.6.1 Genotoxicity

When assessed using a standard battery of assays for genotoxicity, pioglitazone and rosiglitazone have typically given negative results; nonetheless, there are exceptions. Certain metabolites of pioglitazone and rosiglitazone have given positive results in the assay for gene mutation in mouse lymphoma cells and, more recently, pioglitazone has been reported to increase the frequency of chromosomal aberration, sister chromatid exchange, and formation of 8-oxodeoxyguanosine in human peripheral blood lymphocytes, and both pioglitazone and rosiglitazone gave positive results in comet assays in liver cells and peripheral blood lymphocytes from rats. Thus, while perhaps not the primary mechanism, the contribution of genotoxicity to the carcinogenic activity of pioglitazone or rosiglitazone in the urothelium of rats cannot presently be excluded.

4.6.2 Agonist cytotoxicity

Pioglitazone and rosiglitazone are lipophilic drugs that are excreted to a limited extent in the urine of rats. Since urothelial carcinogenesis is typically considered to be mediated by direct urinary exposure to the drugs or their metabolites, rather than through systemic distribution in the blood, a mechanism involving cytotoxicity as a result of direct exposure to the agonists or their metabolites appeared unlikely.

4.6.3 Urolithiasis

The induction of tumours of the urinary bladder in rodents as a consequence of the formation of urinary solids has been documented for several compounds, including carbonic anhydrase inhibitors, HIV protease inhibitors, and sulfonamides. PPARγ agonists are known to cause fluid accumulation, oedema, cardiac enlargement, and heart failure, effects that can lead to significant changes in urine composition. The administration of pioglitazone to rats results in the formation of urinary solids. This occurs to a greater extent in rats than in mice, and in male rats than in female rats; these trends correspond to the greater susceptibility of rats compared with mice, and of male rats compared with female rats, to the induction of urothelial tumours upon the administration of pioglitazone. Further support for a urolithiasis-based mechanism comes from the observation that tumours arising from pioglitazone occur predominantly on the ventral surface of the bladder, the region where urinary solids would settle in rat bladders,

and that acidifying the urine through the administration of ammonium chloride in the diet decreases the amount of urinary solids and the extent of tumorigenesis in the urinary bladder. Urinary acidification did not alter the expression of PPARα, PPARγ, or epidermal growth factor receptor in the rat bladder urothelium, which suggests that a receptor-mediated mechanism is not involved in the tumorigenic response. A similar urolithiasis-based mechanism has been proposed for muraglitazar, a dual-action PPARα and PPARγ agonist (Achanzar *et al.*, 2007).

4.6.4 Receptor-mediated effect

Although a urolithiasis-based mechanism appears plausible for induction of tumours of the bladder in rats treated with pioglitazone, such a mechanism cannot explain the tumours of the bladder observed in rats given rosiglitazone after initiation with BBN (because urinary solids were not observed; Lubet *et al.*, 2008), the promotion of intestinal neoplasms in susceptible mouse strains given pioglitazone, rosiglitazone, or other PPARγ agonists such as troglitazone or NID525 (Lefebvre *et al.*, 1998; Pino *et al.*, 2004), the induction of tumours of the kidney in mice exposed to mainstream cigarette smoke and then pioglitazone (La Maestra *et al.*, 2013), or the induction of tumours of the urinary bladder in rats treated with naveglitazar, a γ-dominant PPARα and PPARγ agonist (Long *et al.*, 2008).

The promoting activity of rosiglitazone in the rat bladder has been attributed to an increased expression of Egr-1, ribosomal S6 protein phosphorylation, and c-Jun transcription factor phosphorylation, which can lead to hypertrophy, hyperplasia, and subsequently urothelial-cancer progression. While these responses appear to be greater with the dual-acting PPARα and PPARγ agonist ragaglitazar, a modest response does occur with rosiglitazone (Egerod *et al.*, 2005, 2009b, 2010). Furthermore, pioglitazone also shows modest PPARα agonist activity that may contribute to the mechanism of induction of tumours of the bladder (Sakamoto *et al.*, 2000). The induction of intestinal neoplasms in susceptible mouse strains treated with PPARγ agonists may be a consequence of increased expression of β-catenin protein, which activates transcription factors associated with colon tumorigenesis (Lefebvre *et al.*, 1998; Pino *et al.*, 2004).

5. Summary of Data Reported

5.1 Exposure data

Thiazolidinediones are a unique class of synthetic oral drug that exert direct effects on the mechanisms of insulin resistance, and result in improved insulin action and reduced hyperglycaemia. Two thiazolidinediones, rosiglitazone and pioglitazone, initially showed great promise as receptor-mediated oral therapy for type 2 diabetes mellitus.

Pioglitazone hydrochloride is approved in some countries for the treatment of type 2 diabetes mellitus. It is available both as a single agent and in combination with other oral medications for diabetes. Until 2009, pioglitazone was among the most widely used oral drugs for the treatment of type 2 diabetes mellitus. Use of pioglitazone hydrochloride has declined following studies suggesting links to cancer of the bladder, heart failure, and bone fractures. While regulatory agencies in France and Germany banned pioglitazone in 2011, global sales remained substantial at US\$ 3.3 billion in 2012.

Rosiglitazone maleate is approved in some countries for the treatment of type 2 diabetes mellitus. It is available both as a single agent and in combination with other oral medications for diabetes. Until 2007, rosiglitazone was among the most widely used oral drugs for treatment of type 2 diabetes. Use of rosiglitazone has declined over the last few years following studies suggesting links to heart attack, heart failure,

and bone fractures. While this agent is banned in Europe and restricted in the USA, substantial use continues in some countries, including China (global sales of US\$ 41 million).

5.2 Human carcinogenicity data

5.2.1 Cancer of the bladder

The risk of cancer of the bladder associated with the use of pioglitazone and rosiglitazone was assessed in several studies, some with overlapping populations, from Europe, North America and Asia. Some subjects may have received both drugs (in sequence) at some time during treatment for diabetes.

Information for pioglitazone was evaluated in one large randomized controlled trial, four cohort studies, and three case–control studies, some with overlapping study populations. Ever-use of pioglitazone was associated with an increased risk of cancer of the bladder in all studies except one case–control study from Taiwan, China, across all study designs and geographical regions, with risk ratios that ranged from 1.2 in the observational studies to a nearly threefold statistically significant increase in the randomized controlled trial. In this trial, the Working Group noted the excess occurrence of these cancers (14 in the treatment group versus 5 in the placebo group) within a short follow-up time (11 of the bladder cancers occurred within 1 year of randomization), and the large number of patients enrolled, and double-blind experimental design resulting in the balance of confounding factors at baseline.

Dose–response relationships were assessed in five studies, three of which were high-quality population-based studies (which adjusted for smoking or chronic obstructive pulmonary disease in the absence of data on smoking) conducted within the large health insurance databases from the USA, United Kingdom, and Taiwan, China. Greater risks were reported with higher dosage or longer use in the case–control study in the United Kingdom, and in the cohort study in the USA. Observation of a dose–response relationship helped to mitigate concerns about potential confounding by most risk factors; nevertheless, the magnitude of the excess risks observed was modest and some estimates were imprecise.

Among ever-users of rosiglitazone, with data available from two case–control studies and two cohort studies, risk ratios for cancer of the bladder were close to the null in all except one study from the United Kingdom.

The Working Group was unable to consistently rule out confounding, selection bias, detection bias, and bias related to indication or severity of disease in the populations studied as potential explanations for positive associations with pioglitazone. Most of the studies were based on medical databases, which allowed for adjustment for potential confounding by medical factors, but did not permit direct control for cigarette smoking and other risk factors. However, for pioglitazone, increased risks were consistently seen in the studies that adjusted for smoking (one cohort study from the USA, two studies from the United Kingdom, and one study from Taiwan, China that adjusted for chronic obstructive pulmonary disease), as well as those that did not. The potential for confounding by smoking is also mitigated by the fact that, in the same studies, there was no consistent evidence of cancer of the lung and elevated risks were not found among rosigilitazone users in the same studies. Furthermore, an excess of cancer of the bladder among pioglitozone users, and not cancer of the lung, was observed in the trial that randomized for potential confounders including smoking.

5.2.2 Other cancer sites

The risk of cancers at several other sites, including the liver, kidney, colorectum, lung, prostate, and breast, among patients using pioglitazone and rosiglitazone has also been evaluated in studies using cohort and case–control designs. No consistent pattern of increased risk was reported for any other specific cancer site, or for all cancers combined for either drug.

5.3 Animal carcinogenicity data

5.3.1 Pioglitazone

In a 2-year study in mice treated by gavage, pioglitazone produced increases in the incidence of benign pheochromocytoma of the adrenal gland in males and increases in the incidence of leiomyosarcoma of the uterine cervix in females. Administration of pioglitazone in the feed caused a significant increase in the incidence of large intestine adenoma in one study in genetically engineered male mice sensitive to intestinal carcinogenesis. In a study in male and female neonatal mice, pioglitazone in the feed promoted mainstream cigarette smoke-induced kidney adenoma in females.

In a first 2-year study in rats treated by gavage, pioglitazone induced a significant positive trend in the incidence of transitional cell carcinoma of the urinary bladder and a significant positive trend in the incidence of subcutaneous fibrosarcoma of the subcutis in males. It also caused a significant positive trend in the incidence of subcutaneous lipoma in females. In a second 2-year study in male rats treated by gavage, pioglitazone caused a significant increase in the incidence of transitional cell papilloma of the urinary bladder.

5.3.2 Rosiglitazone

Administration of diets containing rosiglitazone caused a significant increase in the incidence of large intestine adenoma in one study in genetically engineered male mice sensitive to intestinal carcinogenesis. In a 2-year study in male and female mice treated by gavage, a significant increase in the incidence of liver haemangiosarcoma was observed in males, but this was not treatment-related.

In a 2-year study in rats treated by gavage, rosiglitazone induced significant increases in the incidence of subcutaneous lipoma in males and females.

In two studies in female mice, coexposure to *N*-butyl-*N*-(4-hydroxybutyl)nitrosamine plus rosiglitazone significantly increased the incidences of *N*-butyl-*N*-(4-hydroxybutyl) nitrosamine-induced carcinoma of the urinary bladder.

5.4 Mechanistic and other relevant data

Pioglitazone and rosiglitazone undergo extensive phase I metabolism. Although pioglitazone and rosiglitazone have typically given negative results when assessed in standard batteries of genotoxicity assays, exceptions have been noted. Certain pioglitazone metabolites and rosiglitazone have given positive results in assays in the mouse lymphoma cells; pioglitazone increased the levels of chromosomal aberration, sister chromatid exchange, and 8-oxodeoxy-guanosine in human peripheral blood lymphocytes; and both pioglitazone and rosiglitazone gave positive results in comet assays in liver cells and peripheral blood lymphocytes from rats. Four mechanisms have been considered for the induction of bladder tumours in rats administered pioglitazone (genotoxicity of pioglitazone metabolites; cytotoxicity, urolithiasis, and PPARγ and α receptor-mediated effects). While not mutually exclusive, data supporting urolithiasis and receptor-mediated mechanisms appear to be the strongest. Likewise, receptor-mediated effects may play a role in the tumorigenic response observed in other experimental models (e.g. intestinal neoplasia in mice).

6. Evaluation

6.1 Cancer in humans

There is *limited evidence* in humans for the carcinogenicity of pioglitazone. A positive association has been observed between pioglitazone and cancer of the bladder.

There is *inadequate evidence* in humans for the carcinogenicity of rosiglitazone.

6.2 Cancer in experimental animals

There is *sufficient evidence* in experimental animals for the carcinogenicity of pioglitazone.

There is *limited evidence* in experimental animals for the carcinogenicity of rosiglitazone.

6.3 Overall evaluation

Pioglitazone is *probably carcinogenic to humans (Group 2A)*.

Rosiglitazone is *not classifiable as to its carcinogenicity to humans (Group 3)*.

References

Achanzar WE, Moyer CF, Marthaler LT, Gullo R, Chen SJ, French MH *et al.* (2007). Urine acidification has no effect on peroxisome proliferator-activated receptor (PPAR) signalling or epidermal growth factor (EGF) expression in rat urinary bladder urothelium. *Toxicol Appl Pharmacol*, 223(3):246–56. doi:10.1016/j.taap.2007.06.015 PMID:17663016

AFFSAPS (2013). Use of medications containing pioglitazone (Actos, Competact) suspended June 9th 2011. Press release. Available from: http://ansm.sante.fr/var/ansm_site/storage/original/application/4e293bcd0814c025b94d46d7502a0958.pdf. Accessed 10 July 2014.

Al-Ghamdi AF, Hefnawy MM (2012). Electrochemical determination of rosiglitazone by square-wave adsorptive stripping voltammetry method. *Arab J Chem*, 5:383–389. doi:10.1016/j.arabjc.2011.07.011

Alzoubi K, Khabour O, Hussain N, Al-Azzam S, Mhaidat N (2012). Evaluation of vitamin B12 effects on DNA damage induced by pioglitazone. *Mutat Res*,

748(1–2):48–51. doi:10.1016/j.mrgentox.2012.06.009 PMID:22790087

Avandia (2010). Rosiglitazone maleate. Tablet, film coated. Anonymous. Total physicians care Inc. 1–27. Available from: http://dailymed.nlm.nih.gov/dailymed/lookup.cfm?setid=ec682aec-e98f-41a1-9d21-eb7580ea3a8a. Accessed 1 October 2014.

Azoulay L, Yin H, Filion KB, Assayag J, Majdan A, Pollak MN *et al.* (2012). The use of pioglitazone and the risk of bladder cancer in people with type 2 diabetes: nested case-control study. *BMJ*, 344(may30 3):e3645 doi:10.1136/bmj.e3645 PMID:22653981

BDdrugs (2013). Online drug index of Bangladesh. Available from: http://www.bddrugs.com/

Bedir A, Aliyazicioglu Y, Bilgici B, Yurdakul Z, Uysal M, Suvaci DE *et al.* (2008). Assessment of genotoxicity in rats treated with the antidiabetic agent, pioglitazone. *Environ Mol Mutagen*, 49(3):185–91. doi:10.1002/em.20365 PMID:18213655

Bedir A, Aliyazicioglu Y, Kahraman H, Yurdakul Z, Uysal M, Suvaci DE *et al.* (2006). Genotoxicity in rats treated with the antidiabetic agent, rosiglitazone. *Environ Mol Mutagen*, 47(9):718–24. doi:10.1002/em.20261 PMID:17078099

Bosetti C, Rosato V, Buniato D, Zambon A, La Vecchia C, Corrao G (2013). Cancer risk for patients using thiazolidinediones for type 2 diabetes: a meta-analysis. *Oncologist*, 18(2):148–56. doi:10.1634/theoncologist.2012-0302 PMID:23345544

BrFAM (2011). Important safety information on the use of medicinal products containing pioglitazone. Press release: Available from: http://www.bfarm.de/SharedDocs/Risikoinformationen/Pharmakovigilanz/EN/RHB/2011/rhb-pioglitazon.pdf?__blob=publicationFile&v=3. Accessed 8 July 2014.

Budde K, Neumayer HH, Fritsche L, Sulowicz W, Stompôr T, Eckland D (2003). The pharmacokinetics of pioglitazone in patients with impaired renal function. *Br J Clin Pharmacol*, 55(4):368–74. doi:10.1046/j.1365-2125.2003.01785.x PMID:12680885

Bulliman S, Allen A, Harris AM *et al.* (1995). The influence of food on the pharmacokinetics of BRL 49653 in healthy male volunteers. *Br J Clin Pharmacol*, 40:517

Calixto LA, de Oliveira AR, Jabor VA, Bonato PS (2011). In vitro characterization of rosiglitazone metabolites and determination of the kinetic parameters employing rat liver microsomal fraction. *Eur J Drug Metab Pharmacokinet*, 36(3):159–66. doi:10.1007/s13318-011-0039-8 PMID:21499911

Cantello BC, Cawthorne MA, Cottam GP *et al.* (1994). [[omega-(Heterocyclylamino)alkoxy]benzyl]-2,4-thiazolidinediones as potent antihyperglycemic agents. *J Med Chem*, 37:3977–3985. doi:10.1021/jm00049a017 PMID:7966158

Cayman SDS (2013). Safety data sheet. Cayman Chemical Company.

Chan LY, Yeung JH, Lau TK (2005). Placental transfer of rosiglitazone in the first trimester of human pregnancy. *Fertil Steril*, 83(4):955–8. doi:10.1016/j.fertnstert.2004.10.045 PMID:15820806

Chang CH, Lin JW, Wu LC, Lai MS, Chuang LM, Chan KA (2012). Association of thiazolidinediones with liver cancer and colorectal cancer in type 2 diabetes mellitus. *Hepatology*, 55(5):1462–72. doi:10.1002/hep.25509 PMID:22135104

Chapelsky MC, Thompson-Culkin K, Miller AK, Sack M, Blum R, Freed MI (2003). Pharmacokinetics of rosiglitazone in patients with varying degrees of renal insufficiency. *J Clin Pharmacol*, 43(3):252–9. doi:10.1177/0091270002250602 PMID:12638393

ChemicalBook (2013). Available from: http://www.chemicalbook.com/ProductMSDSDetailCB9257580_EN.htm. Accessed 08 July 2014.

ChemSpider (2013). ChemSpider: The free chemical database. Royal Society of Chemistry. Available from: http://www.chemspider.com. Accessed 10 July 2014.

Christensen ML, Meibohm B, Capparelli EV, Velasquez-Mieyer P, Burghen GA, Tamborlane WV (2005). Single- and multiple-dose pharmacokinetics of pioglitazone in adolescents with type 2 diabetes. *J Clin Pharmacol*, 45(10):1137–44. doi:10.1177/0091270005279578 PMID:16172178

Chu KM, Hu OY, Pao LH, Hsiong CH (2007). Pharmacokinetics of oral rosiglitazone in Taiwanese and post hoc comparisons with Caucasian, Japanese, Korean, and mainland Chinese subjects. *J Pharm Pharm Sci*, 10(4):411–9. PMID:18261363

Colmers IN, Bowker SL, Johnson JA (2012a). Thiazolidinedione use and cancer incidence in type 2 diabetes: a systematic review and meta-analysis. *Diabetes Metab*, 38(6):475–84. doi:10.1016/j.diabet.2012.06.003 PMID:23041441

Colmers IN, Bowker SL, Majumdar SR, Johnson JA (2012b). Use of thiazolidinediones and the risk of bladder cancer among people with type 2 diabetes: a meta-analysis. *CMAJ*, 184(12):E675–83. doi:10.1503/cmaj.112102 PMID:22761478

Cox PJ, Ryan DA, Hollis FJ, Harris AM, Miller AK, Vousden M *et al.* (2000). Absorption, disposition, and metabolism of rosiglitazone, a potent thiazolidinedione insulin sensitizer, in humans. *Drug Metab Dispos*, 28(7):772–80. PMID:10859151

DHHS/FDA (2007). Electronic Orange Book-Approved Drug Products with Therapeutic Equivalence Evaluations. Available from: http://www.fda.gov/cder/ob/

Dormandy JA, Charbonnel B, Eckland DJ, Erdmann E, Massi-Benedetti M, Moules IK *et al.*; PROactive investigators (2005). Secondary prevention of macrovascular events in patients with type 2 diabetes in the PROactive

Study (PROspective pioglitAzone Clinical Trial In macroVascular Events): a randomised controlled trial. *Lancet*, 366(9493):1279–89. doi:10.1016/S0140-6736(05)67528-9 PMID:16214598

Drugbank (2013). Drug Bank: Open Data Drug & Drug Target Database. Available from: http://www.drugbank.ca/

Egerod FL, Bartels A, Fristrup N, Borre M, Ørntoft TF, Oleksiewicz MB *et al.* (2009a). High frequency of tumor cells with nuclear Egr-1 protein expression in human bladder cancer is associated with disease progression. *BMC Cancer*, 9(1):385 doi:10.1186/1471-2407-9-385 PMID:19878561

Egerod FL, Brünner N, Svendsen JE, Oleksiewicz MB (2010). PPARalpha and PPARgamma are co-expressed, functional and show positive interactions in the rat urinary bladder urothelium. *J Appl Toxicol*, 30(2):151–62. PMID:19757489

Egerod FL, Nielsen HS, Iversen L, Thorup I, Storgaard T, Oleksiewicz MB (2005). Biomarkers for early effects of carcinogenic dual-acting PPAR agonists in rat urinary bladder urothelium in vivo. *Biomarkers*, 10(4):295–309. doi:10.1080/13547500500218682 PMID:16240504

Egerod FL, Svendsen JE, Hinley J, Southgate J, Bartels A, Brünner N *et al.* (2009b). PPAR α and PPAR γ coactivation rapidly induces Egr-1 in the nuclei of the dorsal and ventral urinary bladder and kidney pelvis urothelium of rats. *Toxicol Pathol*, 37(7):947–58. doi:10.1177/0192623309351723 PMID:20008548

EMA; European Medicines Agency (2010). European Medicines Agency recommends suspension of Avandia, Avandamet and Avaglim. Available from: http://www.ema.europa.eu/ema/index.jsp?curl=pages/news_and_events/news/2010/09/news_detail_001119.jsp&mid=WC0b01ac058004d5c1

EMA CHMP (2012). Assessment report Pioglitazone Accord. PM: EPA (2011). Estimation Program Interface (EPI). United States, Environmental Protection Agency.

EMEA; European Medecines Agency (2005). Rosiglitazone. Available from: http://www.ema.europa.eu/docs/en_GB/document_library/EPAR_-_Scientific_Discussion/human/000522/WC500028918.pdf. Accessed 20 June 2014.

EMEA; European Medicines Agency (2012). European Public Assessment Report. Pioglitazone. Available from: http://www.ema.europa.eu/docs/en_GB/document_library/EPAR_-_Public_assessment_report/human/002277/WC500126045.pdf. Accessed 10 July 2014.

Enzo PDS (2012). Product data sheet: Enzo life sciences.

FDA (1999a). Review and evaluation of pharmacology and toxicology data: Pioglitazone. Pharmacology Reviews Application Number: 021073. Center for Drug Evaluation and Research. Available from: http://www.accessdata.fda.gov/drugsatfda_docs/nda/99/021073A_Actos.cfm. Accessed 1 July 2014.

FDA (1999b). Review and evaluation of pharmacology and toxicology data: Rosiglitazone. Pharmacology Reviews Application Number: 021071. Center for Drug Evaluation and Research. Available from: http://www.accessdata.fda.gov/drugsatfda_docs/nda/99/21071_Avandia.cfm. Accessed 1 July 2014.

FDA (2013a). Actos Product Information. Available from: http://www.accessdata.fda.gov/drugsatfda_docs/label/2011/021073s043s044lbl.pdf. Accessed 10 July 2014.

FDA (2013b). Actos Risk Evaluation and Mitigation Strategy. Available from: http://www.accessdata.fda.gov/drugsatfda_docs/appletter/2012/021073s045,021842s016,022024s009,021925s012ltr.pdf. Accessed 10 July 2014.

FDA (2013c). Joint Meeting of the Endocrinologic and Metabolic Drugs Advisory Committee and the Drug Safety and Risk Management Advisory Committee Meeting Announcement Committee. Available from: http://www.fda.gov/AdvisoryCommittees/CommitteesMeetingMaterials/Drugs/EndocrinologicandMetabolicDrugsAdvisoryCommittee/ucm331504.htm. Accessed 11 June 2013.

FDA Drug Approval Package (1999a). Actos (Pioglitazone Hydrochloride) Tablets, Application No. 021073.

FDA Drug Approval Package (1999b). Avandia (Rosiglitazone Maleate) Tablets, Application No. 21-071.

Ferrara A, Lewis JD, Quesenberry CP Jr, Peng T, Strom BL, Van Den Eeden SK *et al.* (2011). Cohort study of pioglitazone and cancer incidence in patients with diabetes. *Diabetes Care*, 34(4):923–9. doi:10.2337/dc10-1067 PMID:21447664

Ferwana M, Firwana B, Hasan R, Al-Mallah MH, Kim S, Montori VM *et al.* (2013). Pioglitazone and risk of bladder cancer: a meta-analysis of controlled studies. *Diabet Med*, 30(9):1026–32. doi:10.1111/dme.12144 PMID:23350856

Freed MI, Allen A, Jorkasky DK, DiCicco RA (1999). Systemic exposure to rosiglitazone is unaltered by food. *Eur J Clin Pharmacol*, 55(1):53–6. doi:10.1007/s002280050592 PMID:10206085

Fujimoto K, Hamamoto Y, Honjo S, Kawasaki Y, Mori K, Tatsuoka H *et al.* (2013). Possible link of pioglitazone with bladder cancer in Japanese patients with type 2 diabetes. *Diabetes Res Clin Pract*, 99(2):e21–3. doi:10.1016/j.diabres.2012.11.013 PMID:23228390

Fujita Y, Yamada Y, Kusama M, Yamauchi T, Kamon J, Kadowaki T *et al.* (2003). Sex differences in the pharmacokinetics of pioglitazone in rats. *Comp Biochem Physiol C Toxicol Pharmacol*, 136(1):85–94. doi:10.1016/S1532-0456(03)00194-7 PMID:14522601

Giaginis C, Theocharis S, Tsantili-Kakoulidou A (2007). Investigation of the lipophilic behaviour of some thiazolidinediones. Relationships with PPAR-γ activity. *J Chromatogr B Analyt Technol Biomed Life*

Sci, 857:181–187. doi:10.1016/j.jchromb.2007.07.013 PMID:17660053

Gowramma B, Babu B, Meyyanathan SN *et al.* (2012a). New chiral normal phase HPLC method for determination of pioglitazone enantiomers on its marketed formulation. *J Pharm Res*, 5:72

Gowramma B, Babu B, Meyyanathan SN *et al.* (2012b). Chiral HPLC Method for the Enantioselective Analysis of Rosiglitazone Maleate in Formulations. *J Pharm Res*, 5(1):79–81.

GSK (2012). AVANDIA product monograph: GlaxoSmithKline Inc.

Hassan MM, Curley SA, Li D, Kaseb A, Davila M, Abdalla EK *et al.* (2010). Association of diabetes duration and diabetes treatment with the risk of hepatocellular carcinoma. *Cancer*, 116(8):1938–46. doi:10.1002/cncr.24982 PMID:20166205

Hillaire-Buys D, Faillie JL, Montastruc JL (2011). Pioglitazone and bladder cancer. *Lancet*, 378(9802):1543–4, author reply 1544–5. doi:10.1016/S0140-6736(11)61662-0 PMID:22035550

IMS Health (2012a). Multinational Integrated Data Analysis (MIDAS). Plymouth Meeting, Pennsylvania: IMS Health.

IMS Health (2012b). National Disease and Therapeutic Index (NDTI) 2004–2012. Plymouth Meeting, Pennsylvania: IMS Health.

Jaakkola T, Laitila J, Neuvonen PJ, Backman JT (2006). Pioglitazone is metabolised by CYP2C8 and CYP3A4 in vitro: potential for interactions with CYP2C8 inhibitors. *Basic Clin Pharmacol Toxicol*, 99(1):44–51. doi:10.1111/j.1742-7843.2006.pto_437.x PMID:16867170

Jain D, Jain S, Jain D, Amin M (2008). Simultaneous estimation of metformin hydrochloride, pioglitazone hydrochloride, and glimepiride by RP-HPLC in tablet formulation. *J Chromatogr Sci*, 46(6):501–4. doi:10.1093/chromsci/46.6.501 PMID:18647470

Jedlicka A, Klimes J, Grafnetterová T (2004). Reversed-phase HPLC methods for purity test and assay of pioglitazone hydrochloride in tablets. *Pharmazie*, 59(3):178–82. PMID:15074587

Julie NL, Julie IM, Kende AI, Wilson GL (2008). Mitochondrial dysfunction and delayed hepatotoxicity: another lesson from troglitazone. *Diabetologia*, 51(11):2108–16. doi:10.1007/s00125-008-1133-6 PMID:18726085

Kirchheiner J, Roots I, Goldammer M, Rosenkranz B, Brockmöller J (2005). Effect of genetic polymorphisms in cytochrome p450 (CYP) 2C9 and CYP2C8 on the pharmacokinetics of oral antidiabetic drugs: clinical relevance. *Clin Pharmacokinet*, 44(12):1209–25. doi:10.2165/00003088-200544120-00002 PMID:16372821

Krieter PA, Colletti AE, Doss GA, Miller RR (1994). Disposition and metabolism of the hypoglycemic agent pioglitazone in rats. *Drug Metab Dispos*, 22(4):625–30. PMID:7956739

Krishna SR, Rao B *et al.* (2008). Isolation, synthesis and characterization of rosiglitazone maleate impurities. *E-Journal of Chemistry*, 5:562–566. doi:10.1155/2008/308724

Kumar YR, Reddy AR, Eswaraiah S, Mukkanti K, Reddy MS, Suryanarayana MV (2004). Structural characterization of impurities in pioglitazone. *Pharmazie*, 59(11):836–9. PMID:15587582

La Maestra S, Micale RT, De Flora S, D'Agostini F, Ganchev G, Iltcheva M *et al.* (2013). DNA damage in exfoliated cells and histopathological alterations in the urinary tract of mice exposed to cigarette smoke and treated with chemopreventive agents. *Carcinogenesis*, 34(1):183–9. doi:10.1093/carcin/bgs314 PMID:23042096

Langchem (2013). Langchem material safety data sheet. China Langchem Inc.

Lefebvre A-M, Chen I, Desreumaux P, Najib J, Fruchart JC, Geboes K *et al.* (1998). Activation of the peroxisome proliferator-activated receptor γ promotes the development of colon tumors in C57BL/6J-APCMin/+ mice. *Nat Med*, 4(9):1053–7. doi:10.1038/2036 PMID:9734399

Lewis JD, Ferrara A, Peng T, Hedderson M, Bilker WB, Quesenberry CP Jr *et al.* (2011). Risk of bladder cancer among diabetic patients treated with pioglitazone: interim report of a longitudinal cohort study. *Diabetes Care*, 34(4):916–22. doi:10.2337/dc10-1068 PMID:21447663

Lewis JD, Strom BL, Bilker W, Nessel L, Vaughn DJ, Ferrara A, et al. (2012). Pioglitazone HCl (ACTOS) Clinical Study No. 01–03-TL-OPI-524. Cohort Study of Pioglitazone and Bladder Cancer in Patients with Diabetes Fourth Interim Analysis (8-Year). Report with Data from 1 January 1997 to 31 December 2010. Available from: http://general.takedapharm.com/Trial-Disclosure/01-03-TL-OPI-524-8-year-Interim-Report.pdf. Accessed 2 March 2012.

Lin ZJ, Ji W, Desai-Krieger D, Shum L (2003). Simultaneous determination of pioglitazone and its two active metabolites in human plasma by LC-MS/MS. *J Pharm Biomed Anal*, 33(1):101–8. doi:10.1016/S0731-7085(03)00344-3 PMID:12946536

Loke YK, Singh S, Furberg CD (2009). Long-term use of thiazolidinediones and fractures in type 2 diabetes: a meta-analysis. *CMAJ*, 180(1):32–9. doi:10.1503/cmaj.080486 PMID:19073651

Long GG, Reynolds VL, Lopez-Martinez A, Ryan TE, White SL, Eldridge SR (2008). Urothelial carcinogenesis in the urinary bladder of rats treated with naveglitazar, a γ-dominant PPAR α/γ agonist: lack of evidence for urolithiasis as an inciting event. *Toxicol Pathol*, 36(2):218–31. doi:10.1177/0192623307311757 PMID:18474944

Lu YC, Li YC (2013). How doctors practice evidence-based medicine. *J Eval Clin Pract*, 19:44–49. doi:10.1111/j.1365-2753.2011.01765.x PMID:21883721

Lubet RA, Fischer SM, Steele VE, Juliana MM, Desmond R, Grubbs CJ (2008). Rosiglitazone, a PPAR gamma agonist: potent promoter of hydroxybutyl(butyl) nitrosamine-induced urinary bladder cancers. *Int J Cancer*, 123(10):2254–9. doi:10.1002/ijc.23765 PMID:18712722

Luzy A-P, Orsini N, Linget J-M, Bouvier G (2012). Evaluation of the GADD45α-GFP GreenScreen HC assay for rapid and reliable in vitro early genotoxicity screening. *J Appl Toxicol*, n/a doi:10.1002/jat.2793 PMID:22806210

Madivada LR, Anumala RR, Gilla G, Alla S, Charagondla K, Kagga M *et al.* (2009). An improved process for pioglitazone and its pharmaceutically acceptable salt. *Org Process Res Dev*, 13(6):1190–4. doi:10.1021/op900131m

Martín J, Buchberger W, Santos JL, Alonso E, Aparicio I (2012). High-performance liquid chromatography quadrupole time-of-flight mass spectrometry method for the analysis of antidiabetic drugs in aqueous environmental samples. *J Chromatogr B Analyt Technol Biomed Life Sci*, 895–896:94–101. doi:10.1016/j.jchromb.2012.03.023 PMID:22483984

Milne GWA (2000). Drugs: Synonyms & Properties. Ashgate Publ Co.

Monami M, Lamanna C, Marchionni N, Mannucci E (2008). Rosiglitazone and risk of cancer: a meta-analysis of randomized clinical trials. *Diabetes Care*, 31(7):1455–60. doi:10.2337/dc07-2308 PMID:18375416

Mostafa GA, Al-Majed A (2008). Characteristics of new composite- and classical potentiometric sensors for the determination of pioglitazone in some pharmaceutical formulations. *J Pharm Biomed Anal*, 48(1):57–61. doi:10.1016/j.jpba.2008.04.029 PMID:18555633

National Library of Medicine (2010). Avandia (rosiglitazone maleate) tablet, film coated. Bethesda (MD): National Institutes of Health, Health & Human Services. Available from: http://dailymed.nlm.nih.gov/dailymed/lookup.cfm?setid=ef14122b-7fff-45fa-b13b-0ea9e48bd57d. Accessed 20 June 2014.

Neumann A, Weill A, Ricordeau P, Fagot JP, Alla F, Allemand H (2012). Pioglitazone and risk of bladder cancer among diabetic patients in France: a population-based cohort study. *Diabetologia*, 55(7):1953–62. doi:10.1007/s00125-012-2538-9 PMID:22460763

Nissen SE, Wolski K (2007). Effect of rosiglitazone on the risk of myocardial infarction and death from cardiovascular causes. *N Engl J Med*, 356:2457–2471. doi:10.1056/NEJMoa072761 PMID:17517853

NLM (2013). Hazardous Substances Data Bank: National library of medicine.

Nowak SN, Edwards DJ, Clarke A, Anderson GD, Jaber LA (2002). Pioglitazone: effect on CYP3A4 activity. *J Clin Pharmacol*, 42(12):1299–302. doi:10.1177/0091270002042012009 PMID:12463723

O'Maille G, Pai SM, Tao X, Douglas GT Jr, Jenkins RG (2008). An improved LC-ESI-MS-MS method for simultaneous quantitation of rosiglitazone and N-desmethyl rosiglitazone in human plasma. *J Pharm Biomed Anal*, 48(3):934–9. doi:10.1016/j.jpba.2008.08.001 PMID:18818043

O'Neil (2006). Pioglithazone. The Merck Index - An Encyclopedia of Chemicals, Drugs, and Biologicals. Whitehouse Station (NJ): Merck & Co., Inc.

Palem CR, Gannu R, Yamsani SK, Yamsani VV, Yamsani MR (2011). Development of a high-performance liquid chromatography method for simultaneous determination of pioglitazone and felodipine in pig serum: application to pharmacokinetic study. *Biomed Chromatogr*, 25(8):952–8. doi:10.1002/bmc.1553 PMID:21058416

Pang W, Yang H, Wu Z *et al.* (2009). LC-MS-MS in MRM mode for detection and structural identification of synthetic hypoglycemic drugs added illegally to 'natural' anti-diabetic herbal products. *Chromatographia*, 70:1353–1359. doi:10.1365/s10337-009-1344-0

Perez AT (2013). Pioglitazone and risk of bladder cancer: clarification of the design of the French study. *Diabetologia*, 56(1):227 doi:10.1007/s00125-012-2767-y PMID:23135221

Physicians Desk Reference (2012) Pioglitazone. 66th ed. Montvale (NJ): PDR Network.

Piccinni C, Motola D, Marchesini G, Poluzzi E (2011). Assessing the association of pioglitazone use and bladder cancer through drug adverse event reporting. *Diabetes Care*, 34(6):1369–71. doi:10.2337/dc10-2412 PMID:21515844

Pino MV, Kelley MF, Jayyosi Z (2004). Promotion of colon tumors in C57BL/6J-APC(min)/+ mice by thiazolidinedione PPARgamma agonists and a structurally unrelated PPARgamma agonist. *Toxicol Pathol*, 32(1):58–63. doi:10.1080/01926230490261320 PMID:14713549

Pubchem (2013). Pubchem Databases: National Center for Biotechnology, Pioglitazone. In CID.4829 U.S. National Library of Medicine. Available from: http://pubchem.ncbi.nlm.nih.gov/summary/summary.cgi?q=all&cid=4829#ec. Accessed 10 July 2014.

Pubchem Substance (2013). Rosiglitazone (SID 46504556). Available from: http://pubchem.ncbi.nlm.nih.gov/summary/summary.cgi?sid=46504556

Radhakrishna T, Satyanarayana J, Satyanarayana A (2002b). LC determination of rosiglitazone in bulk and pharmaceutical formulation. *J Pharm Biomed Anal*, 29:873–880. doi:10.1016/S0731-7085(02)00209-1 PMID:12093521

Radhakrishna T, Sreenivas Rao D, Om Reddy G (2002a). Determination of pioglitazone hydrochloride in bulk and pharmaceutical formulations by HPLC and MEKC methods. *J Pharm Biomed Anal*, 29(4):593–607. doi:10.1016/S0731-7085(02)00036-5 PMID:12093488

Ravikanth CH, Kumar AA, Kiran VU (2011). Sensitive and rapid HPLC method for the determination of pioglitazone in rat serum. *Int J Pharmaceutical Sciences Drug Research*, 3(1):38–41.

Richter J, Jirman J, Havlícek J, Hrdina R (2007). Pioglitazone impurities. *Pharmazie*, 62(8):580–4. doi:10.1691/ph.2007.8.6720 PMID:17867551

Ruiter R, Visser LE, van Herk-Sukel MP, Geelhoed-Duijvestijn PH, de Bie S, Straus SM *et al.* (2012). Prescribing of rosiglitazone and pioglitazone following safety signals: analysis of trends in dispensing patterns in the Netherlands from 1998 to 2008. *Drug Saf*, 35:471–480. doi:10.2165/11596950-000000000-00000 PMID:22540371

Rx List (2013). RxList - The internet drug index. Available from: http://www.rxlist.com

Sakamoto J, Kimura H, Moriyama S, Odaka H, Momose Y, Sugiyama Y *et al.* (2000). Activation of human peroxisome proliferator-activated receptor (PPAR) subtypes by pioglitazone. *Biochem Biophys Res Commun*, 278(3):704–11. doi:10.1006/bbrc.2000.3868 PMID:11095972

Sato K, Awasaki Y, Kandori H, Tanakamaru ZY, Nagai H, Baron D *et al.* (2011). Suppressive effects of acid-forming diet against the tumorigenic potential of pioglitazone hydrochloride in the urinary bladder of male rats. *Toxicol Appl Pharmacol*, 251(3):234–44. doi:10.1016/j.taap.2011.01.006 PMID:21255596

SciFinder (2013). SciFinder Databases. Registry, Chemcats. American Chemical Society.

Seedher N, Kanojia M (2008). Micellar solubilization of some poorly soluble antidiabetic drugs: a technical note. *AAPS PharmSciTech*, 9:431–436. doi:10.1208/s12249-008-9057-5 PMID:18431666

Seedher N, Kanojia M (2009). Co-solvent solubilization of some poorly-soluble antidiabetic drugs. *Pharm Dev Technol*, 14:185–192. doi:10.1080/10837450802498894 PMID:19519190

Singh S, Loke YK, Furberg CD (2007a). Thiazolidinediones and heart failure: a teleo-analysis. *Diabetes Care*, 30(8):2148–53. doi:10.2337/dc07-0141 PMID:17536074

Singh S, Loke YK, Furberg CD (2007b). Long-term risk of cardiovascular events with rosiglitazone: A meta-analysis. *JAMA*, 298:1189–1195. doi:10.1001/jama.298.10.1189 PMID:17848653

Sireesha MR Chandan S, Gurupadayya BM, Aswani Kumar CH (2011). Selective and validated spectrophotometric methods for determination of rosiglitazone and pioglitazone with 2, 4-DNP. Department of Pharmaceutical Analysis, JSS College of Pharmacy, JSS University, Mysore, India. Available from: http://www.ijptonline.com/wp-content/uploads/2009/10/1554-1564.pdf. Accessed 1 October 2014.

Smith U (2001). Pioglitazone: mechanism of action. *Int J Clin Pract Suppl*, (121):13–8. PMID:11594239

Song SO, Kim KJ, Lee BW, Kang ES, Cha BS, Lee HC (2012). The risk of bladder cancer in korean diabetic subjects treated with pioglitazone. *Diabetes Metab J*, 36(5):371–8. doi:10.4093/dmj.2012.36.5.371 PMID:23130322

Souri E, Jalalizadeh H, Saremi S (2008). Development and validation of a simple and rapid HPLC method for determination of pioglitazone in human plasma and its application to a pharmacokinetic study. *J Chromatogr Sci*, 46(9):809–12. doi:10.1093/chromsci/46.9.809 PMID:19007483

Sripalakit P, Neamhom P, Saraphanchotiwitthaya A (2006). High-performance liquid chromatographic method for the determination of pioglitazone in human plasma using ultraviolet detection and its application to a pharmacokinetic study. *J Chromatogr B Analyt Technol Biomed Life Sci*, 843(2):164–9. doi:10.1016/j.jchromb.2006.05.032 PMID:16815107

Sultana N, Arayne MS, Shafi N, Siddiqui FA, Hussain A (2011). Development and validation of new assay method for the simultaneous analysis of diltiazem, metformin, pioglitazone and rosiglitazone by RP-HPLC and its applications in pharmaceuticals and human serum. *J Chromatogr Sci*, 49(10):774–9. doi:10.1093/chrsci/49.10.774 PMID:22080805

Sweetman SC (2011) Monographs on drugs and ancillary substances. In: Martindale: The Complete Drug Reference. 37th ed. Vol. A. London, UK: Pharmaceutical Press, pp.494.

Takeda Pharmaceuticals (2013). Actos Product Information. Deerfield (Il): Takeda Pharmaceuticals America, Inc. Available from: http://www.takeda.us/products. Accessed 19 June 2014.

Thevis M, Geyer H, Schänzer W (2005). Identification of oral antidiabetics and their metabolites in human urine by liquid chromatography/tandem mass spectrometry–a matter for doping control analysis. *Rapid Commun Mass Spectrom*, 19(7):928–36. doi:10.1002/rcm.1875 PMID:15747323

Tseng CH (2011). Diabetes and risk of prostate cancer: a study using the National Health Insurance. *Diabetes Care*, 34(3):616–21. doi:10.2337/dc10-1640 PMID:21273499

Tseng CH (2012a). Pioglitazone and bladder cancer: a population-based study of Taiwanese. *Diabetes Care*, 35(2):278–80. doi:10.2337/dc11-1449 PMID:22210574

Tseng CH (2012b). Diabetes, metformin use, and colon cancer: a population-based cohort study in Taiwan. *Eur J Endocrinol*, 167(3):409–16. doi:10.1530/EJE-12-0369 PMID:22778198

Tseng CH (2012c). Thyroid cancer risk is not increased in diabetic patients. *PLoS ONE*, 7(12):e53096 doi:10.1371/journal.pone.0053096 PMID:23300866

Tseng CH (2012d). Pioglitazone and bladder cancer in human studies: is it diabetes itself, diabetes drugs, flawed analyses or different ethnicities? *J Formos Med*

Assoc, 111(3):123–31. doi:10.1016/j.jfma.2011.10.003 PMID:22423665

Tseng CH (2013a). Rosiglitazone is not associated with an increased risk of bladder cancer. *Cancer Epidemiol*, 37(4):385–9. doi:10.1016/j.canep.2013.03.013 PMID:23619142

Tseng CH (2013b). Benign prostatic hyperplasia is a significant risk factor for bladder cancer in diabetic patients: a population-based cohort study using the National Health Insurance in Taiwan. *BMC Cancer*, 13(1):7 doi:10.1186/1471-2407-13-7 PMID:23286275

Tseng CH (2013c). Oral cancer in Taiwan: is diabetes a risk factor? *Clin Oral Investig*, 17(5):1357–64. doi:10.1007/s00784-012-0820-3 PMID:22895832

Venkatesh P, Harisudhan T, Choudhury H *et al.* (2006). Simultaneous estimation of six anti-diabetic drugs– glibenclamide, gliclazide, glipizide, pioglitazone, repaglinide and rosiglitazone: development of a novel HPLC method for use in the analysis of pharmaceutical formulations and its application to human plasma assay. *Biomed Chromatogr*, 20:1043–1048. doi:10.1002/bmc.635 PMID:16506282

Wang M, Miksa IR (2007). Multi-component plasma quantitation of anti-hyperglycemic pharmaceutical compounds using liquid chromatography-tandem mass spectrometry. *J Chromatogr B Analyt Technol Biomed Life Sci*, 856:318–327. doi:10.1016/j.jchromb.2007.06.037 PMID:17689303

Wei L, MacDonald TM, Mackenzie IS (2013). Pioglitazone and bladder cancer: a propensity score matched cohort study. *Br J Clin Pharmacol*, 75(1):254–9. doi:10.1111/j.1365-2125.2012.04325.x PMID:22574756

WHO (2007). Cumulative List No. 14 of INN in Latin, English, French, Spanish, Arabic, Chinese and Russian (in alphabetical order of Latin name), with supllementary information. World Health Organisation.

Woodcock J, Sharfstein JM, Hamburg M (2010). Regulatory action on rosiglitazone by the U.S. Food and Drug Administration. *N Engl J Med*, 363(16):1489–91. doi:10.1056/NEJMp1010788 PMID:20942663

Xavier CM, Basavaiah K (2012). Implementation of Quality by Design for the Development and Validation of Pioglitazone Hydrochloride by RP-UPLC with Application to Formulated Forms *Int School Res Network*, 1–11.

Xue YJ, Turner KC, Meeker JB, Pursley J, Arnold M, Unger S (2003). Quantitative determination of pioglitazone in human serum by direct-injection high-performance liquid chromatography mass spectrometry and its application to a bioequivalence study. *J Chromatogr B Analyt Technol Biomed Life Sci*, 795(2):215–26. doi:10.1016/S1570-0232(03)00575-0 PMID:14522026

Yamashita K, Murakami H, Okuda T, Motohashi M (1996). High-performance liquid chromatographic determination of pioglitazone and its metabolites in human serum and urine. *J Chromatogr B Biomed Appl*, 677(1):141–6. doi:10.1016/0378-4347(95)00440-8 PMID:8925086

Yardımcı C, Ozaltın N, Gürlek A (2007). Simultaneous determination of rosiglitazone and metformin in plasma by gradient liquid chromatography with UV detection. *Talanta*, 72(4):1416–22. doi:10.1016/j.talanta.2007.01.042 PMID:19071778

Zhong WZ, Lakings DB (1989). Determination of pioglitazone in dog serum using solid-phase extraction and high-performance liquid chromatography with ultra-violet (229 nm) detection. *J Chromatogr A*, 490(2):377–85. doi:10.1016/S0378-4347(00)82795-4 PMID:2768410

Zhu Z, Shen Z, Lu Y, Zhong S, Xu C (2012). Increased risk of bladder cancer with pioglitazone therapy in patients with diabetes: a meta-analysis. *Diabetes Res Clin Pract*, 98(1):159–63. doi:10.1016/j.diabres.2012.05.006 PMID:22705039

DIGOXIN

1. Exposure Data

Digoxin is a cardiac glycoside isolated from plants of the genus *Digitalis*. The use of preparations of cardiac glycoside (synonyms: digitalis, cardiac steroids) dates back to 1785, when William Withering published his monograph "An account of the foxglove and some of its medical uses" (Withering, 1785; Albrecht & Geiss, 2000). Isolated digoxin has been used since the early 20th century (Cheng & Rybak, 2010).

The Working Group noted that only four of the many digitalis glycosides present in the plant remain important in the marketplace. These are digoxin, digitoxin, β-acetyldigoxin and methyldigoxin (Kleemann, 2012). Furthermore, the term "digitalis use" found in many reports probably refers not to the use of plant material, which is not commercially available as a medicinal product, but to the use of the isolated compounds. Of the four medicinally available compounds, digoxin is the most important and is exclusively available in some countries, such as the USA (see Section 1.3). The Working Group estimated that digoxin represents at least 90% of the world market for digitalis glycosides.

While use of digitoxin worldwide is much less than that of digoxin, it may be significant in individual countries. Thus, studies reporting use of "digitalis" should be carefully scrutinized since the agent to which people were actually exposed could have been any one of the four digitalis glycosides.

The Working Group noted that most of what has been used under the term "digitalis" in North America and Europe has been digoxin; however, there may be parts of the world where crude extract of the digitalis plant is still in use. No data on the use of digitalis extract were available to the Working Group.

1.1 Chemical and physical data

1.1.1 Nomenclature

Chem. Abstr. Serv. Reg. No.: 20830-75-5 (SciFinder, 2013)

Chem. Abstr. Serv. Name: Card-20(22)-enolide, 3-[(*O*-2,6-dideoxy-β-D-*ribo*-hexopyranosyl--(1→4)-*O*-2,6-dideoxy-β-D-*ribo*-hexopyranosyl-(1→4)-2,6-dideoxy-β-D-*ribo*-hexopyranosyl)oxy]-12,14-dihydroxy-, (3β,5β,12β)- (SciFinder, 2013)

IUPAC Systematic Name: 3-[(3S,5R,8R,9S,10S,12R,13S,14S,17R)-3-[(2R,4S,5S,6R)-5-[(2S,4S,5S,6R)-5-[(2S,4S,5S,6R)-4,5-dihydroxy-6-methyloxan-2-yl]oxy-4-hydroxy-6-methyloxan-2-yl]oxy-4-hydroxy-6-methyloxan-2-yl]oxy-12,14-dihydroxy-10,13-dimethyl-1,2,3,4,5,6,7,8,9,11,12,15,16,17-tetradecahydrocyclopenta[*a*]phenanthren-17-yl]-2*H*-furan-5-one (PubChem, 2013)

Synonyms: 12β-hydroxydigitoxin

Proprietary names for digoxin: Cardigox; Cardiogoxin; Cardioxin; Cardixin; Cardoxin; Chloroformic digitalin; Coragoxine; Cordioxil; Davoxin; Digacin; Digicor; Digitek; Digomal; Digon; Digosin; Digoxin Nativelle; Dilanacin; Dixina; Dokim; Dynamos; Eudigox; Fargoxin; Grexin; Homolle's digitalin; Lanacordin; Lanacrist; Lanicor; Lanikor; Lanocardin; Lanorale; Lanoxicaps; Lanoxin; Lanoxin PG; Lenoxicaps; Lenoxin; Longdigox; Mapluxin; NSC 95 100; Natigoxin; NeoDioxanin; Novodigal-Amp.; Purgoxin; Rougoxin; Stillacor; Toloxin; Vanoxin (from SciFinder, 2013).

1.1.2 Structural and molecular formulae and relative molecular mass

From USP (2007)

$C_{41}H_{64}O_{14}$
Relative molecular mass: 780.94

1.1.3 Chemical and physical properties of the pure substance

Description: Odourless, colourless to white crystals, or white crystalline powder, radially arranged four- and five-sided triclinic plates from dilute alcohol or pyridine (British Pharmacopoeia, 2009; PubChem, 2013)

Melting point: Digoxin melts and decomposes between 230 °C and 265 °C (Foss & Benezra, 1980; ChemicalBook, 2013)

Density: 1.36 ± 0.1 g/cm³ (temperature, 20 °C; pressure, 760 Torr) (SciFinder, 2013)

Spectroscopy data: Specific optical rotation, ultraviolet, infrared, nuclear magnetic resonance, and mass spectral data were reported in the literature (Foss & Benezra, 1980; British Pharmacopoeia, 2009; HSDB, 2013)

Solubility: In water, 64.8 mg/L at 25 °C; soluble in dilute alcohol, pyridine, or mixture of chloroform and alcohol; almost insoluble in ether, acetone, ethyl acetate, chloroform; slightly soluble in diluted alcohol, and very slightly soluble in 40% propylene glycol; (PubChem, 2013)

Stability data: Digoxin is indefinitely stable when kept in the dark in a tightly closed container. No degradation is noted in tablets after 5 years when stored in tightly closed containers. A solution of digoxin hydrolyses in the presence of acid, yielding digoxigenin bis-digitoxoside, digoxigenin mono-digitoxoside and digoxigenin. A neutral solution in ethanol and propylene glycol is stable for up to 5 years. Digoxin solutions are relatively stable to light, except when stored under intense light for long periods of time (Foss & Benezra, 1980)

Storage: Digoxin preparations should be protected from light and stored at 15–25 °C (HSDB, 2013)

Octanol/water partition coefficient (log P): 1.26 (HSDB, 2013)

Dissociation constant: pK_a, basic = −3; pK_a, acidic = 7.15 (DrugBank, 2013)

Vapour pressure: 3.3×10^{-30} mm Hg at 25 °C (PubChem, 2013)

Flash point: 278.5 ± 27.8 °C (SciFinder, 2013)

1.1.4 Technical products and impurities

Since digoxin is isolated from plant materials, at least 21 other cardiac glycosides, including digitoxin, may occur as impurities (British Pharmacopoeia, 2009). The purity of digoxin is typically at least 95% (see Section 1.5). According to the European Pharmacopoeia (2008), not more than 0.5% digitoxin in relation to digoxin may be present as impurity.

(a) Nomenclature for digitoxin

Chem. Abstr. Serv. Reg. No.: 71-63-6 (SciFinder, 2013)

Chem. Abstr. Serv. Name: 3β-[(O-2,6-dideoxy-β-D-ribo-hexopyranosyl-(1→4)-O-2,6-dideoxy-β-D-ribo-hexopyranosyl-(1→4)-2,6-dideoxy-β-D-ribo-hexopyranosyl)oxy]-14-hydroxy-4β,14β-card-20(22)-enolide.

Proprietary names for digitoxin: Crystodigin, Digimed, Digimerck.

(b) Structural and molecular formulae and relative molecular mass of digitoxin

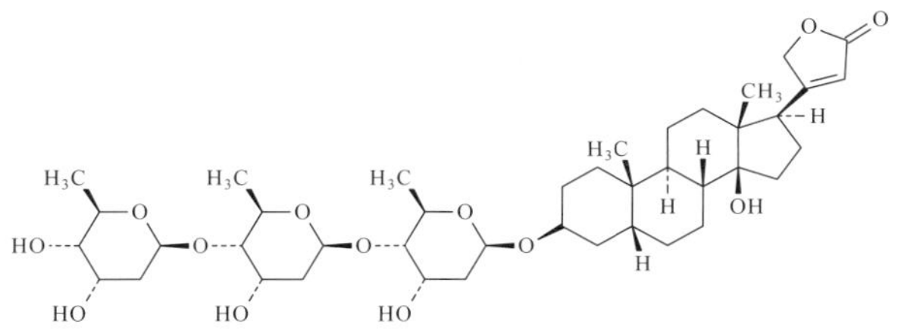

$C_{41}H_{64}O_{13}$

Relative molecular mass: 764.94

1.2 Analysis

Compendial methods to determine digoxin and digitoxin in pharmaceutical preparations are typically based on liquid chromatography with ultraviolet detection. For detection in human plasma or urine, liquid chromatography with mass spectrometric detection is required to achieve the necessary lower detection limits. The analytical methods are summarized in Table 1.1.

1.3 Production and use

1.3.1 Production

Digoxin is isolated from *Digitalis lanata* Ehrh., the woolly foxglove, from the *Scrophulariaceae* family. For the isolation of the therapeutically important secondary glycosides, the finely ground material is moisturized and exposed to glucosidase enzymes at 30–37 °C until glucose is completely removed. Extraction procedures, usually followed by precipitation of tannic acid and related phenolic products with lead salts, afford a crude mixture of cardioactive compounds, which is further purified by chromatography and/or crystallization. Originally, mixtures of glycosides or crude plant extracts were used in therapy; these have been replaced by chemically pure drugs today, which allow better control of therapy. Total syntheses of cardiac steroids and their corresponding glycosides have been accomplished but are not used commercially (Albrecht & Geiss, 2000).

Digitoxin is isolated by extraction of the leaves and seeds of *Digitalis purpurea* L. (purple foxglove) with 50% ethanol and subsequent treatment with the enzyme digilanidase, which effects cleavage of the β-D-glucose moiety at the chain end of the main glycoside, purpureaglycoside A (Kleemann, 2012).

β-Acetyldigoxin is prepared from digoxin by acetylation with acetic acid. Methyldigoxin can be prepared by methylation of digoxin, e.g. with dimethyl sulfate (Kleemann, 2012).

1.3.2 Use

(a) Indications

Digoxin and digitoxin are therapeutically the most widely used digitalis glycosides. Table 1.2 lists the most commonly reported clinical indications for digoxin in the USA. While digoxin was once regarded as the drug of choice for congestive heart failure with reduced left ventricular

Table 1.1 Analytical methods for digoxin

Sample matrix	Sample preparation	Assay method	Detection limit	Reference
Compendial methods				
Digoxin injection, digoxin Tablet and digoxin oral solution	–	LC-UV Column: Packing L1 Mobile phase: water and acetonitrile Flow rate: 3 mL/min Wavelength: 218 nm	NR	USP (2007)
Digoxin injection, paediatric digoxin injection, paediatric digoxin oral solution, and digoxin tablets	–	LC-UV Column: C_{18} Mobile phase: acetonitrile:water (10:90) and water:acetonitrile (10:90) Flow rate: 1.5 mL/min Wavelength 220 nm	NR	BP (2009)
Non-compendial methods				
Human plasma, rat plasma and rat brain	Addition of DMA, addition of NaCl saturated 0.1 mol/L NaOH, collection of organic layer, centrifugation	LC-MS-MS Column: C_{18} Mobile phases: ammonium carbonate, and methanol pH 9.0 Flow rate: 0.7 mL/min SRM: 779.4 *m/z*, 649.4 *m/z*	0.1 ng/mL (LLOQ)	Hirabayashi *et al.* (2011)
Human plasma	Deproteinization with perchloric acid in water, mixing and centrifugation	LC-ESI-MS Column: C_{18} Mobile phase: mixture of methanol and formic acid in sodium acetate Flow rate: 1 mL/min SIM: 803.5 *m/z*	0.5 ng/mL (LLOQ)	Vlase *et al.* (2009)
Human blood and tissues	Mixing with sodium acetate buffer pH 7, homogenization, centrifugation, loaded on SPE column conditioned with methanol, water, and sodium acetate buffer, washing with sodium acetate buffer, dried under vacuum, second wash with 20% isopropyl alcohol, drying, addition of acetone, vacuum drying, elution with acetone	LC-ESI-MS Column: C_8 Mobile phase: 0.1% formic acid in a mixture of 55% methanol and 45% water Flow rate: 0.2 mL/min SIM: 803.4 *m/z*	0.2 ng/g (LLOQ)	Frommherz *et al.* (2008)

Table 1.1 (continued)

Sample matrix	Sample preparation	Assay method	Detection limit	Reference
Human serum	Addition of methyl *tert*-butyl ether, centrifugation, evaporation, and reconstitution in methanol	LC-ESI-MS Column: C_{18} Mobile phase: 10 mM ammonium acetate/0.1% formic acid in water and 0.1% formic acid in acetonitrile Flow rate: 0.3 mL/min SRM transition: 798.6 *m/z*, 651.5 *m/z*	0.1 ng/mL (LLOQ)	Li *et al.* (2010)
Human blood	Mixing with ammonium carbonate buffer, extraction (ethyl acetate/hepatene/dichloromethane = 3 : 1 : 1), centrifugation, collection of organic layer, evaporation, reconstitution in acetonitrile:water	LC-ESI-MS Column: C_{18} Mobile phase: 10 mM ammonium formate and acetonitrile pH 3.1 Flow rate: 0.3 mL/min MRM transitions: 798.4 *m/z*, 651.3 *m/z*; 798.4 *m/z*, 633.3 *m/z*	0.08 ng/mL (LLOQ) 0.032 ng/mL (LOD)	Oiestad *et al.* (2009)
Human plasma	Mixing with 10% ammonium hydroxide, addition of chloroform, centrifugation, evaporation, reconstitution in 1 mM trifluoroacetic acid and acetonitrile (7 : 3).	LC-ESI-MS Column: UPLC˚ AQUITY˚ Mobile phase: 30% 1mM ammonium trifluoroacetate in acetonitrile and 100% water Flow rate: 0.1 mL/min SIM transition: 780.94 *m/z*, 893.5 *m/z*	0.1 ng/mL (LLOQ)	Grabowski *et al.* (2009)
Human plasma	Addition of concentrated NaOH and methyl *t*-butyl ether, shaking, centrifugation, evaporation, reconstitution in mobile phase	LC-ESI-MS Column: C_8 Mobile phase: 0.25 mM sodium acetate in water and 0.25 mM sodium acetate in methanol Flow rate: 0.25 mL/min SIM: 803.4 *m/z* (positive mode)	0.05 ng/mL (LLOQ) 0.025 ng/mL (LOD)	Kirby *et al.* (2008)
Human plasma	Addition of buffer solution pH 6.0, loading into oasis HLB30 mg 96-well plate preconditioned with methanol:water (40:60), elution of analyte with pure methanol, evaporation and reconstitution in methanol	LC-ESI-MS Column: C_{18} Mobile phase: 10 mmol/L ammonium hydrogen carbonate/methanol (1 : 9) and 10 mmol/L ammonium hydrogen carbonate/methanol (9 : 1) Flow rate: 0.6 mL/min SRM transition: 798.5 *m/z*, 651 *m/z*	0.04 ng/mL (LLOQ)	Hashimoto *et al.* (2008)

Table 1.1 (continued)

Sample matrix	Sample preparation	Assay method	Detection limit	Reference
Human plasma and urine	Addition of buffer solution pH 6, loading into oasis HLB30 mg 96-well plate preconditioned with methanol:water (40:60), elution of analyte with pure methanol, evaporation, reconstitution in methanol	LC-ESI-MS Column: C_{18} Mobile phase: 5 mM ammonium acetate and acetonitrile Flow rate: 250 µL/min SRM transition: 798.5 *m/z*, 651.4 *m/z* (positive mode)	0.2 ng/mL (LLOQ) 1 ng/mL (LLOQ)	Salvador *et al.* (2006)
Drinking-water, ground water, surface water, and waste water	SPE by using oasis HLB cartridge	LC-MS-TOF Column: C_8 Mobile phase: acetonitrile, water with 0.1% formic acid	1–1000 ng/L (LOD)	Ferrer & Thurman (2012)
Water, soil, sediment, and biosolids	Extraction with solvents, and SPE	LC-MS-MS	50 ng/L in water (LOD)	EPA (2007)
Plant extract	Extracted from herbaceous plants of the genus *Digitalis*	LC-ESI-MS Column: C_{18} Mobile phase: aqueous ammonium formate/methanol (40/60% v/v), pure methanol Flow rate: 0.3 mL/min SRM transition: 798.5 *m/z*, 780.4 *m/z*	38–936 pg/g in solution (LOD)	Josephs *et al.* (2010)
Rat plasma	Addition of ammonium chloride buffer, acetonitrile and methylene chloride, vortexing, centrifugation, evaporation of organic layer, reconstitution	LC-ESI-MS Column: C_{18} Mobile phase: acetonitrile/ammonium formate Flow rate: 0.2 mL/min SRM transition: 798.60 *m/z*, 651.6 *m/z*	0.1 ng/L (LOQ)	Yao *et al.* (2003)
Human serum	Incubation, centrifugation, supernatant loaded into a vial and frozen	IC Colloidal gold mAb probe-colloidal gold conjugate with IgG	Visual detection limit, 2 ng/mL Detection time, 2–5 min	Omidfar *et al.* (2010)
Human blood and urine	Addition of water and ammonium acetate buffer (2 M, pH 9.5), centrifugation, collection of supernatant, clean-up by SPE	LC-ESI-MS Column: C_{18} Mobile phase: 20% acetonitrile in 80% 2 mM ammonium formate and 80% acetonitrile in 20% 2 mM ammonium formate Flow rate: 0.2 mL/min SRM transition: 799.4 *m/z*, 651.4 *m/z*	0.05 ng/mL (LLOQ)	Guan *et al.* (1999)

Table 1.1 (continued)

Sample matrix	Sample preparation	Assay method	Detection limit	Reference
Rat intestinal perfusion samples	NR	LC-UV Column: C_{18} Mobile phase: 10 mM ammonium acetate, methanol, acetonitrile (50 : 25 : 25) Flow rate: 0.5 mL/min pH 3.0 Wavelength: 220 nm	25 ng/mL (LOQ)	Varma *et al.* (2004)
Human plasma	NR	LC-ESI-MS Column: C_{18} Mobile phase: acetonitrile and 2 mM ammonium acetate pH 3.0 Flow rate: 0.2 mL/min SRM transition:7 99 *m/z*	NR	Tracqui *et al.* (1997)

DMA, *N,N*-dimethylacetamide; IC, immunochromatography; IgG, immunoglobulin G; LC-ESI-MS, liquid chromatography electrospray ionization mass spectrometry; LC-MS-MS, liquid chromatography tandem mass spectrometry; LC-TOF-MS, liquid chromatography time of flight mass spectrometry; LC-UV, liquid chromatography ultraviolet spectroscopy; LLOQ, lower limit of quantification; LOD, limit of detection; LOQ, limit of quantification; mAb, monoclonal antibody; min, minute; MRM, multiple reaction monitoring; *m/z*, mass/charge; NaCl, sodium chloride; NaOH, sodium hydroxide; NR, not reported; SIM, selected ion monitoring; SPE, solid-phase extraction; SRM, selected reaction monitoring

Table 1.2 Most commonly reported clinical indications for digoxin in the USA, 2011–2012

Diagnosis	ICD-9 code[a]	Drug uses (in 1000s)	Percentage of total
Atrial fibrillation	427.301	1595	42.3
Hypertensive heart disease, other	402.901	621	16.5
Congestive heart failure	428.001	501	13.3
Other primary cardiomyopathy, NOS	425.402	113	3.0
Chronic ischaemic disease, unspecified	414.901	81	2.1
Essential hypertension, NOS	401.901	65	1.7
Surgery after heart disease treatment	V67.038	53	1.4
Medical follow-up after atherosclerotic heart disease	V67.533	50	1.3
Paroxysmal supraventricular tachycardia	427.001	50	1.3
Chronic ischaemic disease, unspecified, with hypertension	414.501	50	1.3
All other diagnoses	–	593	15.7
Total with reported diagnoses	–	3771	100.0

[a] ICD-9 codes are a more detailed, proprietary version developed by IMS Health.
Prepared by the Working Group on the basis of data from IMS Health (2012b)
ICD-9, International Classification of Diseases Revision Nine; NOS, not otherwise specified

ejection fraction and for atrial fibrillation, it has been largely supplanted by other medications (Sleeswijk *et al.*, 2007). Digitoxin is useful for maintenance therapy because its long half-life (5 – 9 days) provides a sustained therapeutic effect even if a dose is missed. For the same reason toxic reactions are not easy to manage. Elimination is independent of renal function (Albrecht & Geiss, 2000).

For congestive heart failure, use of digoxin fails to improve survival (Digitalis Investigation Group, 1997) when compared with placebo, unlike other leading therapies. It does, however, provide symptomatic benefits in some cases and is associated with reduced risk of hospitalization. USA guidelines suggest its use in situations where recommended therapies (diuretics, angiotensin-converting-enzyme inhibitors and β-blockers) fail to produce adequate symptom relief (Hunt *et al.*, 2009). European guidelines continue to recommend digoxin as one of several therapies used in combination for the management of congestive heart failure (Dickstein *et al.*, 2008).

As for congestive heart failure, use of digoxin for atrial fibrillation has also declined in preference for other medications, particularly β-blockers and non-dihydropyridine calcium-channel blockers. Digoxin is generally less effective than other drugs in producing consistent reduction of heart rate, particularly during exertion (McNamara *et al.*, 2003). Joint USA/European Union guidelines recommend against use of digoxin as a first-line agent in most cases of atrial fibrillation (Fuster *et al.*, 2006).

(b)   Dosage

Administration is typically oral, although preparations for intravenous administration exist. Typically, digoxin is used orally for months to years, while intravenous use requires careful medical monitoring and is given only in the short-term. The absorption ratio was found to be 70%, the decay ratio is 20%, the effective dose level is 2 mg, and the maintenance dose is 0.5 mg (Albrecht & Geiss, 2000).

For the treatment of heart failure, atrial fibrillation, the loading-dose regimen for intravenous administration is a single dose of 0.4–0.6 mg, with additional doses of 0.1–0.3 mg every 6–8 hours to be given with caution until there is clinical evidence of adequate effect, and the total dose should not exceed 0.008–0.015 mg/kg bw. The oral dosage for this indication is a single dose of 0.5–0.75 mg, then additional doses of 0.125–0.375 mg may be given cautiously every 6–8 hours until clinical evidence of adequate effect, up to a total dose of 0.75–1.25 mg (for a patient weighing 70 kg). The maintenance dose is 0.125–0.5 mg/day, intravenous or oral (Medscape (2013).

Most generic tablet preparations of digoxin average 70–80% oral bioavailability, with 90–100% oral bioavailability for digoxin elixir and the encapsulated gel preparation. Parenteral digoxin is available for intravenous administration, and is of value in patients who are unable to take oral formulations. Caution to avoid over-dosing is necessary in elderly patients or those with renal impairment (Li-Saw-Hee & Lip, 1998). In general, the therapeutic index for digoxin is narrow (Ehle *et al.*, 2011).

When digoxin is indicated, suggested thera-peutic ranges of serum concentrations of digoxin are lower now than in the past (Hunt *et al.*, 2009), particularly given the report that mortality among digoxin users was associated with higher serum concentrations of this drug (Rathore *et al.*, 2003). In a study of post-mortem cases, the range of serum digoxin concentrations in cases of over-dose was 2.7–6.8 nmol/L (mean, 4.7 nmol/L) [2.1–5.3 ng/L (mean, 3.7 ng/L)] (Eriksson *et al.*, 1984).

Country-dependent differences in formula-tions may be correlated to the range of available tablet strengths. For example, the dosage was significantly higher in some hospitals in the USA and France than in the United Kingdom, and significantly higher in France than in the USA (Saunders *et al.*, 1997).

(c)   Trends in use

Use of digoxin in the USA has declined substantially for treatment of congestive heart failure (Banerjee & Stafford, 2010) and of atrial fibrillation (Stafford *et al.*, 1998; Fang *et al.*,

2004). Trends in the European Union may have lagged behind those in the USA, but use for both conditions has declined (Sturm *et al.*, 2007). Use of digoxin may have been reduced between 1991 and 2004 in the USA, but not in the United Kingdom (Haynes *et al.*, 2008).

The Food and Drug Administration (FDA) reported that digitoxin and acetyldigitoxin are no longer manufactured in the USA (FDA, 2013).

Globally, there are 160 licensed products containing digoxin, while there are only seven licensed products containing digitoxin in Germany, Austria, Hungary, and Norway (Index Nominum, 2013).

Despite the introduction of new therapeutic strategies, cardiac glycosides are still widely used, and digoxin belongs to the 10 most frequently prescribed drugs in the USA (Albrecht & Geiss, 2000). In Estonia, the consumption of digoxin was very high in the times of the former Soviet Union and decreased in the first years of inde-pendence. When problems with drug availability were overcome, the use of digoxin increased by 35% in 1994–97 (Pähkla *et al.*, 1999).

While a rare event, the homicidal use of digoxin has been described. Suicide by digoxin may have been more frequent in continental Europe, but has also occurred in the USA and England (Burchell, 1983).

Total worldwide sales of digoxin were US$ 142 million in 2012, with 33% occurring in the USA (US$ 47 million). Other nations reporting appreciable use of digoxin included Japan (US$ 14 million), Canada (US$ 11 million), and the United Kingdom (US$ 9 million) (IMS Health, 2012a).

In the USA in 2012, digoxin was reported by office-based physicians in 1.85 million drug uses, and was being taken by approximately 700 000 patients (IMS Health, 2012b). The trend in use of digoxin in the USA is shown in Fig. 1.1. According to the IMS Health National Prescription Audit Plus, there were a total of 9.6 million prescriptions for digoxin in 2012, down from 14.6 million prescriptions in 2008 (IMS Health, 2012c).

1.4 Occurrence and exposure

1.4.1 Natural occurrence

The principal natural occurrence of digoxin is in the leaves of *Digitalis lanata* Ehrh., but it may also occur in some other *Digitalis* species (Hollman, 1985). After leaf-tissue damage or plant harvest, the primary glycoside lanatoside C is converted to the secondary glycoside digoxin by the endogenous enzyme, digilanidase, present in the leaves, and by subsequent deacetylation. *D. lanata* leaves were found to contain digoxin at 8.6–13.2 µg/100 mg and its precursor, lanatoside C, at 55.8–153.2 µg/100 mg, depending on the health of the plant material (Pellati *et al.*, 2009). Environmental factors that influence the digoxin content in *D. lanata* are carbon-dioxide enrichment and water stress (Stuhlfauth *et al.*, 1987).

1.4.2 Occupational exposure

No data were available to the Working Group.

1.5 Regulations and guidelines

Digoxin has been assigned classification as a "water hazard" in Germany and as an "environmental hazard" in several USA states (SciFinder (2013). The United States Environmental Protection Agency (EPA) assigned it to the list of "extremely hazardous substances" mandated by Section 302 of the Emergency Planning and Community Right-to-Know Act of 1986 (EPCRA), for which the reportable quantity is 10 lbs [~4.5 kg] and the threshold planning quantity is 10/10 000 lbs [4.5/4536 kg].

Digoxin is specified in several official pharmacopoeias (Table 1.3).

2. Cancer in Humans

Beginning in the late 1970s, several small studies based on case series or chart reviews reported a lower risk of cancer of the breast in women using "digitalis" (see introduction to Section 1) (Stenkvist *et al.*, 1979, 1982; Goldin & Safa, 1984). These reports, mostly in brief correspondence, have been cited as supporting the consideration of digitalis as a possible therapy for cancer of the breast (Stenkvist, 1999; Haux, 1999); however, because so little information was provided and larger studies with stronger designs were available, these early studies were judged to be uninformative and were not considered further.

The studies reviewed by the Working Group included a measure of relative risk, such as odds ratios, hazard ratios, and incidence rate ratios. Varied designs were used in these studies. Some studies evaluated associations between risks of cancers of all types and exposures to a wide range of pharmaceuticals, or to a more restricted range of cardiovascular drugs. Others examined risk factors for specific cancers, typically including prescription drugs together with evaluation of other demographic and health parameters. In recent years, national registries of prescription drug use have yielded large data sets in which follow-up can be linked to cancer outcomes in cohort studies.

Many reports described only "digitalis" exposure, and therefore may refer to either digoxin (much more commonly used, especially in recent years) or digitoxin. Even when some epidemiological studies specified "digoxin," the subjects who were enrolled during years when digitoxin was more widely used might have also used digitoxin (e.g. because of renal failure). The studies describing "digitalis" use are therefore included, with the exposure type digoxin, digitoxin, or digitalis, indicated in the tables. Most

Fig. 1.1 Trends in use of digoxin as a drug in the USA, 2004–2012

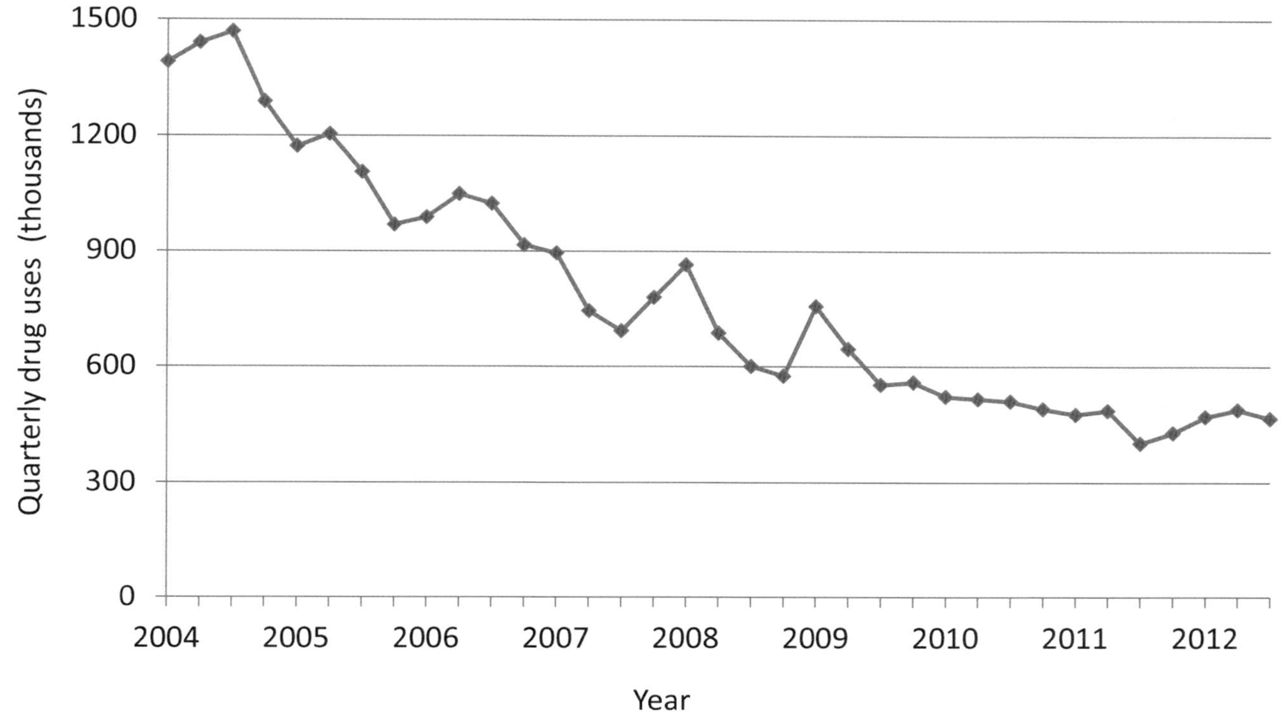

Prepared by the Working Group on the basis of data from IMS Health National Disease and Therapeutic Index, 2004–12 (IMS Health, 2012b).

of what has been used under the term "digitalis" in North America and Europe has been digoxin.

2.1 Cancer of the breast

2.1.1 Case–control studies

See Table 2.1

Studies of the association of risk of cancer with use of digoxin and related drugs have focused mainly on cancer of the breast. Aromaa *et al.* (1976) reported a register-based case–control study in which use of "digitalis" (and many other cardiovascular drugs) in the year before diagnosis was compared in 109 hypertensive women with cancer of the breast and in 109 matched hypertensive women without cancer of the breast. Hypertensive women with cancer of the breast were more likely to be using

digitalis than were women without cancer of the breast (relative risk, RR, 2.67; 95% CI, 0.99–8.33; in the subset restricted to 65 pairs with similar follow-up time.). [Both cases and controls were hypertensive and both were therefore at a high risk of cardiovascular disease. This comparability enhanced internal validity, but it may have reduced generalizability.]

Lenfant-Pejovic *et al.* (1990) described risk factors for cancer of the breast in men in France and Switzerland, comparing 91 cases with 255 controls recruited from hospital cancer clinics in France and a cancer registry in Switzerland, and matched for age and area of residence. Data on risk factors were limited to information available in physician interviews by mail or telephone, and clinical record reviews. Of all prescribed drugs, only use of digitalis for at least 3 months before

Table 1.3 Regulations in pharmacopoeial monographs on digoxin

Regulation	WHO International Pharmacopoeia, 4th edition	United States Pharmacopeial Convention 30	European Pharmacopoeia 7.0	Japanese Pharmacopoeia XVI
Content $C_{41}H_{64}O_{14}$ (dried substance)	95.0–103.0%	95.0–101.0%	96.0–102.0%	96.0–106.0%
Identity tests	Tests ABD or BCD may be applied: A. IR B. TLC C. Colour reaction with dinitrobenzene/ ethanol D. Colour reaction with ferric chloride/ glacial acetic acid/sulfuric acid	A. IR B. HPLC C. TLC	IR	1. Colour reaction with ferric chloride hexahydrate/acetic acid/ sulfuric acid 2. IR
Specific optical rotation	+13.6° to +14.2° (0.10 g/mL in pyridine)	–	+13.9° to 15.9° (0.50 g in 25 mL methanol/methylene chloride 50 : 50)	+10.0 to + 13.0° (0.20 g in 10 mL pyridine)
Sulfated ash	Max. 1.0 mg/g	–	Max. 0.1%	–
Loss on drying	Max. 10 mg/g	Max. 1.0%	Max. 1.0%	Max. 1.0%
Residue on ignition	–	Max. 0.5%	–	Max. 0.5%
Gitoxin	Absorbance at 352 nm, max. 0.22 (about 40 mg/g)	–	–	–
Related substances/ purity	TLC test, absence of spots that are more intense than standard solution at 0.25 mg/mL	TLC test, no spot that is more intensive than gitoxin standard solution (not more than 3% of any related glycoside as gitoxin)	HPLC: specific limits for about 12 related substances are specified	HPLC: total area of peaks of impurities is max. 3%
Organic volatile impurities	–	General requirements, except limits for methylene chloride and chloroform are 2000 µg/g	–	–
Bacterial endotoxins	Max. 200.0 IU of endotoxin per mg	–	–	–

HPLC, high-performance liquid chromatography; IR, infrared; IU, international units; TLC, thin-layer chromatography

Adapted from The United States Pharmacopoeial Convention (2006), European Pharmacopoeia (2008), The International Pharmacopoeia (2011), Pharmaceuticals and Medical Devices Agency (2011)

diagnosis was associated with increased risk (11 users among cases; odds ratio, OR, 4.1; 95% CI, 1.4–12.4). [The data from France and Switzerland were collected in different ways and the Working Group questioned the quality of the data obtained from medical records and physician interviews.]

In another study of risk factors for cancer of the breast in men, Ewertz *et al.* (2001) compared 156 incident cases in men in Norway, Sweden, and Denmark with 468 men matched for year of birth, and country. Many variables were evaluated using self-administered questionnaires, including use of prescribed drugs. Among all drugs assessed, digoxin stood out most strongly, with odds ratios for digoxin of 1.8 (95% CI, 0.7–4.4) in men with < 5 years use and 2.0 (0.9–4.4) for ≥ 5 years use. After adjustment for body mass index determined from self-estimated weight and height 10 years before diagnosis, the association between cancer of the breast and digoxin use was still 1.8 ($P = 0.08$). [Recalculated by the Working Group from observed/expected data to be 1.9 (95% CI, 1.05–3.48).]

Ahern *et al.* (2008) identified 5565 postmenopausal women with incident cancer of the breast who used digoxin with a 10 : 1 birth year- and residence area-matched population-control group in Denmark in 1991–2007. Use of digoxin was ascertained by county-level prescription registry data, and by design, all subjects were required to have used digoxin for ≥ 2 years before diagnosis (and use was likely to be current). Adjustments included age, past use of hormone replacement therapy, nonsteroidal anti-inflammatory drugs (NSAIDs), and anticoagulants including aspirin. Among the cases of cancer of the breast, 324 used digoxin compared with 2546 controls, yielding an adjusted odds ratio of 1.30 (95% CI, 1.14–1.48). Relative to non-users, the odds ratios increased with duration of use from 1.25 (95% CI, 1.03–1.52) with 1–3 years of use to 1.30 (95% CI, 1.05–1.61) with 4–6 years of use to 1.39 (95% CI, 1.10–1.74) with > 6 years of use. The findings persisted after adjustment for exposure to estrogen, use of other

drugs, confounding by indication, and frequency of mammography. [This large study was regarded as being of high quality. However, the Working Group noted that some important risk factors of cancer of the breast, notably parity, obesity, and alcohol drinking, were not controlled in the analysis.]

2.1.2 Cohort studies

See Table 2.2

Using data from persons enrolled in the Kaiser Permanente Medical Care Programme, Friedman & Ury (1980) linked prescription-drug use for 95 drugs and drug classes between 1969 and 1973 to subsequent cancer outcomes (56 types) registered within this health-care system until 1976. The drugs evaluated included "digitalis" as a group. A more detailed presentation of digitalis-related associations used cancer-outcome data for 143 594 subjects updated to 1980 (Friedman, 1984) (results provided in Table 2.2). The age–sex standardized morbidity ratio for cancer of the breast and ever-use of digitalis was 1.2 [95% CI, 0.74–1.87]. [This study was large and was able to examine the association of cancer with many different drugs; however, the precision of specific drug–cancer associations was limited and there was some concern about the large number of comparisons.]

Haux *et al.* (2001) used a database of plasma concentrations of digitoxin for 9271 women and men in Trondheim, Norway, who were undergoing their first treatment with digitoxin between 1986 and 1996. The risk of developing cancer in people receiving their first treatment with digitoxin was compared with the incidence of cancers with at least 30 expected cases (all sites, breast, prostrate, colorectum, lung, kidney/urinary, melanoma, lymphoid/leukaemia) in the national population. Standardized incidence ratios (SIR) for most cancers, including cancer of the breast, were higher (typically by about 25%) among digitoxin users. In an analysis of cancer

Table 2.1 Case–control studies on use of digoxin and cancer of the breast

Reference, study location and period	Subjects	Exposure assessment	Organ site	Exposed cases	Exposure category	Relative risk (95% CI)	Adjustments for potential confounders	Comments
Aromaa et al. (1976), Finland, cases reported in 1973	Women with breast cancers and hypertension (n = 109) compared with matched women with hypertension only (n = 109)	Prescription-acquired cardiovascular drugs	Breast	28	Any digitalis use vs no use	1.33 (0.73–2.48)	Age, geographical area	Digitalis use was a secondary outcome, but the strongest association seen among prescription drug used; probably included some digitoxin users.
				16	Any digitalis use vs no use (case–control pairs with comparable treatment duration)	2.67 (0.99–8.33)		
Lenfant-Pejovic et al. (1990), Switzerland, 1970–86, and France, 1975–88	Men with breast cancer (n = 91) identified in hospital or by tumour registries compared with men with colorectal, haematolymphatic, or skin cancers (n = 255)	Hospital chart abstracts and physician interview; digitalis specified	Breast, adeno-carcinoma	11	Any digitalis use vs no use	4.1 (1.4–12.4)	Controls matched by age and hospital	Digitalis was the only one of many therapeutic drugs for which an association was found. Probably included some digitoxin users.
Ewertz et al. (2001), Norway, Sweden, Denmark, 1987–91	Men with breast cancer (n = 156) compared with men in population registry (n = 468)	Self-reported questionnaires including prescription-drug use and other demographic and health data	Breast	20	Never digoxin Digoxin < 5 yr Digoxin ≥ 5 yr	1.0 (ref.) 1.8 (0.7–4.4) 2.0 (0.9–4.4).	Matched for sex, age; overall analysis adjusted for BMI	Multiple comparisons to diverse demographic, health, and drug-use variables, but association for digoxin appeared to be the strongest among drugs; probably included some digitoxin users. P = 0.08 for overall association between digoxin use and breast cancer

Table 2.1 (continued)

Reference, study location and period	Subjects	Exposure assessment	Organ site	Exposed cases	Exposure category	Relative risk (95% CI)	Adjustments for potential confounders	Comments
Ahern *et al.* (2008), North Jutland and Aarhus Counties, Denmark, 1991–2007	Postmenopausal women with breast cancer (*n* = 5565) compared with matched women from population registry (*n* = 55 650)	County-based pharmacy registries	Breast	5241	Never-user	1.0 (ref.)	Age, location; use of anti-inflammatory drugs, anticoagulants or HRT	Tumour ER status not examined. Association not greatly changed by adjustments; Suggestion of increased risk with longer duration of use. May have included some digitoxin users in early years, although described as digoxin users. Adjusted for age, county of residence, and past receipt of HRT, anticoagulants, high- and low-dose aspirin, and NSAIDs.
				324	Ever used digoxin (restricted to case–control pairs with comparable treatment duration)	1.30 (1.14–1.48)		
				128	1–3 yr	1.25 (1.03–1.52)		
				103	4–6 yr	1.30 (1.05–1.61)		
				93	7–18 yr	1.39 (1.10–1.74)		

BMI, body mass index; ER, estrogen receptor; HRT, hormone replacement therapy; NSAIDs; non-steroidal anti-inflammatory drugs; ref., reference; vs, versus; yr, year incidence in people before their first use of digitoxin, odds ratios for most cancers were similarly increased. An analysis of the relationship between risk of cancer and serum concentration of digitoxin did not show a coherent relationship for cancer of the breast. [The Working Group noted that the national population used as comparison group was external to the study population and may differ in its underlying disease risk or in the quality of cancer ascertainment. Elevated risk of cancer in the study population before beginning treatment may be attributable to underlying increases in the frequency of common risk factors for cancer and for cardiovascular disease requiring digitoxin, rather than the use of digitoxin itself. In addition, estimates of digitoxin dose were based on a single measurement at the start of treatment and there was no information about ongoing exposure.]

Biggar *et al.* (2011) reported a nationwide cohort study in Denmark, evaluating incidence of cancer of the breast in women prescribed digoxin. Data were obtained by linking the national Danish prescription-drug database (available since 1995) and the nationwide Danish cancer registry until 2008. Among 104 648 women using digoxin, 2144 developed cancer of the breast. Risks associated with current and former use, and duration of current use among new users only were analysed, with incidence rate ratios for cancer of the breast adjusted for attained age at diagnosis and calendar year. The relative risk (RR) for current use was 1.39 (95% CI, 1.32–1.46), with higher risk for developing estrogen receptor-positive tumours (RR, 1.35; 95% CI, 1.26–1.45) than estrogen receptor-negative tumours (RR, 1.20; 95% CI, 1.03–1.40) among digoxin users. Incidence was not increased in women who had used digoxin in the past (SIR, 0.91; 95% CI, 0.83–1.00). Increased incidence was not associated with duration of use, but declined to baseline within 1 year after use of digoxin had ceased. [This was regarded as a high-quality study, with the capacity to examine risk by estrogen-receptor status being a particular strength. The study did not examine the effect of menopausal status; however, most women included were postmenopausal (median age, 79 years). Information on other covariates was limited. While there are many risk factors for cancer of the breast, the inability to control for alcohol drinking and obesity was likely to be of greatest concern.]

Biggar *et al.* (2013) examined features of cancer of the breast in a case–case comparison of cancers developed in 369 women who were using digoxin at the time of diagnosis with 34 085 cancers in women not using digoxin. Tumours in users were significantly more likely (*P* = 0.002) to be estrogen receptor-positive (85%) than estrogen receptor-negative (79%), and to have low versus high histological grades, features suggesting better prognosis. [The prognostic factors for cancer of the breast in women receiving digoxin and in women receiving estrogen were similar and more favourable, e.g. estrogen receptor-positive tumours, than in women not receiving treatment (IARC, 2012).]

2.2 Cancers of the uterus and ovary

Cohort study

See Table 2.3

In a cohort study in Denmark, Biggar *et al.* (2012) evaluated the risk of cancer of the uterus. The methods and data sources were identical to those in the study of cancer of the breast described in Section 2.1.2 (Biggar *et al.*, 2011). As with cancer of the breast, the incidence of cancer of the uterus (*n* = 461 cases in digoxin users) was increased among current users (RR, 1.48; 95% CI, 1.32–1.65). In addition, this study also evaluated cancers of the ovary (*n* = 277) and cervix (*n* = 117) as "control cancers," finding no increase in the incidence of either cancer (RR for cancer of the ovary, 1.06; 95% CI, 0.92–1.22; RR for cancer of the cervix, 1.00; 95% CI, 0.79–1.25)

Table 2.2 Cohort studies on use of digoxin and cancer of the breast

Reference, location, and period	Subjects	Exposure assessment	Organ site	Exposed cases	Exposure category	Relative risk (95% CI)	Adjustments for potential confounders Comments
Friedman (1984), Kaiser Permanente Medical Care Program (USA), 1969–80	Members of a private health-care insurance programme (*n* = 143 594)	Pharmacy database from Health Plan	Lung Colon Breast Prostate	48 35 20 34	Digitalis ever-use (digoxin, digitoxin, digitalis)	1.7 [1.22–2.20] 1.5 [1.02–2.04] 1.2 [0.74–1.87] 1.4 [1.00–2.01]	Age, sex Main summary for all drug-cancer relationships reported by Friedman & Ury (1980). Updated to 1980: Friedman (1984). Multiple comparisons. No association found for other cancers.
Haux *et al.* (2001), Trondheim, Norway, 1986–96	People (*n* = 9 271) undergoing their first digitoxin treatment	Digitoxin in plasma measured in a central laboratory	All sites Female breast Prostate Colorectum Lung Kidney/urinary Melanoma Leukaemia/lymphoma (C81–C 85/C88/92) Breast	641 57 108 127 63 59 61 53	Digitoxin use Digitoxin concentration (ng/mL): < 16 16–22 > 22	1.27 (1.18–1.37) 1.25 (0.95–1.62) 1.25 (1.03–1.50) 1.29 (1.06–1.51) 1.35 (1.04–1.74) 1.14 (0.87–1.47) 1.23 (0.94–1.58) 1.41 (1.06–1.85) 1.00 (ref.) 1.04 (0.59–1.84) 0.90 (0.48–1.67)	Age, year of birth, sex Incidence compared to population incidence when > 30 cases were expected Use based on single assessment of digitoxin. A high risk of cancer diagnosed before digitoxin measurement (not shown) suggested high cancer risk preceded use. Expected numbers of cancers obtained from national registry rates. Dose–response on the cohort on digitoxin users by different levels of digitoxin plasma concentration at first measurement divided in tertiles
Biggar *et al.* (2011), Denmark, 1995–2008	Women aged ≥ 20 yr (*n* = 2 011 381)	Nationwide pharmacy registry for drug exposure	Breast	46 872 2144 454 1690	Never Ever Former Current	1.0 1.24 (1.18–1.30) 0.91 (0.83–1.00) 1.39 (1.32–1.46)	Attained age, calendar-year Association found only with current use of digoxin and stronger when restricted to women with ER-positive tumours. Duration results apply to all breast cancers, regardless of ER status.

Table 2.2 (continued)

Reference, location, and period	Subjects	Exposure assessment	Organ site	Exposed cases	Exposure category	Relative risk (95% CI)	Adjustments for potential confounders Comments
Biggar et al. (2011), Denmark, 1995–2008 (cont.)					Duration of use in new users only (mo):		
				306	0–12	1.65 (1.47–1.86)	
				147	13–24	1.31 (1.12–1.55)	
				92	25–36	1.13 (0.92–1.38)	
				265	37+	1.31 (1.16–1.48)	

ER, estrogen receptor; mo, month; ref., reference; vs, versus; yr, year among current users. Patterns of risk with duration of digoxin use were not consistent by cancer type. For cancer of the uterus, stronger associations were observed for digoxin use of 0–12 months (RR, 1.60; 95% CI, 1.23–2.07) and > 37 months (RR, 1.91; 95% CI, 1.51–2.41) among current users, while for cancer of the ovary the strongest association was for digoxin use of 0–12 months among current users (RR, 1.37; 95% CI, 1.01–1.86) among current users. [The strengths and limitations of this study were the same as for the study of cancer of the breast based on the same cohort (Biggar *et al.*, 2011).]

2.3 Cancer of the prostate

Cohort studies

See Table 2.4

Platz *et al.* (2011) examined the association between incidence of cancer of the prostate and use of digoxin in the USA-based Health Professionals Follow-up Study, following 47 884 men from 1986 until 2006. Data on use of digoxin were obtained by self-administered questionnaire at baseline and at 2-year intervals during follow-up. Ever-users of digoxin had lower incidence of cancer of the prostate compared with never-users, after adjustment for multiple risk factors, including race, body mass index, exercise, and smoking (RR, 0.83; 95% CI, 0.72–0.94), which was not changed by adjustment for other cardiovascular drugs (cholesterol-lowering agents, aspirin). The inverse association was seen regardless of indication for digoxin use (heart failure or arrhythmia), present when digoxin was the only cardiac medication used (other than aspirin), apparent at all stages of cancer of the prostate, and stronger in current than former users. The adjusted risk ratio for cancer of the prostate decreased with duration of use from 0.87 (0.73–1.04) for those with < 5 years of use to 0.54 (0.37–0.79) for those with ≥ 10 years of use (*P* for trend < 0.001). [This was regarded as a

high-quality study with robust findings adjusted for an extensive array of covariates. Although exposure data were self-reported, reports by the health professionals were assumed to be of relatively high quality. Cancer outcomes were also self-reported, but validated by pathology-record review in 95% of cases.]

The association between cancer of the prostate and ever-use of drugs in the digitalis group was examined in the cohort study by Friedman & Ury (1980) and Friedman (1984), described in Section 2.1.2. The standardized morbidity ratio was 1.4 [95% CI, 1.00–2.01; 34 cases].

An increased risk of cancer of the prostate was also reported in the Norwegian cohort study by Haux *et al.*, (2001). The relative risk was 1.25 (95% CI, 1.03–1.50). [As noted in Section 2.1.2, relative risks were elevated for most of the cancers examined, leading to doubts about the appropriateness of the comparison group.]

2.4 Non-Hodgkin lymphoma

Case–control study

See Table 2.5

To determine whether the development of non-Hodgkin lymphoma is associated with medication use, Bernstein & Ross (1992) reviewed prescription-medication use in 619 cases of non-Hodgkin lymphoma in Los Angeles, USA, between 1979 and 1982, that were matched to 619 age, race, sex, and neighbourhood controls. Among 49 medications evaluated (along with many other health conditions and immunizations), the odds ratios for use of digitalis were 1.55 (95% CI, 0.99–2.43) for men and women combined, 2.4 (95% CI, 1.31–4.38) for women and 0.75 (95% CI, 0.36–1.59) for men. A trend with duration of use was found in women, but not in men. [Multiple comparisons were made with many drug- and non-drug-related variables, and the association with digitalis, seen only

Table 2.3 Cohort study on use of digoxin and cancer of the corpus uteri, cervix, and ovary

Reference, location, and period	Subjects	Exposure assessment	Organ sites	Exposed cases	Exposure categories	Relative risk (95% CI)	Adjustments for potential confounders Comments
Biggar et al. (2012), Denmark, 1995–2008	See Table 2.2 and Biggar et al. (2011)	Nationwide pharmacy registry	Corpus uteri	111	Former	1.20 (0.99–1.45)	Attained age, calendar year
				350	Current	1.48 (1.32–1.65)	Association to digoxin found only for uterine cancer and statistically significant only in current users; marginal association for former users.
					Duration of use (mo):		For uterine cancer, increase greatest with prolonged use;
				59	0–12	1.60 (1.23–2.07)	For all, a higher incidence was noted in the first year after diagnosis, which could suggest confounding by indication
				26	13–24	1.19 (0.81–1.75)	
				11	25–36	0.70 (0.39–1.27)	
				71	37+	1.91 (1.51–2.41)	
			Ovary	70	Former	0.95 (0.75–1.21)	
				207	Current	1.06 (0.92–1.22)	
					Duration of use (mo):		
				42	0–12	1.37 (1.01–1.86)	
				20	13–24	1.11 (0.71–1.72)	
				13	25–36	1.01 (0.58–1.74)	
				30	37+	1.02 (0.71–1.46)	
			Cervix uteri	36	Former	1.18 (0.85–1.65)	
				81	Current	1.00 (0.79–1.25)	
					Duration of use (mo):		
				18	0–12	1.44 (0.91–2.30)	
				8	13–24	1.10 (0.55–2.20)	
				5	25–36	0.96 (0.40–2.31)	
				8	37+	0.66 (0.33–1.32)	

mo, month

Table 2.4 Cohort study on use of digoxin and cancer of the prostate

Reference, location, and period	Subjects	Exposure assessment	Organ sites	Exposed cases	Exposure categories	Relative risk (95% CI)	Adjustments for potential confounders Comments
Platz *et al.* (2011), Health Professionals Follow-up Study, USA, 1985–2006	Men aged 40–75 years (*n* = 47 884)	Self-reported questionnaire data about current use of digoxin	Prostate, invasive cancer	4923 243 175	Never Ever Current Duration of use (yr): Never	1.0 0.83 (0.72–0.94) 0.78 (0.67–0.90) 1.0	Age, race, calendar year, BMI, height, smoking, diabetes, diet, exercise, vitamin E supplement Cohort analysis undertaken to assess effects observed in vitro (see Section 4). Cancer self-report supplemented with death-certificate data; pathology-record review: 94.5% complete.
				125 90 28	< 5 5–9.9 ≥ 10	0.87 (0.73–1.04) 0.87 (0.70–1.07) 0.54 (0.37–0.79)	

BMI, body mass index; yr, year

Table 2.5 Case–control study on use of digitalis and non-Hodgkin lymphoma

Reference, location, and period	Subjects	Exposure assessment	Organ sites	Exposure categories	Exposed cases	Relative risk (95% CI)	Adjustments for potential confounders
Bernstein & Ross (1992), Los Angeles County (USA), 1979–82	Cases, 619 Controls, 619 (neighbourhood)	Personal interview and questionnaire including ever-use of "digitalis"	Non-Hodgkin lymphoma	No digitalis	35	1.00	Matched on age, sex, race, and neighbourhood
				Digitalis (all)	52	1.55 (0.99–2.43)	
				Men	12	0.75 (0.36–1.59)	
				Women	40	2.40 (1.31–4.38)	
				All (men and women)			
				No digitalis		1.00	
				Digitalis 1–12 mo	23	1.35 (0.99–2.43)	
				Digitalis ≥ 13 mo	28	1.68 (0.92–3.08)	
				P for trend		0.063	
				Men			
				No digitalis		1.00	
				Digitalis 1–12 mo	7	1.00 (0.35–2.85)	
				Digitalis ≥ 13 mo		0.56 (0.19–1.66)	
				P for trend		0.34	
				Women			
				No digitalis		1.00	
				Digitalis 1–12 mo	16	1.72 (0.76–3.91)	
				Digitalis ≥ 13 mo	23	3.05 (1.35–6.87)	
				P for trend		0.042	

mo, month

in women and not in men, could have been a chance finding.]

2.5 Other cancer sites

See Table 2.2

Elevated relative risks of cancers of the lung and colorectum were observed in the cohort study by Friedman & Ury (1980) and Friedman (1984), and in the cohort study by Haux *et al.* (2001) described in Section 2.1.2. The relative risk of cancer of the lung was 1.7 [95% CI, 1.22–2.20] in the former study, and 1.35 (95% CI, 1.04–1.74) in the latter. For cancer of the colorectum, the relative risks were 1.5 [95% CI, 1.02–2.04] and 1.29 (95% CI, 1.06–1.51) for the same studies, respectively. Haux *et al.* (2001) also reported an increased risk of leukaemia and lymphoma combined (RR. 1.41; 95% CI, 1.06–1.85). [The Working Group considered that the study by Haux *et al.* (2001) may have used an inappropriate comparison group, as noted in Section 2.1.2, and had limited confidence in the results. The elevated relative risk of cancer of the lung could be due to an association between smoking and cardiovascular disease for which digitalis was prescribed.]

3. Cancer in Experimental Animals

No data were available to the Working Group.

4. Mechanistic and Other Relevant Data

4.1 Absorption, distribution, metabolism, and excretion

4.1.1 Humans

(a) Absorption and distribution

Digoxin exhibits first-order kinetics (Ehle *et al.*, 2011). In six healthy volunteers (average age, 20 ± 2.5 years) given a single infusion of digoxin of 750 µg for 20 minutes (Finch *et al.*, 1984), digoxin had a half-life of 37.2 ± 12 hours, an area under the curve (AUC) of concentration–time of 147.7 ± 78.6 ng/mL per hour, a large volume of distribution (311.4 ± 94.0 L) and clearance rate of 108.6 ± 59.1 mL/minute. In a study in four healthy men given 1 mg of tritium-labelled digoxin by intravenous injection (Marcus *et al.*, 1964), the drug disappeared very rapidly from the circulation; 3 minutes and 1 hour after the injection, only 15.9% and 2.8%, of the administered dose, respectively, was detected in the blood. The onset of pharmacological action, after intravenous administration, is detected within 15–30 minutes, and maximum effect within 1–4 hours (Ehle *et al.*, 2011).

The distribution of digoxin follows a two-compartment model (Reuning *et al.*, 1973), comprising plasma and rapidly equilibrating tissues (compartment one [small volume]), and the more slowly equilibrating tissues (compartment two [large volume]) (Currie *et al.*, 2011). Equilibrium between compartments is achieved after a minimum of 6 hours, distribution half-life is 35 minutes, onset of action (oral) approximately 30–120 minutes, and time to peak action (oral) is 6–8 hours (Currie *et al.*, 2011), or 2–6 hours, as reported by Ehle *et al.* (2011). Digoxin is 20–25% bound to plasma proteins (Ehle *et al.*, 2011).

After oral administration of digoxin, half-life and time to steady state vary significantly between individuals, and are also dependent on renal function (Ehle *et al.*, 2011). In healthy subjects, the half-life is 1.5–2 days (Currie *et al.*, 2011; Ehle *et al.*, 2011), and steady state is reached in 5–7 days (Ehle *et al.*, 2011). In anuric patients, half-life is prolonged to 3.5–5 days (Currie *et al.*, 2011; Ehle *et al.*, 2011), and steady state is reached in up to 15–20 days (Ehle *et al.*, 2011). The volume of distribution is 4–7 L/kg in healthy subjects (Ehle *et al.*, 2011), but is decreased in people with renal disease and hypothyroidism, and increased in people with hyperthyroidism (Currie *et al.*, 2011). A study of 32 men and 35 women receiving long-term therapy with digoxin (in doses individualized according to body weight), showed no sex-based differences in serum concentration of digoxin (Lee & Chan 2006).

Oral bioavailability (F) of digoxin varies with formulation, and between individuals. Bioavailability from digoxin capsules, elixirs, or tablets are 90%, 80%, and 70%, respectively (Ehle *et al.*, 2011), and almost 100% from gelatine capsules (Currie *et al.*, 2011). Bioavailability of digoxin is physiologically controlled by the transmembrane transporter, P-glycoprotein, which has efflux pump function (Riganti *et al.*, 2011). P-glycoprotein controls bioavailability from its location on apical (or luminal) membranes of enterocytes of the small intestine, by active extrusion of digoxin, back into the lumen of gastrointestinal tract. A critical factor in intestinal absorption is the rate of apical efflux (Riganti *et al.*, 2011).

(i) Studies supporting an effect of MDR1 polymorphism

A study in 21 Caucasian individuals given a single oral dose of digoxin of 0.25 mg showed a correlation between polymorphism of the *MDR1* gene [the gene encoding P-glycoprotein, standard nomenclature, *ABCB1*] at exon 26 (C3435T) and significantly lower levels of duodenal expression and function of *MDR1*. Polymorphic individuals had higher plasma concentrations of digoxin compared with those with wildtype (C3435C) alleles (Hoffmeyer *et al.*, 2000).

In eight volunteers, pre-treatment with rifampicin, an inducer of P-glycoprotein, altered absorption of digoxin. The rifampicin-induced mean concentration of digoxin in people carrying the T-allele single-nucleotide polymorphism was higher than that of the wildtype (CC) population (Hoffmeyer *et al.*, 2000).

In healthy volunteers (with the TT and CC genotypes [$n = 7$ in each group]) given multiple oral doses of digoxin (0.25 mg per day) to achieve steady-state conditions, a statistically significant difference (mean, 38%) was found in maximum serum concentration of digoxin (C_{max}) between the two groups [read from Figure: CC, ~1.60 µg/L; TT, ~2.15 µg/L]. This may reflect the importance of genotype in determining absorption after oral administration of digoxin (Hoffmeyer *et al.*, 2000).

In 24 healthy Caucasian men who were homozygous carriers of the wildtype exon 26 C3435T (CC), or heterozygous (CT), or homozygous mutant (TT) [$n = 8$ in each group], AUC_{0-4h} ($P = 0.042$) and C_{max} ($P = 0.043$) differed significantly, with higher serum concentrations of digoxin in men with the 3435TT genotype than in those with wildtype C3435T (CC). No influence on digoxin parameters was detected for other single-nucleotide polymorphisms (Johne *et al.*, 2002).

Genotypes deduced from single-nucleotide polymorphism 2677G-T (exon 21) and 3435C-T, substantiated by haplotype analysis, also showed significant differences in AUC_{0-4h} and C_{max}. These analyses indicated that haplotype 12 (2677G/3435T) was associated with high values of AUC_{0-4h} and C_{max} for orally administered digoxin (Johne *et al.*, 2002).

In homozygous carriers of TT, kinetic parameters indicated a faster and more complete absorption of digoxin than in carriers of the wildtype. The digoxin plasma time course was evidenced by a 24% higher C_{max} and by a 22% higher AUC_{0-4h}, considered to result from increased rate (indicated by the steeper ascending phase of the curve in TT individuals) and extent of absorption (and not primarily of distribution) (Johne *et al.*, 2002).

High doses of digoxin are thought to saturate P-glycoprotein transport, triggering additional mechanisms. Thus, it is likely that at low doses, the pharmacokinetics of digoxin will be influenced by P-glycoprotein transport only, and thus would be more greatly perturbed by genetic differences in P-glycoprotein activity (Johne *et al.*, 2002).

A study of elderly patients in the Netherlands (n = 195; mean age, 79.4 years) who were taking digoxin regularly also showed that the common *MDR1* variants, 1236C-T, 2677G-T, and 3435C-T and the associated TTT haplotype were correlated with higher serum concentrations of digoxin (Aarnoudse *et al.*, 2008).

To understand the relative contribution of environmental and genetic factors to the pharmacokinetic variability of oral and intravenous digoxin, Birkenfeld *et al.* (2009) conducted a pilot study in 11 pairs of monozygotic twins (whose genes are almost identical), and 4 pairs of dizygotic twins (control). Measures of peak plasma concentration and T_{max} of digoxin, and calculated AUC, bioavailability, and renal clearance, after oral or intravenous administration, demonstrated strong correlation between monozygotic twins, findings explained largely by inheritance of P-glycoprotein function (Birkenfeld *et al.*, 2009).

(ii) Studies not supporting an effect of MDR1 polymorphism

Other studies have not shown an association between polymorphism in the *MDR1* gene and increased plasma concentrations of digoxin. A study in 114 healthy Japanese people given a single oral dose of digoxin of 0.25 mg (Sakaeda *et al.*, 2001) showed the serum concentration to be lower in those with a mutant allele (C3435T) at exon 26 of the *MDR1* gene. For the wildtype allele (CC), heterozygotes with a mutant T allele (C3435T) (CT), and homozygotes for the mutant allele (TT), values for AUC_{0-4h} (± standard deviation) were 4.11 ± 0.57, 3.20 ± 0.49, and 3.27 ± 0.58 ng/hour per mL, respectively. There was a significant difference between CC and CT or TT.

In a study in 39 Caucasian patients with congestive heart failure given digoxin at 0.25 mg per day for at least 7 days to reach steady state, Kurzawski *et al.* (2007) evaluated the effects of *MDR1* gene polymorphism on serum concentrations of digoxin, and in 24 patients, the effects of coadministration of digoxin with P-glycoprotein inhibitors. Significantly higher (approximately 1.5-fold) ($P < 0.002$) minimum serum concentrations of digoxin at steady state ($C_{min\,ss}$) were shown in patients given inhibitors of P-glycoprotein (0.868 ± 0.348 ng/mL), compared with those not given inhibitors (0.524 ± 0.281 ng/mL); however, in contrast to other studies, no association was found between 3435C > T and 2677G > A,T *MDR1* single-nucleotide polymorphisms and steady-state serum concentrations of digoxin (Kurzawski *et al.*, 2007).

A higher (1 mg) single oral dose of digoxin, without drug pre-treatment, in 50 healthy white men (aged 18–40 years) showed no differences in the AUC_{0-4h}, C_{max}, or t_{max} (as indices of digoxin absorption) among the genotype groups tested (Gerloff *et al.*, 2002). In contrast to previous reports (Hoffmeyer *et al.*, 2000), no differences were seen between homozygous carriers of the C and T allele in exon 26 3435 (AUC_{0-4h}, 9.24 and 9.38 mg/hour; C_{max}, 4.73 and 3.81 µg/L; t_{max}, 0.83 and 1.14 hours, respectively). The *MDR1* single-nucleotide polymorphisms studied, including that in exon 26, did not affect the absorption of a single oral dose of 1 mg of digoxin, and it was suggested that the higher dose (1 mg) of digoxin may have caused saturation of the transport capacity of intestinal P-glycoprotein. The pharmacokinetics of digoxin showed substantial variation within each genotypic group, indicating that factors additional to

P-glycoprotein may influence the absorption of digoxin (Gerloff *et al.*, 2002).

It is likely that passive diffusion (Gerloff *et al.*, 2002) or other transporters (Johne *et al.*, 2002), in addition to P-glycoprotein, contribute to variations in the pharmacokinetics of digoxin. Digoxin is a substrate for OATP8 (a member of the organic anion-transporting polypeptide group), for which genetic variants have been identified (Johne *et al.*, 2002), the effects of which, have not yet been elucidated. In addition, genetic variation in regulatory proteins, for example, the pregnane X receptor, involved in regulation of P-glycoprotein, may also affect digoxin disposition (Birkenfeld *et al.*, 2009). The absorption of digoxin may also be influenced by environmental factors (such as diet) by induction or inhibition of P-glycoprotein activity (Johne *et al.*, 2002; Gerloff *et al.*, 2002), or by genetic variants governing its distribution and elimination (Gerloff *et al.*, 2002).

(b)   Metabolism

Gault *et al.* (1984) demonstrated a major metabolic sequence of digoxin hydrolysis, oxidation, and conjugation, leading to polar end-metabolites. In this study, 10 patients with end-stage renal failure (who were dependent on dialysis), and 5 patients with comparatively normal renal function were given digoxin (as an oral dose of 150 µCi of [³H]digoxin-12α) and the metabolites were analysed by high-performance liquid chromatography (HPLC). Of these patients, 13 were receiving maintenance therapy with digoxin and were at steady state. The extent and time course of metabolism of digoxin varied between subjects, but variation was not significant between the two groups with different renal function. For all 15 patients, at 6 hours after drug administration, 26% (range, 7–76%) of the radiolabel was in the form of polar metabolites (quantitatively the most abundant metabolites), and 60% (range, 11–88%) was unchanged digoxin. Metabolites usually found albeit in small amounts were

3β-digoxigenin and its mono- and bis-digitoxosides, and 3-keto and 3α(epi)-digoxigenin.

This metabolic route comprised initial hydrolysis to 3β-digoxigenin with release of sugars in the stomach or liver, followed rapidly by oxidation to 3-keto-digoxigenin, epimerization to 3α(epi)-digoxigenin and finally glucuronide conjugation to polar species, 3-epi-glucuronide and 3-epi-sulfate. Results also indicated that conjugation of the mono-digitoxoside may occur, with steroid-ring hydroxylation, producing two isomers. In individuals demonstrating extensive metabolism, the lactone ring may be opened (possibly by a lactonase), forming a highly polar metabolite, or reduced, forming dihydro-metabolites (Gault *et al.*, 1984).

In studies using suspensions of freshly isolated human hepatocytes in vitro, metabolism of [³H]digoxin-12α has been shown to be very low (Lacarelle *et al.*, 1991); after a 2-hour incubation, extracellular radiolabel represented largely unchanged digoxin (up to 93%), with a minor (5% of the total extracellular radiolabel) unidentified polar metabolite. Similar results were obtained over a 24-hour exposure time in cultured human hepatocytes, and also in human liver microsomal fractions, indicating that cleavage of digoxin sugars is not dependent on the cytochrome P450 (CYP) system that requires reduced nicotinamide adenine dinucleotide phosphate (NADPH) (Lacarelle *et al.*, 1991; also see Fig. 4.1).

Digoxigenin mono-digitoxoside was extensively metabolized by human cultured hepatocytes to a single, more polar metabolite, which was subsequently completely hydrolysed by β-D-glucuronidase, and thus identified as the glucuronide of digoxigenin mono-digitoxoside. The extent of glucuronidation analysed in human liver microsomal fractions prepared from 13 different subjects was shown to vary among individuals by a factor of 3 (Lacarelle *et al.*, 1991).

Digoxigenin was also extensively biotransformed by cultured human hepatocytes. HPLC peaks were shown for one or more glucuronides,

3-epi-digoxigenin, unchanged digoxigenin, and possibly for unidentified metabolites. The intracellular concentration of 3-epi-digoxigenin decreased, due to conversion to polar compounds, which effluxed from the cells as formed. In human liver microsomes, no metabolites were observed in the absence of cofactor (NADPH or uridine 5'-diphospho-glucuronic acid, UDPGA); however, with NADPH present, "pre-digoxigenin" was detected. Formation of "pre-digoxigenin" therefore appeared to be CYP-dependent, with a large variability observed among individuals (Lacarelle *et al.*, 1991; also see Fig. 4.1).

In contrast, formation of 3-epi-digoxigenin did not depend on microsomal enzymes; it was only observed after incubation of digoxigenin with hepatocytes, and not with microsomes. In the presence of both NADPH and UDPGA, only small quantities of polar compounds were observed. These findings confirmed that 3-epi-digoxigenin is formed before synthesis of polar compounds. Thus, the main metabolic route for digoxigenin in vitro is the formation of 3-epi-digoxigenin, which is conjugated to a glucuronide (Lacarelle *et al.*, 1991; also see Fig. 4.1).

(c)   Elimination

Recovery of digoxin in the urine was reported as 70–85% (Currie *et al.*, 2011) and 50–70% (Ehle *et al.*, 2011). Drug recovery in the faeces was, on average, 14.8% of the administered dose, of which 14% comprised metabolic products (Marcus *et al.*, 1964).

In a study of the mechanisms of intestinal and biliary transport of digoxin, eight healthy men (aged 21–37 years), were given segmental intestinal perfusion of a P-glycoprotein inhibitor (quinidine) or inducer (rifampin), with intravenous administration of digoxin (1 mg). Results showed that intestinal P-glycoprotein mediates the elimination of intravenously administered digoxin from the systemic circulation into the gut lumen, as well as the control of absorption of orally administered digoxin from the gastrointestinal tract. These data also demonstrated a non-renal mechanism of elimination of digoxin, entailing direct secretion into the small intestine from the systemic circulation, which had greater importance than elimination via bile (Drescher *et al.*, 2003).

The organic anion transporter in human kidney (OATP4C1) may have an initial role in the transport of digoxin to the kidney. These transporters have been isolated, and shown by immunohistochemical analysis to be localized at the basolateral membrane of the proximal tubule cell in the kidney. Both human OATP4C1 and rat OATP4C1 transport digoxin in a sodium-independent manner (Mikkaichi *et al.*, 2004).

The role of OATPs in the disposition of digoxin has not been clearly defined. Data from various in-vitro systems have indicated that digoxin is not a substrate for human OATP1A2, OATP1B1, OATP1B3, or OATP2B1, although OATP4C1 may facilitate active uptake of digoxin into human kidney and liver. Digoxin is a substrate for a sodium-dependent transporter, shown to be endogenously expressed in a human kidney cell line (HEK29), and may, by its location in proximal tubular cells, partially facilitate renal clearance of digoxin (Taub *et al.*, 2011).

(d)   Interactions

The bioavailability of digoxin is affected by concurrent administration of many drugs which compete for binding to P-glycoprotein. Thus, digoxin auto-regulates its absorption. Many lipophilic P-glycoprotein-inducing drugs also promote CYP3A activity, and so a complex, and poorly understood, network of interactions between drugs or endogenous metabolites may affect transport and metabolic inactivation of digoxin (Riganti *et al.*, 2011).

Fig. 4.1 Structure of digoxin and proposed metabolic pathways

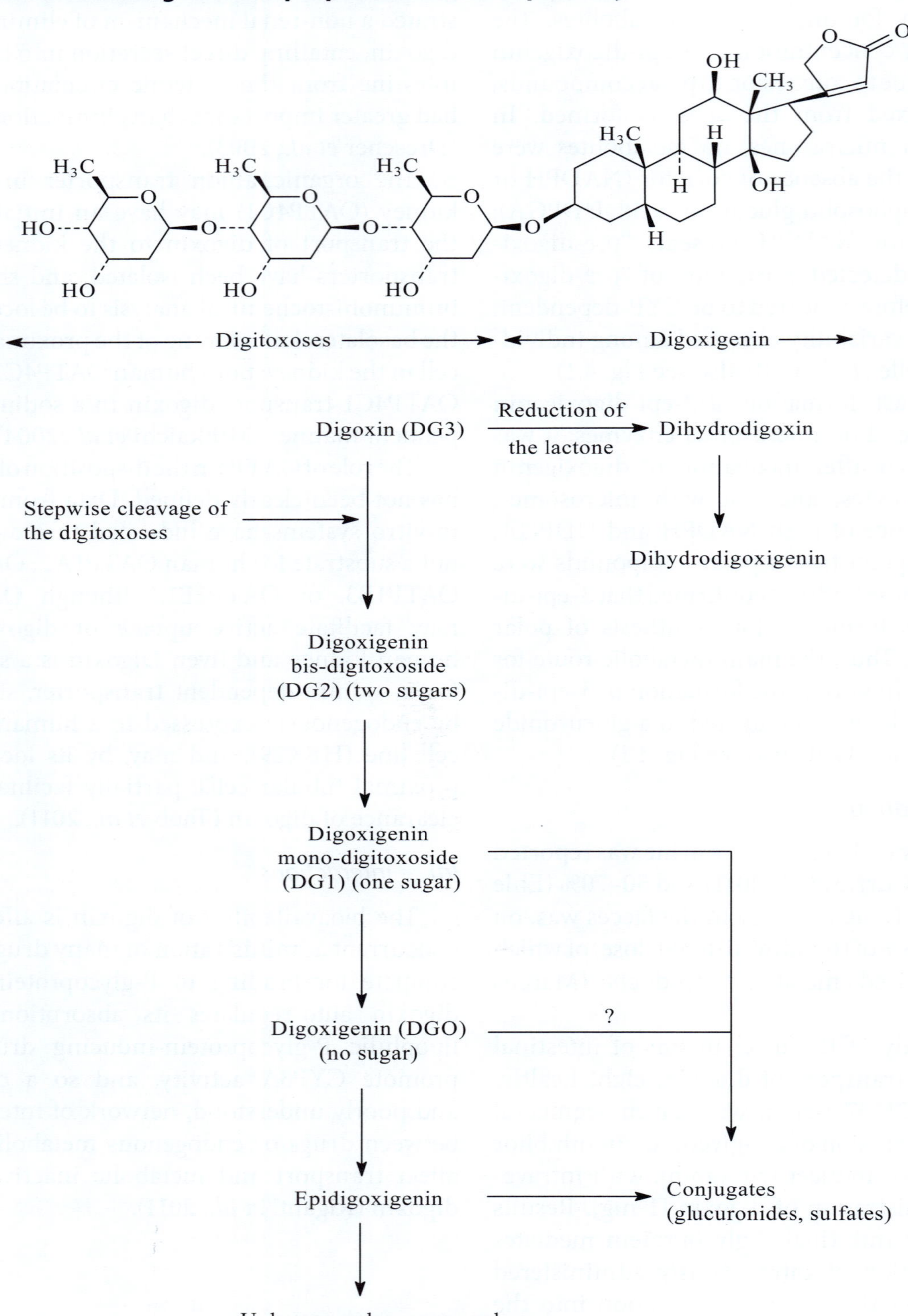

From Lacarelle *et al.* (1991), Copyright © 1991, John Wiley and Sons

4.1.2 Experimental systems

(a)   Absorption

The pharmacokinetics of digoxin was studied in male Sprague-Dawley rats given an intravenous bolus dose at 1 mg/kg bw. Plasma and urine samples were analysed by thin-layer chromatography to separate digoxin and its metabolites. Digoxin concentrations were described as a two-compartment model. Parent drug was rapidly eliminated from the plasma, with half-life of 2.5 hours, a volume of distribution of 3.6 L/kg, and a total body clearance of 5.77 mL/minute. Bile-duct ligation produced comparable pharmacokinetic parameters (with the exception of the total body clearance, 5.18 mL/minute). In rats with bilateral ureter ligation, the plasma half-life of digoxin was increased to 4 hours (Harrison & Gibaldi, 1976).

The function of P-glycoprotein in vivo has been investigated pharmacokinetically, using *mdr1a* (–/–) mice [*Abcb1a* (–/–)] (Schinkel *et al.*, 1995; Mayer *et al.*, 1996; Kawahara *et al.*, 1999). These mice show no major pathology, but their intestinal epithelium and brain endothelial cells have no detectable P-glycoprotein (Schinkel *et al.* 1995). Schinkel *et al.* (1995) demonstrated that concentrations of [3H]digoxin in plasma and most tissues were twofold, and in brain were 35-fold, in *mdr1a* (–/–) mice given [3H]digoxin intravenously compared with *mdr1a* (+/+) mice. Similarly, Kawahara *et al.* (1999) reported that digoxin accumulation in the brain was 68-fold higher. Mayer *et al.* (1996) further demonstrated that the brain concentrations of [3H]digoxin continued to increase over 3 days after injection in *mdr1a* (–/–) mice, resulting in a 200-fold higher concentration than in *mdr1a* (+/+) mice. However, Kawahara *et al.* (1999) reported that disruption of the *mdr1a* gene did not to change plasma-protein binding or the blood-to-plasma partition coefficient.

Inhibition studies in vitro have shown that anionic transporters, in addition to P-glycoproteins, are involved in the absorption of digoxin (Yao & Chiou, 2006).

An additional non-*MDR1* component may contribute to active secretion of digoxin back into the lumen, to limit its intestinal absorption. In support of this, *MDR1*-transfected Madin-Darby canine kidney (MDCKII) cell monolayers showed reduced secretion of digoxin by the *MDR1* inhibitor cyclosporin A, but not by the *MDR1* inhibitor MK-571 (Lowes *et al.*, 2003).

(b)   Metabolism

A proposed metabolic pathway for digoxin is shown in Fig. 4.1 (Lacarelle *et al.*, 1991).

In humans, more than 73% of an intravenous dose is excreted unchanged via the kidneys. In contrast, the rat metabolizes approximately 60% of an intraperitoneal dose, and approximately 30% is excreted via biliary and urinary routes (Harrison & Gibaldi, 1976).

Metabolism of digoxin follows a similar metabolic pathway in humans and rats, i.e. stepwise cleavage of the sugar residues to form the digoxigenin bis- and mono-digitoxoside and the aglycone digoxigenin before conjugation and elimination, but the rate is faster in rats (Harrison & Gibaldi, 1976).

The three sequential steps of oxidative metabolism of digoxin (to digoxigenin bis-digitoxoside, digoxigenin mono-digitoxoside, and digoxigenin) were studied in rat liver microsomes (Salphati & Benet, 1999). Inhibition of the CYP3A subfamily with ketoconazole or triacetyloleandomycin, or with antibodies specific to rat CYP3A2, affected oxidative metabolism; the formation of digoxigenin bis-digitoxoside and digoxigenin mono-digitoxoside decreased by up to 90%, and the rate of oxidation of digoxin and digoxigenin bis-digitoxoside was decreased by up to 85%, respectively. These oxidation reactions were unaffected by chemical or immunological inhibition of CYP2E1, CYP2C or CYP1A2. The subsequent metabolic step, i.e. oxidation of digoxigenin mono-digitoxoside, was not inhibited by triacetyloleandomycin or by antibodies to CYP3A2, CYP2C11, CYP2E1, CYP2B1/2B2 or CYP1A2, but was however reduced (by > 80%) by inhibitors of human CYP3A. In summary, these results indicated that CYP3A, most likely CYP3A2, is the primary enzyme responsible for metabolism of digoxin and digoxigenin bis-digitoxoside in rat liver microsomes, but the enzyme that metabolizes digoxigenin mono-digitoxoside remains to be identified (Salphati & Benet, 1999).

(c) Elimination

Digoxin is eliminated primarily via the kidney through glomerular filtration and tubular secretion. P-glycoprotein has a role in the elimination of digoxin. Studies in vitro have demonstrated that mouse *mdr1a* and human *MDR1* P-glycoprotein actively transport digoxin across a polarized kidney epithelial cell layer (Schinkel *et al.*, 1995). Furthermore, experiments in vivo showed that *mdr1a* (–/–) mice eliminated [³H] digoxin-12α more slowly (Schinkel *et al.*, 1995). The total body clearance was lower in *mdr1a* (–/–) mice than in the wildtype (+/+) mice; however, disruption of the *mdr1a* gene did not change the contributions of renal and bile clearances to total clearance (Kawahara *et al.*, 1999).

Digoxin is partly excreted via the biliary system. In male Sprague-Dawley rats, total body clearance values for digoxin were 10% lower in rats with bile-duct ligation, and were reduced by a further 30% by bilateral ureter ligation. The approximately 60% of total body clearance unaffected by ligations of bile duct or ureter were considered due to biotransformation of digoxin. A main excretory route for digoxigenin bis-digitoxoside was shown to be biliary as indicated by high levels of this metabolite in plasma and urine of rats with ligated bile ducts (Harrison & Gibaldi, 1976).

Intestinal P-glycoprotein in mice has been shown to contribute to excretion of [³H]digoxin via the gastrointestinal epithelium. Mayer *et al.* (1996) demonstrated a shift in balance of excretion in *mdr1a* (–/–) mice given [³H]digoxin (0.2 mg/kg bw) as a single intravenous or oral bolus, i.e. lower faecal elimination of [³H]digoxin. This was due to reduced drug excretion via intestinal epithelium, since biliary excretion was not decreased in *mdr1a* (–/–) mice, and suggested that other transporters could be involved in the biliary excretion of digoxin. Indeed, the capacity for renal excretion remained substantial, and cumulative urinary excretion of digoxin in *mdr1a* (–/–) mice was greater than in wildtype (+/+) mice. Thus, intestinal P-glycoprotein acts by directly excreting digoxin into the intestinal lumen, and also limiting the rate of its re-uptake from the intestine by biliary excretion, thus directing faecal excretion (Mayer *et al.*, 1996). [P-glycoprotein seems to have important roles in elimination of digoxin from the systemic circulation, and also in decreasing intestinal re-uptake of digoxin after biliary excretion.]

4.2 Genetic and related effects

No data were available to the Working Group.

4.3 Other mechanistic data relevant to carcinogenicity

4.3.1 Effects on cell physiology

The physiological action of digoxin involves binding to and inhibition of the α-subunit of the Na⁺/K⁺ ATPase pump on the myocyte plasma membrane. This causes an increase in intracellular concentrations of sodium and calcium ions. Digoxin shares some structural homology with steroid hormones, suggesting functional similarities (Schussheim & Schussheim, 1998; Newman *et al.*, 2008). There is evidence that digitoxin at concentrations of $0.5–2.0 \times 10^{-6}$ M competes with estrogen for the estrogen cytosolic receptor in the rat uterus; however, no evidence for competition by digoxin was obtained (Rifka *et al.*, 1976; Rifka *et al.* 1978).

Other intriguing evidence for digoxin includes a case report of gynaecomastia (Aiman *et al.*, 2009), an increased relative risk of uraemic cancer in digoxin users (RR, 1.48; 45% CI: 1.32–1.65; $n = 350$) (Biggar, 2012), and lower relative risks of cancer of the prostate (RR, 0.76; 95% CI, 0.61–0.95) among regular users versus non-users (Platz *et al.*, 2011).

4.3.2 Effects on cell function

Digoxin reduces synthesis of the TP53 protein in human cancer cell lines; this appears to be triggered by activation of Src/mitogen-activated protein kinase signalling as a consequence of inhibition of the Na^+/K^+ ATPase pump (Wang *et al.*, 2009). Digoxin also inhibits the action of cellular DNA topoisomerases in MCF-7 cells (Bielawski *et al.*, 2006), and inhibits synthesis of hypoxia-inducible factor 1α (HIF-1α) in human Hep3B-c1 hepatoblastoma cells (Zhang *et al.*, 2008). Digoxin may inhibit synthesis of steroids (Kau *et al.*, 2005).

4.4 Susceptibility

4.4.1 Effects of age on elimination

Since young children require higher doses of digoxin per kilogram of body weight than adults to achieve pharmacological effects, there has been interest in whether expression of P-glycoprotein is age-dependent. Pinto *et al.* (2005) have studied *mdr1a* and *mdr1b* and the clearance rates of digoxin (dose, 7 μg/kg bw) in FVB mice of different ages (at birth, and age 7, 14, 21, 28 or 45 days). At birth and day 7, gene expression of *mdr1a* and *mdr1b* was very low, but mdr1b levels were significantly higher at day 21 than at days 14 or 28. Digoxin clearance rates correlated significantly with expression of P-glycoprotein, showing highest clearance values at day 21. It was concluded that increases in digoxin clearance rates after weaning may be attributed, at least

in part, to similar increases in P-glycoprotein expression (Pinto *et al.*, 2005).

Evans *et al.*, (1990) showed that age affects the clearance of digoxin in rats. In male Fischer 344 rats (age, 4, 14, or 25 months) given [³H]digoxin and unlabelled digoxin at a dose of 1 mg/kg bw as an intravenous bolus dose, total body clearance was 14.2, 12.1, and 7.5 mL/minute per kg, respectively, indicating a significant decrease in clearance ($P < 0.05$). No difference was seen in the terminal elimination half-life (2.0, 2.3, and 2.5 hours respectively) or steady-state volume of distribution (1.51, 1.49, and 1.27 L/kg, respectively) in rats aged 4, 14, and 25 months. Serum protein binding did not change with age; the average percentage of unbound digoxin for all rats was 61.3 ± 5.3% (mean ± standard deviation; $n = 15$) (Evans *et al.*, 1990).

4.4.2 Effects of renal failure on elimination

Tsujimoto *et al.* (2008) showed that, in contrast to normal serum, 10% uraemic serum inhibited the hepatic uptake of digoxin by human isolated hepatocytes (by 23%) and by rat hepatocytes (by 50%). It was further shown that the uraemic toxins 3-carboxy-4-methyl-5-propyl-2-furanpropanoic acid (CMPF), *p*-cresol, (both at 400 mM, which is within the plasma concentration range for patients with renal failure) and hippuric acid (at 3000 μM) significantly inhibited the uptake of digoxin. CMPF and *p*-cresol inhibited the uptake of digoxin into rat hepatocytes by 27% and 23%, respectively, and into human hepatocytes by 23% and 28%, respectively. These toxins were, however, not wholly responsible for inhibition of uptake. Indeed, 10% uraemic serum from patients contained these toxins at concentrations (CMPF, 37.6 mM; hippuric acid, 26.8 mM; and *p*-cresol, 19.5 mM) that may not have been sufficient to inhibit the uptake of digoxin. Additionally, the mechanism of inhibition of these toxins was competitive, while the inhibition shown by 10% uraemic serum was non-competitive. Thus, the inhibitory effects of 10% uraemic serum cannot be fully explained by the three major uraemic toxins studied (Tsujimoto *et al.*, 2008).

4.5 Mechanistic considerations

The increase in the incidence of cancers of the breast and uterus after long-term treatment with digoxin (Biggar, 2012), and the observed estrogen-like side-effects of digoxin and digitoxin (Rifka *et al.*, 1976, 1978; Schussheim & Schussheim, 1998), suggested that digoxin and digitoxin act via estrogen-signalling pathways to increase cell proliferation in the mammary gland, potentially contributing to tumour development. However, mechanistic evidence was limited to a demonstration that digitoxin inhibited the binding of estradiol to specific, saturable binding sites in the rat uterine cytosol. Mammary epithelial cells contain several estrogen-binding proteins, including estrogen receptors (ERα and ERβ) and estrogen-related receptors (ERRα and ERRβ), and the signalling pathways linking receptor activation to cellular proliferation are complex (Gibson & Saunders, 2012). The molecular targets associated with the carcinogenic properties of digoxin and digitoxin have not yet been defined.

5. Summary of Data Reported

5.1 Exposure data

Digoxin is a glycoside isolated from *Digitalis lanata* and is used in the treatment of chronic heart failure and irregular heart rhythm. While use may have declined over the past 30 years, digoxin is still frequently prescribed. Global sales of digoxin were US$ 142 million in 2012, with 33% occurring in the USA. Other countries with appreciable use included Japan, Canada, and the United Kingdom.

Digitoxin, another glycoside isolated from *D. purpurea*, is used for the same indications as digoxin in certain countries; it is also found as an impurity in preparations of digoxin.

In most countries, use of "digitalis" would in practice almost always correspond to digoxin, unless digitoxin were specified.

Specifications for digitalis glycosides are provided in several international and national pharmacopoeia. In some countries, digoxin has been classified as a "hazard to water," an "environmental hazard," or as an "extremely hazardous substance."

5.2 Human carcinogenicity data

Studies in humans have assessed the risk of cancer in patients who may have used digoxin, digitoxin, or digitalis drugs as a group. The principal cancer of interest is cancer of the breast. Although risk of some other cancers has been found to be increased, the literature on other cancers was insufficient to establish patterns of increased risk.

5.2.1 Cancer of the breast

Information about the association of cancer of the breast with use of digoxin and digitoxin is available from four case–control studies (including two studies in men) conducted in four Nordic countries, France, and Switzerland, and a nationwide cohort study of women in Denmark, and other cohort studies in the USA and Norway.

Statistically significant increases in the occurrence of cancer of the breast in users of digoxin were seen in three case–control studies; in one study in women, the odds ratio was 1.3, while odds ratios were two- and fourfold in the two studies in men. The largest study, which included all women using digitalis in Denmark, reported an increased risk for current users (hazard ratio, 1.39). The positive associations with exposure to digoxin in this study were due to increased risk in current users only: there was no association in former users and the number of new tumours declined after discontinuing drug use. Dose–response effects were difficult to examine because of the narrow dose range, and trends in risk with duration of exposure were generally not observed. In a case–case comparison among a subset of the same population, tumours occurring in digitalis users were reported to have more favourable prognostic features (estrogen receptor-positive) than in non-users. Data on the association of cancer of the breast with use of digitoxin were available from one cohort study in women in Denmark, which reported a positive association (relative risk, 1.39). These studies had limited ability to account for other risk factors for cancer of the breast, with obesity and alcohol drinking being of greatest concern.

5.2.2 Other cancer sites

Increases in the incidence of cancer of the uterus in current users of digoxin were found in one cohort study in Denmark. The same study found no increase in risk of cancers of the cervix and ovary. The risk of cancer of the prostate, another cancer that is influenced by hormones, was reduced in one high-quality cohort study from the USA, but increased in two others (one study with methodological weaknesses from Norway, and the other a very large database-screening programme from a health plan in northern California, USA). The increased risk of cancer of the uterus, and decreased risk of cancer of the prostate, is also consistent with a hormone-related mechanism, adding to the plausibility of the epidemiological findings.

Excess risks of cancers of the lung and colorectum were also observed in the cohort studies in Norway and northern California. The cohort study in Norway reported a positive association with leukaemia and lymphoma combined.

In a case–control study from southern California, USA, a positive association was observed with non-Hodgkin lymphoma in women, but not in men.

5.2.3 Synthesis

Statistically significant associations of cancer of the breast with use of digoxin were observed consistently in women and men, across different geographical regions, and with different study designs. Cancer of the breast is rare in men and strengthens the validity of association observed for cancer of the breast in women. The record-linkage studies that provided key evidence were not able to adjust for many of the recognized risk factors for cancer of the breast, notably obesity and alcohol drinking, although there was no reason to believe these would be associated with use of digoxin. Although clear effects with duration and dose were not observed, a decline in the detection of new tumours after cessation of exposure was seen in the largest study from Denmark, consistent with a possible promoting effect of digoxin. The association was specific to estrogen receptor-positive tumours of the breast in the same study.

5.3 Animal carcinogenicity data

No data were available to the Working Group.

5.4 Mechanistic and other relevant data

Oral bioavailability of digoxin is generally high, but varies due to interindividual genetic differences in expression of the efflux pump, P-glycoprotein.

The metabolism of digoxin in rats and humans involves stepwise hydrolytic cleavage of the digitoxoses to form digoxigenin bis- and mono-digitoxosides and the aglycone digoxigenin before conjugation and renal elimination.

No data were available on genetic effects of digoxin or its metabolites.

Digoxin has structural homology with steroid hormones, suggesting functional similarities. The structurally related glycoside digitoxin competes with estrogen for the rat uterine estrogen cytosolic receptor; however, no evidence for competition by digoxin was found.

Digoxin reduces synthesis of the TP53 protein in human cancer cells, inhibits cellular DNA topoisomerases, inhibits the synthesis of hypoxia-inducible factor 1α, and may inhibit synthesis of steroids.

The possible association between use of digoxin and an increased incidence of endocrine-related human cancers (primarily breast) suggests a mechanism that is estrogen receptor-mediated. However, evidence that digoxin and digitoxin act through estrogen-signalling pathways was limited to a demonstration that digitoxin inhibited the binding of estradiol to specific, saturable binding sites in rat uterine cytosol. The molecular targets associated with the carcinogenic properties of digoxin and digitoxin have not yet been identified.

6. Evaluation

6.1 Cancer in humans

There is *limited evidence* in humans for the carcinogenicity of digoxin. A positive association has been observed between use of digoxin and cancer of the breast.

6.2 Cancer in experimental animals

There is inadequate evidence in experimental animals for the carcinogenicity of digoxin.

6.3 Overall evaluation

Digoxin is *possibly carcinogenic to humans (Group 2B).*

The Working Group recognized a possible association between digoxin and an increased incidence of endocrine-related human cancers. However, the evidence that digoxin and digitoxin act through an estrogen-receptor mediated mechanism was limited.

Favouring a *Group 2A* classification, the epidemiological data associating increased risk of cancer of the breast with use of digoxin were compelling. Consistent with an endocrine-mediated mechanism, the increase in risk was largely for estrogen receptor-positive tumours; further, risk of uterus cancer was increased and cancer of the prostate was decreased. The evidence in humans favoured a promoter effect that is seen only in current users.

Favouring a *Group 2B* classification, not all potential confounders were eliminated in the epidemiological studies, in particular, obesity. In addition, there were no available data from studies in experimental animals, and no known molecular mechanism by which digoxin might be a carcinogen. The weak evidence supporting an endocrine-mediated mechanism was noted as a problem.

References

Aarnoudse AJ, Dieleman JP, Visser LE, Arp PP, van der Heiden IP, van Schaik RH *et al.*(2008). Common ATP-binding cassette B1 variants are associated with increased digoxin serum concentration. *Pharmacogenet Genomics*, 18(4):299–305. doi:10.1097/FPC.0b013e3282f70458 PMID:18334914

Ahern TP, Lash TL, Sørensen HT, Pedersen L (2008). Digoxin treatment is associated with an increased incidence of breast cancer: a population-based case-control study. *Breast Cancer Res*, 10(6):R102 doi:10.1186/bcr2205 PMID:19055760

Aiman U, Haseeen MA, Rahman SZ (2009). Gynecomastia: An ADR due to drug interaction. *Indian*

J Pharmacol, 41(6):286–7. doi:10.4103/0253-7613.59929 PMID:20407562

Albrecht HP, Geiss KH (2000). Cardiac glycosides and synthetic cardiotonic drugs. In: Ullmann's Encyclopedia of Industrial Chemistry. Weinheim, Germany: Wiley-VCH Verlag GmbH & Co. KGaA; pp. 1–18. http://dx.doi.org/10.1002/14356007.a05_271 doi:10.1002/14356007.a05_271

Aromaa A, Hakama M, Hakulinen T, Saxén E, Teppo L, Idä lan-Heikkilä J (1976). Breast cancer and use of rauwolfia and other antihypertensive agents in hypertensive patients: a nationwide case-control study in Finland. *Int J Cancer*, 18(6):727–38. doi:10.1002/ijc.2910180603 PMID:992904

Banerjee D, Stafford RS (2010). Lack of improvement in outpatient management of congestive heart failure in the United States. *Arch Intern Med*, 170(15):1399–400. doi:10.1001/archinternmed.2010.270 PMID:20696970

Bernstein L, Ross RK (1992). Prior medication use and health history as risk factors for non-Hodgkin's lymphoma: preliminary results from a case-control study in Los Angeles County. *Cancer Res*, 52(19):Suppl: 5510s–5s. PMID:1394165

Bielawski K, Winnicka K, Bielawska A (2006). Inhibition of DNA topoisomerases I and II, and growth inhibition of breast cancer MCF-7 cells by ouabain, digoxin and proscillaridin A. *Biol Pharm Bull*, 29(7):1493–7. doi:10.1248/bpb.29.1493 PMID:16819197

Biggar RJ (2012). Molecular pathways: digoxin use and estrogen-sensitive cancers–risks and possible therapeutic implications. *Clin Cancer Res*, 18(8):2133–7. doi:10.1158/1078-0432.CCR-11-1389 PMID:22368159

Biggar RJ, Andersen EW, Kroman N, Wohlfahrt J, Melbye M (2013). Breast cancer in women using digoxin: tumor characteristics and relapse risk. *Breast Cancer Res*, 15(1):R13 doi:10.1186/bcr3386 PMID:23421975

Biggar RJ, Wohlfahrt J, Melbye M (2012). Digoxin use and the risk of cancers of the corpus uteri, ovary and cervix. *Int J Cancer*, 131(3):716–21. doi:10.1002/ijc.26424 PMID:21913187

Biggar RJ, Wohlfahrt J, Oudin A, Hjuler T, Melbye M (2011). Digoxin use and the risk of breast cancer in women. *J Clin Oncol*, 29(16):2165–70. doi:10.1200/JCO.2010.32.8146 PMID:21422417

Birkenfeld AL, Jordan J, Hofmann U, Busjahn A, Franke G, Krüger N et al.(2009). Genetic influences on the pharmacokinetics of orally and intravenously administered digoxin as exhibited by monozygotic twins. *Clin Pharmacol Ther*, 86(6):605–8. doi:10.1038/clpt.2009.170 PMID:19776737

British Pharmacopoeia (2009) British Pharmacopoeia. London, UK: Medicines and healthcare products regulatory agency.

Burchell HB (1983). Digitalis poisoning: historical and forensic aspects. *J Am Coll Cardiol*, 1(2 Pt 1):506–16. doi:10.1016/S0735-1097(83)80080-1 PMID:6338083

ChemicalBook (2013). ChemicalBook-Chemical Search Engine. Available from: http://www.chemicalbook.com/, accessed 10 February 2015.

Cheng JW, Rybak I (2010). Use of digoxin for heart failure and atrial fibrillation in elderly patients. *Am J Geriatr Pharmacother*, 8(5):419–27. doi:10.1016/j.amjopharm.2010.10.001 PMID:21335295

Currie GM, Wheat JM, Kiat H (2011). Pharmacokinetic considerations for digoxin in older people. *Open Cardiovasc Med J*, 5(1):130–5. doi:10.2174/1874192401105010130 PMID:21769303

Dickstein K, Cohen-Solal A, Filippatos G, McMurray JJ, Ponikowski P, Poole-Wilson PA et al.; ESC Committee for Practice Guidelines (CPG)(2008). ESC Guidelines for the diagnosis and treatment of acute and chronic heart failure 2008: the Task Force for the Diagnosis and Treatment of Acute and Chronic Heart Failure 2008 of the European Society of Cardiology. Developed in collaboration with the Heart Failure Association of the ESC (HFA) and endorsed by the European Society of Intensive Care Medicine (ESICM). *Eur Heart J*, 29(19):2388–442. doi:10.1093/eurheartj/ehn309 PMID:18799522

Digitalis Investigation Group(1997). The effect of digoxin on mortality and morbidity in patients with heart failure. *N Engl J Med*, 336(8):525–33. doi:10.1056/NEJM199702203360801 PMID:9036306

Drescher S, Glaeser H, Mürdter T, Hitzl M, Eichelbaum M, Fromm MF (2003). P-glycoprotein-mediated intestinal and biliary digoxin transport in humans. *Clin Pharmacol Ther*, 73(3):223–31. doi:10.1067/mcp.2003.27 PMID:12621387

DrugBank (2013). DrugBank: Open Data Drug & Drug Target Database. Available from: http://www.drugbank.ca/, accessed 10 February 2015.

Ehle M, Patel C, Giugliano RP (2011). Digoxin: clinical highlights: a review of digoxin and its use in contemporary medicine. *Crit Pathw Cardiol*, 10(2):93–8. doi:10.1097/HPC.0b013e318221e7dd PMID:21988950

EPA (2007). Method 1694: Pharmaceuticals and Personal Care Products in Water, Soil, Sediment, and Biosolids by HPLC/MS/MS. Washington (DC): U.S. Environmental Protection Agency.

Eriksson M, Lindquist O, Edlund B (1984). Serum levels of digoxin in sudden cardiac deaths. *Z Rechtsmed*, 93(1):29–32. doi:10.1007/BF00202981 PMID:6495885

European Pharmacopoeia (2008). Digoxin. 7th ed. Strasbourg, France: European Directorate for the Quality of Medicines & HealthCare.

Evans RL, Owens SM, Ruch S, Kennedy RH, Seifen E (1990). The effect of age on digoxin pharmacokinetics in Fischer-344 rats. *Toxicol Appl Pharmacol*, 102(1):61–7. doi:10.1016/0041-008X(90)90083-7 PMID:2296772

Ewertz M, Holmberg L, Tretli S, Pedersen BV, Kristensen A (2001). Risk factors for male breast cancer–a case-control study from Scandinavia. *Acta Oncol*, 40(4):467–71. doi:10.1080/028418601750288181 PMID:11504305

Fang MC, Stafford RS, Ruskin JN, Singer DE (2004). National trends in antiarrhythmic and antithrombotic medication use in atrial fibrillation. *Arch Intern Med*, 164(1):55–60. doi:10.1001/archinte.164.1.55 PMID:14718322

FDA (2013). Drugs@FDA. FDA Approved Drug Products. Available from: http://www.accessdata.fda.gov/scripts/cder/drugsatfda/, accessed 8 September 2014

Ferrer I, Thurman EM (2012). Analysis of 100 pharmaceuticals and their degradates in water samples by liquid chromatography/quadrupole time-of-flight mass spectrometry. *J Chromatogr A*, 1259:148–57. doi:10.1016/j.chroma.2012.03.059 PMID:22487190

Finch MB, Johnston GD, Kelly JG, McDevitt DG (1984). Pharmacokinetics of digoxin alone and in the presence of indomethacin therapy. *Br J Clin Pharmacol*, 17(3):353–5. doi:10.1111/j.1365-2125.1984.tb02353.x PMID:6712868

Foss PRB, Benezra SA (1980). Digoxin. In: Florey K, editor. Analytical Profiles of Drug Substances. Academic press, vol 9, pp. 207–243.

Friedman GD (1984). Digitalis and breast cancer. *Lancet*, 324(8407):875 doi:10.1016/S0140-6736(84)90915-2 PMID:6148608

Friedman GD, Ury HK (1980). Initial screening for carcinogenicity of commonly used drugs. *J Natl Cancer Inst*, 65(4):723–33. PMID:6932525

Frommherz L, Köhler H, Brinkmann B, Lehr M, Beike J (2008). LC-MS assay for quantitative determination of cardio glycoside in human blood samples. *Int J Legal Med*, 122(2):109–14. doi:10.1007/s00414-007-0175-5 PMID:17569072

Fuster V, Rydén LE, Cannom DS, Crijns HJ, Curtis AB, Ellenbogen KA *et al.*; American College of Cardiology/American Heart Association Task Force on Practice Guidelines; ; European Society of Cardiology Committee for Practice Guidelines; ; European Heart Rhythm Association; ; Heart Rhythm Society(2006). ACC/AHA/ESC 2006 Guidelines for the Management of Patients with Atrial Fibrillation: a report of the American College of Cardiology/American Heart Association Task Force on Practice Guidelines and the European Society of Cardiology Committee for Practice Guidelines (Writing Committee to Revise the 2001 Guidelines for the Management of Patients With Atrial Fibrillation): developed in collaboration with the European Heart Rhythm Association and the Heart Rhythm Society. *Circulation*, 114(7):e257–354. PMID:16908781

Gault MH, Longerich LL, Loo JC, Ko PT, Fine A, Vasdev SC *et al.*(1984). Digoxin biotransformation. *Clin Pharmacol Ther*, 35(1):74–82. doi:10.1038/clpt.1984.11 PMID:6690172

Gerloff T, Schaefer M, Johne A, Oselin K, Meisel C, Cascorbi I *et al.*(2002). MDR1 genotypes do not influence the absorption of a single oral dose of 1 mg digoxin in healthy white males. *Br J Clin Pharmacol*, 54(6):610–6. doi:10.1046/j.1365-2125.2002.01691.x PMID:12492608

Gibson DA, Saunders PT (2012). Estrogen dependent signalling in reproductive tissues - a role for estrogen receptors and estrogen related receptors. *Mol Cell Endocrinol*, 348(2):361–72. doi:10.1016/j.mce.2011.09.026 PMID:21964318

Goldin AG, Safa AR (1984). Digitalis and cancer. *Lancet*, 323(8386):1134 doi:10.1016/S0140-6736(84)92556-X PMID:6144872

Grabowski T, Świerczewska A, Borucka B, Sawicka R, Sasinowska-Motyl M, Gumułka SW *et al.*(2009). A rapid chromatographic/mass spectrometric method for digoxin quantification in human plasma. *Pharm Chem J*, 43(12):710–5. doi:10.1007/s11094-010-0384-y

Guan F, Ishii A, Seno H, Watanabe-Suzuki K, Kumazawa T, Suzuki O (1999). Identification and quantification of cardiac glycosides in blood and urine samples by HPLC/MS/MS. *Anal Chem*, 71(18):4034–43. doi:10.1021/ac990268c PMID:10500489

Harrison LI, Gibaldi M (1976). Pharmacokinetics of digoxin in the rat. *Drug Metab Dispos*, 4(1):88–93. PMID:3407

Hashimoto Y, Shibakawa K, Nakade S, Miyata Y (2008). Validation and application of a 96-well format solid-phase extraction and liquid chromatography-tandem mass spectrometry method for the quantitation of digoxin in human plasma. *J Chromatogr B Analyt Technol Biomed Life Sci*, 869(1–2):126–32. doi:10.1016/j.jchromb.2008.05.026 PMID:18515196

Haux J (1999). Digitoxin is a potential anticancer agent for several types of cancer. *Med Hypotheses*, 53(6):543–8. doi:10.1054/mehy.1999.0985 PMID:10687899

Haux J, Klepp O, Spigset O, Tretli S (2001). Digitoxin medication and cancer; case control and internal dose-response studies. *BMC Cancer*, 1(1):11 doi:10.1186/1471-2407-1-11 PMID:11532201

Haynes K, Heitjan D, Kanetsky P, Hennessy S (2008). Declining public health burden of digoxin toxicity from 1991 to 2004. *Clin Pharmacol Ther*, 84(1):90–4. doi:10.1038/sj.clpt.6100458 PMID:18091761

Hirabayashi H, Sugimoto H, Matsumoto S, Amano N, Moriwaki T (2011). Development of a quantification method for digoxin, a typical P-glycoprotein probe in clinical and non-clinical studies, using high performance liquid chromatography-tandem mass spectrometry: the usefulness of negative ionization mode to avoid competitive adduct-ion formation. *J Chromatogr B Analyt Technol Biomed Life Sci*, 879(32):3837–44. doi:10.1016/j.jchromb.2011.10.031 PMID:22098716

Hoffmeyer S, Burk O, von Richter O, Arnold HP, Brockmöller J, Johne A *et al.*(2000). Functional polymorphisms of the human multidrug-resistance gene:

multiple sequence variations and correlation of one allele with P-glycoprotein expression and activity in vivo. *Proc Natl Acad Sci USA*, 97(7):3473–8. doi:10.1073/pnas.97.7.3473 PMID:10716719

Hollman A (1985). Plants and cardiac glycosides. *Br Heart J*, 54(3):258–61. doi:10.1136/hrt.54.3.258 PMID:4041297

HSDB (2013). Hazardous substance databank. National library of medicine. Available from: http://toxnet.nlm.nih.gov/cgi-bin/sis/htmlgen?HSDB, accessed 10 February 2015.

Hunt SA, Abraham WT, Chin MH, Feldman AM, Francis GS, Ganiats TG et al.(2009). 2009 focused update incorporated into the ACC/AHA 2005 Guidelines for the Diagnosis and Management of Heart Failure in Adults: a report of the American College of Cardiology Foundation/American Heart Association Task Force on Practice Guidelines: developed in collaboration with the International Society for Heart and Lung Transplantation. *Circulation*, 119(14):e391–479. doi:10.1161/CIRCULATIONAHA.109.192065 PMID:19324966

IARC (2012). Pharmaceuticals. Volume 100 A. A review of human carcinogens. *IARC Monogr Eval Carcinog Risks Hum*, 100:Pt A: 1–401. PMID:23189749

IMS Health (2012a). Multinational Integrated Data Analysis (MIDAS). Plymouth Meeting, Pennsylvania: IMS Health; 2012.

IMS Health (2012b). National Disease and Therapeutic Index (NDTI). Plymouth Meeting, Pennsylvania: IMS Health; 2004–12.

IMS Health (2012c). National Prescription Audit Plus (NPA). Plymouth Meeting, Pennsylvania: IMS Health; 2008–12.

Index Nominum (2013). International Drug Directory. Edited by the Swiss Pharmaceutical Society. Stuttgart, Germany: Medpharm Scientific Publishers.

Johne A, Köpke K, Gerloff T, Mai I, Rietbrock S, Meisel C et al.(2002). Modulation of steady-state kinetics of digoxin by haplotypes of the P-glycoprotein MDR1 gene. *Clin Pharmacol Ther*, 72(5):584–94. doi:10.1067/mcp.2002.129196 PMID:12426522

Josephs RD, Daireaux A, Westwood S, Wielgosz RI (2010). Simultaneous determination of various cardiac glycosides by liquid chromatography-hybrid mass spectrometry for the purity assessment of the therapeutic monitored drug digoxin. *J Chromatogr A*, 1217(27):4535–43. doi:10.1016/j.chroma.2010.04.060 PMID:20537342

Kau MM, Kan SF, Wang JR, Wang PS (2005). Inhibitory effects of digoxin and ouabain on aldosterone synthesis in human adrenocortical NCI-H295 cells. *J Cell Physiol*, 205(3):393–401. doi:10.1002/jcp.20415 PMID:15887230

Kawahara M, Sakata A, Miyashita T, Tamai I, Tsuji A (1999). Physiologically based pharmacokinetics of digoxin in mdr1a knockout mice. *J Pharm Sci*, 88(12):1281–7. doi:10.1021/js9901763 PMID:10585223

Kirby BJ, Kalhorn T, Hebert M, Easterling T, Unadkat JD (2008). Sensitive and specific LC-MS assay for quantification of digoxin in human plasma and urine. *Biomed Chromatogr*, 22(7):712–8. doi:10.1002/bmc.988 PMID:18317988

Kleemann A (2012). Cardiovascular Drugs. In: Ullmann's Encyclopedia of Industrial Chemistry. Weinheim, Germany: Wiley-VCH Verlag GmbH & Co. KGaA, pp. 1–18. http://dx.doi.org/10.1002/14356007.a05_289 doi:10.1002/14356007.a05_289

Kurzawski M, Bartnicka L, Florczak M, Górnik W, Droździk M (2007). Impact of ABCB1 (MDR1) gene polymorphism and P-glycoprotein inhibitors on digoxin serum concentration in congestive heart failure patients. *Pharmacol Rep*, 59(1):107–11. PMID:17377214

Lacarelle B, Rahmani R, de Sousa G, Durand A, Placidi M, Cano JP (1991). Metabolism of digoxin, digoxigenin digitoxosides and digoxigenin in human hepatocytes and liver microsomes. *Fundam Clin Pharmacol*, 5(7):567–82. doi:10.1111/j.1472-8206.1991.tb00746.x PMID:1778535

Lee LS, Chan LN (2006). Evaluation of a sex-based difference in the pharmacokinetics of digoxin. *Pharmacotherapy*, 26(1):44–50. doi:10.1592/phco.2006.26.1.44 PMID:16509025

Lenfant-Pejovic MH, Mlika-Cabanne N, Bouchardy C, Auquier A (1990). Risk factors for male breast cancer: a Franco-Swiss case-control study. *Int J Cancer*, 45(4):661–5. doi:10.1002/ijc.2910450415 PMID:2323842

Li S, Liu G, Jia J, Miao Y, Gu S, Miao P et al.(2010). Therapeutic monitoring of serum digoxin for patients with heart failure using a rapid LC-MS/MS method. *Clin Biochem*, 43(3):307–13. doi:10.1016/j.clinbiochem.2009.09.025 PMID:19833118

Li-Saw-Hee FL, Lip GY (1998). Digoxin revisited. *QJM*, 91(4):259–64. doi:10.1093/qjmed/91.4.259 PMID:9666948

Lowes S, Cavet ME, Simmons NL (2003). Evidence for a non-MDR1 component in digoxin secretion by human intestinal Caco-2 epithelial layers. *Eur J Pharmacol*, 458(1–2):49–56. doi:10.1016/S0014-2999(02)02764-4 PMID:12498906

Marcus FI, Kapadia GJ, Kapadia GG (1964). The metabolism of digoxin in normal subjects. *J Pharmacol Exp Ther*, 145:203–9. PMID:14214418

Mayer U, Wagenaar E, Beijnen JH, Smit JW, Meijer DK, van Asperen J et al.(1996). Substantial excretion of digoxin via the intestinal mucosa and prevention of long-term digoxin accumulation in the brain by the mdr 1a P-glycoprotein. *Br J Pharmacol*, 119(5):1038–44. doi:10.1111/j.1476-5381.1996.tb15775.x PMID:8922756

McNamara RL, Tamariz LJ, Segal JB, Bass EB (2003). Management of atrial fibrillation: review of the evidence for the role of pharmacologic therapy, electrical cardioversion, and echocardiography. *Ann Intern Med*, 139(12):1018–33.

doi:10.7326/0003-4819-139-12-200312160-00012 PMID:14678922

Medscape (2013). Medscape Drugs & Disease. Available from: http://reference.medscape.com/drug/lanoxin-digoxin-342432, accessed 5 June 2013.

Mikkaichi T, Suzuki T, Onogawa T, Tanemoto M, Mizutamari H, Okada M et al.(2004). Isolation and characterization of a digoxin transporter and its rat homologue expressed in the kidney. *Proc Natl Acad Sci USA*, 101(10):3569–74. doi:10.1073/pnas.0304987101 PMID:14993604

Newman RA, Yang P, Pawlus AD, Block KI (2008). Cardiac glycosides as novel cancer therapeutic agents. *Mol Interv*, 8(1):36–49. doi:10.1124/mi.8.1.8 PMID:18332483

Oiestad EL, Johansen U, Stokke Opdal M, Bergan S, Christophersen AS (2009). Determination of digoxin and digitoxin in whole blood. *J Anal Toxicol*, 33(7):372–8. doi:10.1093/jat/33.7.372 PMID:19796507

Omidfar K, Kia S, Kashanian S, Paknejad M, Besharatie A, Kashanian S et al.(2010). Colloidal nanogold-based immunochromatographic strip test for the detection of digoxin toxicity. *Appl Biochem Biotechnol*, 160(3):843–55. doi:10.1007/s12010-009-8535-x PMID:19224402

Pähkla R, Irs A, Oselin K, Rootslane L (1999). Digoxin: use pattern in Estonia and bioavailability of the local market leader. *J Clin Pharm Ther*, 24(5):375–80. doi:10.1046/j.1365-2710.1999.00239.x PMID:10583701

Pellati F, Bruni R, Bellardi MG, Bertaccini A, Benvenuti S (2009). Optimization and validation of a high-performance liquid chromatography method for the analysis of cardiac glycosides in Digitalis lanata. *J Chromatogr A*, 1216(15):3260–9. doi:10.1016/j.chroma.2009.02.042 PMID:19268961

Pharmaceuticals and Medical Devices Agency (2011). The Japanese Pharmacopoeia Sixteenth Edition, English Version. Tokyo, Japan: Ministry of Health, Labour and Welfare. Available from: http://jpdb.nihs.go.jp/jp16e/jp16e.pdf, accessed 10 February 2015.

Pinto N, Halachmi N, Verjee Z, Woodland C, Klein J, Koren G (2005). Ontogeny of renal P-glycoprotein expression in mice: correlation with digoxin renal clearance. *Pediatr Res*, 58(6):1284–9. doi:10.1203/01.pdr.0000188697.99079.27 PMID:16306209

Platz EA, Yegnasubramanian S, Liu JO, Chong CR, Shim JS, Kenfield SA et al.(2011). A novel two-stage, transdisciplinary study identifies digoxin as a possible drug for prostate cancer treatment. *Cancer Discov*, 1(1):68–77. doi:10.1158/2159-8274.CD-10-0020 PMID:22140654

PubChem (2013). Pubchem database. NCBI. Available from: https://pubchem.ncbi.nlm.nih.gov/, accessed 10 February 2015.

Rathore SS, Curtis JP, Wang Y, Bristow MR, Krumholz HM (2003). Association of serum digoxin concentration and outcomes in patients with heart failure. *JAMA*, 289(7):871–8. doi:10.1001/jama.289.7.871 PMID:12588271

Reuning RH, Sams RA, Notari RE (1973). Role of pharmacokinetics in drug dosage adjustment. I. Pharmacologic effect kinetics and apparent volume of distribution of digoxin. *J Clin Pharmacol New Drugs*, 13(4):127–41. doi:10.1002/j.1552-4604.1973.tb00074.x PMID:4487163

Rifka SM, Pita JC Jr, Loriaux DL (1976). Mechanism of interaction of digitalis with estradiol binding sites in rat uteri. *Endocrinology*, 99(4):1091–6. doi:10.1210/endo-99-4-1091 PMID:976189

Rifka SM, Pita JC, Vigersky RA, Wilson YA, Loriaux DL (1978). Interaction of digitalis and spironolactone with human sex steroid receptors. *J Clin Endocrinol Metab*, 46(2):338–44. doi:10.1210/jcem-46-2-338 PMID:86546

Riganti C, Campia I, Kopecka J, Gazzano E, Doublier S, Aldieri E et al.(2011). Pleiotropic effects of cardioactive glycosides. *Curr Med Chem*, 18(6):872–85. doi:10.2174/092986711794927685 PMID:21182478

Sakaeda T, Nakamura T, Horinouchi M, Kakumoto M, Ohmoto N, Sakai T et al.(2001). MDR1 genotype-related pharmacokinetics of digoxin after single oral administration in healthy Japanese subjects. *Pharm Res*, 18(10):1400–4. doi:10.1023/A:1012244520615 PMID:11697464

Salphati L, Benet LZ (1999). Metabolism of digoxin and digoxigenin digitoxosides in rat liver microsomes: involvement of cytochrome P4503A. *Xenobiotica*, 29(2):171–85. doi:10.1080/004982599238722 PMID:10199593

Salvador A, Sagan C, Denouel J (2006). Rapid quantitation of digoxin in human plasma and urine using isotope dilution liquid chromatography-tandem mass spectrometry. *J Liquid Chromatogr Relat Technol*, 29(13):1917–32. doi:10.1080/10826070600757821

Saunders KB, Amerasinghe AK, Saunders KL (1997). Dose of digoxin prescribed in the UK compared with France and the USA. *Lancet*, 349(9055):833–6. doi:10.1016/S0140-6736(96)09057-5 PMID:9121258

Schinkel AH, Wagenaar E, van Deemter L, Mol CA, Borst P (1995). Absence of the mdr1a P-Glycoprotein in mice affects tissue distribution and pharmacokinetics of dexamethasone, digoxin, and cyclosporin A. *J Clin Invest*, 96(4):1698–705. doi:10.1172/JCI118214 PMID:7560060

Schussheim DH, Schussheim AE (1998). Is digoxin a designer oestrogen? *Lancet*, 351(9117):1734 doi:10.1016/S0140-6736(05)77771-0 PMID:9734913

SciFinder (2013). Digoxin: Regulatory Information. Columbus (OH): American Chemical Society. Available from: http://www.chemnet.com/cas/en/20830-75-5/digoxin.html, accessed 8 September 2014.

Sleeswijk ME, Van Noord T, Tulleken JE, Ligtenberg JJ, Girbes AR, Zijlstra JG (2007). Clinical review: treatment of new-onset atrial fibrillation in medical intensive care patients–a clinical framework. *Crit Care*, 11(6):233 doi:10.1186/cc6136 PMID:18036267

Stafford RS, Robson DC, Misra B, Ruskin J, Singer DE (1998). Rate control and sinus rhythm maintenance in atrial fibrillation: national trends in medication use, 1980–1996. *Arch Intern Med*, 158(19):2144–8. doi:10.1001/archinte.158.19.2144 PMID:9801182

Stenkvist B (1999). Is digitalis a therapy for breast carcinoma? *Oncol Rep*, 6(3):493–6. PMID:10203580

Stenkvist B, Bengtsson E, Dahlqvist B, Eriksson O, Jarkrans T, Nordin B (1982). Cardiac glycosides and breast cancer, revisited. *N Engl J Med*, 306(8):484 doi:10.1056/NEJM198202253060813 PMID:7057849

Stenkvist B, Bengtsson E, Eriksson O, Holmquist J, Nordin B, Westman-Naeser S (1979). Cardiac glycosides and breast cancer. *Lancet*, 1(8115):563 doi:10.1016/S0140-6736(79)90996-6 PMID:85158

Stuhlfauth T, Klug K, Fock HP (1987). The production of secondary metabolites by Digitalis lanata during CO2 enrichment and water stress. *Phytochemistry*, 26(10):2735–9. doi:10.1016/S0031-9422(00)83581-5

Sturm HB, van Gilst WH, Veeger N, Haaijer-Ruskamp FM (2007). Prescribing for chronic heart failure in Europe: does the country make the difference? A European survey. *Pharmacoepidemiol Drug Saf*, 16(1):96–103. doi:10.1002/pds.1216 PMID:16528759

Taub ME, Mease K, Sane RS, Watson CA, Chen L, Ellens H *et al.*(2011). Digoxin is not a substrate for organic anion-transporting polypeptide transporters OATP1A2, OATP1B1, OATP1B3, and OATP2B1 but is a substrate for a sodium-dependent transporter expressed in HEK293 cells. *Drug Metab Dispos*, 39(11):2093–102. doi:10.1124/dmd.111.040816 PMID:21849517

The International Pharmacopoeia (2011) 4th Edition. Geneva, Switzerland: World Health Organization.

Tracqui A, Kintz P, Ludes B, Mangin P (1997). High-performance liquid chromatography-ionspray mass spectrometry for the specific determination of digoxin and some related cardiac glycosides in human plasma. *J Chromatogr B Biomed Sci Appl*, 692(1):101–9. doi:10.1016/S0378-4347(96)00462-8 PMID:9187389

Tsujimoto M, Kinoshita Y, Hirata S, Otagiri M, Ohtani H, Sawada Y (2008). Effects of uremic serum and uremic toxins on hepatic uptake of digoxin. *Ther Drug Monit*, 30(5):576–82. doi:10.1097/FTD.0b013e3181838077 PMID:18708994

United States Pharmacopoeial Convention (2006) United States Pharmacopeial Convention, 30. Rockville (MD): The United States Pharmacopoeia Convention.

USP; US Pharmacopeia (2007) United States Pharmacopeial Convention. Rockville (MD), USA: United States Pharmacopeial Convention.

Varma MVS, Kapoor N, Sarkar M, Panchagnula R (2004). Simultaneous determination of digoxin and permeability markers in rat in situ intestinal perfusion samples by RP-HPLC. *J Chromatogr B Analyt Technol Biomed Life Sci*, 813(1–2):347–52. doi:10.1016/j.jchromb.2004.09.047 PMID:15556552

Vlase L, Popa D-S, Muntean D, Mihu D, Leucuta S (2009). A new, high-throughput high-performance liquid chromatographic/mass spectrometric assay for therapeutic level monitoring of digoxin in human plasma. *J AOAC Int*, 92(5):1390–5. PMID:19916377

Wang Z, Zheng M, Li Z, Li R, Jia L, Xiong X *et al.*(2009). Cardiac glycosides inhibit p53 synthesis by a mechanism relieved by Src or MAPK inhibition. *Cancer Res*, 69(16):6556–64. doi:10.1158/0008-5472.CAN-09-0891 PMID:19679550

Withering W (1785) An account of the foxglove and some of its medical uses: with practical remarks on dropsy, and other diseases. London, UK: G.G.J. and J. Robinson.

Yao HM, Chiou WL (2006). The complexity of intestinal absorption and exsorption of digoxin in rats. *Int J Pharm*, 322(1–2):79–86. doi:10.1016/j.ijpharm.2006.05.030 PMID:16781832

Yao M, Zhang H, Chong S, Zhu M, Morrison RA (2003). A rapid and sensitive LC/MS/MS assay for quantitative determination of digoxin in rat plasma. *J Pharm Biomed Anal*, 32(6):1189–97. doi:10.1016/S0731-7085(03)00050-5 PMID:12907263

Zhang H, Qian DZ, Tan YS, Lee K, Gao P, Ren YR *et al.* (2008). Digoxin and other cardiac glycosides inhibit HIF-1α synthesis and block tumor growth. *Proc Natl Acad Sci USA*, 105(50):19579–86. doi:10.1073/pnas.0809763105 PMID:19020076

LIST OF ABBREVIATIONS

5-ASA	5-aminosalicylic acid
ACBS	2-amino-4-chloro-1,3-benzenedisulfonamide
AUC	area under the curve
BBN	American Cancer Society
bw	body weight
CI	confidence interval
CMPF	3-carboxy-4-methyl-5-propyl-2-furanpropanoic acid
CYP	cytochrome P450
DDD	defined daily doses
EPA	Environmental Protection Agency
ELS	evaporative light scattering
ESI-MS	body mass index
FDA	United States Food and Drug Administration
GC	gas chromatography
HbA1c	glycated haemoglobin
HCTZ	hydrochlorothiazide
^{1}H-NMR	proton nuclear magnetic resonance
HPLC	high-performance liquid chromatography
HPLC/UV	high-performance liquid chromatography/ultraviolet
HPTLC	high-performance thin-layer chromatography
IBD	inflammatory bowel disease
ICD	International Classification of Diseases
KPNC	Kaiser Permanente Northern California
LOQ	limit of quantitation
MRT	mean residence time
MS	mass spectrometry
NADPH	reduced nicotinamide adenine dinucleotide phosphate
NMR	nuclear magnetic resonance
NQO	NAD(P)H quinone oxidoreductase
NTP	National Toxicology Program
OAT	organic anion transporter
OTC	over the counter
PEMA	phenylethyl malonamide
PPARγ	peroxisome proliferator-activated receptor γ

SMR	standardized morbidity ratio
SSL	solar simulated light
TLC	thin-layer chromatography
TSH	thyroid-stimulating hormone
UGT	UDP glycosyltransferase
USP	United States Pharmacopeia
UV	Ultraviolet
v/v	volume for volume
w/w	weight for weight